KU-261-574

THE HANDBOOK OF ADULT LANGUAGE DISORDERS

Second Edition

Edited by Argye E. Hillis

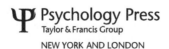
Psychology Press
Taylor & Francis Group
NEW YORK AND LONDON

Second Edition published 2015
by Psychology Press
711 Third Avenue, New York, NY 10017

and by Psychology Press
27 Church Road, Hove, East Sussex BN3 2FA

Psychology Press is an imprint of the Taylor & Francis Group, an informa business

© 2015 Taylor & Francis

The right of the editor to be identified as the author of the editorial
material, and of the authors for their individual chapters, has been asserted
in accordance with sections 77 and 78 of the Copyright, Designs and
Patents Act 1988.

All rights reserved. No part of this book may be reprinted or
reproduced or utilised in any form or by any electronic, mechanical,
or other means, now known or hereafter invented, including photocopying
and recording, or in any information storage or retrieval system, without
permission in writing from the publishers.

Trademark notice: Product or corporate names may be trademarks or
registered trademarks, and are used only for identification and explanation
without intent to infringe.

First edition published by Psychology Press 2002

Library of Congress Cataloging-in-Publication Data
The handbook of adult language disorders / [edited by] Argye E.
Hillis. — Second edition.
p. ; cm.
Includes bibliographical references and index.
I. Hillis, Argye Elizabeth, editor.
[DNLM: 1. Adult. 2. Language Disorders—therapy. 3. Aphasia—
therapy. 4. Cognition—physiology. 5. Language Disorders—
physiopathology. 6. Models, Theoretical. WL 340.2]
RC423
616.85'5—dc23
2014045753

ISBN: 978-1-84872-685-7 (hbk)
ISBN: 978-1-84872-686-4 (pbk)
ISBN: 978-1-315-71355-7 (ebk)

Typeset in Bembo
by Apex CoVantage, LLC

Printed and bound in Great Britain by
CPI Group (UK) Ltd, Croydon, CR0 4YY

This book is dedicated to my mentees, including many who have contributed to chapters in this book, and others who have contributed to research that is cited herein. All of my mentees have taught me a great deal, have challenged me to think more innovatively, and have made the work fun, interesting, and much more important.

CONTENTS

Contents

ABOUT THE EDITOR

Argye E. Hillis is a Professor of Neurology, with joint faculty appointments in Physical Medicine and Rehabilitation and in Cognitive Science at Johns Hopkins University. Dr. Hillis serves as the Executive Vice Chair of the Department of Neurology and Director of the Cerebrovascular Division of Neurology. Prior to medical training and neurology residency, she trained in the fields of speech-language pathology and cognitive neuropsychology, spent a decade in rehabilitation of aphasia, and conducted clinical research focusing on understanding and treating aphasia. Her current research combines longitudinal task-related and task-free functional imaging and structural imaging from the acute stage of stroke through the first year of recovery, with detailed cognitive and language assessments to improve our understanding of how language and other cognitive functions recover after stroke. Her other avenue of research involves developing novel treatment strategies for aphasia.

CONTRIBUTORS

Pélagie M. Beeson
Department of Speech, Language, and Hearing Sciences
University of Arizona, USA

Dana Boatman
Department of Neurology
Johns Hopkins University, USA

Bonnie Breining
Department of Cognitive Science
Johns Hopkins University, USA

Martha W. Burton
Department of Neurology
University of Maryland, USA

David Caplan
Neuropsychology Lab
Massachusetts General Hospital, USA

Jenny Crinion
Institute of Cognitive Neuroscience
University College London, England

Yasmeen Faroqi-Shah
Department of Hearing and Speech Services
University of Maryland at College Park, USA

Simon Fischer-Baum
Department of Psychology
Rice University, USA

Rhonda B. Friedman
Department of Neurology
Georgetown University, USA

Elaine Funnell
Psychology Department
University of London, England

Michael Grosvald
Department of English Literature and Linguistics, College of Arts and Sciences
Qatar University, Qatar

Trevor A. Harley
School of Psychology
University of Dundee, Scotland

Jacqueline J. Hinckley
Communication Sciences and Disorders
University of South Florida, USA

Audrey L. Holland
Department of Speech and Hearing Sciences
University of Arizona, USA

Swathi Kiran
Aphasia Research Laboratory
Boston University, USA

Matti Laine
University of Turku, Finland

Jiyeon Lee
Department of Communication Sciences and Disorders
Northwestern University, USA

Chia-Ming Lei
Department of Communication Science and Disorders
University of Pittsburgh, USA

Daniel A. Llano
Department of Molecular and Integrative Physiology
University of Illinois at Urbana-Champaign, USA

Susan Nitzberg Lott
Department of Neurology
Georgetown University Medical Center, USA

Jane Marshall
Department of Language and Communication Science
City University at London, England

Nadine Martin
Department of Communication Sciences and Disorders
Temple University College of Public Health, USA

Randi C. Martin
Department of Psychology
Rice University, USA

Stephanie Nagle
Department of Audiology, Speech-Language Pathology and Deaf Studies
Towson University, USA

Jeremy J. Purcell
Department of Cognitive Science
Johns Hopkins University, USA

David C. Race
Department of Neurology
Johns Hopkins University School of Medicine, USA

Deepti Ramadoss
Department of Neurology
Johns Hopkins University School of Medicine, USA

Elliott Ross
Pharmacology, Green Center for Systems Biology
University of Texas Southwestern Medical Center, USA

Steven Z. Rapcsak
Department of Neurology
University of Arizona, USA

Brenda Rapp
Department of Cognitive Science
Johns Hopkins University, USA

Anastasia M. Raymer
Department of Communication Disorders & Special Education
Old Dominion University, USA

Teresa M. Schubert
Department of Cognitive Science
Johns Hopkins University, USA

Rajani Sebastian
Department of Neurology
Johns Hopkins University School of Medicine, USA

Steven L. Small
Department of Neurology
University of California at Irvine, USA

Yingying Tan
Division of Linguistics and Multilingual Studies
Nanyang Technological University, Singapore

Cynthia K. Thompson
Communication Sciences and Disorders
Northwestern University, USA

Donna C. Tippett
Departments of Otolaryngology, Neurology, and Physical Medicine and Rehabilitation
Johns Hopkins University Hospital, USA

Connie A. Tompkins
Communication Science and Disorders
University of Pittsburgh, USA

Kyrana Tsapkini
Department of Neurology
Johns Hopkins University, USA

Sofia Vallila-Rohter
Aphasia Research Laboratory, Boston University, USA
Massachusetts Institute of Technology, USA

Alexandra Zezinka
The Ohio State University, USA

PREFACE

Aphasiology, or the science of aphasia, is a field dedicated to understanding how language breaks down after focal injury to the brain and how it recovers. The cognitive and neural mechanisms underlying language as revealed by aphasia have been investigated by neurophysiologists, neurologists, neuropsychologists, linguists, speech-language pathologists, and other researchers in cognitive science and neuroscience. There are strong scientific and clinical motivations for studying aphasia. Because language is among the most important human functions, scientists have sought to understand how language is represented and processed in the brain for more than 150 years. Furthermore, aphasia is one of the most common and disabling consequence of stroke, affecting more than a million people (1 in every 250) in the United States alone. Characterizing the cognitive and neural processes that account for each variant of aphasia provides a first step toward developing effective rehabilitation. This book was designed to provide a unique perspective on the field, by bringing together investigators and clinicians from a variety of backgrounds, to summarize recent advances in the field. Importantly, for each domain of language, one chapter summarizes research that provides evidence for the cognitive mechanisms, or architecture, underlying that language task (e.g., naming or sentence production). The next chapter reports studies on the neural mechanisms underlying the same language task. The third chapter describes investigations of treatment for impairments in that domain of language. In addition, there are chapters that describe approaches to investigation of language or treatment more generally, rather than specific to a given domain of language. For example, Nadine Martin and colleagues in Chapter 20 describe how computational models have contributed to studying aphasia and developing treatment strategies for aphasia. Daniel Llano and Steven Small in Chapter 21 report on studies of pharmacological approaches to aphasia treatment, and Jenny Crinion in Chapter 22 reports on how transcranial direct current stimulation can augment speech and language therapy for aphasia. Jacqueline Hinckley and Audrey Holland in Chapter 23 describe a life participation approach to aphasia rehabilitation. Connie Tompkins and colleagues in Chapter 24 summarize research on communication disorders in individuals with right hemisphere lesions, and Donna Tippett and Elliott Ross in Chapter 25 focus more specifically on impairments of prosody after right hemisphere lesions.

The authors of this book represent all of the various disciplines that study aphasia, and many chapters are the products of interdisciplinary collaborations. Furthermore, several of the authors have training in two or more scientific disciplines (e.g., David Caplan: linguistics and neurology;

Dana Boatman: linguistics and audiology; Steven Small: computational science and neurology). The book is not meant for a single discipline or course. Rather, it is meant to be useful to a broad range of investigators and clinicians interested in understanding how language breaks down after focal brain damage, what patterns of impairment reveal about normal language, and how recovery can be optimally facilitated.

PART 1

Reading

1

ACQUIRED IMPAIRMENTS IN READING

Jeremy J. Purcell, Teresa M. Schubert, and Argye E. Hillis

The act of reading—converting light reflected from printed text into both understanding and speech—is a complex cognitive endeavor. In modern society, it has become a critically valuable skill for learning and communication. Therefore, understanding the mechanisms that underlie how specific aspects of reading are robbed from individuals with acquired neurological impairments is of critical scientific interest. Commensurate with this interest, there has been an explosion of recent scientific query into acquired reading deficits, spanning a broad range of fields such as neuropsychology, experimental psychology, and computational neuroscience.

One major attraction to this field of study is that reading is a highly specialized skill that, unlike other cognitive skills such as spoken language, is not known to have developed through evolutionary pressures. Instead, it has been proposed that the ability to discern the phonological and semantic content from written words co-opts neuronal structures that were originally developed for different functions (e.g., non-orthographic object processing, spoken language processing, working memory processing) prior to learning to read (Dehaene & Cohen, 2007). For further discussion of this "neuronal recycling hypothesis" see Castles and Friedmann (2014), Coltheart (2014), Dehaene (2014), Downey (2014), and Menary (2014). Another attraction to the study of reading is that a variety of reading disorders can be expressed after brain damage. The study of these different forms of reading disorders has allowed for the delineation of distinct cognitive component processes of reading. This in turn has contributed to the development of cognitive architecture models that conceptualize the reading system as a set of interacting yet discrete cognitive mechanisms.

From the perspective of studying individuals with acquired reading disorders, there is practical utility in employing a cognitive architecture that allows for the description of discrete cognitive mechanisms. First, the acquired reading disorder can be categorized by type and severity, which is useful for diagnoses and potential focused therapy for the disorder. Second, discrete mental representations and processes schemata of reading can provide a valuable theoretical scaffold upon which to describe and scientifically study—that is, test specific hypotheses regarding—the cognitive architecture of reading.

In this chapter, we explore the underlying mental structure of reading via studies of individuals with damage to their reading system. The reading system involves the flow of information from the input of light rays reflected off a page or screen, to the discernment of visual letters, to comprehension of a word's meaning, to the articulators associated with spoken output. Deficits in these different aspects of reading processing can be characterized by delineating different *levels*

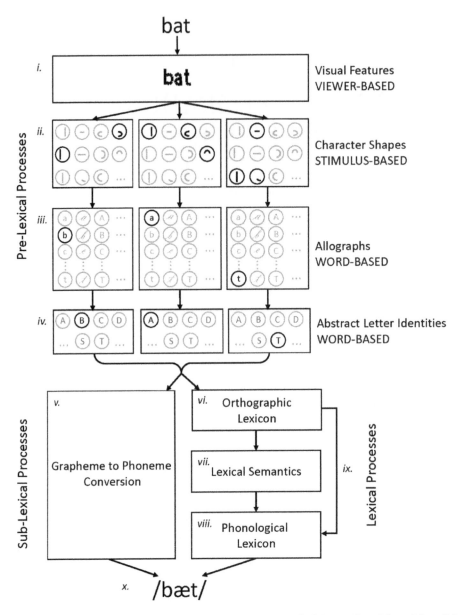

Figure 1.1 A schematic representation of the cognitive processes underlying reading. Adapted from Schubert and McCloskey (2013).

of mental representation as well as different *frames of reference* within which these representations operate. The levels of mental representation or mechanisms that we will discuss in this chapter are depicted as boxes in Figure 1.1. The frames of reference within which these representations operate, when they are known, are depicted in uppercase text alongside the levels. The organization of the boxes indicates an order of cognitive operation between visual word input *bat* and comprehension and/or spoken-word output /bæt/. It is worth stating that the information does not necessarily proceed in a stepwise or linear manner across different levels of the architecture; that is, the characterizations of the representations at a given level are not necessarily the inputs or outputs from adjacent levels in this architecture. Instead this model claims that as one explores reading via the characterization of acquired reading disorders, processing proceeds through different stages. The inputs to these levels and their underlying nature are likely far more complex than we have depicted here.

In the remainder of the chapter, evidence will be presented from neurologically impaired patients whose pattern of performance in reading and other cognitive tasks results from selective damage to one or more component processes of reading. The particular component(s) discussed will be denoted by Roman numerals corresponding to processing stages depicted in Figure 1.1.

First, let us outline the basic computational requirements of reading a word. Initially, the basic visual features (Figure 1.1.*i*) that comprise individual letters or strings of letters must be resolved at early levels of visual processing into character shape maps (Figure 1.1.*ii*). Next is an allograph level that represents the different letter shape forms that are font or case specific (Figure 1.1.*iii*). The allograph level is followed by a level of abstract letter identities (ALIs) (Figure 1.1.*iv*); at this level letters are represented independently of their visual form. For example, TEAR and tear and *tear* are strings that contain the same letter identities in the same order.

This ALI level precedes higher-level sub-lexical grapheme-to-phoneme mapping and orthographic lexical mechanisms. Via sub-lexical processes (Figure 1.1.*v*), both novel (pseudo-words or uncommon proper names) and familiar words can be "sounded out" through the mapping of graphemes (single- or multi-letter pronounceable units of orthography, e.g., P, PH)[1] to phonemes. Via this route, a plausible pronunciation is assigned without accessing stored orthographic, semantic, or phonological representations. For example, the editor's first name Argye has elicited a variety of equally plausible pronunciations based on its constituent graphemes (including: /argaI/, /ard3i/, /ard3ai/), although just as often it is mispronounced as "Argyle" or "argue."

Turning to lexical processing, the orthographic lexicon allows the recognition of strings of ALIs as familiar words stored in long-term memory (Figure 1.1.*vi*). Via the lexical route, familiar words that do not adhere to the typical grapheme-phoneme correspondence conventions can be read. For example, if its pronunciation is familiar, the name Argye can be read expertly (/argi/) via orthographic lexical mechanisms. The recognition of a word in the orthographic lexicon enables access to a stored meaning, or semantic representation, appropriate to the context (Figure 1.1.*vii*). The word *tear*, for instance, is understood differently in the context *a tear dropped* versus *tear the paper*. Whichever discrete semantic representation is activated (e.g., <a droplet from the eye> versus <to rip>) is then used to access the stored pronunciation, or phonological representation, corresponding to that meaning in the phonological lexicon (Figure 1.1.*viii*). Thus, the word *tear* in *tear the paper* will be pronounced such that it rhymes with *bear* and not *fear*. Furthermore, in some schema, words without homographs may access a phonological representation directly without semantic access via a direct orthographic lexicon to phonological lexicon mapping (Figure 1.1.*ix*). At some point in this process, either parallel to, or prior to, accessing a phonological representation, information about the syntactic role of the word is also activated, so that we know that the word *tear* is a noun in the context of the phrase *a tear dropped*, but is a verb in the context of the phrase *tear the paper*. Lastly, this phonological representation serves as the basis for activating particular motor programs for articulation that lead to spoken output (Figure 1.1.*x*).

It is worth noting that the model of reading used in this chapter is not universally accepted. For example, alternative models assume that many of the proposed representations are activated in parallel (Plaut & Shallice, 1993) or in cascade (Humphreys, Riddoch, & Quinlan, 1988), or that there are not separate mechanisms for reading familiar and unfamiliar words (Seidenberg & McClelland, 1989). These alternative interpretations of specific acquired reading disorders will be discussed further in section 6.

1 Pre-Lexical Representations

1.1 Early Visual Representations (Figure 1.1.i)

The initial stage of reading involves the generation of a low-level visual feature map in the early visual cortex. Such low-level features include, but are not limited to, oriented bars and dots. These features, along with their retinal position, determine properties of the stimulus, such as the spatial frequency. Damage to the visual feature map is not reading specific, but is common to general visual processing. Severe damage at this early stage of visual processing will lead to an anopia, which is characterized by the inability to process any visual information regarding all or part of the visual field. A milder deficit at this level of processing can lead to impairments in low-level processing of visual stimuli that can affect reading.

Some work has proposed that mild damage at this level may lead to deficits that have a cascading effect, leading to impairments that can be detected at (and possibly confused with) higher-level object and letter processing. For instance, damage at this level of processing has been associated with a pattern of letter-by-letter reading, which is characterized by slower read-ing for longer versus shorter words and is thought to be due to the inability to process words in "parallel" (Price & Humphreys, 1992; Shallice & Saffran, 1986). One group of researchers has reported on a series of individuals who express a letter-by-letter reading pattern and who also show reduced sensitivity to high spatial frequencies and impaired processing of highly com-plex novel visual objects; this was determined by observing impaired performance on visual discrimination tasks involving checker displays and Japanese characters (Roberts et al., 2012). This group suggests that impairment to the processing of high spatial frequencies can lead to both reading impairment and impaired processing of non-orthographic objects. This work highlights the importance of determining the underlying cause of impairments in reading. In order to more fully understand the panoply of reading disorders it is important to distinguish a lower-level deficit with downstream consequences at higher levels from a deficit in higher-level processing.

Other works have found that damage at this level can lead to impairments in processing words in a viewer-centered frame of reference. A viewer-centered frame of reference may be retinotopic, based on the position of eye fixation, or it may be any other egocentric frame. To elaborate, when a word is read, the first representation takes the form of edges, intersections, blobs and other variations in light intensities that are represented with respect to the viewer, with letters to the left of the viewer represented distinctly from letters to the right of the viewer (Marr & Nishihara, 1978; Monk, 1985). Therefore, computation at this level of representation will be disrupted by viewer-centered hemispatial neglect, such as in the patients CS, AS, and AWR (Hillis, Rapp, Benzing, & Caramazza, 1998). All three failed to read words correctly if they were presented on the left side of their view. Furthermore, all three patients made more errors on letters that were further to the left of their view, whether the letters comprised the initial letters of the word (in standard text) or the final letters (in upside-down or mirror-reversed text). Furthermore, they made no errors on words that were presented non-visually (e.g., rec-ognizing words spelled orally to them), indicating that the deficit involved visual computations. It is important to note that this deficit is considered to be selective to the left side of the *intact visual field*. That is, AWR had a left homonymous hemianopia and therefore, could not see anything in the left visual field; it was confirmed that the reported impairments were specific to the left side of the intact visual field (i.e., the right visual field) when compared to the right side of the intact visual field. This work strongly suggests that the representations expressed at the earliest stages of reading have a viewer-centered frame of reference, as opposed to purely a retinotopic-centered one.

1.2   Character-Shape Representations (Figure 1.1.ii)

Low-level visual feature maps feed into a higher level of processing associated with representing character shapes. Processing at this level involves stimulus-based representations, composed of distinct character shapes. For example, the shape of each individual letter in the word *bat* is considered to be composed of a distinct set of activated shape features. It is at this point that visual features are grouped into a single representation for each letter-shape object. It is worth noting that the representations at this level of processing distinguish shapes, but not the identity of the letters; therefore, real or known letters are not distinguished from false letters (or digits).

The representations at this level are considered to have a stimulus-based frame of reference. This is supported by evidence from patients who make reading errors on the left side of words, irrespective of where the word is presented in their view. To illustrate, patients RW (Hillis & Caramazza, 1991b) and BPN (Hillis & Caramazza, 1995a) made errors on the initial letters of words (the left side of the visual stimulus) in reading standard text, but on the final letters of words (again, the left side of the visual stimulus) in reading mirror-reversed print. This occurred regardless of whether the stimuli were presented on the left or right side of the body or visual field. For example, *bear* was read as "fear" in standard text and as "bead" in mirror-reversed text. Therefore, their errors seem to concern one side of the visuospatial representation defined by the coordinates of the stimulus, rather than location with respect to the viewer. We have called this level of representation the "stimulus-centered representation" because errors increase as a function of the distance (in this case, to the left) in the visual stimulus (Caramazza & Hillis, 1990a; Hillis & Caramazza, 1995d).

To further illustrate, when a suffix was added to a word (e.g., sad, sadness), the initial letter of the word was "pushed" further leftward in the stimulus, and RW and BPN were more likely to make errors on the initial letter in this condition. That is, both were more likely to make errors on the *s* in *sadness* (e.g., *sadness* → "badness") than on the *s* in *sad*. Furthermore, if a prefix was added to the word, pushing the initial letter of the root word closer to the center of the word, fewer errors were made on the initial letter of the root word. For instance, both RW and BPN were more likely to make an error on the *c* in *cook* (e.g., *cook* → "look") than on the *c* in *precook*. Neither RW nor BPN made left-sided errors in recognizing words that were spelled aloud to them, indicating that their deficit concerned visuospatial representations rather than abstract grapheme or word-level representations. However, both patients made more errors in identifying/copying left sides of picture stimuli, irrespective of where the stimuli were presented with respect to the viewer. These results indicated that the deficit in RW and BPN concerned stimulus-centered representations of not only words, but also visual/spatial stimuli more generally (see Costello & Warrington, 1987; Haywood & Coltheart, 2000; Patterson & Wilson, 1990 for cases of similar hemispatial errors in reading but not in non-lexical visuospatial tasks). Other patients with patterns of performance indicating neglect at the level of stimulus-centered representations have been reported by Subbiah and Caramazza (2000), Haywood and Coltheart (2000), and Nichelli, Venneri, Pentore, and Cubelli (1993).

1.3   Stored Allograph and Letter Representations

Here we will discuss the allograph stage of processing and a relatively later abstract letter identity stage. It is at these levels of processing that representational properties emerge that can be considered particularly relevant to visual letters as opposed to different classes of visual objects.

Deficits at these two levels of representation are thought to have a word-centered frame of reference (e.g., Caramazza & Hillis, 1990a; Schubert & McCloskey, 2013). First, we will consider evidence for allograph representations and their reference frame, followed by abstract letter identities.

1.3.1 Allograph Representations (Figure 1.1.iii)

Allographs are representations of the basic shapes of letters. Although a number of studies have presented evidence in support of an allographic level of representations in reading (Brunsdon, Coltheart, & Nickels, 2006; Caplan & Hedley-Whyte, 1974; Chanoine, Teixeira Ferreira, Demonet, Nespoulous, & Poncet, 1998; Dalmás & Dansilio, 2000; Miozzo & Caramazza, 1998; Rapp & Caramazza, 1989; Volpato, Bencini, Meneghello, Piron, & Semenza, 2012), we will focus on the work of Schubert and McCloskey (2013) with LHD, an individual with acquired dyslexia. LHD expressed a clear word length effect in reading and made high rates of single letter substitution errors. This deficit was also evident in naming the letters in random letter strings (e.g., kgnyq), suggesting that the deficit was rooted in an impairment of letter-level processing rather than of later reading processes. LHD's intact ability to copy pseudoletter characters suggested that she successfully constructed visual feature maps and character shape representations (example in Figure 1.2.i). These two levels of representation are utilized for both letter and non-letter characters, and the results narrowed the location of her deficit to between the character shape and abstract letter identity levels.

To probe her processing at letter-specific levels the authors administered two tasks on identical stimuli: strings containing half pseudoletter characters and half letters (see Figure 1.2.ii). On one run through the stimuli, LHD was asked to distinguish between the pseudoletter and letter characters, which she performed with near-perfect accuracy (99.8% correct). Subsequently, she was asked to name the letters, and displayed impaired performance (6% error rate, a significant difference). Two conclusions follow from these results: LHD accessed stored letter representations, allowing her to discriminate between pseudoletters and real letters, but this does not entail access to abstract letter identities needed for letter naming.

On the basis of the evidence that LHD had intact access to stored letter representations, along with the accumulation of similar evidence presented by previous authors, Schubert and McCloskey (2013) concluded that an allograph level intervenes between character shape and abstract letter identity levels. To further explore the properties of allograph representations, they utilized four same/different tasks (for a similar approach, see Rapp & Caramazza, 1989).

In all of these tasks LHD was presented with a pair of three-letter strings and asked to decide whether they contained the same letters. Each task included physically identical pairs, on which LHD was unimpaired. Impaired performance on cross-case pairs (e.g., htf—HTF) confirmed that LHD was impaired at matching lower and uppercase letter forms, and that these forms are represented with distinct allographs. Cross-style pairs (e.g., izt—*izt*) also resulted in impaired performance, suggesting that distinct forms of letters are represented separately, even when occurring

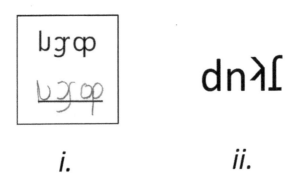

i.   *ii.*

Figure 1.2 Pseudoletter task stimuli. (i) Example of a pseudoletter string and LHD's copy response. (ii) Example of a half pseudoletter and half letter stimulus. Adapted from Schubert and McCloskey (2013).

within a single case (e.g., z and *ℊ*). However, allographs do not seem to separately represent every physical difference in letter form. Rather, LHD was intact at making same/different judgments on cross-size (36 point and 52 point font) and cross-font (Courier New and Consolas) pairs. These stimuli differ in scaling or small visual differences (e.g., serifs), which seem to be abstracted over at the allograph level: r and r activate the same allograph. This finding is somewhat surprising considering that the size of the serifs that differentiate these stimuli approaches the size of the visual difference that distinguishes the letters c and e. Thus, the allograph level does not uniformly discard information about visual differences; rather it encodes (only) those visual differences which inform letter identity.

1.3.2   Abstract Letter Identity Representations (Figure 1.1.iv)

Clearly, letters that have the same identity can have drastically different visual form (e.g., q and Q), and for reasons of computational efficiency, it is unlikely that the ability to recognize these various letter forms rests on direct mappings of character shapes or allographic representations to orthographic word forms. This is just one of many reasons that reading researchers have supported a representational level of abstract letter identities, or ALIs, as the final letter-based representation prior to lexical and sub-lexical processing (Bowers, 2000; Coltheart, 1981; Evett & Humphreys, 1981; Humphreys, Evett, & Quinlan, 1990; R.C. Martin & Caramazza, 1982; Peressotti, Job, Rumiati, & Nicoletti, 1995; Polk & Farah, 1997; Rapp & Caramazza, 1989; Rynard & Besner, 1987).

Within pre-lexical letter processing, there is increasing abstraction as visual information proceeds from the retina to low- and then higher-level cortical areas of the ventral visual stream. This progression abstracts away from low-level visual features, from location, from size, from small alterations in letter shapes, and at the level of ALIs from various allographic forms of the same letter. The abstract letter identity level represents a letter's identity regardless of the visual form. Additionally, it is assumed that ALIs can be accessed via other modalities such as spoken letter names or tactile letter input (Brunsdon et al., 2006; Caramazza & Hillis, 1990a; Rapp & Caramazza, 1989; Schubert & McCloskey, 2013). The strongest evidence from the deficit literature for ALI representations are reading deficits that are found not to be due to impaired orthographic word knowledge or impaired processing of allographs. For example, LHD, who was impaired at accessing letter identities, could activate ALIs from tactile letter input or spoken letter input (Schubert & McCloskey, 2013). Two other examples of similar cases include JGE (Rapp & Caramazza, 1997) and GV (Miozzo & Caramazza, 1998). All of these individuals demonstrated impairments in accessing letter identities from visual input, but were able to recognize words when spelled orally to them (e.g., "B-A-T," "bat"). This task involves abstract letter identities and subsequently activates lexical and sub-lexical reading processes (Coltheart, Masterson, Byng, Prior, & Riddoch, 1983; Forde & Humphreys, 2005; Greenwald & Gonzalez Rothi, 1998; Hanley & Kay, 1992; Patterson & Kay, 1982; Tainturier & Rapp, 2003).[2] Evidence for a word-based frame of reference at the ALI level comes from LHD (Schubert & McCloskey, 2013) and from patient NG (Caramazza & Hillis, 1990a, 1990b). NG made reading errors on the right side of written words. More generally, her errors were a function of the letter position in the canonical representation of the word: she made errors on the *final* letters of words, whether words were presented in standard print, mirror-reversed print, or vertical print (Caramazza & Hillis, 1990a, 1990b). She also made errors on the final letters of words when they were spelled aloud to her for recognition or when she spelled aloud or wrote the word, as shown in Table 1.1. These errors indicate that her deficit concerned the final portion of an abstract representation of the word in its canonical orientation, independent of the orientation or modality of the stimulus. Also, as described for RW and BPN, NG's error rate in reading

Table 1.1 Example of NG's Errors in Various Lexical Tasks

Task	Stimulus	NG's Response	
Oral reading: standard print	stripe	strip	
	study	stud	
	humid	human	
	chin	chew	
	sprinter	sprinkle	
Oral reading: vertical print (top-to-bottom)	rang	ran	
	forced	force	
	blending	blemish	
	risks	rich	
	common	comet	
Oral reading: vertical print (bottom-to-top)	friend	fright	
	candid	candle	
	agency	agenda	
	repeat	reply	
	barbeque	barbell	
Oral reading: mirror-reversed print	common	comet	
	greenish	greenery	
	joint	join	
	discovery	disco	
	dashes	dash	
Recognition of orally spelled words	j-o-y-o-u-s	joy	
	f-i-x-e-d	fix	
	w-o-r-e	work	
	t-a-1-e-n-t	tall	
	e-a-r-n-s	earring	
Written spelling	pretty	pret	
	fact	fac	
	blame	bland	
	crow	croy	
	sneeze	sneed	
Oral spelling	spoke	s-p-o-k	(spok)
	priest	p-r-i-e-s	(pries)
	jury	j-u-r-i-o-n	(jurion)
	event	e-v-e-n-i-s	(evenis)
	soft	s-o-f-e	(sofe)
Backward oral spelling	absorb	n-w-o-s-b-a	(absown)
	sky	k-i-k-s	(skik)
	church	r-u-h-c	(chur)
	garbage	i-s-b-r-a-g	(garbsi)
	oyster	e-t-s-y-o	(oyste)

words was a function of the distance from the center of the word; she made more errors on the final letter of a root word when a prefix was added (pushing the final letter further to the right from the center) and fewer errors when a suffix was added (pushing the final letters closer to the center of the word (Caramazza & Hillis, 1990a, 1990b). Additional patients have been reported whose patterns of performance on reading and/or spelling (Barbut & Gazzaniga, 1987; Baxter & Warrington, 1983; Hillis & Caramazza, 1995d) and non-lexical tasks (Bisiach & Berti, 1987; Bisiach & Luzzatti, 1978) indicated damage at the level of object-centered representations. These results provide evidence that a word/object-centered representation is computed from the visual stimulus and is used to access stored orthographic or canonical object representations.

In general, ALI units provide a computationally efficient way to map a set of identities regardless of visual form complexity, position, size, format, case, or even modality of letter into a feature space that represents higher-order orthographic units. These latter units can range in size from graphemes to larger whole word lexical units; these will be discussed in the next section.

2 Orthographic Sub-Lexical and Lexical Representations

Acquired reading disorders at higher levels of reading processing are expressed in fundamentally different manners than those of pre-lexical processing. Although the processing up to individual ALIs may be intact, impairments in processing can involve later orthographic units such as graphemes or whole words. Graphemes are distinguished from ALIs in that a grapheme necessarily corresponds to a single phoneme and is associated with grapheme-to-phoneme mapping mechanisms. Importantly, it needs to be demonstrated that these types of impairments are not due to deficits in more general semantic or phonological processing, but are, in fact, driven by impairments in processing mechanisms involving orthography. A prevalent and practical way for characterizing these deficits within the context of acquired reading disorders is to divide them into two broad category types: sub-lexical and lexical processing deficits.

Combined, these profiles can be interpreted as evidence for distinct cognitive mechanisms for reading familiar versus unfamiliar words (or pseudowords). Familiar words are thought to be read via the orthographic lexicon, and pseudowords or unfamiliar words are read via orthographic to phonological correspondence (OPC) mechanisms (Coltheart, Patterson, & Marshall, 1980).

2.1 Sub-Lexical Representations (Figure 1.1.v)

Inherent to the processing of sub-lexical representations is the mapping of graphemes to their phonological counterparts, phonemes. These mapping mechanisms involve the most common correspondence between a grapheme and a phoneme and have been termed orthographic-to-phonological correspondences (OPCs). The study of OPCs and the underlying sub-lexical units is primarily focused on case studies of acquired dyslexic reading performance that is characterized by better reading of familiar, irregular words (i.e., real words that have uncommon mappings of orthography to phonology, e.g., *eye* or *yacht*) than pseudowords (a pronounceable nonword, e.g., *fodap* or *lurat*). This profile is sometimes referred to as "deep dyslexia." Pseudoword reading performance probes processing of the mappings between orthography and phonemic units. If there is an impaired ability to map between known orthographic and phonemic units, it is difficult or impossible to read a pseudoword; on the other hand, the ability to read a known word is spared because this instead requires lexical units accessed from long-term memory.

An exploration of reading deficits associated with sub-lexical processing has revealed a complex system that extends beyond simple one-to-one mappings between graphemes and phonemes. For instance, some studies have reported on intact pseudoword reading, yet impaired single letter reading (e.g., Dickerson, 1999; Funnell, 1983). The case study of Funnell (1983) reported on an individual FL who could read pseudowords with moderate accuracy (74%), but could only produce the sound of single written letters 33% of the time. This was not due to impaired spoken output because the pronunciations of the letters in pseudowords were relatively intact. This indicates that when letters were grouped into higher-level units they could be read, but not read at the level of individual graphemes.

Conversely, there have been cases of individuals who have had difficulty reading orthographic units that are larger than individual graphemes (e.g., Beauvois & Derouesne, 1981; Holmes, 1978; Marshall & Newcombe, 1973; Newcombe & Marshall, 1985). For example, consider the case study of RG who was 100% accurate at reading nouns but only 10% correct at reading pseudowords.

The errors with pseudoword reading led to a failure to identify the correct phonemes or an attempt to state a similar word (e.g., RG, a French reader, responded to the pseudoword "vina" by stating that it looked almost like "vinaigre," the French word for vinegar). The researchers determined that this was not a deficit at the phonetic production level of processing, as RG was 100% accurate at repeating pseudowords. Interestingly, when the letters of a word were read individually, RG was relatively accurate (87%), but when two letters or four/five letter nonwords were read the accuracy dropped dramatically (42% and 10%, respectively). These researchers further found that RG had a deficit at the level of syllable processing in pseudowords. For instance, when asked to read pseudowords with a simple syllabic composition (i.e., for V = Vowel and C = Consonant: V, CV, VC, or CVC syllables) RG had an accuracy rate of 55%, but when the syllabic composition was complex, (e.g., CCV) the accuracy rate dropped significantly to 32%. This work suggests that RG had a deficit in processing written words when they could not be read as a whole lexical unit, that is, if they were pseudowords that did not have any lexical representations to rely on. Further, the impairment was prominent when mapping of graphemes to phonemic representations involved multi-letter graphemic units. Interestingly, the pseudoword reading performance was better when the syllabic units were simpler, suggesting that there may be some structure to the mappings of graphemes to phonemes that utilizes syllabic information and may have provided some syllabic features that contributed to the higher performance.

Further work has suggested that there may be syllabic units in reading. This comes from the work of Lesch and Martin (1998) who described the case of ML, who demonstrated excellent word reading (100%) but impaired nonword reading (38% accuracy). Interestingly, ML was unimpaired at tasks that involved parsing a word into its syllables (e.g., CO-PY), but was impaired at separating words into their graphemic units (e.g., CH-AI-R). Furthermore, ML was impaired at pronouncing the onsets of words (e.g., SN-) or the bodies of words (e.g., —ACK) alone (14% and 20% accuracy, respectively). In contrast, ML was able to read the syllables on their own, but only if they actually appeared in real words (e.g., FLUT from FLUTTER; 71% accuracy). ML was impaired at pronouncing syllables that do not actually occur in any word (e.g., FLUB). This work suggests that there was a selective deficit in nonword reading that impaired units at the sub-syllabic level.

The study of individuals with impaired pseudoword reading suggests that there is a nonlinear structure to units of pronunciation in reading that can vary by size and structure and can range from single letters, to graphemes, to syllables (e.g., Berndt, 1996; Shallice & McCarthy, 1985; Warrington & Shallice, 1980).

2.2 *Orthographic Lexical Representations (Figure 1.1.vi)*

The orthographic lexicon is a long-term memory repository of familiar words. This knowledge of word spellings is obligatorily used to read words that do not conform to the typical orthography to phonology correspondence (OPC) rules, such as *colonel* (sub-lexical procedures might read this as /ko-lo-nɛl/ rather than /ker-nɛl/).

There have been a large number of cases of reading impairments characterized by impaired orthographic lexical processing. The study of orthographic lexical deficits has primarily focused on case studies of acquired dyslexic reading performance, in which there is better reading of pseudowords than irregular words (sometimes referred to as "input surface dyslexia"). In many of these cases, patients cannot distinguish real words from pseudowords. This latter ability can be examined with a lexical decision task that simply requires individuals to determine if a stimulus is either a word or a novel word (pseudoword). Impaired performance on this task is typically diagnostic of impaired orthographic lexical processing because it requires the ability to determine whether a string of letters is stored in long-term memory.

Most of the earliest cases of orthographic lexical deficits (see Marshall & Newcombe, 1973; McCarthy & Warrington, 1990; Patterson, Marshall, & Coltheart, 1985) involved spared reading of pseudowords and patients who could "sound out" words and pseudowords according to common OPC rules. If the orthographic lexical processing stream is impaired, then an individual must rely on mappings of sub-lexical orthographic units in order to read. Reading only via sub-lexical mappings can allow for reading of "regular" words (i.e., words with common orthography to phonology mappings, like "dot") and pseudowords (pronunciations of pseudowords, based on OPC rules, are always accurate since they cannot be irregular), but it does not allow one to accurately read words that have irregular or uncommon orthography to phonology mappings. Such cases have been interpreted as manifesting impaired access to orthographic lexical representations, but intact access to OPC procedures.

Consider patient PS who read pseudowords more accurately than words and regular words significantly better than irregular words (Hillis, 1993). His errors in reading seemed to result from an over-dependence on OPC rules. For example, he read *threat* as "threet" (rhyming with *beet*) and *stood* as "stewed." He also understood words based on the pronunciation he gave, even when it was incorrect, indicating that he did not access semantics from the orthographic representation but rather from the phonological representation activated by his application of OPC mechanisms. So, for example, he read the word *bear* as "beer" and defined it as something to drink at the bar. Consequently, he had a great deal of trouble distinguishing homophones, such as *beet* and *beat*. Therapy designed to reestablish orthographic representations of words, or access to them, in order to activate the corresponding semantic representations led to improved reading of irregular words, homophones, and words with ambiguous pronunciations, such as *bear* (Hillis, 1993).[3]

The strength of entries in the mental lexicon are thought to be modulated by reading experience; words that have a higher frequency (i.e., are read more often) will have stronger memory traces than those that occur at a lower frequency. Therefore, impairments in reading at the level of orthographic lexical processing are often characterized by differential accuracy on high-frequency relative to low-frequency words, high-frequency words being less susceptible to damage due to the strength of their representations.

Additional work studying orthographic lexical processing has reported on deficits that affect the mapping from orthographic lexicon representations to semantics. Take the case of DPT, who expressed a selective deficit in reading and spelling (Tsapkini & Rapp, 2010). In extensive testing DPT demonstrated normal performance in many cognitive areas, such as verbal working memory, visual perception and memory, fine motor speed and precision, spoken-word naming and fluency, single word auditory comprehension, and recognition memory for words and face (for further details see Tsapkini & Rapp, 2010). This case is interesting because the reading deficit was relatively subtle: accuracy on reading was unimpaired but reading speed for irregular and low-frequency words was significantly slower than a control group; this is characteristic of a mild deficit in orthographic lexical processing. Furthermore, DPT was slower than controls on visual word synonym judgments and visual semantic priming (i.e., a visual lexical decision task with semantic primes). Critically, DPT was unimpaired on comparable tasks in the auditory domain (i.e., an auditory word synonym judgment task and auditory lexical decision semantic prime task). These researchers concluded that DPT suffered from a deficit in mapping from orthographic lexical representations to lexical-semantic processes, and vice versa (Tsapkini & Rapp, 2010). This case study highlights the fact that precisely characterizing reading deficits can require sensitive measures such as reaction time in order to detect subtle deficits that may not be evident with accuracy measures.

Overall, these studies indicate that not only can orthographic lexical processing be impaired, but also the communication of orthographic representations to (and from) lexical-semantic processing may be disrupted. The next section will discuss impairments in lexical-semantic processing in reading.

3   Lexical-Semantic Processing (Figure 1.1.vii)

At minimum, in order to read a word one must be able to interpret the meaning of a written word. Disorders of reading comprehension can be driven by impairments in lexical-semantic processing. Such impairments tend to also be associated with impairments in lexical-semantic processing in other modalities, such as spoken-word retrieval.

Individuals with acquired reading disorders that impair lexical-semantic processing tend to make "regularization" errors in reading but can still distinguish words from pseudowords, and they can often extract at least some meaning from familiar words. Moreover, their understanding of words is no better when the word is read aloud correctly. Consider, for example, JJ (Hillis & Caramazza, 1991a, 1991c). He made regularization errors, such as reading *pear* as "pier"; in this instance the mispronunciation of *pear* is a regularization error because the "pier" pronunciation utilizes a different yet typical mapping of the "ea" grapheme (e.g., as in *ear, clear, tear,* etc.). Such regularization errors, along with his relatively accurate reading of pseudowords, indicated that JJ could read aloud via OPC mechanisms (at least when he failed to understand the words at all). Interestingly, most printed words were partially understood. For example, he typically selected the correct printed word or a semantically related word to match a picture (e.g., JJ matched a pictured chair to the word *bed*). His rates and types of errors in word-picture matching were identical with spoken and written word stimuli, indicating that both forms accessed an incomplete semantic representation. JJ also made semantically related word errors in spoken and written naming (e.g., JJ named a picture of a boat as "motorcycle") with approximately the same frequency as his errors in comprehension tasks. JJ's pattern of performance across lexical tasks can therefore be explained by selective damage to the lexical semantic system, which is assumed to be shared by reading, writing, naming, and comprehension tasks.

Although the semantic component is crucial in correctly reading homographs, such as *tear* in appropriate contexts, and in reading irregular words, the semantic component is not required for reading regular words by relying on OPC mechanisms. The reliance on OPC mechanisms alone results in the correct oral reading of regular words. However, irregular words, such as *one*, are misread (as "own" in this example) when using OPC alone, as reported in JJ's case. Nevertheless, it was noted that JJ read aloud some irregular words correctly. Many of these words were probably read correctly via the partially intact semantic component, since he also understood these words. It was found that the only irregular words that JJ read aloud accurately were words that he understood at least partially. For example, he read *one* correctly and defined it as "the number of ears I have"; although this is an incorrect definition, it was partially intact in that he knew it was a low number. Irregular words that he failed to understand at all were misread as phonologically plausible errors. For instance, he read *quay* as /kweI/ or "kway" (rhyming with *kay*) and defined it as "I have no idea; it looks like a type of bird." It was therefore hypothesized that phonological representations for output can be accessed by a "summation" of partial information from the semantic component and partial information from OPC mechanisms (Hillis & Caramazza, 1991c, 1995c; see Patterson & Hodges, 1992 for a similar proposal about the interaction of semantics and OPC mechanisms). Additional evidence for this hypothesis is that the rare semantic errors JJ made in oral reading were all phonologically related, as well as semantically related, to the target. For example, JJ misread *skirt* as "shirt." Other authors have proposed that correct oral reading of irregular words that are not understood provides evidence that phonological representations for output can be activated directly from orthographic representations; that is, that there is a "direct route" from the orthographic (input) lexicon to the phonological (output) lexicon (Coslett, 1991; Schwartz, Marin, & Saffran, 1979). Indeed, there have been cases reported in which irregular words are pronounced correctly without any apparent evidence of comprehension of the words (but see

Hillis & Caramazza, 1991c for discussion). Obviously, reliance on this "nonsemantic route" would not allow one to read homographs, such as *lead, read*, or *tear*, correctly in various contexts.

Other patients with impairment at the level of the semantic representation do not produce regularization errors. Rather, they make errors that are semantically related to the target. To illustrate, patient KE made semantically related errors in reading, oral naming, written naming, spoken-word comprehension, and written word comprehension (e.g., *onion* named as "carrot"; *jacket* read as "belt"; Hillis, Rapp, Romani, & Caramazza, 1990). He showed no ability to use OPC mechanisms to read aloud familiar or unfamiliar words or pseudowords. If his OPC mechanisms had been spared at all, the phonological information yielded by OPC would likely have "blocked" the production of semantically related words in oral reading. The production of semantically related word errors in oral reading, along with the inability to read pseudowords, is a pattern sometimes referred to as "deep dyslexia." However, it will be shown below that this pattern can be a consequence of damage to different components of the reading system, making it a heterogeneous class of disorders.

4 Phonological Representation Processing (Figure 1.1.viii)

The semantic representation of a word activates a phonological representation for spoken output. As noted above, it is also possible that OPC mechanisms and/or orthographic lexical representations alone can activate a phonological representation for spoken output. Normally, only the target phonological representation is selected for output. However, in cases of reading impairment the target phonological representation may be unavailable. There are at least two possible consequences of impaired access to the target phonological representations. First, if the patient has intact OPC mechanisms, he or she might rely on these mechanisms and produce phonologically plausible errors. Consider, for example, patient HG (Hillis, 1991). HG was unable to access correct phonological representations in any spoken task (spontaneous speech, oral naming, repetition, or oral reading). Her spontaneous speech consisted of fluent, low-volume jargon, with virtually no content. However, her OPC mechanisms were intact (at least after some brief training), and so she sounded out words slowly in oral reading tasks. For example, she read *feet* correctly and read *comb* as "sombe" (/soUmb/). In contrast, HG had relatively preserved access to orthographical representations for written output. Thus, in naming tasks she often wrote the correct word, but read aloud her own written word incorrectly (e.g., *comb* as "sombe"). Furthermore, at times she would produce a phonologically plausible rendition of the orthographic stimulus, even though no written name was available. That is, she named *comb* as "sombe" in response to the object, even though she did not write or have available the written word. In conversation, her rare content words were often phonologically plausible renditions of the written form of the word. For example, she named *Broad St.* as "brode sssst" (/brod st/). She apparently had no recollection that the abbreviation *St.* represented the word *street*. When *street* was written out, she pronounced it correctly, indicating that her mispronunciations were not due to motor programming or articulation problems. HG was able to learn the correct pronunciations of words (i.e., to develop, or restore access to, phonological representations) only if they were spelled for her phonetically. Thus, learning to say *pizza* correctly was accomplished by spelling it as *peetsa* (Hillis, 1991). HG's case demonstrates that regularization errors can occur as a result of damage not only at the levels of the orthographic input lexicon or the semantic system, but also at the level of the phonological output lexicon; that is, damage anywhere along the lexical route, sparing the OPC route.

A second reported pattern of errors that can result from impaired access to phonological representations for output is the production of semantically related words in oral reading and naming. In these cases, there has been severe impairment of OPC mechanisms, as well as impaired access to some phonological representations. One illustrative case is that of RGB (Caramazza & Hillis, 1990c; Hillis & Caramazza, 1995e). RGB had fluent, grammatical speech, with frequent circumlocutions and semantic paraphasias. However, in contrast to patients JJ and KE, who made semantic errors in both oral naming and comprehension, RGB had perfectly intact comprehension of written and spoken words (as indicated by his 100% accurate word/picture verification, his accurate definitions of words, and so on). Nevertheless, he read aloud words as semantically related words. For instance, he read the word *red* as "yellow" but defined it as "the color of blood." RGB's oral reading and naming could not be improved by providing the phonetically spelled word, since he had no ability to use OPC mechanisms to read familiar or unfamiliar words. However, his oral reading and naming improved with a cuing hierarchy that increased production of the correct word. That is, it is thought that the availability of a phonological representation is dependent on its "threshold of activation," which is a function of the frequency of production of a word. Thus, cued production of the word likely increased its frequency of production and perhaps lowered its threshold of activation.

Why did RGB make semantic errors, rather than phonological errors, in reading and naming, if his semantic component was intact (as indicated by preserved comprehension)? One account for the production of semantic errors in the face of spared comprehension is the following: semantic representations are composed of all the semantic features that together define the meaning of the word, and each of these features activates every phonological representation to which it corresponds. For example, the semantic representation of *mitten* might be composed of semantic features, such as <clothing>, <for hands>, <for cold weather>, <woolen or weather-resistant material>, <without separate parts for each digit>. These features would also activate corresponding phonological representations. To illustrate, the feature <clothing> would activate phonological representations of *skirt, shirt, pants, sock, mitten*, and so on, whereas the feature <for hands> would activate phonological representations of words such as *mitten, glove, hand lotion*, and so on. Normally, only the target phonological representation would receive the most activation (from all of the semantic features) and would thus be selected for output. However, if that representation were to be unavailable (e.g., in the case of RGB), one of the other representations (e.g., *glove*) activated by one or more of the semantic features, might be activated instead (see Hillis & Caramazza, 1995b, 1995e). In this way, the production of semantic errors in reading, along with impaired OPC mechanisms (the pattern known as "deep dyslexia"), can result from damage to either the phonological lexicon or the semantic component. In the latter case, semantic errors are likely to arise when there is damage to one or more features of the semantic representations such that the impoverished semantic representation is equally compatible with (and equally activates) several phonological representations. For instance, if the semantic representation of *mitten* were missing the feature <for hands> the remaining features might equally activate *mitten* and *sock*. Whichever phonological representation had a lower threshold of activation (e.g., higher frequency) would be selected for output. This account explains the inconsistent production of semantic errors and correct names in oral reading and naming by patients with semantic impairments (e.g., KE, described earlier).

Others propose a "direct" or "third" route from orthographic to phonological lexicon, bypassing semantics (see Figure 1.1.*ix.*) (e.g., Coslett, 1991). Schwartz, Saffran, and Marin (1980) describe the case of patient WLP, who, despite a severe deficit in semantic processing, was able to read both regular and irregular words. WLP's semantic deficit was evidenced by impairment in tasks tapping knowledge of semantic properties accessed through reading. She had difficulty in matching written words to pictures, as well as sorting written words by semantic category (e.g., sort a card with the word *elephant* into the "animals" category). Despite these difficulties, WLP was able to correctly produce the phonological form of each word, reading them correctly but not accessing the corresponding semantic representation. This pattern persisted even for irregular words, which should obligatorily require use of the lexical reading route. Schwartz and colleagues suggest that these results are best accounted for by a pathway from the orthographic lexicon that leads directly to the phonological lexicon, bypassing the lexical semantic system (Figure 1.1.*ix*).

5   Output Processing (Figure 1.1.x)

5.1   *Phonetic Selection*

After brain damage, many patients fail to read aloud or name words correctly, even though they seem to know the correct pronunciation. That is, they appear to access the target phonological representation, but then produce either a phonologically similar word (e.g., *mitten* → "kitten"; Martin, Dell, Saffran, & Schwartz, 1994) or non-word (e.g., *mitten* → "titten"). They may attempt to self-correct the phonological error. A case in point is that of JBN (Hillis, Boatman, Hart, & Gordon, 1999). JBN had fluent, grammatical speech, but with frequent phonological errors. Her comprehension of written words was intact, as indicated by printed word/picture verification tasks with both phonologically and semantically related foils and by matching printed words to synonyms. She also seemed to access the correct phonological representation, as indicated by her ability to match rhyming words or pictures. Nevertheless, in oral reading (and oral naming), she made frequent phonological errors in producing the words. The problem was not in motor planning or articulation, since JBN correctly repeated nonsense syllables. Rather, her performance was explained by assuming impaired selection of the sequence of phonemes (or sub-lexical phonological units) to articulate.

5.2   *Motor Programming and Articulation*

Once the sequence of phonemes (or phonetic segments) is selected for output it must be translated into the appropriate sequence of movements through programming and coordination of the lips, tongue, jaw, soft palate, and vocal cords. Since this handbook concerns language (rather than speech production) disorders, a full discussion of the variety of motor deficits that can interfere with accurate oral reading is beyond the scope of this chapter. However, it is important to note that either dysarthria or apraxia can result in impaired, or difficult-to-understand, oral reading. Dysarthria is an impairment in the range, strength, rate, or coordination of movements of the articulators, due to upper and/or lower cranial nerve deficits or damage to the basal ganglia and/ or cerebellum. Apraxia of speech is an impairment in programming or sequencing these complex movements in the face of normal range, strength, and rate of movements.

6   A Connectionist Approach to Reading Impairments

It should be stated that the aforementioned account of reading deficits has been opposed by authors who posit that impairments in reading are needlessly categorized into distinct streams of processing. Instead, these researchers contend that the underlying neural processing is far more complex and rich than can be described by positing deficits in discrete streams of processing.

Such views often refer to computer simulations of reading, in which both words and pseudowords can be correctly pronounced without postulating distinct cognitive mechanisms or streams of processing associated with any particular type of written word (Seidenberg & McClelland, 1989). Some typical patterns of impaired reading performance, such as better reading of pseudowords than words or vice versa, can be simulated by creating damage to such a neural network (Plaut & Shallice, 1993). For example, plausible pronunciations of words (reported in cases of "surface dyslexia") and a pattern in which errors include visually similar words (e.g., *ford* for *fork*) and semantically similar words (e.g., *spoon* for *fork*), as reported in cases of "deep dyslexia," have been simulated.

There are advantages to being able to implement a comprehensive computational model that facilitates the description of reading impairments. It would facilitate a mechanistically simplistic characterization of the underlying reading impairments (i.e., it need not posit separate lexical and sub-lexical processing mechanisms) and also allow for assessments of the degree of damage to the connections between component processes in the model (Woollams, 2013). However, current simulations fail to reproduce certain reported patterns of performance, such as the production of only semantically related words (e.g., by RGB in Caramazza & Hillis, 1990c) or the production of only phonologically or visually similar words (e.g., Hillis et al., 1999). Thus, currently, only models that postulate separate cognitive mechanisms for lexical representations and OPC can account for the full spectrum of impaired reading patterns due to focal brain injury. Nevertheless, certain features of these connectionist models or neural networks of the reading process, such as the interaction between separate levels of processing, are likely to capture important features of the reading system.

Summary

This review of the components of the reading process (schematically represented in Figure 1.1) was meant to provide the reader with an overview of some of the major levels of representations and cognitive mechanisms underlying reading that have been identified through the study of neurologically impaired subjects. It is not comprehensive. For instance, some investigators would add a level of representation—the lemma—that mediates between semantics and phonological representations (Roelofs, 1992). This level of representation is further discussed in chapters 7 and 17. Furthermore, a number of investigators would add more (or less) interaction between levels of representation. This topic, of the degree and type (feedforward, feedback, or both) of interaction, and between what levels of representation has been discussed elsewhere (e.g., Rapp & Goldrick, 2000). Most computational models have assumed both feedforward and feedback interaction between all levels of representation (see N. Martin et al., chapter 20, this volume), whereas most "serial" models have assumed virtually no interaction between components (but see Hillis & Caramazza, 1991c, 1995c; Humphreys et al., 1988). Recent investigations indicate that the hypothesis of limited interaction between specific levels of representation may best account for the empirical evidence (Rapp & Goldrick, 2000).

Still other investigators would question the existence of one or more of the levels of representation or processing specified in Figure 1.1. For example, many computational models have accounted for at least a subset of data from neurologically impaired subjects without proposing independent lexical and sub-lexical (OPC) mechanisms. It is not clear, however, how these models could be revised to account for patients like HG, who relied solely on OPC mechanisms, even to pronounce printed words that she understood. Nor could they account for the fact that HG could only learn correct pronunciations of printed irregular words when she was presented with the printed word misspelled phonetically. As mentioned, these computational models also fail to account for patients who make strictly one sort of error (either phonologically/visually similar errors or semantically related errors) in reading. Computational models that do specify lexical levels (or a lemma level) of representation separate from a semantic component can better account for the observed patterns of performance, but only if selective components of the system are "lesioned" (see chapter 7 in this volume). Other computational models would do away with an "object-centered" level of spatial representation (Mozer & Behrmann, 1990), but in so doing cannot account for patients, like NG, who make errors on one side of the "canonical" representation of a word, irrespective of its orientation or modality of presentation.

Although the components of the reading system are represented by discrete boxes in Figure 1.1, it is highly likely that these functional entities consist of distributed representations in the brain. That is, a "semantic representation" almost certainly consists of co-activation of numerous regions of the brain (let alone thousands or millions of neurons) that represent separate features that jointly define the meaning of a given word. Similarly, an orthographic representation might be best thought of as co-activation of the component graphemes, together with ordering information, which may or may not be represented in a unified brain region. Nevertheless, there does seem to be a certain amount of localization of these separate cognitive components to specific brain regions, although there is assuredly not a single region of the brain that carries out the entire reading task. The localization of distinct operations in the reading process is discussed in chapter 2.

It was noted in this chapter that patients with selective damage to specific components of the reading system responded to different types of therapy to improve their reading. Specific remediation strategies for a number of the patients described in this chapter, along with other patients with damage to one or more levels of processing in reading, are described in more detail elsewhere (e.g., in Beeson & Hillis, 2001; Hillis & Caramazza, 1994). More important, discussion of how a model of the reading task can focus therapy for patients with a variety of reading disorders is discussed in detail by Rhonda B. Friedman in chapter 3.

It is safe to conclude from the cases of impaired reading described in this chapter and elsewhere that reading is a complex process that entails activation of a number of different mental representations and operations that can be selectively impaired by focal brain damage. Many of these representations and operations are shared by other language tasks, such that damage—say, to the semantic component—is reflected not only in reading, but also in oral and written naming and in comprehension tasks. Thus, pinpointing and characterizing the level of impairment in reading often requires assessment of a variety of lexical tasks, with different input and output modalities. Reading sentences and narratives recruits additional processes, such as short-term memory and syntactic processes. Even so, evidence of the type reported in this chapter, that single word reading consists of a number of functionally distinct components carried out by various regions of the brain, has played a crucial role in the development of cognitive neuroscience. Such evidence has been pivotal in further investigation of the neural substrates of reading and other lexical processes and investigation into the types of therapeutic interventions (see chapter 3) that might restore language function after brain damage.

Notes

1 The distinction between graphemes and ALIs is based on two criteria. (1) Whereas graphemes necessarily map to individual phonemes, ALIs do not. For instance the grapheme PH maps to a single phoneme /f/, but is composed of two separate ALIs (P and H). (2) An individual letter (e.g., P) is considered a grapheme when discussed within the context of orthography-to-phonology mapping mechanisms, but is considered an ALI when discussed within the context of mechanisms that abstract away from its visual form.

2 Some researchers have suggested that recognition of oral spelling recruits spelling rather than reading processes (Cipolotti & Warrington, 1996; Shallice & McCarthy, 1985; Warrington & Langdon, 2002). However, it is unclear how recognition of oral spelling could proceed via spelling processes. Furthermore, in the case of LHD, recognizing orally spelled words could not ostensibly utilize the spelling system because LHD also had an impairment to orthographic lexical processing in spelling. A reading model that posits abstract letter identities that can be accessed via different modalities (e.g., spoken letter names) provides a straightforward explanation for these findings. Readers are referred to Schubert and McCloskey (Submitted) for details.

3 Early after his brain damage, PS also had an impairment at the level of semantics, but this deficit only affected the semantic representations of animals and vegetables (Hillis & Caramazza, 1991a).

References

Barbut, D., & Gazzaniga, M.S. (1987). Disturbances in conceptual space involving language and speech. *Brain, 110(Pt 6)*, 1487–1496.

Baxter, D.M., & Warrington, E.K. (1983). Neglect dysgraphia. *Journal of Neurology, Neurosurgery, and Psychiatry, 46*(12), 1073–1078.

Beauvois, M.F., & Derouesne, J. (1981). Lexical or orthographic agraphia. *Brain, 104*(Pt 1), 21–49.

Beeson, P.M., & Hillis, A. (2001). Comprehension and production of written words. In R. Chapey (Ed.), *Comprehension and production of written words* (4th ed.). Baltimore: Williams and Wilkin.

Berndt, R.S. (1996). An investigation of nonlexical reading impairments. *Cognitive Neuropsychology, 13*(6), 763–801. doi:10.1080/026432996381809

Bisiach, E., & Berti, A. (1987). Dyschiria. An attempt at its systemic explanation. In M. Jeannerod (Ed.), *Neurophysiological and neuropsychological aspects of spatial neglect* (pp. 183–201). New York: Elsevier Science Publishing Company.

Bisiach, E., & Luzzatti, C. (1978). Unilateral neglect of representational space. *Cortex, 14*(1), 129–133.

Bowers, J.S. (2000). In defense of abstractionist theories of repetition priming and word identification. *Psychonomic Bulletin & Review, 7*(1), 83–99.

Brunsdon, R., Coltheart, M., & Nickels, L. (2006). Severe developmental letter-processing impairment: A treatment case study. *Cognitive Neuropsychology, 23*(6), 795–821. doi:10.1080/02643290500310863

Caplan, L.R., & Hedley-Whyte, T. (1974). Cuing and memory dysfunction in alexia without agraphia. *Brain, 97*, 251–262.

Caramazza, A., & Hillis, A. (1990a). Levels of representation, coordinate frames, and unilateral neglect. *Cognitive Neuropsychology, 7*(5/6), 391–445.

Caramazza, A., & Hillis, A. (1990b). Spatial representation of words in the brain implied by studies of a unilateral neglect patient. *Nature, 346*(6281), 267–269. doi:10.1038/346267a0

Caramazza, A., & Hillis, A. (1990c). Where do semantic errors come from? *Cortex, 26*(1), 95–122.

Castles, A., & Friedmann, N. (2014). Developmental dyslexia and the phonological deficit hypothesis. *Mind & Language, 29*(3), 270–285. doi:10.1111/mila.12050

Chanoine, V., Teixeira Ferreira, C., Demonet, J.-F., Nespoulous, J., & Poncet, M. (1998). Optic aphasia with pure alexia: a mild form of visual associative agnosia? A case study. *Cortex, 34*(3), 437–448. doi:10.1093/neucas/6.4.273-a

Cipolotti, L., & Warrington, E.K. (1996). Does recognizing orally spelled words depend on reading? An investigation into a case of better written than oral spelling. *Neuropsychologia, 34*(5), 427–440.

Coltheart, M. (1981). Disorders of reading and their implications for models of normal reading. *Visible Language, 15*(3), 245–286.

Coltheart, M. (2014). The neuronal recycling hypothesis for reading and the question of reading universals. *Mind & Language, 29*(3), 255–269. doi:10.1111/mila.12049

Coltheart, M., Masterson, J., Byng, S., Prior, M., & Riddoch, J. (1983). Surface dyslexia. *The Quarterly Journal of Experimental Psychology Section A, 35*(3), 469–495. doi:10.1080/14640748308402483

Coltheart, M., Patterson, K., & Marshall, J.C. (1980). *Deep dyslexia*. London: Routledge and Kegan Paul.

Coslett, H.B. (1991). Read but not write "idea": evidence for a third reading mechanism. *Brain and Language, 40*(4), 425–443.

Costello, A.D., & Warrington, E.K. (1987). The dissociation of visuospatial neglect and neglect dyslexia. *Journal of Neurology, Neurosurgery, and Psychiatry, 50*(9), 1110–1116.

Dalmás, J.F., & Dansilio, S. (2000). Visuographemic alexia: a new form of a peripheral acquired dyslexia. *Brain and Language, 75*(1), 1–16. doi:10.1006/brln.2000.2321

Dehaene, S. (2014). Reading in the brain revised and extended: response to comments. *Mind & Language, 29*(3), 320–335. doi:10.1111/mila.12053

Dehaene, S., & Cohen, L. (2007). Response to Carreiras et al: the role of visual similarity, feedforward, feedback and lateral pathways in reading. *Trends in Cognitive Science, 11*(11), 456–457. doi:10.1016/j.tics.2007.08.009

Dickerson, J. (1999). Format distortion and word reading: the role of multiletter units. *Neurocase, 5*(1), 31–36. doi:10.1080/13554799908404062

Downey, G. (2014). All forms of writing. *Mind & Language, 29*(3), 304–319. doi:10.1111/mila.12052

Evett, L.J., & Humphreys, G.W. (1981). The use of abstract graphemic information in lexical access. *The Quarterly Journal of Experimental Psychology Section A, 33*(4), 325–350. doi:10.1080/14640748108400797

Forde, E.M.E., & Humphreys, G.W. (2005). Is oral spelling recognition dependent on reading or spelling systems? Dissociative evidence from two single case studies. *Cognitive Neuropsychology, 22*(2), 169–181. doi:10.1080/02643290442000040

Funnell, E. (1983). Phonological processes in reading: new evidence from acquired dyslexia. *British Journal of Psychology (London, England: 1953), 74*(Pt 2), 159–180.

Greenwald, M.L., & Gonzalez Rothi, L.J. (1998). Lexical access via letter naming in a profoundly alexic and anomic patient: a treatment study. *Journal of the International Neuropsychological Society: JINS, 4*(6), 595–607.

Hanley, J.R., & Kay, J. (1992). Does letter-by-letter reading involve the spelling system? *Neuropsychologia, 30,* 237–256.

Haywood, M., & Coltheart, M. (2000). Neglect dyslexia and the early stages of visual word recognition. *Neurocase, 6,* 33–44. doi:10.1080/13554790008402755

Hillis, A. (1991). Effects of separate treatments for distinct impairments within the naming process. Retrieved from http://aphasiology.pitt.edu/archive/00000120/

Hillis, A. (1993). The role of models of language processing in rehabilitation of language impairments. *Aphasiology, 7*(1), 5–26. doi:10.1080/02687039308249497

Hillis, A., Boatman, D., Hart, J., & Gordon, B. (1999). Making sense out of jargon: a neurolinguistic and computational account of jargon aphasia. *Neurology, 53*(8), 1813–1824.

Hillis, A., & Caramazza, A. (1991a). Category-specific naming and comprehension impairment: a double dissociation. *Brain: A Journal of Neurology, 114*(Pt 5), 2081–2094.

Hillis, A., & Caramazza, A. (1991b). Deficit to stimulus-centered, letter shape representations in a case of "unilateral neglect." *Neuropsychologia, 29*(12), 1223–1240.

Hillis, A., & Caramazza, A. (1991c). Mechanisms for accessing lexical representations for output: evidence from a category-specific semantic deficit. *Brain and Language, 40*(1), 106–144.

Hillis, A., & Caramazza, A. (1994). Theories of lexical processing and theories of rehabilitation. In M.J. Riddoch & G.W. Humphreys (Eds.), *Cognitive neuropsychology and cognitive rehabilitation* (pp. 449–482). Hillsdale, NJ: Lawrence Erlbaum Associates.

Hillis, A., & Caramazza, A. (1995a). A framework for interpreting distinct patterns of hemispatial neglect. *Neurocase, 1*(3), 189–207. doi:10.1080/13554799508402364

Hillis, A., & Caramazza, A. (1995b). Cognitive and neural mechanisms underlying visual and semantic processing: implications from "optic aphasia." *Journal of Cognitive Neuroscience, 7*(4), 457–478. doi:10.1162/jocn.1995.7.4.457

Hillis, A., & Caramazza, A. (1995c). Converging evidence for the interaction of semantic and sublexical phonological information in accessing lexical representations for spoken output. *Cognitive Neuropsychology, 12*(2), 187–227. doi:10.1080/02643299508251996

Hillis, A., & Caramazza, A. (1995d). Spatially specific deficits in processing graphemic representations in reading and writing. *Brain and Language, 48*(3), 263–308.

Hillis, A., & Caramazza, A. (1995e). The compositionality of lexical semantic representations: clues from semantic errors in object naming. *Memory (Hove, England), 3*(3–4), 333–358. doi:10.1080/09658219508253156

Hillis, A., Rapp, B., Benzing, L., & Caramazza, A. (1998). Dissociable coordinate frames of unilateral spatial neglect: "viewer-centered" neglect. *Brain and Cognition, 37*(3), 491–526. doi:10.1006/brcg.1998.1010

Hillis, A., Rapp, B., Romani, C., & Caramazza, A. (1990). Selective impairment of semantics in lexical processing. *Cognitive Neuropsychology, 7*(3), 191–243. doi:10.1080/02643299008253442

Holmes, J.M. (1978). Regression and reading breakdown. In A. Caramazza (Ed.), *Language acquisition and language breakdown: parallels and divergences* (pp. 87–98). Baltimore: Johns Hopkins University Press.

Humphreys, G.W., Evett, L.J., & Quinlan, P.T. (1990). Orthographic processing in visual word identification. *Cognitive Psychology, 22*(4), 517–560.

Humphreys, G.W., Riddoch, J., & Quinlan, P. (1988). Cascade processes in picture identification. *Cognitive Neuropsychology, 5*(1), 67–104. doi:10.1080/02643298808252927

Lesch, M.F., & Martin, R.C. (1998). The representation of sublexical orthographic-phonologic correspondences: evidence from phonological dyslexia. *The Quarterly Journal of Experimental Psychology Section A, 51*(4), 905–938. doi:10.1080/713755790

Marr, D., & Nishihara, H. (1978). Representation and recognition of the spatial organization of three-dimensional shapes. *Proceedings of the Royal Society of London, 200*(1140), 269–294.

Marshall, J.C., & Newcombe, F. (1973). Patterns of paralexia: a psycholinguistic approach. *Journal of Psycholinguistic Research, 2*(3), 175–199.

Martin, N., Dell, G.S., Saffran, E.M., & Schwartz, M.F. (1994). Origins of paraphasias in deep dysphasia: testing the consequences of a decay impairment to an interactive spreading activation model of lexical retrieval. *Brain and Language, 47*(4), 609–660. doi:10.1006/brln.1994.1061

Martin, R.C., & Caramazza, A. (1982). Short-term memory performance in the absence of phonological coding. *Brain and Cognition, 1*(1), 50–70.

McCarthy, R.A., & Warrington, E.K. (1990). *Cognitive neuropsychology: a clinical introduction* (1st ed.). San Diego: Academic Press.

Menary, R. (2014). Neural plasticity, neuronal recycling and niche construction. *Mind & Language, 29*(3), 286–303. doi:10.1111/mila.12051

Miozzo, M., & Caramazza, A. (1998). Varieties of pure alexia: the case of failure to access graphemic representations. *Cognitive Neuropsychology, 15*(1), 203–238. doi:10.1080/026432998381267

Monk, A. (1985). Theoretical note: coordinate systems in visual word recognition. *Quarterly Journal of Experimental Psychology, 37*(4), 613–625.

Mozer, M.C., & Behrmann, M. (1990). On the interaction of selective attention and lexical knowledge: a connectionist account of neglect dyslexia. *Journal of Cognitive Neuroscience, 2*(2), 96–123. doi:10.1162/jocn.1990.2.2.96

Newcombe, F., & Marshall, J.C. (1985). Reading and writing by letter sounds. *Surface dyslexia: cognitive and neuropsychological studies of phonological reading.* Hove: Lawrence Erlbaum Associates.

Nichelli, P., Venneri, A., Pentore, R., & Cubelli, R. (1993). Horizontal and vertical neglect dyslexia. *Brain and Language, 44*(3), 264–283.

Patterson, K., & Hodges, J.R. (1992). Deterioration of word meaning: implications for reading. *Neuropsychologia, 30*(12), 1025–1040.

Patterson, K., & Kay, J. (1982). Letter-by-letter reading: psychological descriptions of a neurological syndrome. *Quarterly Journal of Experimental Psychology, 34A*, 411–441.

Patterson, K., Marshall, J.C., & Coltheart, M. (1985). *Surface dyslexia: neuropsychological and cognitive studies of phonological reading.* Hillsdale, NJ: Lawrence Erlbaum Associates.

Patterson, K., & Wilson, B. (1990). A rose is a rose or a nose: a deficit in initial letter identification. *Cognitive Neuropsychology, 7*(5/6), 447–477.

Peressotti, F., Job, R., Rumiati, R., & Nicoletti, R. (1995). Levels of representation in word processing. *Visual Cognition, 2*(4), 421–450. doi:10.1080/13506289508401740

Plaut, D.C., & Shallice, T. (1993). Deep dyslexia: A case study of connectionist neuropsychology. *Cognitive Neuropsychology, 10*(5), 377–500.

Polk, T.A., & Farah, M.J. (1997). A simple common contexts explanation for the development of abstract letter identities. *Neural Computation, 9*(6), 1277–1289. doi:10.1162/neco.1997.9.6.1277

Price, C., & Humphreys, G.W. (1992). Letter-by-letter reading? Functional deficits and compensatory strategies. *Cognitive Neuropsychology, 9*(5), 427–457. doi:10.1080/02643299208252067

Rapp, B., & Caramazza, A. (1989). Letter processing in reading and spelling: some dissociations. *Reading and Writing, 1*(1), 3–23. doi:10.1007/BF00178834

Rapp, B., & Caramazza, A. (1997). From graphemes to abstract letter shapes: levels of representation in written spelling. *Journal of Experimental Psychology: Human Perception and Performance, 23*(4), 1130–1152.

Rapp, B., & Goldrick, M. (2000). Discreteness and interactivity in spoken word production. *Psychological Review, 107*(3), 460–499.

Roberts, D.J., Woollams, A.M., Kim, E., Beeson, P.M., Rapcsak, S.Z., & Lambon Ralph, M. A. (2012). Efficient visual object and word recognition relies on high spatial frequency coding in the left posterior fusiform gyrus: evidence from a case-series of patients with ventral occipito-temporal cortex damage. *Cerebral Cortex*, (2002). doi:10.1093/cercor/bhs224

Roelofs, A. (1992). A spreading-activation theory of lemma retrieval in speaking. *Cognition, 42*(1–3), 107–142.

Rynard, D., & Besner, D. (1987). Basic processes in reading: on the development of cross-case letter matching without reference to phonology. *Bulletin of the Psychonomic Society, 25*(5), 361–363.

Schubert, T., & McCloskey, M. (2013). Prelexical representations and processes in reading: evidence from acquired dyslexia. *Cognitive Neuropsychology, 30*(6), 360–395. doi:10.1080/02643294.2014.880677

Schwartz, M.F., Marin, O.S., & Saffran, E.M. (1979). Dissociations of language function in dementia: a case study. *Brain and Language, 7*(3), 277–306.

Schwartz, M.F., Saffran, E.M., & Marin, O.S.M. (1980). Fractionating the reading process in dementia: evidence for word-specific print-to-sound associations. In M. Coltheart, K. Patterson, & J.C. Marshall (Eds.), *Deep dyslexia* (pp. 259–269). London: Routledge & Kegan Paul.

Seidenberg, M.S., & McClelland, J.L. (1989). A distributed, developmental model of visual word recognition and naming. *Psychological Review, 96*(4), 523–568.

Shallice, T., & McCarthy, R. (1985). Phonological reading: from patterns of impairment to possible procedures. In K.E. Patterson, J.C. Marshall, & M. Colheart (Eds.), *Surface dyslexia: neuropsychological and cognitive studies of phonological reading* (pp. 361–398). London: Lawrence Erlbaum.

Shallice, T., & Saffran, E. (1986). Lexical processing in the absence of explicit word identification: evidence from a letter-by-letter reader. *Cognitive Neuropsychology, 3*(4), 429–458. doi:10.1080/02643298608252030

Subbiah, I., & Caramazza, A. (2000). Stimulus-centered neglect in reading and object recognition. *Neurocase, 6*, 13–31.

Tainturier, M.-J., & Rapp, B.C. (2003). Is a single graphemic buffer used in reading and spelling? *Aphasiology, 17*(6–7), 537–562. doi:10.1080/02687030344000021

Tsapkini, K., & Rapp, B. (2010). The orthography-specific functions of the left fusiform gyrus: evidence of modality and category specificity. *Cortex, 46*(2), 185–205.

Volpato, C., Bencini, G., Meneghello, F., Piron, L., & Semenza, C. (2012). Covert reading of letters in a case of global alexia. *Brain and Language, 120*(3), 217–225. doi:10.1016/j.bandl.2011.12.014

Warrington, E.K., & Langdon, D.W. (2002). Does the spelling dyslexic read by recognizing orally spelled words? An investigation of a letter-by-letter reader. *Neurocase, 8*(3), 210–218. doi:10.1093/neucas/8.3.210

Warrington, E.K., & Shallice, T. (1980). Word-form dyslexia. *Brain, 103*(1), 99–112.

Woollams, A.M. (2013). Connectionist neuropsychology: uncovering ultimate causes of acquired dyslexia. *Philosophical Transactions of the Royal Society of London. Series B, Biological Sciences, 369*. doi:http://dx.doi.org/10.1098/rstb.2012.0398

2

NEUROANATOMICAL ASPECTS OF READING

Kyrana Tsapkini and Argye E. Hillis

In the last two decades there has been a great interest in 'reading in the brain,' as the homonymous seminal book by Stanislas Dehaene instantiates (Dehaene, 2009). As shown in the previous chapter on models of reading, describing the reading process is a complex endeavor, and describing how that occurs in the brain becomes even more complicated. The complication exists because part of the 'how' involves inevitably explaining the 'why,' and that implies an explanation of how anatomy, evolution, culture, and education have affected the process of reading in the brain. The explosion of imaging, in general, and functional neuroimaging techniques, in particular, in both 'normal' and impaired populations such as individuals with developmental or acquired reading disorders has created a new science of reading. We will only tackle a small part of this 'new science of reading' to show the biological (brain) aspect of this complicated process; that is, how particular areas of the brain specialize but also work synergistically to accomplish this linguistic function.

The relationship between brain and behavior in language has generated heated debates since the beginning of the 19th century, such as those between Pierre Paul Broca and Pierre Marie, and over the past few decades the debates have been elevated to new heights with the rise of functional neuroimaging. Functional neuroimaging became a new means to address old questions regarding the biological basis of behavior. Some have theorized that functional neuroimaging is mostly a method to validate our cognitive models in the brain (Caramazza & Mahon, 2003), whereas others have dared to claim that functional neuroimaging, and imaging in general, can pose and answer scientific questions about our cognitive models (Coltheart, 2006; Rothlein & Rapp, 2014).

In this chapter we will present the debate(s) regarding reading, trying to go beyond correlating particular brain areas with each component of cognitive models of reading. We will present data from both lesion-deficit correlation studies and functional imaging studies, and we will discuss the potential contribution of each to understanding the neural substrates of reading, along with conflicting results as well as points of convergence. We will try to show what each approach focuses on and why, and stress how these approaches evolved over time in the quest to answer the big question: how the brain reads.

History and Modernity in Lesion Studies

The discussion about the neural site(s) of reading has a long history dating back to French neurologist Joseph-Jules Dejerine, who in 1892, after studying Mr. C, coined the term 'pure verbal blindness' as the inability to read in the presence of intact spoken language; intact spelling; intact visual recognition of other items, such as objects, faces, drawings, or even digits; and preserved tactile or motor knowledge of letter shapes (Dejerine, 1891, 1892). The inability to read along with the above symptomatology in a subsequent series of individuals with brain lesions confirmed Dejerine's initial observations. The new term used was 'pure alexia' or 'alexia without agraphia.' The term has dominated the neuropsychological literature since, although the profile ranged from complete inability to recognize single letters to increased time to read a word, a pattern of performance labeled 'letter-by-letter reading.' Crucially, Mr. C's lesion revealed post-mortem four years after the initial stroke was very similar to contemporary individuals with pure alexia and involved the regions of the left occipital lobe starting at the base of the cuneus as well the lingual and fusiform lobules. Dejerine used the term 'disconnection syndrome' to emphasize that Mr. C's lesion had also destroyed long-distance connections of the corpus callosum that fed visual information from the right to the left occipito-temporal areas. However, a region he called the 'visual center for letters' located in the angular gyrus was intact, albeit without visual input. Interestingly, most cases with pure alexia had similar lesions involving the left occipito-temporal region and splenium of the corpus callosum, since such lesions frequently result from strokes due to occlusion of the left posterior cerebral artery. Recent magnetic resonance imaging analyses compared individuals with pure alexia to a group of individuals with brain lesions who did not have alexia (Binder & Mohr, 1992; Cohen et al., 2003; Damasio & Damasio, 1983; Leff et al., 2001) by superimposing their lesions and computing the intersections in three-dimensional space. These analyses revealed that the most common area of overlap for pure alexia was located in the left occipito-temporal area, within a groove in the lateral occipito-temporal sulcus. Cohen and Dehaene called it the 'visual word form area,' or VWFA, and reasoned that this is indeed the area where location-independent, font-independent representations of letter strings are computed, rather the angular gyrus where Dejerine assumed the visual images of letters were represented (Cohen et al., 2000; Cohen et al., 2002; Dehaene, Le Clec'H, Poline, Le Bihan, & Cohen, 2002; Dehaene et al., 2004; Gaillard et al., 2006). The term itself and the claim generated a heated debate in the neuropsychological and neuroimaging literature resulting in strongly opposing views (Price & Devlin, 2011; Price, Winterburn, Giraud, Moore, & Noppeney, 2003; Price et al., 2006; Price & Devlin, 2003; Price & Devlin, 2004), as well as more integrative approaches based on neuroanatomical hypotheses that tried to present converging accounts for seemingly non-congruent data (see Hillis, Newhart, Heidler, Barker, Herskovits, & Degaonkar, 2005; Philipose et al., 2007b; Sebastian et al., 2014). One of the main reasons for opposing such a claim was the consistent finding that individuals with post-stroke lesions in the inferior occipito-temporal area often showed deficits in naming objects and/or spelling; therefore, this area could not be dedicated to one single brain function (i.e., reading) (Hillis et al., 2005; Price & Devlin, 2003).

Dejerine may have over-estimated the role of the angular gyrus in reading for several reasons. One is that he did not have the help of recent functional imaging techniques that can show all the areas engaged in a task. Dejerine, as well as other brilliant scientists before the recent neuroimaging advances, had underestimated the complexity of brain processing for reading. They thought in terms of a linear processing chain: words entered the visual cortex in the form of visual patterns, then they were sent to the angular gyrus to find the visual images of words, then to Wernicke's area where the auditory images of words were supposedly located, then to Broca's area where articulation patterns were retrieved in order to finally end up in the motor cortex that controls the mouth muscles. Today we know that several of these operations happen in parallel; brain areas are more interconnected, many times bidirectionally; and brain regions are activated simultaneously in non-linear ways. Unraveling the brain's complexity with recent neuroimaging techniques helped to refine our understanding of brain functioning but at the same time increased the complexity we strive to understand.

Since at least the mid-1800s, conclusions about where language is processed in the brain have been based largely on observations about deficits incurred by circumscribed brain lesions. The reasoning behind this approach is straightforward: if a lesion in a focal area of the brain causes impairment of a particular language process, then that area of the brain must have been necessary for that language process. The lesion approach has led many times to conflicting results. One explanation for the conflicting results of lesion-deficit studies is that the characterization of reading impairment was too gross. As delineated in the previous chapter, reading is a complex process requiring several relatively distinct mechanisms and levels of representation (e.g., the roots of the words, their meaning, their sound patterns, their motor articulation schemes) that might take place in different brain regions. Damage to any one of these components might disrupt the reading task (although in different ways). Hence, it is not surprising that a variety of sites of damage would result in alexia.

Early lesion studies relied on post-mortem autopsies to identify the brain regions affected by a stroke, many times available only several years post-stroke. Subsequent advances in magnetic resonance imaging have allowed investigators to describe pure alexia symptoms and correlate them with brain areas affected without waiting for post-mortem evaluations. Nevertheless, most cases were studied many years post-stroke when reorganization has already taken place. This is a more general limitation of possible conclusions drawn using the lesion approach. There is strong evidence that substantial reorganization of structure-function relationships occurs within weeks of onset of brain injury (Jenkins & Merzenich, 1987; Merzenich et al., 1987). Thus, even if a lesion (e.g., in the frontal lobe) initially caused reading impairment, reading ability may have been recovered prior to studying the individual, due to reorganization, with or without rehabilitation. Therefore, in studying individuals with chronic lesions there may be little correlation between deficits at the time of investigation and the deficits initially caused by the lesion. Furthermore, studies of chronic stroke do not include individuals whose deficits resolved quickly or those who had no deficits after the brain injury. This selection bias precludes determination of the probability that a particular lesion will cause a specific deficit. That is, many individuals who have the particular lesion but do not have the deficit are not included in the study.

To circumvent this problem, a number of investigators have attempted to identify the sites at which temporary lesions (caused by focal electrical stimulation) do or do not cause impaired reading. Such studies involve stimulation of electrodes placed directly on the cortex, used to guide surgery to remove a lesion or an area of the brain thought to be causing intractable epilepsy (Duffau, Gatignol, Mandonnet, Capelle, & Taillandier, 2008; Gil-Robles et al., 2013; Luders, 1991; Ojemann, Ojemann, Lettich, & Berger, 1989; Ojemann, 2003; Schäffler, Lüders, & Beck, 1996). Of course, these cortical stimulation studies can only be carried out in patients with lesions or chronic epilepsy, whose brains may have already undergone substantial reorganization due to the lesion or seizures. Ojemann (Ojemann et al., 1989; Ojemann, 2003) reported that a variety of temporal and parietal sites resulted in impaired reading in these participants. He identified sites involved in the reading process; that is, their stimulation would result in 'speech arrest' in reading, sometimes similar to naming sites. These sites were localized in temporo-parietal as well as frontal areas. Many sites affected both reading and naming, but a larger number of sites affected only one task or the other. Sites that interfered with both naming and reading generally caused slow, effortful reading, while sites that were specific to reading caused morpho-syntactic errors in reading. Of note, cortical stimulation studies investigate only areas of the brain being considered for resection (nearly always temporal and/or parietal regions, more than frontal or occipital), so sites outside of these areas that may be essential for reading cannot be investigated. Interestingly, Schäffler and colleagues (1996) identified in 45 participants with epilepsy cortical sites in basal temporal regions, along with sites in Broca's and Wernicke's areas, that produced reading arrest. Additionally, Roux and colleagues (2004) in their extensive review of brain stimulation studies and their own investigation of 44 left-hemisphere and 10 right-hemisphere participants confirmed previous findings of shared areas for naming/reading as well as specific cortical areas involved in reading, most often in supramarginal, posterior temporal, and angular gyri, very often in the vicinity of naming sites, creating 'cortical patches' of these language functions. In a very recent study of intra-operative mapping devoted to looking at common versus separate areas for reading and naming, Duffau and colleagues (Gil-Robles et al., 2013) reported for the first time a double dissociation between visual recognition of words (and symbols) and picture naming in three participants who underwent cortical and subcortical intra-operative stimulation. They confirmed that after stimulating the left basal posterior temporal cortex participants typically reported 'non-recognition' of the whole word and 'letter-by-letter' reading but no naming impairment. However, two participants did experience a transient object naming difficulty after stimulation of the left fusiform gyrus. The same pattern was elicited by stimulating the inferior left fasciculus, a white matter tract behind the 'visual word form area.' However, stimulating laterally and superior to this area elicited semantic paraphasias in picture naming. This study, thus, confirmed the cortical proximity of areas potentially dedicated specifically to reading and naming and the different white matter pathways that may connect them to other areas of the brain where processing of semantic or phonological features may take place (Gil-Robles et al., 2013). This possibility that integrates previous seemingly conflicting findings in the lesion and even functional magnetic resonance imaging (fMRI) literature is fully fleshed out in a recent integrative account of the role of the VWFA in reading, spelling, and naming (Sebastian et al., 2014), as explained below.

In continuing our discussion on lesion studies, another lesion-deficit approach that largely avoids the problems of reorganization and selection bias is the use of recent advanced imaging techniques to identify sites of lesion and poorly functioning brain regions, along with concurrent evaluation of reading, in individuals with hyperacute stroke. Participants are studied within hours (less than 24 hours) of onset of stroke symptoms to identify which components of the reading process are impaired. Within minutes or hours of this testing they undergo magnetic resonance diffusion-weighted imaging (DWI) and perfusion-weighted imaging (PWI) to identify the structural and functional brain lesions associated with the deficits. DWI is highly sensitive to infarct or densely ischemic tissue within minutes of onset, and PWI shows areas of poor blood flow, or hypoperfusion, that cause tissue dysfunction (Barber et al., 1999; Beaulieu et al., 1999; Hillis, Barker, Beauchamp, Gordon, & Wityk, 2000). By studying all individuals with symptoms of left hemisphere stroke prospectively, it is possible to determine the association between the presence or absence of a lesion and the presence or absence of a particular deficit at the time of onset. This has been the primary method we have used to identify sites of dysfunctional or damaged brain tissue associated with specific deficits in language. Results from individuals who had evaluation of reading, PWI, and DWI within 24 hours of onset of stroke are included in the following sections (see Hillis et al., 2000, for details of the method).

The role of the 'visual word form area' versus the left lateral inferior temporal gyrus, both in left Brodmann area 37 (BA 37), in reading has been studied in acute ischemic stroke before any reorganization (Hillis et al., 2005; Philipose et al., 2007; Sebastian et al., 2014). The first question was whether damage to left BA 37 versus other regions of interest (such as the angular gyrus, the supramarginal gyrus, the inferior frontal gyrus, and the superior temporal gyrus) results in reading deficits and whether impairment was specific to reading (i.e., not associated with deficits in other lexical output tasks such as naming or spelling). Hillis and colleagues (2005) examined 80 individuals within 24 hours post-onset of acute left ischemic stroke. They found that dysfunction, i.e., hypoperfusion of left BA 37, was not associated with impairment of written word comprehension or lexical decision but was associated with all tasks requiring lexical output: oral reading, naming, and spelling. Impaired written comprehension was most strongly associated with hypoperfusion of the left posterior, superior temporal, and angular gyri. These authors suggested that early visual processing and computation of viewer-centered and stimulus-centered representations of written words depend on early visual areas (V1–V4), whereas word-centered pre-lexical representations of words may be subserved by either the right or left VWFA (a finding contrary to Cohen and Dehaene's claim about the uniqueness of the left VWFA for pre-lexical processing in early accounts of their own model), but access to lexical or lemma representations for output depends on the left BA 37. This finding is in line with Cohen and Dehaene's claim about the specialization and subsequent coining of the left mid-fusiform gyrus as the 'visual word form area,' reserving orthography to phonology conversion in the angular gyrus and phonological-articulatory mechanisms to the left posterior inferior frontal gyrus (IFG). Semantic representations were postulated to be distributed throughout the left temporal lobe. Subsequent papers by the same group studying even greater numbers of participants (106 acute stroke participants in Philipose et al., 2007 and 234 participants in Sebastian et al., 2014) confirmed and expanded the suggested model. Additionally, the subsequent papers indicated that there is a shared neural network critical for reading and spelling involving left BAs 37, 40, and 22, as well as 39 and 44/45 to a lesser extent (Philipose et al., 2007). The latter study showed additionally that reading and spelling of words and pseudowords are also associated with dysfunction of BA 37. Other lesion and functional neuroimaging studies by different groups have also shown this association (Beeson et al., 2003; McCandliss, Cohen, & Dehaene, 2003; Purcell, Napoliello, & Eden, 2011; Rapp & Lipka, 2011; Tsapkini & Rapp, 2010). In their last reconciliation paper, the Hillis group built on a previous proposal by Cohen and colleagues (Cohen & Dehaene, 2004; Cohen, Jobert, Le Bihan, & Dehaene, 2004) who claimed that in the left inferotemporal cortex (in left BA 37) there exist two areas with different functions adjacent to each other: the VWFA with orthography-specific specialization for words and the left inferolateral multimodality area (LIMA) area for multimodal, non-orthography-specific processing that links semantic attributes to lexical representations, and thus it is also involved in reading as well as naming. In this way, they were able to reconcile some of the most problematic findings for the specificity of the left inferotemporal cortex (i.e., its involvement in naming) (Price & Devlin, 2011; Price & Devlin, 2003; Price & Devlin, 2004; Price et al., 2006). Hillis and her group studied 234 participants with acute ischemic stroke within 48 hours post-onset in a series of lexical processing tasks such as reading, spelling, and naming (Sebastian et al., 2014). They found that damage to the VWFA would indeed impair processing of written forms of words (i.e., reading and spelling), whereas damage to the LIMA area would impair naming as well. This finding is also in line with other findings from the same group on individuals with primary progressive aphasia (PPA). Longitudinal imaging in PPA showed atrophy in the left fusiform associated with deficits in spelling, whereas atrophy in the inferior lateral temporal cortex associated with decline in naming (Race et al., 2013).

An inherent problem with lesion studies (even with advanced imaging techniques such as perfusion and diffusion imaging at the acute stage before reorganization) is related to the nature of a cerebrovascular accident: tissue dysfunction is guided by the vascular architecture of the brain. In many cases strokes involve large areas, thus making it difficult to delineate the independent contribution of particular regions to specific tasks. Therefore, studies in individuals with highly focal lesions are needed in order to draw more definite conclusions about the specific role of each area (Philipose et al., 2007). A few recent studies have tried to answer these questions by studying participants with small or focal lesions due to surgical resections (Gaillard et al., 2006; Purcell, Shea, & Rapp, 2014; Tsapkini & Rapp, 2010; Tsapkini, Vindiola, & Rapp, 2011). Gaillard and colleagues (2006) studied an individual for whom they had an fMRI before and after surgery that had shown a normal mosaic of ventral visual selectivity for words, faces, houses, and tools. After surgical removal of a small portion of the word responsive occipito-temporal cortex the person developed a marked reading deficit with intact recognition of other visual categories. In the post-surgery fMRI only word-specific activations disappeared. The authors considered these results as direct evidence for the causal role of the left occipito-temporal cortex in the recognition of visual words. In two subsequent papers, Tsapkini and colleagues (Tsapkini & Rapp, 2010; Tsap-kini et al., 2011) studied a man three years after left fusiform resection who showed an impairment in word reading of irregular and low-frequency words that consisted of slowed reaction times but not impaired accuracy, as well as a pronounced impairment in spelling accuracy but not naming (although he complained of word-finding difficulties immediately after his resection). His fMRI revealed a different brain pattern of reorganization for words, pseudowords, faces, and objects. The spatial organization of his activation peaks in the left mid-fusiform gyrus (but not in other reading areas) for word reading was spatially different from a group of matched controls, as measured by Mahalanobis distance. This was not the case for pseudowords or faces or objects, and it corre-sponded to his pronounced slowness in reading words. These results indicate a necessary role of the left mid-fusiform gyrus for efficient orthographic processing. Purcell and colleagues (2014) have expanded on this reasoning using a different methodology of lesion mapping in three participants and provided evidence of topographically distinct areas for access to orthography from semantics (spelling) and access to semantics from orthography (reading) within the basal temporal language area. These studies converge nicely with the integrative attempts discussed earlier and the claims for distinct sub-regions within the basal language area (Cohen & Dehaene, 2004; Cohen et al., 2004; Hillis et al., 2005; Philipose et al., 2007; Sebastian et al., 2014).

Reading in the Advent and Rise of Functional Neuroimaging

The advent of functional neuroimaging a little more than two decades ago provided for the first time the advantage to examine the living brain in action. Despite the limitations and potential for over-interpretation in each functional neuroimaging method (that are not few or negligible), it offered an opportunity to answer a different sort of question from those addressed by lesion studies. While lesion studies can identify the areas that are essential for a function (at least initially) or what areas are essential for recovery of a function, functional imaging studies can identify all of the areas that are engaged during a task. In the last two decades there has been a refinement of our questions that has gone hand-by-hand with refinement of our imaging methods and has shaped what is now called 'a new science of reading.'

Reading is among the first language functions that have ever been investigated with func-tional imaging. The first-ever study of functional neuroimaging was performed by Petersen's group (Petersen, Fox, Posner, Mintun, & Raichle, 1988) using positron emission tomography (PET). Later, fMRI became more instrumental in brain imaging due to its many advantages over PET, such as lower cost, lack of radioactive exposure, and better spatial resolution. Both methods, however, suffer from imprecise temporal resolution, a limitation that is only absent in magnetoencephalography (MEG). The two primary methods of evaluating regions of brain that are 'activated' during specific components of the reading process in normal or brain-damaged subjects have been O^{15} PET and fMRI. Both types of studies have generally relied on the 'subtraction method' to identify activated regions of cortex. In this method, subjects undergo imaging during a baseline task and during an experimental task. Then, areas that are activated during baseline are subtracted from areas that are activated during the experimental task. It is thus hoped that areas activated only during a particular component of the reading task can be isolated. For example, several studies have compared regional activation during viewing of real words versus viewing a checkerboard, and this task has been widely used as a VWFA localizer (e.g., Cohen & Dehaene, 2004; Cohen et al., 2004; Dehaene, Cohen, Sigman, & Vinckier, 2005; Dehaene et al., 2004). In this way, regions of activation associated with primary vision and spatial attention to the black-and-white contrast of letters are 'subtracted out.' The activation associated with the experimental task (viewing real words) minus baseline (viewing a checker-board) thus corresponds to the activation associated with access to orthographic representations in the lexicon. However, it becomes obvious that this may also include 'automatic' access to the meaning of the words and/or the pronunciation of the words.

Results from functional imaging studies (like lesion studies) of reading have often been conflicting. There are many potential reasons for the discordant results. The most important is that many aspects of the particular experimental paradigm can substantially influence the results of functional imaging studies. In the first-ever study of the human living brain for language, Petersen and colleagues (1988) reported results using PET indicating that passive viewing of real words or pronounceable pseudowords, compared to visual fixation of a crosshair, activated left extrastriate areas. In contrast, passive viewing of un-pronounceable letter strings or strings of false fonts compared to visual fixation did not activate these regions. They concluded that access to orthographic representations of words in the lexicon occurs in the left extrastriate cortex as well as a small region at the border of the occipital and temporal cortex that corresponds nicely to Cohen and Dehaene's VWFA. This area was not activated in other tasks, such as spoken-word production, for which anterior regions around Broca's area were activated. In contrast, Howard and coworkers (1992), using PET, found no activation of the left extrastriate cortex in a task designed to isolate access to orthographic lexical representations. They compared an experimental task of reading real words aloud to a baseline task of saying the word *crime* when viewing false fonts. Again, this subtraction should isolate areas activated during access to the orthographic representations with or without 'automatic' access to word meanings. Since the verbal response, early visual processing, and spatial attention were present in both the baseline and the experimental task, activation associated with these processes should have been subtracted out. In this study, access to orthographic lexical representations was associated with activation in the left posterior middle and inferior temporal area (BA 37), not the left extrastriate cortex. C. J. Price and coworkers (1994) noted that the duration of exposure of stimuli was 150 msec in the Peterson et al. study and was 1000 msec in the Howard et al. study. They evaluated whether the conflicting results were due to different exposure durations by using similar tasks as in the previous studies, with exposure durations of both 150 msec and 1000 msec. The results of their PET study indicated that a verbal response to words minus a verbal response to pseudowords activated both left extrastriate and left temporal cortex with exposure duration of 150 msec, but activated neither region with exposure duration of 1000 msec. Furthermore, passive viewing of words compared to false fonts activated left BA 37 with exposure duration of 150 msec or 1000 msec, but did not activate left extrastriate cortex with either exposure duration. Additionally, other regions were activated at one exposure duration or the other. Thus, the results did not replicate either the Peterson et al. study or the Howard et al. study, but did show that exposure duration influenced results. Importantly, these results underscore the complication that functional imaging studies are very sensitive to both task selection and other variables of paradigm design (such as exposure duration) that are irrelevant to the question being studied. This complication is encountered at least equally in fMRI studies as in PET studies and may account for the many failures to replicate findings, especially in the early days of functional neuroimaging (Grabowski & Damasio, 2000).

Additionally, even the most robust results from functional imaging studies about the localization of cognitive mechanisms underlying reading often conflict with the most reliable results from lesion–deficit correlation studies. For example, a large number of PET studies and fMRI studies show activation of the right cerebellum during silent word reading tasks, although large lesions of the right cerebellum are not associated with deficits in silent word reading. One reason for such apparently contradictory results is that, as noted earlier, functional imaging studies show areas that are *active* during a particular task, whereas lesion–deficit studies reveal areas that are *essential* for the task. A broad network of regions as revealed by functional neuroimaging has been implicated in reading.

Despite the foregoing caveats about the methods used to localize specific cognitive functions, there is evidence from functional imaging for proposing that specific brain regions are essential for certain components of the reading process. In functional neuroimaging studies of neurologically intact individuals, an area of the left mid-fusiform gyrus/occipito-temporal sulcus (within BA 37) has been identified as an important component of the reading network (Baker et al., 2007; Binder, Medler, Westbury, Liebenthal, & Buchanan, 2006; Booth et al., 2002a; Booth et al., 2002b; Carreiras, Mechelli, Estévez, & Price, 2007; Cohen & Dehaene, 2004; Cohen, Dehaene, Vinckier, Jobert, & Montavont, 2008; Cohen et al., 2000; Cohen et al., 2002; Cohen et al., 2004; Dehaene et al., 2005; Dehaene et al., 2002; Dehaene et al., 2004; Fiez, Balota, Raichle, & Petersen, 1999; Indefrey et al., 1997; Kronbichler et al., 2007; McCandliss et al., 2003; Mechelli et al., 2005; Moore & Price, 1999; Pugh et al., 1996; Pugh et al., 2001; Rapp & Lipka, 2011). The neuroimaging findings are consistent with lesion/deficit correlation studies of individuals with acquired reading impairments (Behrmann, Nelson, & Sekuler, 1998; Damasio & Damasio, 1983; Gaillard et al., 2006; Hillis et al., 2001a; Leff et al., 2001; Marsh & Hillis, 2005; Marsh & Hillis, 2006; Philipose et al., 2007; Sebastian et al., 2014; Tsapkini et al., 2011).

Since the first papers by Dehaene and Cohen's group and the insights and controversies it raised, several functional neuroimaging studies have found that the left mid-fusiform gyrus in BA 37, coined as the 'visual word form area,' was specially tuned (and thus selectively activated) to processing of words rather than letter-like symbols and unreadable letter-strings and was invariant to a number of visual-only characteristics such as case and language scripts (Baker et al., 2007; Cohen et al., 2000; Cohen et al., 2002; Cohen et al., 2004; Dehaene et al., 2005; Dehaene & Cohen, 2011; Dehaene et al., 2004; Dehaene & Cohen, 2007). Those opposed to the orthographic specificity of the VWFA showed that it was activated in non-reading lexical tasks such as naming (Buchel, Price, Frackowiak, & Friston, 1998; Devlin, Jamison, Gonnerman, & Matthews, 2006; Price & Devlin, 2011; Price et al., 2003; Price & Devlin, 2003; Price & Devlin, 2004; Wright et al., 2007). As reported above, more integrative accounts tried to reconcile and explain the conflicting results (Hillis et al., 2005; Philipose et al., 2007; Sebastian et al., 2014). Cohen, Dehaene, and their colleagues (Cohen & Dehaene, 2004; Cohen et al., 2004) refined their account and proposed two separate areas in the left occipito-temporal cortex: the VWFA responsible for orthographic-specific processing and font- and location-independent graphemic representations, and laterally and more anterior to that, the lateral inferiotemporal multimodal area (LIMA) responsible for modality-independent lexical processing, including naming (Cohen et al., 2004; Sebastian et al., 2014).

An interesting elaboration of the hypothesized role of the occipito-temporal cortex in reading has been put forward (Cohen & Dehaene, 2004; Dehaene et al., 2005; Dehaene & Cohen, 2007; Vinckier et al., 2007). Investigators used fMRI to test whether a hierarchy is present in the left occipito-temporal cortex, at the site of the visual word-form area, and with an anterior-to-posterior progression. They exposed adult readers to (1) false-font strings, (2) strings of infrequent letters, (3) strings of frequent letters but rare bigrams, (4) strings with frequent bigrams but rare quadrigrams, (5) strings with frequent quadrigrams, and (6) real words. A gradient of selectivity was observed through the entire span of the occipito-temporal cortex, with activation becoming more selective for higher-level stimuli toward the anterior fusiform region. A similar gradient was also seen in the left inferior frontoinsular cortex. Those gradients were asymmetrical in favor of the left hemisphere. They concluded that the left occipito-temporal visual word form area, far from being a homogeneous structure, presents a high degree of functional and spatial hierarchical organization for the decoding of meaning.

Other areas usually implicated in reading are areas for accessing semantics from orthography and phonology. There is strong evidence from early PET studies that access to the lexical-semantic representations in response to either words or pictures activates Wernicke's area BA 22 (Demonet et al., 1992; Vandenberghe, Price, Wise, Josephs, & Frackowiak, 1996). These studies also demonstrate activation in surrounding temporal and parietal regions as well. It is likely that BA 22 is not the site at which lexical-semantic representations are *stored*, but a site that is crucial for linking widely distributed lexical-semantic representations to spoken and written words. Chronic lesion studies have also confirmed that lesions in BA 22 result in lexical-semantic impairments (Goodglass & Wingfield, 1997; Hart & Gordon, 1990; Wernicke, 1874). Convergent results have been obtained with cortical stimulation of BA 22, which causes impairment in word comprehension (Lesser et al., 1986). Finally, we found that in hyperacute stroke, lexical-semantic deficits were strongly associated with hypoperfusion of Wernicke's area and less strongly associated with surrounding areas, including the supramarginal gyrus (BA 40), the middle temporal lobe (BA 21 and 37), angular gyrus (BA 39), and visual association cortex (BA 19) (Hillis et al., 2001b). In contrast, hypoperfusion of Wernicke's area was not at all associated with impairment to any other component of the reading process. Furthermore, reperfusion of BA 22 in acute stroke resulted in recovery of lexical-semantic deficits (Hillis, Tuffiash, Wityk, & Barker, 2002; Hillis et al., 2001b). Also, the severity of hypoperfusion of BA 22 was strongly correlated with the severity of word comprehension deficit in 80 participants with acute stroke (Hillis et al., 2001b).

More studies on functional and effective connectivity are apparently needed to make any robust claims with regard to the time course of the reading process and the particular timing of involvement of semantic areas. For this reason, Simos and colleagues (2002) and Tarkiainen and colleagues (Tarkiainen, Helenius, Hansen, Cornelissen, & Salmelin, 1999; Tarkiainen, Cornelissen, & Salmelin, 2002) used MEG, a time-sensitive functional neuroimaging technique, and tracked down the areas involved in each component of the reading process. Both groups, in the US and Finland respectively, found activation in BA 22 after occipito-temporal activations in normal readers.

Finally, the neural substrates of oral reading overlap with those of word production in general (see chapter 7, this volume). For example, impaired access to phonological representations for output was observed when BA 37 was hypoperfused, and recovered access to phonological representations was seen when blood flow was restored to BA 37 (Hillis et al., 2001b; Hillis et al., 2002b). These results are consistent with chronic lesion studies indicating that damage to BA 37 results in anomic aphasia, which reflects impaired retrieval of phonological representations of words. However, these studies may be specific to accessing phonological representations of nouns, since only nouns were tested in our study and in many reports of anomic aphasia (for a discussion see Miceli, Silveri, Nocentini, & Caramazza, 1988). Access to the phonological representation of verbs is likely to occur in the posterior frontal regions (Damasio & Tranel, 1993; Daniele, Giustolisi, Silveri, Colosimo, & Gainotti, 1994; Miceli, Silveri, Villa, & Caramazza, 1984; Perani et al., 1999; K. Shapiro, Pascual-Leone, Mottaghy, Gangitano, & Caramazza, 2001; K.A. Shapiro, Moo, & Caramazza, 2006; Sloan Berndt, Mitchum, Haendiges, & Sandson, 1997). This proposal may account for at least some of the cases of impaired oral reading due to frontal lesions. Reading of unfamiliar words or pseudowords (e.g., *glamp*) cannot be accomplished by accessing stored, orthographic representations alone, since there are no stored representations corresponding to stimuli that have not been previously encountered. Rather, the reader relies on orthography-to-phonology conversion (OPC) mechanisms. Damage at the level of OPC mechanisms results in inability to 'sound out' pseudowords or unfamiliar words. Therefore, reading pseudowords increased activation of the left occipital and nearby temporal and parietal cortices, including angular gyrus (BA 39) and supramarginal gyrus (BA 40) (Small, Flores, & Noll, 1998). Consistent with this proposed posterior temporo-parietal localization of OPC mechanisms, we found that hyperacute impairment of OPC mechanisms was associated with hypoperfusion of the angular gyrus and the supramarginal gyrus within hours of stroke onset (Hillis et al., 2001a). Recent fMRI studies have looked at reading aloud words and pseudowords and confirm a correlation with activation in posterior frontal regions (Gaillard et al., 2006; Henry et al., 2005; Kronbichler et al., 2007; McCandliss et al., 2003; Mechelli, Gorno-Tempini, & Price, 2003; Mechelli, Friston, & Price, 2006; Tsapkini et al., 2011). In one of our studies we looked at pseudoword reading in a group of healthy controls as well as an individual with resection in the mid-fusiform gyrus (Tsapkini et al., 2011). Healthy controls activated the fusiform area more posteriorly than the area activated for words; the participant with a lesion in this region activated adjacent peri-lesional areas as well as the supramarginal gyrus and the inferior frontal gyrus. This pattern allowed him successful pseudoword reading, indicating that the VWFA or the mid-fusiform gyrus is not a necessary structure for grapheme-to-phoneme conversion.

Summary

Functional imaging studies of reading and lesion studies of individuals with acquired reading impairments converge in support of the hypothesis that the network of regions required to support reading overlaps with the network of regions that support other language tasks. Meta-analyses of functional imaging studies of reading revealed that these areas include Wernicke's area (BA 22), angular gyrus (BA 39), supramarginal gyrus (BA 40), Broca's area (BA 44, 45), premotor cortex (BA 6), as well as occipito-temporal/fusiform cortex (BA 37) (Jobard, Crivello, & Tzourio-Mazoyer, 2003; Turkeltaub, Eden, Jones, & Zeffiro, 2002). Some subregions of BA 37 in mid-fusiform cortex may be relatively specific for orthographic processes such as reading and spelling, although the extent to which they are critical for comparable visual perceptual tasks remains a matter of debate (see Starrfelt & Shallice, 2014 for a detailed review).

Acknowledgment

Some of the research reported in this chapter was supported by R01 DC05375.

References

Baker, C.I., Liu, J., Wald, L.L., Kwong, K.K., Benner, T., & Kanwisher, N. (2007). Visual word processing and experiential origins of functional selectivity in human extrastriate cortex. *Proceedings of the National Academy of Sciences of the United States of America, 104*(21), 9087–9092.

Barber, P.A., Darby, D.G., Desmond, P.M., Gerraty, R.P., Yang, Q., Li, T., et al. (1999). Identification of major ischemic change. Diffusion-weighted imaging versus computed tomography. *Stroke, 30*(10), 2059–2065.

Beaulieu, C., De Crespigny, A., Tong, D.C., Moseley, M.E., Albers, G.W., & Marks, M.P. (1999). Longitudinal magnetic resonance imaging study of perfusion and diffusion in stroke: Evolution of lesion volume and correlation with clinical outcome. *Annals of Neurology, 46*(4), 568–578.

Beeson, P., Rapcsak, S., Plante, E., Chargualaf, J., Chung, A., Johnson, S., et al. (2003). The neural substrates of writing: A functional magnetic resonance imaging study. *Aphasiology, 17*(6–7), 647–665.

Behrmann, M., Nelson, J., & Sekuler, E.B. (1998). Visual complexity in letter-by-letter reading: "Pure" alexia is not pure. *Neuropsychologia, 36*(11), 1115–1132.

Binder, J.R., Medler, D.A., Westbury, C.F., Liebenthal, E., & Buchanan, L. (2006). Tuning of the human left fusiform gyrus to sublexical orthographic structure. *NeuroImage, 33*(2), 739–748.

Binder, J.R., & Mohr, J.P. (1992). The topography of callosal reading pathways. A case-control analysis. *Brain, 115*(Pt 6), 1807–1826.

Booth, J.R., Burman, D.D., Meyer, J.R., Gitelman, D.R., Parrish, T.B., & Mesulam, M.M. (2002a). Functional anatomy of intra- and cross-modal lexical tasks. *NeuroImage, 16*(1), 7–22.

Booth, J.R., Burman, D.D., Meyer, J.R., Gitelman, D.R., Parrish, T.B., & Mesulam, M.M. (2002b). Modality independence of word comprehension. *Human Brain Mapping, 16*(4), 251–261.

Buchel, C., Price, C., Frackowiak, R.S., & Friston, K. (1998). Different activation patterns in the visual cortex of late and congenitally blind subjects. *Brain, 121*(Pt 3), 409–419.

Caramazza, A., & Mahon, B.Z. (2003). The organization of conceptual knowledge: The evidence from category-specific semantic deficits. *Trends in Cognitive Sciences, 7*(8), 354–361.

Carreiras, M., Mechelli, A., Estévez, A., & Price, C.J. (2007). Brain activation for lexical decision and reading aloud: Two sides of the same coin? *Journal of Cognitive Neuroscience, 19*(3), 433–444.

Cohen, L., & Dehaene, S. (2004). Specialization within the ventral stream: The case for the visual word form area. *NeuroImage, 22*(1), 466–476.

Cohen, L., Dehaene, S., Naccache, L., Lehericy, S., Dehaene-Lambertz, G., Henaff, M.A., et al. (2000). The visual word form area: Spatial and temporal characterization of an initial stage of reading in normal subjects and posterior split-brain patients. *Brain, 123*(Pt 2), 291–307.

Cohen, L., Dehaene, S., Vinckier, F., Jobert, A., & Montavont, A. (2008). Reading normal and degraded words: Contribution of the dorsal and ventral visual pathways. *NeuroImage, 40*(1), 353–366.

Cohen, L., Jobert, A., Le Bihan, D., & Dehaene, S. (2004). Distinct unimodal and multimodal regions for word processing in the left temporal cortex. *NeuroImage, 23*(4), 1256–1270.

Cohen, L., Lehericy, S., Chochon, F., Lemer, C., Rivaud, S., & Dehaene, S. (2002). Language-specific tuning of visual cortex? Functional properties of the visual word form area. *Brain: A Journal of Neurology, 125*(Pt 5), 1054–1069.

Cohen, L., Martinaud, O., Lemer, C., Lehericy, S., Samson, Y., Obadia, M., et al. (2003). Visual word recognition in the left and right hemispheres: Anatomical and functional correlates of peripheral alexias. *Cerebral Cortex (New York, N.Y.: 1991), 13*(12), 1313–1333.

Coltheart, M. (2006). Perhaps functional neuroimaging has not told us anything about the mind (so far). *Cortex, 42*(3), 422–427.

Damasio, A.R., & Damasio, H. (1983). The anatomic basis of pure alexia. *Neurology, 33*(12), 1573–1583.

Damasio, A.R., & Tranel, D. (1993). Nouns and verbs are retrieved with differently distributed neural systems. *Proceedings of the National Academy of Sciences of the United States of America, 90*(11), 4957–4960.

Daniele, A., Giustolisi, L., Silveri, M.C., Colosimo, C., & Gainotti, G. (1994). Evidence for a possible neuroanatomical basis for lexical processing of nouns and verbs. *Neuropsychologia, 32*(11), 1325–1341.

Dehaene, S. (2009). *Reading in the brain: The new science of how we read.* New York: Penguin.

Dehaene, S., & Cohen, L. (2007). Cultural recycling of cortical maps. *Neuron, 56*(2), 384–398.

Dehaene, S., & Cohen, L. (2011). The unique role of the visual word form area in reading. *Trends in Cognitive Sciences, 15*(6), 254–262.

Dehaene, S., Cohen, L., Sigman, M., & Vinckier, F. (2005). The neural code for written words: A proposal. *Trends in Cognitive Sciences, 9*(7), 335–341.

Dehaene, S., Jobert, A., Naccache, L., Ciuciu, P., Poline, J.B., Le Bihan, D., et al. (2004). Letter binding and invariant recognition of masked words: Behavioral and neuroimaging evidence. *Psychological Science, 15*(5), 307–313.

Dehaene, S., Le Clec'H, G., Poline, J.B., Le Bihan, D., & Cohen, L. (2002). The visual word form area: A prelexical representation of visual words in the fusiform gyrus. *Neuroreport, 13*(3), 321–325.

Dejerine, J. (1891). Sur un cas de cécité verbale avec agraphie, suivi d'autopsie. *Mémoires De La Société De Biologie, 3*, 197–201.

Dejerine, J. (1892). Contribution a l'etude anatomoclinique et clinique des differentes varietes de cecite verbale. *CR Hebdomadaire Des Seances Et Memoires De La Societe De Biologie, 4*, 61–90.

Demonet, J.F., Chollet, F., Ramsay, S., Cardebat, D., Nespoulous, J.L., Wise, R., et al. (1992). The anatomy of phonological and semantic processing in normal subjects. *Brain, 115*(Pt 6), 1753–1768.

Devlin, J., Jamison, H., Gonnerman, L., & Matthews, P. (2006). The role of the posterior fusiform gyrus in reading. *Journal of Cognitive Neuroscience, 18*(6), 911–922.

Duffau, H., Gatignol, P., Mandonnet, E., Capelle, L., & Taillandier, L. (2008). Intraoperative subcortical stimulation mapping of language pathways in a consecutive series of 115 patients with grade II glioma in the left dominant hemisphere. *Journal of Neurosurgery, 109*(3), 461–471.

Fiez, J.A., Balota, D.A., Raichle, M.E., & Petersen, S.E. (1999). Effects of lexicality, frequency, and spelling-to-sound consistency on the functional anatomy of reading. *Neuron, 24*(1), 205–218.

Gaillard, R., Naccache, L., Pinel, P., Clémenceau, S., Volle, E., Hasboun, D., et al. (2006). Direct intracranial, fMRI, and lesion evidence for the causal role of left inferotemporal cortex in reading. *Neuron, 50*(2), 191–204.

Gil-Robles, S., Carvallo, A., Jimenez Mdel, M., Gomez Caicoya, A., Martinez, R., Ruiz-Ocana, C., et al. (2013). Double dissociation between visual recognition and picture naming: A study of the visual language connectivity using tractography and brain stimulation. *Neurosurgery, 72*(4), 678–686.

Goodglass, H., & Wingfield, A. (1997). *Anomia: Neuroanatomical and cognitive correlates.* New York: Academic Press.

Grabowski, T.J., & Damasio, A.R. (2000). Investigating language with functional neuroimaging. In A.W. Toga & J.C. Mazziotta (Eds.), *Brain Mapping: The Systems* (pp. 425–461). New York: Academic Press.

Hart, J., & Gordon, B. (1990). Delineation of single-word semantic comprehension deficits in aphasia, with anatomical correlation. *Annals of Neurology, 27*(3), 226–231.

Henry, C., Gaillard, R., Volle, E., Chiras, J., Ferrieux, S., Dehaene, S., et al. (2005). Brain activations during letter-by-letter reading: A follow-up study. *Neuropsychologia, 43*(14), 1983–1989.

Hillis, A.E., Barker, P.B., Beauchamp, N.J., Gordon, B., & Wityk, R.J. (2000). MR perfusion imaging reveals regions of hypoperfusion associated with aphasia and neglect. *Neurology, 55*(6), 782–788.

Hillis, A.E., Barker, P.B., Beauchamp, N.J., Winters, B.D., Mirski, M., & Wityk, R.J. (2001a). Restoring blood pressure reperfused Wernicke's area and improved language. *Neurology, 56*(5), 670–672.

Hillis, A.E., Kane, A., Tuffiash, E., Beauchamp, N.J., Barker, P.B., Jacobs, M.A., & Wityk, R.J. (2002a). Neural substrates of the cognitive processes underlying spelling: Evidence from MR diffusion and perfusion imaging. *Aphasiology, 16*(4–6), 425–438.

Hillis, A.E., Kane, A., Tuffiash, E., Ulatowski, J.A., Barker, P.B., Beauchamp, N.J., & Wityk. R.J. (2001b). Reperfusion of specific brain regions by raising blood pressure restores selective language functions in subacute stroke. *Brain and Language, 79*(3), 495–510.

Hillis, A.E., Newhart, M., Heidler, J., Barker, P., Herskovits, E., & Degaonkar, M. (2005). The roles of the "visual word form area" in reading. *NeuroImage, 24*(2), 548–559.

Hillis, A.E., Tuffiash, E., Wityk, R.J., & Barker, P.B. (2002b). Regions of neural dysfunction associated with impaired naming of actions and objects in acute stroke. *Cognitive Neuropsychology, 19*(6), 523–534.

Howard, D., Patterson, K., Wise, R., Brown, W.D., Friston, K., Weiller, C., et al. (1992). The cortical localization of the lexicons. Positron emission tomography evidence. *Brain, 115*(Pt 6), 1769–1782.

Indefrey, P., Kleinschmidt, A., Merboldt, K.D., Kruger, G., Brown, C., Hagoort, P., & Frahm, J. (1997). Equivalent responses to lexical and nonlexical visual stimuli in occipital cortex: A functional magnetic resonance imaging study. *NeuroImage, 5*(1), 78–81.

Jenkins, W.M., & Merzenich, M.M. (1987). Reorganization of neocortical representations after brain injury: A neurophysiological model of the bases of recovery from stroke. *Progress in Brain Research, 71*, 249–266.

Jobard, G., Crivello, F., & Tzourio-Mazoyer, N. (2003). Evaluation of the dual route theory of reading: A met-analysis of 35 neuroimaging studies. *NeuroImage, 20*(2), 693–712.

Kronbichler, M., Bergmann, J., Hutzler, F., Staffen, W., Mair, A., Ladurner, G., & Wimmer, H. (2007). Taxi vs. taksi: On orthographic word recognition in the left ventral occipitotemporal cortex. *Journal of Cognitive Neuroscience, 19*(10), 1584–1594.

Leff, A.P., Crewes, H., Plant, G.T., Scott, S.K., Kennard, C., & Wise, R.J. (2001). The functional anatomy of single-word reading in patients with hemianopic and pure alexia. *Brain, 124*(Pt 3), 510–521.

Lesser, R.P., Lüders, H., Morris, H.H., Dinner, D.S., Klem, G., Hahn, J., & Harrison, M. (1986). Electrical stimulation of Wernicke's area interferes with comprehension. *Neurology*, 36(5), 658-663.

Luders, H., Lesser, R.P., Hahn, J., Dinner, D.S., Morris, H.H., Wyllie, E., et al. (1991). Basal temporal language area. *Brain, 114*(Pt.2), 743–754.

Marsh, E.B., & Hillis, A.E. (2005). Cognitive and neural mechanisms underlying reading and naming: Evidence from letter-by-letter reading and optic aphasia. *Neurocase, 11*(5), 325–337.

Marsh, E.B., & Hillis, A.E. (2006). Recovery from aphasia following brain injury: The role of reorganization. *Progress in Brain Research, 157*, 143–156.

McCandliss, B.D., Cohen, L., & Dehaene, S. (2003). The visual word form area: Expertise for reading in the fusiform gyrus. *Trends in Cognitive Sciences, 7*(7), 293–299.

Mechelli, A., Crinion, J.T., Long, S., Friston, K.J., Ralph, M.A.L., Patterson, K., et al. (2005). Dissociating reading processes on the basis of neuronal interactions. *Journal of Cognitive Neuroscience, 17*(11), 1753–1765.

Mechelli, A., Friston, K.J., & Price, C.J. (2006). The effects of presentation rate during word and pseudoword reading: A comparison of PET and fMRI. *Journal of Cognitive Neuroscience, 12*(Suppl 2), 145–156.

Mechelli, A., Gorno-Tempini, M., & Price, C. (2003). Neuroimaging studies of word and pseudoword reading: Consistencies, inconsistencies, and limitations. *Journal of Cognitive Neuroscience, 15*(2), 260–271.

Merzenich, M.M., Nelson, R.J., Kaas, J.H., Stryker, M.P., Jenkins, W.M., Zook, J.M., et al. (1987). Variability in hand surface representations in areas 3b and 1 in adult owl and squirrel monkeys. *Journal of Comparative Neurology, 258*(2), 281–296.

Miceli, G., Silveri, C., Nocentini, U., & Caramazza, A. (1988). Patterns of dissociation in comprehension and production of nouns and verbs. *Aphasiology, 2*(3/4), 351–358.

Miceli, G., Silveri, M.C., Villa, G., & Caramazza, A. (1984). On the basis for the agrammatic's difficulty in producing main verbs. *Cortex, 20*(2), 207–220.

Moore, C.J., & Price, C.J. (1999). Three distinct ventral occipitotemporal regions for reading and object naming. *NeuroImage, 10*(2), 181–192.

Ojemann, G.A. (2003). The neurobiology of language and verbal memory: Observations from awake neuro-surgery. *International Journal of Psychophysiology, 48*(2), 141–146.

Ojemann, G., Ojemann, J., Lettich, E., & Berger, M. (1989). Cortical language localization in left, dominant hemisphere: An electrical stimulation mapping investigation in 117 patients. *Journal of Neurosurgery, 71*(3), 316–326.

Perani, D., Cappa, S.F., Schnur, T., Tettamanti, M., Collina, S., Rosa, M.M., et al. (1999). The neural correlates of verb and noun processing. A PET study. *Brain, 122*(Pt 12), 2337–2344.

Petersen, S.E., Fox, P.T., Posner, M.I., Mintun, M., & Raichle, M.E. (1988). Positron emission tomographic studies of the cortical anatomy of single-word processing. *Nature, 331*(6157), 585–589.

Philipose, L.E., Gottesman, R.F., Newhart, M., Kleinman, J.T., Herskovits, E.H., Pawlak, M.A., et al. (2007). Neural regions essential for reading and spelling of words and pseudowords. *Annals of Neurology, 62*(5), 481–492.

Price, C.J., & Devlin, J.T. (2003). The myth of the visual word form area. *NeuroImage, 19*(3), 473–481.

Price, C.J., & Devlin, J.T. (2004). The pro and cons of labelling a left occipitotemporal region: "The visual word form area." *NeuroImage, 22*(1), 477–479.

Price, C.J., & Devlin, J.T. (2011). The interactive account of ventral occipitotemporal contributions to reading. *Trends in Cognitive Sciences, 15*(6), 246–253.

Price, C.J., McCrory, E., Noppeney, U., Mechelli, A., Moore, C., Biggio, N., et al. (2006). How reading differs from object naming at the neuronal level. *NeuroImage, 29*(2), 643–648.

Price, C.J., Winterburn, D., Giraud, A., Moore, C., & Noppeney, U. (2003). Cortical localisation of the visual and auditory word form areas: A reconsideration of the evidence. *Brain and Language, 86*(2), 272–286.

Price, C.J., Wise, R.J., Watson, J.D., Patterson, K., Howard, D., & Frackowiak, R.S. (1994). Brain activity during reading. The effects of exposure duration and task. *Brain, 117*(Pt 6), 1255–1269.

Pugh, K.R., Mencl, W.E., Jenner, A.R., Katz, L., Frost, S.J., Lee, J.R., et al. (2001). Neurobiological studies of reading and reading disability. *Journal of Communication Disorders, 34*(6), 479–492.

Pugh, K.R., Shaywitz, B.A., Shaywitz, S.E., Constable, R.T., Skudlarski, P., Fulbright, R.K., et al. (1996). Cerebral organization of component processes in reading. *Brain, 119*(Pt 4), 1221–1238.

Purcell, J.J., Napoliello, E.M., & Eden, G.F. (2011). A combined fMRI study of typed spelling and reading. *NeuroImage, 55*(2), 750–762.

Purcell, J.J., Shea, J., & Rapp, B. (2014). Beyond the visual word form area: The orthography–semantics interface in spelling and reading. *Cognitive Neuropsychology*, (ahead-of-print), 1–29.

Race, D.S., Tsapkini, K., Crinion, J., Newhart, M., Davis, C., Gomez, Y., Hillis, A. E., & Faria, A.V. (2013). An area essential for linking word meanings to word forms: Evidence from primary progressive aphasia. *Brain and Language, 127*(2), 167–176.

Rapp, B., & Lipka, K. (2011). The literate brain: The relationship between spelling and reading. *Journal of Cognitive Neuroscience, 23*(5), 1180–1197.

Rothlein, D., & Rapp, B. (2014). The similarity structure of distributed neural responses reveals the multiple representations of letters. *NeuroImage, 89*, 331–344.

Roux, F.E., Lubrano, V., Lauwers-Cances, V., Tremoulet, M., Mascott, C.R., & Demonet, J.F. (2004). Intra-operative mapping of cortical areas involved in reading in mono- and bilingual patients. *Brain, 127*(Pt 8), 1796–1810.

Schäffler, L., Lüders, H.O., & Beck, G.J. (1996). Quantitative comparison of language deficits produced by extraoperative electrical stimulation of Broca's, Wernicke's, and basal temporal language areas. *Epilepsia, 37*(5), 463–475.

Sebastian, R., Gomez, Y., Leigh, R., Davis, C., Newhart, M., & Hillis, A.E. (2014). The roles of occipitotemporal cortex in reading, spelling, and naming. *Cognitive Neuropsychology*, (ahead-of-print), 1–18.

Shapiro, K., Pascual-Leone, A., Mottaghy, F., Gangitano, M., & Caramazza, A. (2001). Grammatical distinctions in the left frontal cortex. *Journal of Cognitive Neuroscience, 13*(6), 713–720.

Shapiro, K.A., Moo, L.R., & Caramazza, A. (2006). Cortical signatures of noun and verb production. *Proceedings of the National Academy of Sciences of the United States of America, 103*(5), 1644–1649.

Simos, P.G., Breier, J.I., Fletcher, J.M., Foorman, B.R., Castillo, E.M., & Papanicolaou, A.C. (2002). Brain mechanisms for reading words and pseudowords: An integrated approach. *Cerebral Cortex (New York, N.Y.: 1991), 12*(3), 297–305.

Sloan Berndt, R., Mitchum, C.C., Haendiges, A.N., & Sandson, J. (1997). Verb retrieval in aphasia. 1. Characterizing single word impairments. *Brain and Language, 56*(1), 68–106.

Small, S.L., Flores, D.K., & Noll, D.C. (1998). Different neural circuits subserve reading before and after therapy for acquired dyslexia. *Brain and Language, 62*(2), 298–308.

Starrfelt, R., & Shallice, T. (2014). What's in a name? The characterization of pure alexia. *Cognitive Neuropsychology, 31*(5–6), 367–377.

Tarkiainen, A., Cornelissen, P.L., & Salmelin, R. (2002). Dynamics of visual feature analysis and object-level processing in face versus letter-string perception. *Brain, 125*(Pt 5), 1125–1136.

Tarkiainen, A., Helenius, P., Hansen, P.C., Cornelissen, P.L., & Salmelin, R. (1999). Dynamics of letter string perception in the human occipitotemporal cortex. *Brain, 122*(Pt 11), 2119–2132.

Tsapkini, K., & Rapp, B. (2010). The orthography-specific functions of the left fusiform gyrus: Evidence of modality and category specificity. *Cortex, 46*(2), 185–205.

Tsapkini, K., Vindiola, M., & Rapp, B. (2011). Patterns of brain reorganization subsequent to left fusiform damage: fMRI evidence from visual processing of words and pseudowords, faces and objects. *NeuroImage, 55*(3), 1357–1372.

Turkeltaub, P.E., Eden, G.F., Jones, K.M., & Zeffiro, T.A. (2002). Meta-analysis of the functional neuroanatomy of single-word reading: Method and validation. *NeuroImage, 16*(3), 765–780.

Vandenberghe, R., Price, C., Wise, R., Josephs, O., & Frackowiak, R. (1996). Functional anatomy of a common semantic system for words and pictures. *Nature, 383*(6597), 254–256.

Vinckier, F., Dehaene, S., Jobert, A., Dubus, J.P., Sigman, M., & Cohen, L. (2007). Hierarchical coding of letter strings in the ventral stream: Dissecting the inner organization of the visual word-form system. *Neuron, 55*(1), 143–156.

Wernicke, C. (1874). Der aphasische symptomencomplex.

Wright, N.D., Mechelli, A., Noppeney, U., Veltman, D.J., Rombouts, S.A., Glensman, J., Haynes, J. D., & Price, C. J. (2007). Selective activation around the left occipito-temporal sulcus for words relative to pictures: Individual variability or false positives? *Human Brain Mapping, 29*(8), 986–1000.

3

CLINICAL DIAGNOSIS AND TREATMENT OF READING DISORDERS

Rhonda B. Friedman and Susan Nitzberg Lott

Assessing the Underlying Cognitive Deficit

Reading depends upon the integration of many component processes, both linguistic and visual. Thus, there are many different ways for reading to break down following injury to the brain (alexia). A thorough assessment of reading begins with an examination of elementary visual processing, and proceeds through analyses of orthographic, phonological, and semantic processing of single written words, to a final assessment of reading comprehension of text.

Visual Processing, Neglect, and Attention

In searching for the cause of a patient's reading deficit, it is important to first ascertain that the written letters and words are being perceived properly. To rule out early perceptual processing impairment, have the patient copy or trace individual letters.

Visual (hemispatial) neglect may interfere with the visual perception of the letters of a word (Kinsbourne & Warrington, 1962). Since hemispatial neglect is usually associated with lesions of the right hemisphere, it most commonly has its effects on the left half of stimuli or stimuli that appear on the left side of the reader's body or field of vision. See chapter 1 of this volume for discussion of various types of hemispatial neglect and how they affect reading.

The presence of a right homonymous hemianopia (RHH), a common accompaniment of pure alexia, can also affect reading ability. Because eye movements in text reading are guided by information to the right of fixation, a RHH can have a marked effect upon text reading. Visual field testing, with computerized perimetry or confrontation testing, can detail the extent of the visual field loss.

Disorders of attention may also affect reading, particularly reading of text. Patients with impaired selective attention may have difficulty segregating words from other words in space. As a result, letters tend to "migrate" from adjacent words (Shallice & Warrington, 1977). Deficits in sustained attention could lead to impairments in comprehension of text, even when single word and sentence reading remain intact. Tests of attention should be administered if this is suspected.

Letter Knowledge

Naming and Pointing to Letters Named

As an initial test of letter knowledge, individual letters—both upper- and lowercase—should be presented to the patient for naming. The ability to attach a letter's name to its physical form is a good indication that knowledge of the letter's identity remains intact. However, failure to name letters may reflect a problem with word retrieval, not letter identification. Patients who fail to name letters accurately should be given a sheet of paper upon which all twenty-six letters are scattered. The patient is asked to point to each letter as the therapist names it. Success at this task demonstrates that a letter's form is still associated with its name, even if the patient cannot retrieve that name.

Identity

Even if a patient can no longer associate the names of letters with their shapes, it might still be possible to demonstrate intact knowledge of letters' abstract identities. This can be done with a cross-case matching task. Two letters, one uppercase and one lowercase, appear together, and the patient determines whether they represent the same letter. Patients who can perform this task, even for letters with different upper- and lowercase shapes (for example, Rr), retain information about the letters' identities. This is important, as it is letters' identities, and not their names, that are the foundation of successful reading in most situations.

Recognition

The simplest level of letter knowledge is recognition; that is, knowing that a particular written symbol is an actual letter of the alphabet. One easy way to test for this knowledge is with a forced-choice task in which the patient must distinguish correct letters from mirror-reversed letters. This task does not require explicit identification of letters, only recognition of the correct shapes of real letters of the alphabet. Patients who cannot perform this task adequately are not likely to be good candidates for alexia treatment.

Access to the Lexicon through the Visual Modality

Orthographic representations and other aspects of lexical knowledge may remain intact in patients whose reading is impaired because they cannot access that knowledge through the visual modality. In these patients, whose reading disorder is known as pure alexia (or "alexia without agraphia" or "letter-by-letter reading"), the integrity of orthographic representations can be demonstrated through intact spelling or through intact recognition of orally spelled words. These patients often spontaneously compensate for their deficit by naming each letter of the word aloud or silently, which often allows them to recognize the word (hence "letter-by-letter reading").

Length Effect

Not all patients with pure alexia show outward signs of letter-by-letter reading. A second means of assessing difficulty with processing whole words as single units (or accessing the orthographic lexicon) is to examine for an effect of length on reading accuracy and/or reading speed. Patients should be asked to read a list of words that vary systematically in letter length. Words should be matched for frequency and part of speech across length, and should range from three letters to at least eleven letters. Substantial differences in accuracy as letter length increases is diagnostic of difficulty with accessing the orthographic representation. A more sensitive means of assessing length effects, for patients whose accuracy is high given unlimited time, is to look for increasing time required to read longer words. While normal readers will show a slight increase in time to read longer words, simply because longer words take more time to articulate, patients with pure alexia will require considerably more time to read the longer words.

Spelling

A patient's writing and spelling will likely be assessed as part of a comprehensive aphasia battery. For the purposes of demonstrating intact orthographic representations in the face of inability to access these representations visually, patients should be asked to write or orally spell words and pseudowords (PWs) that s/he has been asked to read (preferably in a separate testing session). Most patients with an alexic disturbance will perform more poorly on spelling than reading. Patients with pure alexia will show the opposite pattern: relatively better spelling than reading.

Recognition of Orally Spelled Words

Another means of ascertaining intact orthographic representations in a patient who cannot access these representations visually is to spell the words aloud to the patient, one letter at a time. Again, words and PWs that the patient has been asked to read should be used for this task. Words should not be so long as to exceed a normal verbal short-term memory span (approximately seven letters). Patients with pure alexia will perform normally on this task, recognizing words without regard to part of speech, and PWs as well. Importantly, performance on this task will exceed performance on reading these same words for pure alexic patients but not for patients with damage to the reading process at a level beyond access to the orthographic lexicon.

Integrity of Orthographic Representations

Lexical Decision

A disturbance of the internal orthographic representations of words may be revealed with a lexical decision task in which the word and nonword stimuli are carefully chosen. The real words should include words with regular spelling-to-sound correspondences—for example, *mint*—and words with irregular spelling-to-sound correspondences (orthography-to-phonology conversion)—for example, *pint*. The nonwords should include pseudowords that are homophonic with real words—for example, *sope*. Patients whose orthographic representations are not adequately activated tend to read all letter strings as they would be pronounced according to spelling-to-sound rules. Hence, they will have difficulty with such a lexical decision task. They will incorrectly accept the pseudohomophones (for example, *sope*) as being real words, because they sound like real words when pronounced, and they will incorrectly reject irregular words as being nonwords, because they do not sound like real words when pronounced according to spelling-to-sound rules ("/pInt/; that's not a word").

Homophones

A second means of assessing inadequate orthographic activation, related to the above lexical decision task, is a homophone definition task. Words that have homophones (for example, *oar, whole*) are presented one at a time, and the patient is asked to both read and define the words. Patients who are relying on the phonological code derived from the orthography, rather than the orthographic representation itself, will have no way to distinguish *tacks* from *tax* or *pray* from *prey*. This will be manifest in the patient's reading the word correctly, but defining it as its homophone (for example, defining *tacks* as money collected from people by the government).

Superior reading of regular words compared with irregular words, and poor homophone comprehension, are the hallmarks of the reading disorder known as surface alexia.

Phonological Processing

Reading Pseudowords

To evaluate the ability to access the phonology of written letter strings without regard to semantic processing, patients should be asked to read pseudowords (PWs); that is, orthographically legal, pronounceable nonwords. PW reading should be compared to the reading of words that are similar in length and structure. Difficulty reading PWs (called phonological alexia) is never a modality-specific problem: a PW reading deficit seen for written words will also be apparent if PWs are spelled aloud to the patient.

Pseudoword Repetition

Impaired PW reading may reflect a deficit that is specific to reading, or it may be part of a more general phonological processing deficit. The most sensitive means of testing this is to ask the patient to repeat multisyllabic pseudowords. Impaired performance on this task suggests a general phonological processing deficit. Additionally, such a deficit may be picked up by asking patients to read or repeat real words of increasing syllable length and phonological complexity.

Digit Span

Patients with reduced short-term phonological memory may experience difficulty reading text, while showing relatively intact single word reading. This disorder, termed phonological text alexia (Friedman, 1996), is accompanied by difficulty reading PWs. To assess a patient's ability to hold multiple phonological codes in short-term memory, variations of a standard digit span test, such as that contained in the Wechsler Memory Scale, should be administered. This includes normal digits forward and backward, single noun span, single functor word span, and single PW span.

Semantic Representation

Word-Picture Matching

The most direct method of testing access to semantics from the written word (that is, comprehension of written words) is to use a word-picture matching task. The task is to choose the picture, from an array, that matches a given written word; no verbal output is required. If the foils are pictures that are unrelated to the target, the patient may choose the correct picture even if only partial semantic information is activated. To test for more precise information about the word's meaning, picture foils should be chosen from the same superordinate category as the target.

Other Semantic Tasks

Milder impairments of semantic processing may affect only words of low imageability, or abstract words. Such semantic impairments may not be picked up with the word–picture matching task, which uses only words that are high in imageability (that is, they are picturable). Other semantic decision tasks may be helpful in these instances. In the odd-man-out test three words are presented (for example, *faith, belief, anger*), and the patient must point to the word that does not belong with the other two words. Alternatively, the patient may be asked whether the referent of a written word belongs to a particular category (for example, "Is the word *sadness* an emotion?") or whether two written words are similar in meaning.

Concreteness Effects in Oral Reading

When semantic processing is impaired concurrently with phonological reading, the result may be an effect of concreteness in oral reading. Words with less stable or accessible semantic value—that is, words of lower concreteness—are read more poorly than words of high concreteness. To test for this effect, patients should be asked to read a list of words, half of which are high in concreteness and half of which are low in concreteness. High- and low-concreteness words should be matched for frequency and length. A significant advantage for reading highly concrete words is consistent with an impairment in semantic reading, although concreteness effects may also occur as a result of damage at different levels of processing, for different reasons (see chapter 1).

Semantic Paralexias

The production of a word that is related in meaning to the target word (for example, *dog* read as "cat") is known as a semantic paralexia. These errors may occur when the incorrect semantic representation is activated from the written word or when an impoverished semantic representation is activated. However, they also can occur as a result of difficulty accessing the correct phonological representation of the word from the appropriate semantic representation. One may attempt to tease apart these possibilities (Friedman & Perlman, 1982) by having the patient read aloud a written word and then point to its referent from among four pictures in which the foils are highly semantically related to the target. Error responses might suggest a weakened phonological activation for the word (incorrect word reading but correct picture identification) or an inaccurate activation of the semantic representation (incorrect word reading and incorrect picture identification). An alternative method for evaluating access to semantics in the presence of semantic paralexias, in patients with adequate speech production, is to ask the patient to define the word that s/he just read aloud. For example, patient RGB (Caramazza & Hillis, 1990) read aloud *red* as "yellow" but defined it as "the color of blood." He apparently accessed an intact semantic representation, but then activated the incorrect phonological representation for output.

Patients who make semantic paralexias in reading often are observed to also show several other features of impaired reading: a concreteness effect, difficulty reading PWs, part-of-speech effects (nouns read better than verbs or functors), and morphological errors (for example, *write* → "wrote"). This collection of characteristics has been labeled "deep alexia." However, the label does not pin down the level of disruption in the reading process, since (as just discussed) semantic paralexias may arise at the level of semantics or at the level of access to the phonological representation. Furthermore, some of these features have been observed in patients who do not produce semantic paralexias. Most patients with deep alexia, and some patients with phonological alexia, exhibit selective difficulty reading functors, and these patients may or may not show an advantage of nouns over verbs. Thus, understanding what component processes are impaired in an individual patient, based on convergence of evidence from error types, parameters that do and do not affect reading (word class, concreteness, frequency, word length), and performance across various reading and semantic tasks, is more useful than applying a label.

Part of Speech Effects

Difficulty reading words of certain form class can be uncovered by asking the patient to read a list of words containing nouns, verbs, adjectives, and functors (prepositions, conjunctions, pronouns, auxiliary verbs). Words of the different form classes should be matched for letter length. It is difficult to match for frequency, as functors tend to be higher in frequency than other words. However, one should at least ensure that all nonfunctor words have the highest frequency possible.

The finding of a part of speech effect has typically been interpreted in a manner similar to that of the concreteness effect, with which it is commonly associated. That is, functors are not as strongly represented within the semantic lexicon as nouns are, and hence are less likely to be accessed in reading by the "lexical-semantic route," particularly if there is an impairment within the semantic lexicon. However, selective impairment in accessing one grammatical class of words (for example, nouns or verbs) can also occur as a result of damage at the level of the phonological lexicon. In such cases, the patient reads aloud and orally names one class of words (say, verbs) poorly, but has no trouble comprehending written verbs or in written naming of verbs (see Tippett & Hillis, chapter 7, this volume, for illustrative cases and discussion). Furthermore, a part of speech effect may be the result of a syntactic processing deficit, particularly when the effect is seen solely within the context of text reading, a phenomenon that has been called phonological text alexia (Friedman, 1996). When a part of speech effect is seen in reading, one should always evaluate it within the context of the patient's speech: the deletion of functors (agrammatism) likely indicates a grammatical processing deficit.

Morphological Paralexias

Closely tied to the part of speech effects seen in certain alexic patients is the phenomenon of the production of morphological paralexias. These errors typically involve the substitution of one affix for another (for example, *lovely* for *loving*), or simply the deletion or addition of an affix (for example, *play* for *playing*). As with errors on functor words, morphological paralexias are often attributed to a deficit in accessing phonology directly from orthography; the semantic pathway is simply unable to deal with these semantically weak morphemes. However, these errors may also be seen as orthographic errors; that is, errors in which the word produced is similar in spelling to the target word (and thus may occur as a result of hemispatial neglect or other visual processing deficit). Likewise, these errors may be seen as semantic paralexias; the meaning of *play* is certainly semantically similar to the meaning of *playing*. And, as with the part of speech effect, morphological errors may be a reflection of a more pervasive grammatical problem.

As with all types of paralexias, it is difficult to devise a task specifically to elicit these errors. It is even more problematic to assess their prevalence, as it is difficult to know how many of such errors one should expect for a given set of words. One is best advised to include words with different affixes in a list of words presented to the patient and to keep track of such errors (including additions of affixes to nonaffixed words) in all lists of words that the patient is asked to read. For details on how one might assess morphological errors in reading, see Badecker and Caramazza (1987).

Sentence and Text Reading

It is clearly the case that most patients who have difficulty reading single words will have difficulty reading text, although some patients may read text more accurately due to the contextual cues provided by the text. However, it is more common to encounter a patient who complains of difficulty reading text yet appears to have no difficulty reading single words. This dissociation may be a reflection of grammatical difficulties, and can be examined by presenting sentences of increasing grammatical complexity. Difficulty with text reading may also be caused by hemispatial neglect or other visual processing/eye movement impairments, attentional deficits, or phonological processing deficits (which may result in increased difficulty with increasing sentence length).

Most patients with pure alexia also have a partial or complete right homonymous hemianopia; this visual field cut may further impair text reading. Indeed, "hemianopic alexia" was identified more than one hundred years ago (Wilbrand, 1907, as cited in Zihl 1995). Pure hemianopic alexia may be difficult to document. Single word reading is intact, and there is no word length effect.

Reading speed is reduced, but this may be ascertainable only by the patient's report, since there is no way to determine premorbid reading speed.

Clinical Assessment Tools

The previous section of this chapter suggested ways to assess those aspects of reading that are most likely to be disturbed in patients with acquired alexia. Here, we review some of the best known of the clinical assessment tools that may be useful in performing such an evaluation.

Aphasia Tests

The Psycholinguistic Assessment of Language Processing in Aphasia (PALPA; Kay, Lesser, and Coltheart, 1992), a test of language function, contains a fairly comprehensive assessment of reading function. The PALPA contains sixty subtests, many devoted to written language processing. Each subtest has normative data, clear descriptions of the parameters being assessed, and well-organized answer sheets. A large number of the assessments discussed in the previous section are represented in the PALPA.

One disadvantage to using the PALPA is that it was normed only for British English; thus, some of the items are not appropriate for speakers of American English (for example, *pram, hosepipe*). Another potential disadvantage is the brevity of the word lists. This is desirable as a screening for potential deficits, but is somewhat inadequate for definitive affirmation of the presence of a particular deficit. Longer lists controlled for various parameters such as part-of-speech, word length, frequency, concreteness, and regularity are found in the Johns Hopkins University Dyslexia Battery (Goodman & Caramazza, 1986; published with permission in Beeson & Hillis, 2001).

The Boston Diagnostic Aphasia Exam (BDAE), 3rd Edition (Goodglass, Kaplan, and Barresi 2000) contains several subtests of reading that may be of some use in evaluating possible alexias, including single letter and short word matching across case and font. This test of letter identity contains too few items to make any real determination about the patient's abilities, however.

Also included in the BDAE are subtests dealing with morphology. One advantage of these subtests is that they do not require the patient to produce verbal output; a word is spoken by the examiner, and the patient points to the corresponding word from a multiple-choice list. Included are functors and words with bound grammatical and derivational morphemes. However, performance on these items is not compared with performance on nongrammatical words, making it difficult to identify a relative deficit for grammatical words. Further, as this is a screening test of reading embedded within a much larger language test, the number of items are insufficient to be sensitive to milder problems.

Reading Tests

The Weschler Test of Adult Reading (WTAR; Wechsler, 2001) was designed as a measure of premorbid IQ in patients with brain damage. It consists of fifty words with irregular spelling-to-sound correspondences. The words in the test are arranged to decrease in word frequency, making the later words less likely to be read correctly than the earlier words. Other tests of this ilk include the National Adult Reading Test (NART; Nelson, 1982) and the North American Adult Reading Test (NAART; Blair and Spreen, 1989). These tests may be a useful source of irregular words if surface alexia is suspected. However, the number of irregular words that a reader of normal IQ would be expected to read correctly is rather limited, diminishing the usefulness of the test.

The Gates-MacGinitie Reading Tests (Gates & MacGinitie, 1965) were designed to assess single word comprehension, comprehension of short paragraphs of increasing difficulty, and speed and accuracy of reading one- to two-sentence paragraphs. The single words were not chosen on the basis of any psycholinguistic parameters, so this part of the test is of limited value. The speed and accuracy subtest evaluates accuracy with a forced-choice sentence completion test. It assesses speed by measuring how many paragraphs can be completed in four minutes. This subtest, and the slightly longer paragraph subtest, can be useful in assessing oral reading and reading comprehension of text.

The Reading Comprehension Battery for Aphasia, 2nd Edition (RCBA-2; LaPointe and Horner, 1998) assesses functional silent reading, letter knowledge, lexical decision, and oral reading. Letter knowledge is assessed with a physical matching task; the subject decides whether two uppercase letters are identical or not. Tests for neglect are incorporated into a test of letter naming and a test of pointing to the letter named.

In the lexical decision task, the subject is asked to choose the real word from among a triad of one word and two pseudowords. The PWs are not created to be pseudohomophones of real words, and the real words are not chosen to assess regularity; thus this test will not be adequate to completely determine the integrity of orthographic representations.

In the single word comprehension task, a single picture must be matched to one of three words that is either orthographically similar, phonologically similar (and possibly orthographically similar as well), or semantically similar. A synonym matching task is included as well. There is also an assessment of "functional reading," which includes different formats, such as labels, signs, and entries in phone books.

Oral reading of single words is assessed for nouns only. Oral reading of sentences is assessed for sentences of subject-verb-object structure only. The effect of context is incorporated into this task by including words from the single word oral reading task.

In a sentence comprehension task, the subject chooses one of three pictures that corresponds to a written sentence. In one subtest, the sentences are chosen to assess morphosyntactic reading. Another task tests short paragraph comprehension. Longer paragraphs are presented for comprehension in a test containing both factual and inferential questions.

The Gray Oral Reading Tests, Fifth Edition (GORT-5; Wiederholt and Bryant, 2012) is normed to age twenty-three. It has two equivalent forms, each consisting of sixteen increasingly difficult passages, which are each followed by five passage-dependent multiple-choice questions. The test evaluates oral reading rate, accuracy, and comprehension. The two forms are useful in evaluating post-treatment changes.

Treatment of the Alexias

Controlled studies of treatments for the alexias have only begun to appear in the last few decades, following the development of cognitive neuropsychological models of reading and reading disorders. Prior to the 1970s, alexic disorders were not well differentiated (aside from pure alexia), and so clinical treatments did not take into account the nature of the specific deficit. The identification of various types of alexias, such as surface alexia and phonological alexia (Marshall & Newcombe, 1973), changed the way that many speech-language pathologists consider remediating reading. The current trend, then, is to identify the specific cognitive deficits that underlie the reading problem in an individual patient, and to devise a treatment program accordingly. A description of some of the treatment studies that have been published in the last three decades follows.

Treatment of Attentional Deficits Affecting Reading

Coelho (2005) described a person with mild anomic aphasia subsequent to a left temporoparietal stroke who complained of difficulty reading, although single word and sentence reading were relatively normal. Reading rate and reading comprehension were found to be impaired on formal testing. Further testing revealed deficits in attention, and an eight-week treatment based on Sohlberg et al.'s (1994) Attention Process Training-II was administered. At the end of treatment, reading comprehension scores improved. This was a single case study, and the participant was less than one year post stroke when it was carried out, so results should be interpreted with caution. Nevertheless, if the dominant complaint is difficulty reading, no deficit specific to the reading process can be demonstrated, and cognitive testing reveals impairments in attention, one might do well to direct treatment strategies to attention training.

Treatment for Impaired Text Reading Due to Hemianopia

Moving Text

One approach that has been taken to improve scanning into the impaired visual field in people with RHH involves the use of moving text (Kerkhoff et al., 1992; Spitzyna et al., 2007). The words of sentences are read aloud as they move from right to left across the screen. Velocity of text movement increases gradually. Following treatment, increased reading speed was found under normal reading conditions.

Oculomotor Training

In a treatment involving simple instruction, a word appears on the screen and the patient is instructed to intentionally shift his gaze to the end of the word (Schuett et al., 2008). Words of different length were used, and the presentation time was gradually decreased. Following treatment, reading speed was increased. Similar improvements were found when the stimuli were composed of numbers rather than words.

Treatment for Letter Recognition Deficit in Pure Alexia

As mentioned above, patients with pure alexia may recover some reading function by learning to read in a serial letter-by-letter fashion. Use of letter-by-letter reading may be taught by the therapist (see, for example, Daniel, Bolter, & Longs, 1992), though it is often discovered by the patients themselves. However, some patients with pure alexia also have difficulty recognizing individual letters. If letters are misidentified, it follows that the word in which they are contained will be misread. A fairly successful remedy for this problem involves *tactile-kinesthetic (T-K)* letter identification (Greenwald & Gonzalez Rothi, 1998; Kashiwagi & Kashiwagi, 1989; Kim, Rapcsak, Andersen, & Beeson, 2011; Lott, Friedman, & Linebaugh, 1994; Lott & Friedman, 1999; Lott, Carney, Glezer, & Friedman, 2010; Maher, Clayton, Barrett, Schober-Peterson, & Gonzalez Rothi, 1998; Sage, Hesketh, & Lambon Ralph, 2005). The rationale for this technique is straightforward. Because the deficit in pure alexia is one of access to the orthographic lexicon when stimuli are presented in the visual modality, the T-K technique is designed to provide a means for accessing orthographic lexical representations through other modalities—tactile and/or kinesthetic.

In a typical T-K treatment, the patient is first trained to recognize single letters in isolation. A letter is presented on a computer screen or an index card, and the patient traces or copies the letter, and then names it. Some studies used only kinesthetic feedback by having the patient copy letters onto the table or a piece of paper (Maher et al., 1998; Kashiwagi & Kashiwagi, 1989; Kim et al., 2011), while the Sage et al. (2005) study used only tactile feedback by having the therapist trace letters onto the patient's hand. The Lott et al. studies (1994, 1999, and 2010) invoked both tactile and kinesthetic feedback by having the patient copy the letters onto the palm of his or her other hand. Once the patient has mastered single letter recognition, training proceeds to whole words, and eventually to sentences.

After the patient's accuracy of letter-by-letter reading has reached an acceptable level, training can next be geared toward improving speed of reading. In the Lott and Friedman (1999) study, the patient was first encouraged to use the T-K strategy to name letters aloud as rapidly as possible. Feedback was provided, and training continued until the patient's speed reached a plateau. The next phase involved the naming of letters in a letter string, followed by single word reading. Feedback about speed was given after each block. The result of this treatment was substantial improvement in reading speed, with no sacrifice in accuracy. The Lott et al. (2010) study replicated these successful results in three additional patients. Furthermore, these patients significantly improved accuracy and speed of reading untrained words *even without overt use of the strategy*. This improvement was attributed to continuing to train letter naming beyond the point at which letter naming accuracy was initially achieved, or "overtraining." Two of the three patients became so adept that they were able to read entire sentences.

The Kim et al. (2011) study reported a patient who improved letter-naming accuracy using a T-K strategy, but who did not improve reading of untrained words. The authors attributed this to a concomitant kinesthetic-verbal disconnection. While this additional deficit is not typically seen with pure alexia, this study illustrates the importance of fully evaluating your patient's underlying deficits since a unique constellation of impairments might limit the effectiveness of a particular treatment approach.

Treatment for Impaired Whole Word Recognition in Pure Alexia: A Semantic Approach

It has been reported that some patients with pure alexia may be able to recognize words as wholes if the words are presented rapidly (Coslett & Saffran, 1989; Shallice & Saffran, 1986). The explanation for this finding is that a secondary reading system, based upon semantics, is available to the patients but only becomes available when the patient is prevented from employing a letter-by-letter reading strategy. It has been suggested (Coslett & Saffran, 1989) that patients can be trained to employ this alternate reading mechanism by presenting words tachistoscopically and focusing on tasks that emphasize semantic processing, such as category decision or other semantic judgments. This notion has been put into practice in several treatment studies.

Gonzalez Rothi and Moss (1992) used the semantic approach in treating the reading deficit of a patient with pure alexia. Written words were presented tachistoscopically in three different tasks: homophone decision, semantic category decision, and lexical decision. Results revealed improved accuracy for the stimuli presented in all three tasks. Reading of untrained words showed some improvement in speed, but not accuracy. The authors reported some success with this approach in one subsequent case, but failure in another case.

Further investigations of the training of whole word reading suggest that focusing on semantic processing may not be necessary for this strategy to be successful. Friedman and Lott (2000) used 50 msec presentations of words, presented over many sessions with feedback, to train patient RS to make accurate semantic judgments for trained words. However, their patient also learned to recognize rapidly presented words when the task was simple oral reading, not categorization. Further, the patient learned words of lower semantic value (that is, functors) as rapidly as words high in semantic value (concrete nouns), again suggesting that the mechanism of learning may not be semantically based. This technique has since been used successfully with several other pure alexic patients; one patient failed to benefit from this therapy (Friedman & Lott, unpublished data). Ablinger and Domahs (2009) also successfully trained a patient to recognize rapidly presented words in a simple oral reading task. After several training sessions, reading speed and accuracy of both trained and control words improved significantly. Improved single letter naming and text reading were also reported.

Given that it may be possible to train patients with pure alexia to recognize words rapidly, but that it is unrealistic to attempt to train all words of the language, Friedman and Lott (1997) trained a patient to recognize 125 to 150 of the most frequent words of the language, words that tend to appear repeatedly within typical sentences and paragraphs. Mastery of these words improved her speed of reading sentences composed entirely of the trained sight words, but did not generalize to improvement in reading other sentences, suggesting that the improvement on each sight word might have been too small to affect an overall improvement in sight reading. Further study is needed to evaluate whether "overtraining" a set of sight words such as these might lead to measurable improvement in functional reading material.

It is worth noting that this training paradigm has been implemented successfully on a computer (Friedman & Lott, 2000; Lott & Friedman, 1994) so that the patient can self-train at home between therapy sessions. The program is set up so that a word is flashed on the screen, and the patient reads the word. Following a key press, the computer presents the word auditorily, providing the necessary feedback.

Treatment for Inability to Access Orthographic Representation in Surface Alexia

A patient who consistently reads regular words (*home*) better than irregular words (*come*) and who defines words according to their derived pronunciation (*come* → "you use it to fix your hair") has difficulty accessing lexical orthographic representations of known words. In an attempt to ameliorate this problem in such a surface alexic patient, Byng and Coltheart (1986) developed a technique in which targeted irregular words were paired with semantic cues. For example, the word *through* was presented with an arrow drawn through it. The patient's reading of words paired with semantic cues improved more than his reading of words that were not included in the treatment, but some generalization may have occurred as well. These results were replicated in a subsequent study by Weekes and Coltheart (1996).

Scott and Byng (1989) employed context-rich sentences for training the meanings of homophonic words in a patient with surface alexia. The task was forced-choice sentence completion. The six choices included the correct word, its homophone, and a pseudohomophone of the correct word. Following ten weeks of training, the patient showed improvement of the trained words. However, improvement of the untrained words on two of the three post-tests made interpretation of the results problematic. Hillis (1993) reported improved oral reading and comprehension (and spelling) of trained homophones (for example, *stake* and *steak*) without generalization to untrained homophones in a similar study. Here, the task was to read each trained word and its definition and then write it in a sentence.

Treating a Deficit in Accessing Phonology from Orthography in Phonological and Deep Alexia

Training Grapheme-Phoneme Correspondence Rules

Patients with "deep alexia" have difficulty reading many words that are low in concreteness and are unable to use orthography-to-phonology correspondences to decode these words. One approach to reading remediation in these patients is to retrain the use of such correspondences.

dePartz (1986) successfully taught her patient to use grapheme-to-phoneme correspondence rules by associating a "relay" word with each letter of the alphabet (for example, "boy" for b), then elongating pronunciation of the first phoneme in the relay word, and finally pronouncing only the phoneme. The patient was trained to read aloud short nonwords by sounding out each letter individually, and then to read aloud short real words. After nine months, the patient improved word reading from 28% to 98% correct.

Three subsequent therapy programs for deep alexic patients (Laine & Niemi, 1990; Mitchum & Berndt, 1991; Nickels, 1992), modelled after dePartz's, all met with considerably less success. The patient of Laine and Niemi and the patient of Mitchum and Berndt both learned to produce the appropriate phonemes for given graphemes, but were never able to successfully blend the phonemes into syllables. Integrity of phonological short-term memory and aphasia type (and lesion location) varied across these patients and may be relevant to the success/failure of this therapy technique.

Nickels (1992) used a combination nonlexical and lexical training approach with her patient, who learned to assign the appropriate phonemes to graphemes, but could not learn to blend them into syllables. The patient was then trained to produce the initial phoneme of a word, think about its meaning, and attempt to say the word. Two weeks after therapy ended there was significant improvement in the reading of high imageability words. It is important to note, however, that patients who have trouble decoding phonology from orthography tend to have more trouble with low imageability words than high imageability words, a fact that renders this approach less useful.

Rather than focusing on semantics, Yampolsky and Waters (2002) and Stadie and Rilling (2006) addressed the blending problem by including treatment phases that explicitly targeted blending. Yampolsky and Waters trained phonics and blending skills simultaneously with grapheme-to-phoneme correspondences. Tasks included manipulating single grapheme cards into various CVC (consonant-vowel-consonant) words, tapping a finger for each grapheme, and orally reading CVCs. Patient MO improved her reading of untrained CVC words and pseudowords, but not of words of untrained syllabic structures. Stadie and Rilling (2006) first trained grapheme-to-phoneme correspondences, and then trained blending. Their patient, too, improved her reading of untrained words and nonwords. These results show that successful blending of single phonemes may be achieved with specific training, for some patients.

Training Bigraphs

As discussed in the above section, the greatest challenge of the grapheme-phoneme therapy was learning to blend individual phonemes into syllables. Friedman and Lott (2002) devised a therapy predicated on the premise that grapheme-phoneme conversion is not the most natural way to translate letters into sounds: in particular, many consonantal phonemes cannot actually be produced in isolation; a vowel (usually a schwa) must be produced as well. When blending these sounds, then, the schwa must first be inhibited, and this appears to be difficult for these patients (Berndt, Haendiges, Mitchum, & Wayland, 1996), and for many young children as well (Rozin & Gleitman, 1977).

The Friedman and Lott (2002) therapy was based upon a more natural unit of pronunciation, the bigraph syllable. The patient is first trained to associate a set of bigraphs with their corresponding sounds, using the "relay" procedure, much like the one used by dePartz (1986): when presented with a two-letter bigraph (for example, *ma*), the patient is trained to produce a word that begins with those letters (for example, *match*), then cut it short so that only the appropriate bigraph syllable is produced (/mætʃ/ → /mæ/). After learning consonant-vowel (CV) bigraphs and vowel-consonant (VC) bigraphs, the patient learns to put CVs and VCs together into CVC words; for example, /mæ/ + /æt/ = mat. Two patients were able to learn the trained bigraphs; both were able to combine those bigraphs to read a large number of untrained words. Kim and Beaudoin-Parsons (2007) replicated these successful results with another patient. They further demonstrated significantly improved reading accuracy of low-imageability words and text, as well as improved comprehension of text.

Bowes and Martin (2007) extended the bigraph approach by training both reading of bigraphs and writing of biphones. Patient MQ improved her reading and writing of untrained one-syllable nonwords, two-syllable words, and phrases following this treatment.

These combined studies demonstrate that bigraph training can improve the phonological decoding skills of some alexic patients. However, it does have certain limitations. In any irregular language such as English there are many exceptions to contend with (for example, producing /mæ/ at the beginning of the word *many* would lead to an incorrect reading). In addition, using such a strategy with multisyllabic words may be problematic. Finally, the number of different bigraphs that must be trained is large. Despite these obstacles, providing patients with a means of decoding even short words or syllables may go a long way toward improving their overall reading, particularly if combined with other strategies such as focusing on semantics (Nickels, 1992), training blending (Yampolsky & Waters, 2002; Stadie & Rilling, 2006), or including writing tasks (Bowes & Martin, 2007).

Training General Phonological Processing

Another approach for improving orthography-to-phonology conversion is to train general phonological skills, rather than focusing on reading-specific skills. Kendall, Conway, Rosenbeck, and Gonzalez Rothi (2003) first trained two patients on phoneme discrimination tasks that focused on each phoneme's visual, auditory, and oral kinesthetic unique features. The patients were then trained to use this knowledge to improve phonological awareness through tasks such as segmentation and identification of phonemes within spoken syllables. Ultimately, treatment focused on generalizing these phonological skills to spelling and reading of simple and complex nonwords. One patient demonstrated a treatment effect in word reading, while the second demonstrated only minimal improvement. Neither patient demonstrated improved nonword reading.

Semantic Mediation

Patients with "phonological alexia" (predominant impairment in orthography-to-phonology conversion) often have difficulty reading functors and other words that are low in concreteness, while retaining fairly good reading of concrete words. Friedman, Sample and Lott (2002) made use of two such patients' intact reading of content words to aid in their reading of functors and verbs. Words low in semantic value, and hence poorly read by these patients, are paired with relay words high in semantic value that are phonologically similar. The most perfect case of this type of pairing is the homophone: the word *be* is paired with the relay word *bee*. As most words do not have homophones, near-homophones were used as well (for example, *me, meat*). The phonology of the relay homophones remains accessible because they are supported by rich semantic activation. The phonological activation of the relay homophones primes the phonology of the targets.

The target word (*be*) is printed on the front of an index card; its relay homophone (*bee*), along with a picture of the homophone, appears on the back of the card. The patients in this study learned to pair the targets with their relay homophone or near-homophone, and eventually learned to read the target words before turning over the card.

The requirement that a target word needs a homophone, or a near homophone, obviously limits the potential number of target words that could be trained via this approach. In a follow-up study, Lott, Sample, Oliver, Lacey, and Friedman (2008) demonstrated successful learning of target words trained via relay words of varying degrees of phonological similarity. For example, it might be necessary to drop the final phonemes of the relay word (for example, relay word *bologna* for target *below*), or it might be necessary to drop and then add phonemes (for example, relay word *elk* for target *else*). Target words that were paired with some type of phonologically-related relay word were learned to criterion, while those trained in control conditions (paired with a non-phonologically related relay word, or simply repeated without use of a relay word) were not. These results suggest that virtually any problematic word can be trained via this approach. Selecting the most phonologically related relay word possible will, of course, maximize the likelihood of success.

In this study, greater maintenance of the treatment effect was achieved when items were "overtrained"; that is, they continued to be trained beyond the time when criterion was first achieved. In addition to the behavioral data, Kurland et al. (2008) demonstrated a shift in the neural activation for words that were "overtrained" via this paradigm. Compared with untrained words, reading trained words recruited larger and more significant clusters of activation in the right hemisphere, including right inferior frontal and inferior parietal cortex. Predominate activation shifted to the left hemisphere regions, including perilesional activation in the superior parietal lobe, when reading overtrained words compared with untrained words. These data support the notion that "overtraining" items alters both neural activation and long-term behavioral outcome of this treatment. It is likely that "overtraining" might be beneficial in other treatment paradigms as well.

Treating the Semantic Deficit in Deep Alexia

As in phonological alexia, patients with deep alexia have difficulty reading functors and abstract words; however, they also make frequent semantic errors on concrete words. Some studies have attempted to directly strengthen semantic route reading in patients with deep alexia. Ska and colleagues (2003) trained their patient JH to name fifty pictures by forming a mental association between the picture and the written word. After five sessions, he improved his reading of trained words, but not untrained words. The semantic treatment evaluated by Stadie and Rilling (2006) used a priming task in which a prime word was presented for 300 msec, followed by presentation of the target word 1100 msec later. Primes for nouns and verbs were semantically related words, and primes for adjectives were antonyms. Since function words have little semantic content, they were primed with phonologically similar content words. It is interesting to note that this is the same relationship used in Lott et al.'s semantic treatment discussed above, but presented in a priming paradigm rather than paired associate learning. As in all the semantically-based treatments discussed, reading of trained, but not untrained, words improved. This is in contrast with the treatment effects resulting from the phonologically-based approaches discussed earlier that successfully generalized to untrained words. However, occasionally, semantically-based treatment generalizes to untrained semantically related words (see chapter 12).

Treatment Focusing on Text Reading

Sentence Building

Patients with very mild phonological alexia, or phonological text alexia (Friedman, 1996), make errors on functors and affixes when read in text, but not when read in isolation. It has been suggested that this error pattern is due to incomplete or slowed phonological activation of functors, making them vulnerable to interference from the more richly represented content words during sentence processing. Lott, Sperling, Watson, and Friedman (2009) developed a treatment based on repetition priming that aimed to speed and strengthen phonological activation when reading text. The patient was trained to use a strategy that she could employ whenever reading, which involved building sentences in steps. For example, when presented with the following sentence in its entirety, "*The employees at the zoo know not to tease the animals*," the patient first read "*The*," then "*The employees*," then "*The employees at*," and so on until the entire sentence was read. Patient

NYR learned to use this "sentence building" strategy to accurately read practiced sentences. More importantly, after twenty-four treatment sessions (two-hour sessions twice per week for twelve weeks), she independently used the strategy to read unpracticed sentences with improved accuracy and comprehension. Due to its tedious nature, this strategy has limited functional application for reading lengthy text, such as an article or a book, but is quite functional for short yet important text such as driving directions or medical instructions.

The Multiple Oral Rereading Approach

The multiple oral rereading (MOR) technique was developed by Moyer (1979) in an attempt to improve the reading speed of her pure alexic patient. The patient read aloud a simple (sixth grade level) 600-word passage, then practiced reading it aloud for thirty minutes a day for one week. A new selection was introduced each week. Speed of reading the practiced selection and speed of reading an unpracticed selection were recorded each week. At the end of three months, the patient's speed of reading new selections had improved significantly.

Tuomainen and Laine (1991) found the MOR technique to be successful with two of their three pure alexic patients. Only one of the patients showed increased speed of reading single words, leading the authors to conclude that MOR does not affect the "underlying defect in pure alexia," but rather serves to improve top-down processing strategies in text reading.

Beeson (1998), Beeson, Magloire, and Robey (2005), and Moody (1988) replicated the findings of the previous study. The patient with pure alexia in each of these studies showed improved speed of reading text following MOR therapy. The patient in Beeson et al. (2005) also showed improvement in single word reading, while the patient in Beeson (1998) did not.

Moody (1988) and Cherney (2004) both tested the efficacy of the MOR technique with patients with phonological alexia. The results were equivocal. One of Moody's phonological alexic patients showed improvement reading unpracticed text, while the other patient did not. Cherney's (2004) patient improved her reading rate and comprehension of novel text.

Beeson and Insalaco (1998) also tested the efficacy of MOR with patients with phonological alexia, one of whom also demonstrated a significant word length effect. MOR treatment was followed by practice reading text that was divided into phrases. Following the treatments, both patients showed improved reading speed, and particular improvement with functors. The first patient no longer showed a word length effect. The authors concluded that this patient showed "a generalized improvement in whole word recognition and a specific improvement in associating written functors to their corresponding phonological representations." Because multiple treatments were administered, it is impossible to know which of these treatments produced the increased reading speed for functors.

The study by Lacey, Lott, Snider, Sperling, and Friedman (2010) was designed to clarify the role of MOR therapy in the rehabilitation of pure alexia and phonological alexia. Unique to this study was the control over the trained functors, content words, and phrases used in the untrained passages, and assessing generalization by timing participants' reading of these passages before and after each week of MOR therapy. Therapy was provided for one two-hour session per week for eight weeks, with a different training passage practiced each week. Feedback regarding accuracy was provided as needed. For the rest of the week, the patients practiced the passage at home six times per day. Two patients with pure alexia and four with mild phonological alexia participated. All patients read novel passages faster only when they contained a critical mass of words that were read repeatedly in the practice passages; they did *not* get faster reading passages that included only a minimal number of practiced words. These results support the hypothesis that MOR works by improving bottom-up processing (that is, single word reading), rather than top-down processing (that is, using the semantic and syntactic context of the text). If MOR improved top-down processing, the patients would have improved on all passages, regardless of whether individual words had been practiced. The results further support the notion that the source of improvement in pure alexia is different than that in phonological alexia. The patients with pure alexia improved their speed of reading all novel passages that contained a critical mass of practiced words regardless of their part of speech. The patients with phonological alexia, however, got faster reading only the novel passages containing trained functors and/or phrases, but importantly not the passages with practiced content words.

The MOR approach has been modified to include additional training modalities. Originally developed to improve reading comprehension, the Oral Reading for Language in Aphasia (ORLA) approach includes choral reading, in which the patient reads text aloud in unison with the therapist, before reading it aloud independently. Cherney (2004) reported improved oral reading of trained, but not untrained sentences, by a patient with deep alexia and improved reading comprehension on other untrained stimuli.

Orjada and Beeson (2005) combined Oral Rereading Treatment (ORT), a modified form of ORLA, with a concurrent spelling treatment for a patient with phonological alexia. Here, the text was composed of personally relevant scripts that were written specifically for the patient. The target words for the spelling treatment were selected from the trained reading stimuli. After ten weeks of treatment, patient BB improved reading accuracy and speed of the trained scripts. Consistent with the findings of the Lacey et al. study (2010), the greatest improvement was on functors. Reading accuracy on the GORT-3 also improved, but reading rate remained slow. A large effect size was reported for improvement in spelling trained words. Improvement in spoken language as measured by the WAB was also noted.

Therapy of this kind, whose beneficial effect is primarily in speed rather than accuracy of reading, is appropriate for patients whose reading is already at a fairly high level of competence.

Summary

Reading is a complex process that requires a number of relatively independent processing components. Individuals with focal brain damage often have impaired reading as a result of disruption of one or more of these processing components. A number of tests have been reviewed that allow the clinician to pinpoint which processing components are impaired in each case. Once the level of disruption has been identified, therapy can focus on specifically treating the impaired component, or can focus on using intact processing mechanisms to compensate for the impaired mechanism or level of representation. More recent studies have invoked multiple treatment modalities to maximize the likelihood of success, such as training grapheme-to-phoneme correspondences in conjunction with general phonological skills (Stadie & Rilling, 2006; Yampolsky & Waters, 2002), adding choral reading to MOR (Cherney, 2004), and adding spelling tasks to reading treatments (Bowes & Martin, 2007; Orjada & Beeson, 2005). Whether the success of these studies can be attributed to training via multiple modalities has not yet been systematically evaluated within a single study. One aspect of treatment design that has been demonstrated to be effective in a variety of treatment approaches is "overtraining," or training items beyond the point at which criterion is first achieved (Kurland et al., 2008; Lott et al., 2008; Lott et al., 2010).

References

Ablinger, I., & Domahs, F. (2009). Improved single-letter identification after whole-word training in pure alexia. *Neuropsychological Rehabilitation, 19*(3), 340–363.

Badecker, W., & Caramazza, A. (1987). The analysis of morphological errors in a case of acquired dyslexia. *Brain and Language, 32*, 278–305.

Beeson, P.M. (1998). Treatment for letter-by-letter reading: A case study. In N.H. Estabrooks & A. Holland (Eds.), *Approaches to the treatment of aphasia*. San Diego: Singular Publishing Group.

Beeson, P.M., & Hillis, A.E. (2001). Comprehension and production of written words. In R. Chapey (Ed.), *Language intervention strategies in adult aphasia* (4th ed.). Baltimore: Lippincott, Williams and Wilkens.

Beeson, P.M., & Insalaco, D. (1998). Acquired alexia: Lessons from successful treatment. *Journal of the International Neuropsychological Society, 4*(6), 621–635.

Beeson, P.M., Magloire, J.G., and Robey, R.R. (2005). Letter-by-letter reading: Natural recovery and response to treatment. *Behavioral Neurology, 16*, 191–202.

Berndt, R.S., Haendiges, A.N., Mitchum, C.C., & Wayland, S.C. (1996). An investigation of nonlexical-reading impairments. *Cognitive Neuropsychology, 13*(6), 763–801.

Blair, J.R., & Spreen, O. (1989). Predicting premorbid IQ: A revision of the National Adult Reading Test. *The Clinical Neuropsychologist, 3*(2), 129–136.

Bowes, K., & Martin, N. (2007). Longitudinal study of reading and writing rehabilitation using a bigraph-biphone correspondence approach. *Aphasiology, 21*(6/7/8), 687–701.

Byng, S., & Coltheart, M. (1986). Aphasia therapy research: Methodological requirements and illustrative results. *Advances in Psychology, 34*, 191–213.

Cherney, L. R. (2004). Aphasia, alexia, and oral reading. *Topics in Stroke Rehabilitation, 11*(1), 22–36.

Coelho, C. (2005). Direct attention training as a treatment for reading impairment in mild aphasia. *Aphasiology, 19*(3/4/5), 275–283.

Coslett, H.B., & Saffran, E.M. (1989). Evidence for preserved reading in "pure alexia." *Brain, 112*, 327–359.

Daniel, M.S., Bolter, J.F., & Longs, C.J. (1992). Remediation of alexia without agraphia: A case study. *Brain Injury, 6*(6), 529–542.

dePartz, M.-P. (1986). Re-education of a deep dyslexic patient: Rationale of the method and results. *Cognitive Neuropsychology, 3*(2), 149–177.

Friedman, R.B. (1996). Phonological text alexia: Poor pseudoword reading plus difficulty reading functors and affixes in text. *Cognitive Neuropsychology, 13*(6), 869–885.

Friedman, R.B., & Lott, S.N. (1997). Treatment for pure alexia employing two distinct reading mechanisms. *Brain and Language, 60*(1), 118–120.

Friedman, R.B., & Lott, S.N. (2000). Rapid word identification in pure alexia is lexical but not semantic. *Brain and Language, 72*(3), 219–237.

Friedman, R.B., & Lott, S.N. (2002). Successful blending in a phonologic reading treatment for deep dyslexia. *Aphasiology, 16*(3), 355–372.

Friedman, R.B., & Perlman, M.B. (1982). On the underlying causes of semantic paralexias in a patient with deep dyslexia. *Neuropsychologia, 20*(5), 559–568.

Friedman, R.B., Sample, D.M., & Lott, S.N. (2002). The role of level of representation in the use of paired associate learning for rehabilitation of alexia. *Neuropsychologia, 40*(2), 223–234.

Gates, A.I., & MacGinitie, W.H. (1965). *Gates-MacGinitie reading tests.* New York: Teachers College Press.

Gonzalez Rothi, L.J., & Moss, S. (1992). Alexia without agraphia: Potential for model assisted therapy. *Clinics in Communication Disorders, 2*(1), 11–18.

Goodglass, H., & Kaplan, E., & Barresi, B. (2000). *The assessment of aphasia and related disorders* (3rd ed.). Philadelphia: Lea & Febiger.

Goodman, R.A., & Caramazza, A. (1986). *The Johns Hopkins dyslexia battery.* Baltimore: Johns Hopkins University Press.

Greenwald, M.L., & Gonzalez Rothi, L.J. (1998). Lexical access via letter naming in a profoundly alexic and anomic patient: A treatment study. *Journal of the International Neuropsychological Society, 4*(6), 595–607.

Hillis, A.E. (1993). The role of models of language processing in rehabilitation of language impairments. *Aphasiology, 7*(1), 5–26.

Kashiwagi, T., & Kashiwagi, A. (1989). Recovery process of a Japanese alexic without agraphia. *Aphasiology, 3*(1), 75–91.

Kay, J., Lesser, R., & Coltheart, M. (1992). *PALPA: Psycholinguistic assessments of language processing in aphasia.* London: Lawrence Erlbaum Associates.

Kendall, D.L., Conway, T., Rosenbeck, J., & Gonzalez Rothi, L. (2003). Phonological rehabilitation of acquired phonologic alexia. *Aphasiology, 17*(11), 1073–1095.

Kerkhoff, G., Munßinger, U., Eberle-strauss, G., & Stögerer, E. (1992). Rehabilitation of hemianopic alexia in patients with postgeniculate visual field disorders. *Neuropsychological Rehabilitation, 2*(1), 21–42.

Kim, M., & Beaudoin-Parsons, D. (2007). Training phonologic reading in deep alexia: Does it improve reading words with low imageability? *Clinical Linguistics and Phonetics, 21*(5), 321–351.

Kim, E.S., Rapcsak, S.Z., Andersen, S., & Beeson, P.M. (2011). Multimodal alexia: Neuropsychological mechanisms and implications for treatment. *Neuropsychologia, 49*(13), 3551–3562.

Kinsbourne, M., & Warrington, E.K. (1962). A variety of reading disability associated with right hemisphere lesions. *Journal of Neurology, Neurosurgery, and Psychiatry, 25*(4), 339–344.

Kurland, J., Cortes, C.R., Wilke, M., Sperling, A.J., Lott, S.N., Tagamets, M.A., VanMeter, J., & Friedman, R.B. (2008). Neural mechanisms underlying learning following semantic mediation treatment in a case of phonologic alexia. *Brain Imaging and Behavior, 2*(3), 147–162.

Lacey, E.H., Lott, S.N., Snider, S.F., Sperling, A.J., & Friedman, R.B. (2010). Multiple Oral Re-reading treatment for alexia: The parts may be greater than the whole. *Neuropsychological Rehabilitation, 20*(4), 601–623.

Laine, M., & Niemi, J. (1990). Can the oral reading skills be rehabilitated in deep dyslexia? In M. Hietanen, J. Vilkki, M.-L. Niemi, & M. Korkman (Eds.), *Clinical neuropsychology: Excursions into the field in Finland.* Rauma, Finland: Suomen Psykologinen Seura.

LaPointe, L.L., & Horner, J. (1998). *Reading comprehension battery for aphasia, Second Edition (RCBA-2).* Austin, TX: PRO-ED, Inc.

Lott, S.N., Carney, A.S., Glezer, L.J., & Friedman, R.B. (2010). Overt use of a tactile-kinesthetic strategy shifts to covert processing in rehabilitation of letter-by-letter reading. *Aphasiology, 24(11)*, 1424–1442.

Lott, S.N., & Friedman, R.B. (1994). Treatment for pure alexia via the information superhighway. *Brain and Language, 47*, 524–527.

Lott, S.N., & Friedman, R.B. (1999). Can treatment for pure alexia improve letter-by-letter reading speed without sacrificing accuracy? *Brain and Language, 67*(3), 188–201.

Lott, S.N., Friedman, R.B., & Linebaugh, C.W. (1994). Rationale and efficacy of a tactile-kinaesthetic treatment for alexia. *Aphasiology, 8*(2), 181–195.

Lott, S.N., Sample, D.M., Oliver, R. T., Lacey, E.H., & Friedman, R.B. (2008). A patient with phonologic alexia can learn to read "much" from "mud pies." *Neuropsychologia, 46*(10), 2515–2523.

Lott, S.N., Sperling, A.J., Watson, N.L., & Friedman, R.B. (2009). Repetition priming in oral text reading: A therapeutic strategy for phonological text alexia. *Aphasiology, 23*(6), 659–675.

Maher, L.M., Clayton, M. C, Barrett, A.M., Schober-Peterson, D., & Gonzalez Rothi, L.J. (1998). Rehabilitation of a case of pure alexia: Exploiting residual abilities. *Journal of the International Neuropsychological Society, 4*(6), 636–647.

Marshall, J. C., & Newcombe, F. (1973). Patterns of paralexia: A psycholinguistic approach. *Journal of Psycholinguistic Research, 2*(3), 175–199.

Mitchum, C.C., & Berndt, R.S. (1991). Diagnosis and treatment of the non-lexical route in acquired dyslexia: an illustration of the cognitive neuropsychological approach. *Journal of Neurolinguistics, 6*(2), 103–137.

Moody, S. (1988). The Moyer Reading Technique re-evaluated. *Cortex, 24*(3), 473–476.

Moyer, S.B. (1979). Rehabilitation of alexia: A case study. *Cortex, 15*(1), 139–144.

Nelson, H.E. (1982). The National Adult Reading Test (NART): Test manual. London: NFER-Nelson.

Nickels, L. (1992). The autocue? Self-generated phonemic cues in the treatment of a disorder of reading and naming. *Cognitive Neuropsychology, 9*, 155–182.

Orjada, S.A., & Beeson, P.M. (2005). Concurrent treatment for reading and spelling in aphasia. *Aphasiology, 19*(3/4/5), 341–351.

Rozin, P., & Gleitman, L.R. (1977). The structure and acquisition of reading II: The reading process and the acquisition of the alphabetic principle. In A.S. Reber & D.L. Scarborough (Eds.), *Toward a psychology of reading.* Hillsdale, NJ: Lawrence Erlbaum Associates.

Sage, K., Hesketh, A., & Ralph, MA. (2005). Using errorless learning to treat letter-by-letter reading: Contrasting word versus letter-based therapy. *Neuropsychological Rehabilitation, 15*(5), 619–642.

Schuett, S., Heywood, C., Kentridge, R., & Zihl, J. (2008). Rehabilitation of hemianopic dyslexia: Are words necessary for re-learning oculomotor control? *Brain, 131*(Pt 12), 3156–3168.

Scott, C., & Byng, S. (1989). Computer assisted remediation of a homophone comprehension disorder in surface dyslexia. *Aphasiology, 3*(3), 301–320.

Shallice, T., & Saffran, E. (1986). Lexical processing in the absence of explicit word identification: Evidence from a letter-by-letter reader. *Cognitive Neuropsychology, 3*(4), 429–458.

Shallice, T., & Warrington, E.K. (1977). The possible role of selective attention in acquired dyslexia. *Neuropsychologia, 15*(1), 31–41.

Ska, B., Garneau-Beaumont, D., Chesneau, S., & Damien, B. (2003). Diagnosis and rehabilitation attempt of a patient with acquired deep dyslexia. *Brain and Cognition, 53*(2), 359–363.

Sohlberg, M., Johnson, L., Paule, L., et al. (1994). Attention Process Training II: A program to address attentional deficits for persons with mild cognitive dysfunction. Puyallup, WA: Association for Neuropsychological Research and Development.

Spitzyna, G., Wise, R., McDonald, S., Plant, G., Kidd, D., Crewes, H., & Leff, A. (2007). Optokinetic therapy improves text reading in patients with hemianopic alexia. *Neurology, 68*(22), 1922–1930.

Stadie, N., & Rilling, E. (2006). Evaluation of lexically and nonlexically based reading treatment in a deep dyslexic. *Cognitive Neuropsychology, 23*(4), 643–672.

Tuomainen, J., & Laine, M. (1991). Multiple oral rereading technique in rehabilitation of pure alexia. *Aphasiology, 5*(4–5), 401–409.

Wechsler, D. (2001). *Wechsler Test of Adult Reading: WTAR*. Upper Saddle River, NJ: Pearson Education, Inc.

Weekes, B., & Coltheart, M. (1996). Surface dyslexia and surface dysgraphia: Treatment studies and their theoretical implications. *Cognitive Neuropsychology, 13*(2), 277–315.

Wiederholt, J., & Bryant, B. (2012). Gray Oral Reading Test, Fifth Edition. Austin, TX: Pro-Ed, Inc.

Wilbrand, H. (1907). Uber die makular-hemianopische Lesestorung und die von Monakow'sche Projektion der Makula auf die Sehsphare. *Klin Mbl Augenheilk, 45*, 1–39 (as cited in Zihl).

Yampolsky, S., & Waters, G. (2002). Treatment of single word oral reading in an individual with deep dyslexia. *Aphasiology, 16*(4/5/6), 455–471.

Zihl, J. (1995). Eye movement patterns in hemianopic dyslexia. *Brain, 118*(Pt 4), 891–912.

PART 2

Spelling

4

UNCOVERING THE COGNITIVE ARCHITECTURE OF SPELLING

Brenda Rapp and Simon Fischer-Baum

A variety of different patterns of spelling impairment may be observed subsequent to neurological damage. For example, *"sauce"* might be spelled as SOSS or as SOUCF or as GRAVY. Errors such as these, as well as other aspects of the spelling performance of dysgraphic individuals, have made fundamental contributions to our understanding of the nature and organization of the mental operations that are normally involved in spelling words. In this chapter we will first provide an overview of our current understanding of the normal spelling process. We will then illustrate, through a series of case studies, how the performance of dysgraphic individuals has been used in uncovering this cognitive architecture of spelling. In a final section we review what we have learned from the study of acquired dysgraphia about the structure and organization of the representations of word spellings themselves.

A Cognitive Architecture of the Spelling Process

The term *cognitive architecture* is used to describe the organization of the various mental operations that are involved in a skill such as spelling. A cognitive architecture specifies not only the functions of the various cognitive processes but also the relationships amongst them. In this context it is important to distinguish between cognitive functions and behavioral tasks. A cognitive function is a mental operation or process that can be used in a number of tasks. For example, if cognitive function A involves searching memory for the spelling of a word, then we assume that cognitive function A is used in any task that requires that function: searching memory for the spelling of a word is required for tasks such as spelling a word in response to a picture stimulus, spelling a word to dictation, or spelling a word in the course of writing a business letter. These tasks are similar in that they all make use of function A; however, they also differ in that each requires other cognitive processes that are not shared by all of the tasks. What is important to note is that there is not a one-to-one relationship between tasks and cognitive functions.

Figure 4.1 is a schematic depiction of the cognitive architecture of the spelling process that is assumed in most current work on spelling. In this section we will describe each of the cognitive components or functions that are assumed in this theory of spelling, grouping the functions into the categories of lexical, sub-lexical, and post-lexical. While these functions are specifically used in spelling, there may be similarities with functions that are used in other cognitive domains. For example, like many other cognitive systems, spelling relies on both long-term memory and working memory processes.

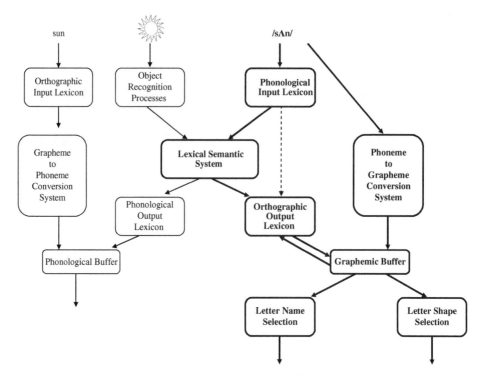

Figure 4.1 A schematic depiction of lexical, post-lexical, and sub-lexical cognitive processes. Those processes specifically involved in spelling are bolded.

Lexical Processes

Lexical processes refer to those functions that involve processing single words. It is generally assumed that, as a result of repeated experiences in hearing a spoken word, a memory trace of the word's phonological form is laid down in long-term memory. The collection of the long-term memory traces of phonological word forms is referred to as the **phonological lexicon**. A distinction is often drawn between an input and an output lexicon. The phonological input lexicon is involved in processing phonological input, in recognizing spoken words. By contrast, the phonological output lexicon is involved in producing spoken words.

The phonological input lexicon plays a role in the spelling process when the stimulus for spelling is a spoken word. When a person is asked to spell a word to dictation (or is taking notes in class or messages on the phone), the spoken stimulus is subjected to a series of pre-lexical auditory and phonological input processes that translate the acoustic stimulus to a phonological form. Subsequently, a process "searches" the phonological input lexicon for a stored memory trace that matches the phonological representation of the stimulus. If the search is successful it can be said that an entry in the phonological input lexicon has been "addressed" or "accessed." The phonological input lexicon is involved in a large number of tasks—in effect, in any task that includes (among other processes) hearing a word and determining whether the word form is familiar. Examples of such tasks would include: spelling to dictation, spoken language comprehension, spoken-word picture matching, and so forth.

The **lexical semantic system** is the long-term memory store of all the word meanings that an individual is familiar with. We assume that the same store of word meanings is involved regardless of the modality of presentation of a word (spoken, written, or pictorial) and regardless of the modality of production (spoken or spelled). After a word is accessed in the phonological input lexicon, and in order for the word to be understood, the long-term memory of its meaning must be contacted in the lexical semantic system. This will be true of tasks that involve simply understanding a spoken word as well as tasks such as spelling to dictation where the word must first be understood and then spelled. The lexical semantic system is, therefore, required for virtually all word comprehension and production tasks.

The **orthographic output lexicon** is the repository for the long-term memory representations of all familiar word spellings and is, therefore, sometimes referred to as "orthographic long-term memory" (Buchwald & Rapp, 2009). It is assumed to be specifically involved in the production of word spellings. By contrast, the recognition of word spellings, in tasks such as reading, is often assumed to make use of the orthographic input lexicon. Figure 4.1 depicts both orthographic input and output lexicons. However, there has been considerable controversy regarding whether reading and spelling actually depend on different lexical stores, with some researchers proposing a single-lexicon model (e.g., Allport & Funnel, 1981; Behrmann & Bub, 1992; Coltheart & Funnel, 1987). The single-lexicon model predicts that lexical orthographic damage should necessarily result in an association of impairments in reading and spelling, while the two-lexicon model predicts that there need not be such an association. This debate is ongoing and unresolved, and while the weight of current evidence favors a common orthographic lexicon for reading and spelling (see Hillis & Rapp, 2004 for a review), we have chosen here to present the two-lexicon model, which, given this chapter's focus on spelling, is somewhat easier to depict schematically. (Note that none of the arguments we present in the chapter are affected by the one- vs. two-lexicon distinction.)

As Figure 4.1 indicates, once a word's meaning has been accessed or activated, its semantic representation can serve as the basis for searching orthographic long-term memory for the corresponding spelling. According to this architecture, it is not necessary to go from a word's meaning to its phonological form in order to retrieve its spelling; instead, orthographic word forms can be retrieved independently of their corresponding phonological forms. In other words, phonological mediation between word meaning and orthographic form is not required. The evidence supporting this claim will be discussed in detail below.

Thus, the orthographic output lexicon is required for any task that involves going from the long-term memory representations of word meanings to long-term memory representations of word spellings, regardless of the form of the input. This includes the task of spelling to dictation, but is not limited to it since accessing the orthographic output lexicon will also be necessary if one simply writes down a word whose meaning one has in mind while writing a letter, a poem, or a grocery list. In addition, addressing the orthographic output lexicon from the lexical semantic system will be necessary if the stimulus for spelling is a picture or an object. For spelling the name of a picture or a visually presented object (the task of written naming) additional cognitive components are required for processing the visual stimulus and then accessing the lexical semantic system (see Figure 4.1).

Some theorists posit a direct connection between the phonological input lexicon and the orthographic output lexicon (Patterson, 1986; Roeltgen, Rothi, & Heilman, 1986). This is sometimes referred to as the "direct route" or the "nonsemantic route." This proposal is based on the finding that some individuals with dysgraphia can correctly spell words with highly irregular spellings (e.g., YACHT) despite the fact that they apparently do not understand the meanings of the words. This pattern suggests that there is a way to retrieve the spellings of words from the orthographic long-term memory (orthographic lexicon) without relying on the lexical semantic system. This issue has not been resolved as alternative accounts of the data have been proposed that do not require positing a direct, non-semantic route for word spelling (Hillis & Caramazza, 1991; Brown & Loosemore, 1994).

Post-Lexical Processes

A number of processes are required for going from the point at which a word's spelling is contacted in the orthographic output lexicon to actually producing a spelling. Spelling knowledge can be expressed in a variety of ways or "formats": written spelling, oral spelling, typing, squirting icing onto a cake, arranging shells on the beach or toothpicks in the shapes of letters and words, and so on. Here we will be concerned with the two most common means of spelling: oral and written. In oral spelling, a word's orthography is expressed by saying the names of letters (e.g., *cat* → /si, eI, ti/), whereas in written spelling it is expressed by producing letter shapes (e.g., *cat* → CAT). In written spelling there are a number of types of letter shapes that may be used: CAT, cat, *cat*.

Given that spelling knowledge can be expressed in such a wide range of formats, the following question arises: In what format are word spellings represented in long-term memory in the orthographic output lexicon? Based on a body of research findings, it is generally assumed that information about word spellings is stored in the orthographic output lexicon in an abstract format-independent manner. That is, our memories of the letter combinations that make up word spellings do not consist of letter shapes or letter names; instead, they consist of **abstract letter representations**, or graphemes.

The abstract graphemic representations stored in the orthographic output lexicon are given form by post-lexical processes that are dedicated to translating graphemes into specific letter shapes (in written spelling) or letter names (in oral spelling), as the situation requires. Post-lexically, therefore, there is a bifurcation of processes into those that are specific to written spelling and those that are specific to oral spelling (and other modalities, such as typing, etc.).

For written spelling, the **letter-shape selection process** (sometimes referred to as the allographic conversion process) translates each grapheme of a word's spelling into a letter-shape representation. These letter-shape representations specify the case (upper/lower) and font (print/cursive) corresponding to each grapheme and serve as the "blueprint" for complex motor processes that send commands to specific muscles that generate the movements required to produce the target shapes.

For oral spelling, the **letter-name selection process** translates abstract, graphemic representations into their corresponding letter names. The phonological representations that are the output of the letter-name selection process serve as the basis for the motor, articulatory plans that produce the movements of the oral articulators necessary for pronouncing the target letter names. (Note that the letter-name selection process yields phonological representations corresponding to letter names, such as /si/ /eI/ /ti/ for CAT, and not the names of the words themselves.)

Producing a word's spelling (either orally or in writing) is a time-consuming, serially executed process. Abstract letter codes need to be converted into letter shapes or letters names one at a time, in the correct order. In order to do this, the spelling system relies on an **orthographic working memory** system—commonly called the **graphemic buffer**. This system is dedicated to maintaining the correct sequence of abstract letter codes active throughout the production process. Graphemic buffering is required for both written and oral spelling and, as a result, is active after the retrieval of a word's spelling from the orthographic output lexicon and prior to the letter-name and letter-shape selection processes. Recent research (Costa et al., 2011) shows that orthographic working memory (OWM) is not a single process but rather involves multiple processes that are dedicated to such things as maintaining the activity level and distinctiveness of the letter codes over time to ensure temporal stability as well as coordinating the process of serially selecting each letter for production so that letters can be produced in the correct order. Although to date there has been relatively little research on this topic, the evidence indicates that these subcomponents of orthographic working memory can be selectively affected by brain damage (Costa et al., 2011).

Sub-Lexical Processes

In addition to being able to spell familiar words, we are also able to produce plausible spellings for words that we have never heard before (e.g., unfamiliar proper names). Thus, if you take a phone message from a Mrs. /f l i p/, you may write down a note that a Mrs. Flepe, Fleep, Fleap, or Phlepe called. The cognitive system containing the knowledge required to derive a plausible spelling for an unfamiliar phonological form is referred to as the **phoneme-grapheme conversion system** (or PG system).

It is typically assumed that the PG system consists of at least two processes: phonological parsing and phoneme-grapheme assignment. The phonological parsing process takes the output of pre-lexical auditory and phonological processes and parses (or organizes) the phonological information into smaller phonological units (perhaps individual phonemes or syllabically defined units). The phoneme-grapheme assignment process then operates on this representation, selecting a plausible spelling for each phoneme. Table 4.1 reports the possible phoneme-to-grapheme mappings for the phonemes in the unfamiliar word /f l i p/, as well as the frequencies of each mapping. Thus the PG system contains the knowledge of the regularities in the relationship between sounds and letters in English. It is referred to as a sub-lexical system because the units that are represented and manipulated are smaller than the whole-word or morpheme-sized units that are manipulated by the lexical system. Presumably, PG conversion knowledge is laid down as a result of each individual's accumulated experience in spelling the words of the language.

Interestingly, evidence from cognitively intact subjects as well as from dysgraphic individuals indicates that the PG system contains knowledge of the multiple ways in which the sounds of English may be spelled; that is, it does not simply encode that /f/ may be spelled with F, but rather it encodes that it may be spelled with F or PH. Furthermore, the evidence indicates that these multiple PG mappings (e.g., /f/ → F) are weighted in the PG system according to their frequency in the language. For example, as is shown in Table 4.1, 85 percent of all the words of English with syllable-initial /f/ are spelled with an initial F, while only 11 percent of such words are spelled with PH. There is some evidence that PG mappings are selected according to their frequency or mapping probability. Given this, the PG system is far more likely to generate a spelling for Mrs. /f l i p/ that begins with F than with PH.

As seen in Figure 4.1, the PG system shares with the lexical system not only the early pre-lexical components involved in processing an auditory stimulus, but also the post-lexical processes. The PG system relies on the orthographic working memory system to maintain the sequence of abstract graphemic codes generated by the PG system as well as on the letter-shape and letter-name conversion processes required to translate abstract graphemic codes into letter names or letter shapes

Table 4.1 Possible phoneme-to-grapheme mappings for the spoken unfamiliar word /f l i p/, as well as the frequency of those mappings.

Phoneme	Possible Grapheme	PG Mapping Frequency★
/f/	F	0.85
	PH	0.11
/l/	L	0.99
/i/	EA	0.30
	EA	0.28
	E_E	0.10
/p/	P	0.89
	PP	0.11

★ PG mapping frequencies from Hanna, Hanna, Hodges, & Rudorf Jr. (1966).

for the written or oral spelling of unfamiliar words (sometimes also referred to as nonwords or pseudowords).

How Patterns of Dysgraphic Performance Have Revealed the Functional Architecture of the Spelling Process

In the case of the spelling system, patterns of performance of dysgraphic individuals have formed the primary source of evidence regarding the organization of the system depicted in Figure 4.1. In the next sections, we review a number of case studies that specifically illustrate how dysgraphic performance has contributed to the development of the cognitive architecture just described.

The Question of Orthographic Autonomy: RGB (Caramazza & Hillis, 1990)

A long-standing issue in written language research has been the relationships amongst orthographic, phonological, and semantic systems. In the context of spelling, the specific question has been: If we have the meaning of a word in mind, do we need to access the word's spoken form in order to retrieve its spelling? According to the hypothesis of **obligatory phonological mediation**, the retrieval of a word's spelling requires the prior retrieval of its phonological form (see Figure 4.2[a]). According to this hypothesis, activation of a word's meaning is followed by activation of its spoken form, and only then can one gain access to its written form. This hypothesis is based on the traditional assumption that written language knowledge is entirely dependent on spoken language knowledge (Brown, 1972; Frith, 1979; Geschwind, 1969; Grashey, 1885; Head, 1926; Hecaen & Angelergues, 1965; Hotopf, 1980; Lichtheim, 1885; Luria, 1966; Van Orden, Johnston, & Hale, 1988; Wernicke, 1886). An alternative hypothesis, **orthographic autonomy**, proposes that, although orthography builds on phonology in the course of written language acquisition, in the fully developed system orthography can be retrieved directly from meaning, without phonological mediation (see Figure 4.2[b]). This direct relationship between orthography and semantics is assumed in the spelling architecture depicted in Figure 4.1.

Dysgraphic performance has been especially useful in adjudicating between these two hypotheses, because the two make clearly different predictions regarding the performance patterns that should be possible subsequent to damage. According to the hypothesis of obligatory phonological mediation, a deficit that affects the ability to access the phonological output lexicon should necessarily also disrupt spelling. In contrast, according to the hypothesis of orthographic autonomy, a deficit that affects phonological retrieval need not have any consequences for spelling. In order to evaluate these hypotheses, it is necessary to consider cases of individuals with damage affecting the phonological output lexicon or access to it. According to the obligatory phonological mediation hypothesis, in such cases spelling should also be affected, while, according to the orthographic autonomy hypothesis, it need not be.

The case of RGB (Caramazza & Hillis, 1990) provided a strong test of these predictions. RGB was an English-speaking, 62-year-old, right-handed retired personnel manager with a high school education. He suffered a left middle cerebral artery occlusion four years prior to the research study, with CT scans revealing a large, left frontoparietal infarct.

RGB showed intact access to semantic knowledge in comprehension tasks from both spoken and written word stimuli as well as from pictures. This was demonstrated by flawless performance on comprehension tasks requiring him to provide definitions for printed words or verifying whether written or spoken words matched pictures (Table 4.2). This performance indicates that RGB's lexical semantic system was intact.

A.

B.

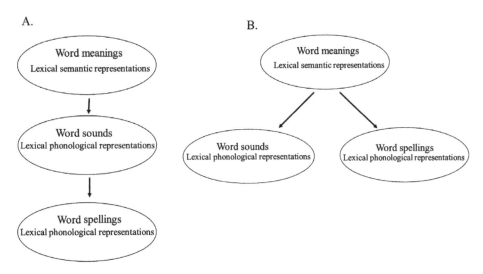

Figure 4.2 A schematic depiction of: (A) the hypothesis of obligatory phonological mediation and (B) the hypothesis of orthographic autonomy.

Interestingly, however, RGB had a clear impairment (68 to 89 percent accuracy) in spoken production tasks, such as oral naming of pictures and oral reading (Table 4.2). He made frequent semantic errors in these tasks; for example, he named a picture of a kangaroo as "raccoon," mittens as "socks," and clam as "octopus"; similarly, he read *kangaroo* as "giraffe," *mittens* as "gloves," and *banana* as "pineapple." The fact that his lexical semantic system was intact rules it out as the source of the errors; the fact that semantic errors (rather than phonological errors) were produced makes a post-lexical phonological deficit unlikely. This indicates that the semantic errors in spoken naming arose from difficulties in activating the correct phonological representation in the phonological output lexicon. To account for the occurrence of semantic errors at this level of the system, Caramazza and Hillis (1990) proposed that a semantic representation (e.g., [pronged + eating utensil + for spearing]) serves as the basis for the activation of a set of representations in the phonological output lexicon to varying degrees depending upon the extent to which they match the semantic features of the target (e.g., "fork," "spoon," "knife," "pitchfork"). The most active representation, normally the correct word, is selected for output. If for some reason (e.g., neurological damage) the target word is not available, the most highly activated member of the set will be produced, and a semantic error will be observed (e.g., *fork* named as "spoon").

For RGB, a post-semantic deficit affecting access to phonological representations is consistent with the fact that in oral reading, on the same trials that RGB produced semantic errors, he was able to correctly define the target word. For example, *records* was read as "radio" but defined as "you play 'em on a phonograph . . . can also mean notes you take and keep"; *volcano* was read as "lava" and defined as "fire comes of it . . . a big thing . . . a mountain." Thus, RGB constitutes an individual for whom neurological damage interrupted access to correct lexical phonological forms—a case with just the characteristics for testing the predictions of the orthographic autonomy and phonological mediation hypotheses.

RGB's spelling accuracy was critical for adjudicating between these two hypotheses. As Table 4.2 indicates, contrary to the prediction of the obligatory phonological mediation hypothesis, RGB's accuracy was excellent on written production tasks and, importantly, RGB never produced semantic errors in either writing to dictation or written picture naming tasks. In these

Table 4.2 RGB's Performance on Comprehension, Spoken Production, and Written Production Tasks

Task	Correct* (%)	Semantic (%)	Definitions (%)	Morph (%)	Other (%)
Defining printed words (n = 200)	100				
Auditory word/picture matching (n = 144)	100				
Printed word/picture matching (n = 144)	100				
Oral reading (n = 144)	69	12	14	5	
Spoken picture naming (n = 144)	68	15	16	1	
Writing to dictation (n = 144)	94				6
Written picture naming (n = 144)	94				6

*For written responses this includes clearly recognizable responses such as SQUAH for "squash."

tasks, he sometimes produced recognizable misspellings (e.g., "donkey" spelled as DOKNY or a picture of celery spelled as CELEY), but "full" errors occurred on 6 percent of items for which he was able to provide only the initial letter.

In order to account for RGB's pattern of good spelling in the face of semantic errors in spoken production, it is necessary to assume a cognitive architecture in which lexical orthographic forms can be retrieved directly from semantic representations without a mediating role for phonology. Thus, the hypothesis of orthographic autonomy can account for the data, while the hypothesis of obligatory phonological mediation cannot. In this way, RGB's performance serves to uncover a very basic aspect of the organization of the cognitive processes within the architecture of the spelling system.

A number of other cases have also provided evidence for the orthographic autonomy hypothesis (Rapp, Benzing, & Caramazza, 1997; Nickels, 1992; Basso, Taborelli, & Vignolo, 1978; Hillis & Caramazza, 1995b; Miceli, Benvegnu, Capasso, & Caramazza, 1997; Hanley & McDonnell, 1997; Bub & Kertesz, 1982; Hier & Mohr, 1977; Levine, Calvanio, & Popovics, 1982; Cuentos & Labos, 2001; Tainturier et al., 2001; Law, Wong & Kong, 2006; Piras & Marangolo, 2004; Kemmerer, Tranel & Manzel, 2005). Interestingly, the individuals reported in these case studies had a variety of language backgrounds, including users of languages in which there is a highly transparent relationship between orthography and phonology, such as Spanish (Cuentos & Labos, 2001), Welsh (Tainturier et al., 2001), and Italian (Miceli et al., 1997), as well as users of languages in which the relationship between orthographic and phonological forms is highly opaque, such as Chinese (Law, Wong, & Kong, 2006). Therefore, at least with regard to orthographic autonomy, the organization of the cognitive processes within the architecture of the spelling system does not appear to depend on the transparency/predictability of the phonology-orthography mappings across different languages; instead, the possibility of retrieving a word's spelling directly from its meaning without obligatory access to the word's sounds seems to be a characteristic of the cognitive architecture of the adult spelling system.

The Distinction between Lexical and Sub-Lexical Processing: RG (Beauvois & Derouesne, 1981) and PR (Shallice, 1981)

The architecture depicted in Figure 4.1 assumes that different processes are involved in the spelling of familiar and unfamiliar words (or pseudowords). An alternative hypothesis is that words and pseudowords are spelled making use of the same cognitive functions. Although the hypothesis of a common set of procedures for the processing of familiar words and pseudowords has not been extensively discussed in the context of spelling, it has played a central role in debates and research on reading (Seidenberg & McClelland, 1989; Harm & Seidenberg, 2004; Glushko, 1979; Plaut, McClelland, Seidenberg, & Patterson, 1996; Marcel, 1980). Evidence for the independence of processes involved in spelling familiar words and pseudowords comes from observations indicating that neurological damage may affect one of these skills and not the other.

Beauvois and Derouesne (1981) described the case of RG, a French-speaking, right-handed man who had been an agricultural machinery sales manager until undergoing surgery for a left parieto-occipital angioma. Post-surgery, RG's IQ remained in the average range and, except for reading and spelling deficits and difficulties in naming tactile stimuli, his language comprehension and production were normal.

With regard to spelling, RG's ability to spell pseudowords was unaffected: he was accurate with both short two-phoneme pseudowords (e.g., *ka*) as well as longer six-phoneme ones. In contrast, he had considerable difficulty correctly spelling words (see Table 4.3). This pattern (often referred to as surface dysgraphia) is difficult to understand without assuming that processes for spelling words are sufficiently distinct from those for spelling nonwords that they can be selectively affected by neurological damage. In this way, these findings support a distinction between lexical and sub-lexical spelling processes (for other similar cases see also Baxter & Warrington, 1987; Behrmann & Bub, 1992; De Partz, Seron, & Van der Linden, 1992; Goodman & Caramazza, 1986; Goodman-Shulman & Caramazza, 1987; Hatfield & Patterson, 1983; Iribarren, Jarema, & Lecours, 2001; Luzzi et al., 2003; Parkin, 1993; Sanders & Caramazza, 1990; Weekes & Coltheart, 1996; Weekes, Davies, Parris, & Robinson, 2003).

Within the lexical route (see Figure 4.1), RG's difficulties in word spelling could not be attributed to a deficit in processing the phonological input in writing to dictation, as both word repetition and spoken-word comprehension were intact. Furthermore, the same spelling difficulties he experienced in writing to dictation were observed in spontaneous writing where there is no phonological input. Peripheral difficulties with letter-shape selection were ruled out as he exhibited the same difficulties in written and oral spelling. The absence of an effect of word length also ruled out a deficit at the level of graphemic buffering. On this basis, RG's deficit was best described as affecting his ability to retrieve word spellings from the orthographic output lexicon. Damage of this sort is almost invariably sensitive to the frequency of the stored information, with higher frequency words (more common words) being less susceptible to disruption than lower frequency words. Consistent with this, RG's spelling exhibited a significant effect of lexical frequency: high-frequency words were 70 percent correct; low-frequency words were 53 percent correct.

There are a number of other very specific characteristics of the spelling errors that RG produced that provide further support for the spelling architecture depicted in Figure 4.1. The errors that RG produced when attempting to spell words consisted entirely of nonwords that had the

Table 4.3 Contrasting Patterns of Word and Nonword Spelling Accuracy for RG (Beauvois & Derouesne, 1981) and PR (Shallice, 1981)

	Words (%)	Nonwords (%)
RG	61	99
PR	94	18

same pronunciation as the target word (e.g., "rameau" spelled as RAMO; an English-language example would be spelling "sauce" as SOSS). Such errors are generally referred to as **phonologically plausible errors**, or PPEs. These kinds of errors can be understood if we assume that they are generated by the sub-lexical system subsequent to a failure in accessing the word's spelling from the orthographic output lexicon. The sub-lexical system should generate a plausible spelling for phonological stimuli, treating words and pseudowords in the same manner. In addition, if we are correct in assuming that the sub-lexical system is sensitive to the frequency with which a phoneme-grapheme relationship occurs in the language, the sub-lexical system should actually produce correct spellings for words with very common (high-frequency) phoneme-grapheme mappings (also referred to as high-probability PG mappings). This should manifest itself in greater accuracy with words containing only high-probability mappings, which are sometimes called "regular" words (e.g., in English, words such as *cat, fender, town*), than with words containing low-probability PG mappings, which are sometimes called "irregular" words (e.g., *once, yacht, aisle*). Indeed, as indicated in Table 4.4, RG's accuracy in spelling words containing only high-probability PG mappings was very high (91 percent), while his accuracy with low-probability PG words was only 30 percent.

It is important to note that while the *lexical* frequency effect mentioned above reflects the fact that high-frequency words are, at the level of the orthographic output lexicon, less susceptible to damage, the PG probability effect is not a reflection of the robustness of the *lexical* representations. Instead, this effect is based simply on the likelihood that the sub-lexical process will generate a spelling that happens to correspond to the lexical spelling. As a result of these properties of the lexical and sub-lexical systems, we should expect to see an accuracy interaction between word frequency and PG probability. Specifically, although low-frequency words should be comparably affected in the orthographic output lexicon regardless of their PG mapping probabilities, they will surface as errors depending on their PG mapping probabilities. Thus, frequency effects should be masked for words with only high PG mappings, but clearly visible for words containing low PG mappings. This interaction is clearly depicted in Table 4.4. The fact that as many as 44 percent of high-frequency, low-probability words resulted in errors suggests that there was considerable damage to the orthographic lexicon. The fact that 92 percent of high-frequency, high-probability words were correctly written indicates that the sub-lexical system was intact and able to produce appropriate spellings. The most vulnerable category of words is the set of low-frequency, low-probability words. Because of their low lexical frequency, these words have a higher likelihood of having been affected by the damage affecting the orthographic output lexicon; because of their low PG mapping status, they have very little chance of being correctly spelled via the sub-lexical system.

The proposed distinction between lexical and sub-lexical processes predicts that it should be possible to observe a dissociation complementary to the one exhibited by RG; namely, impaired pseudoword spelling in the face of preserved word spelling. Just such a pattern was reported by Shallice (1981). PR was an English-speaking patient whose spelling of words was excellent, with 94 percent accuracy (Table 4.3). His word spelling was not affected by word frequency or PG probability. In contrast, his spelling of pseudowords was severely impaired (18 percent correct).

Table 4.4 RG's Spelling Accuracy, Revealing a Probability-by-Frequency Interaction

	Low Frequency (%)	*High Frequency (%)*	*Total (%)*
Low probability	19	44	30
High probability	90	92	91
Total	53	70	

The pattern of essentially intact word spelling in the face of severely affected pseudoword spelling is sometimes referred to as phonological dysgraphia. PR's difficulties in pseudoword spelling were not readily attributable to difficulties in processing or remembering the pseudoword stimulus given that although he was able to correctly spell only 27 percent of the pseudowords, he was able to correctly repeat 77 percent of them after misspelling them. Further, he experienced important difficulties (30 percent correct) in writing even short (vowel-consonant) pseudowords, and his performance was comparable in oral and written spelling. On this basis his deficit was localized to the sub-lexical spelling system (for other cases demonstrating this double dissociation see Bub & Kertesz, 1982; Goodman-Shulman & Caramazza, 1987; Henry et al., 2007; Iribarren, Jarema, & Lecours, 2001; Rapcsak & Beeson, 2004; Roeltgen, 1985; Roeltgen, Sevush, & Heilman, 1983).

PR's ability to spell both high- and low-PG probability words also has important implications for debates concerning the content of the orthographic output lexicon. One possibility is that only those words that cannot be correctly derived by the sub-lexical system are stored in the orthographic lexicon. Under that scenario, low-PG-probability words would be spelled through the lexical system but high-PG-probability words would rely on the sub-lexical system. This leads to the prediction that an individual with a deficit to the sub-lexical system should have difficulty spelling *both* pseudowords and highly regular words. The fact that this was not observed with PR provides support for the hypothesis that the orthographic output lexicon stores the spellings of all familiar words, regardless of their regularity.

Another debate that these cases contribute to concerns the question of whether an orthographic lexicon exists at all in highly transparent orthographies (Spanish, Italian, Turkish, German, etc.). The possibility has been raised that literate individuals using these languages need not store word spellings in long-term memory, as they can always derive them from the application of the sub-lexical system (e.g., Ardila, 1991). If that were the case, then we should find that individuals with damage to the sub-lexical system used in spelling should necessarily be impaired in spelling both pseudowords and real words, as all rely on the sublexical system. However, a number of cases have been reported in which individuals who write in a highly transparent language, although highly impaired in spelling pseudowords, are, nonetheless, highly accurate in their word spelling (e.g., Spanish: Iribarrren, Jarema, & Lecours, 2001; Italian: Miceli, Capasso, & Caramazza, 1994; Turkish: Raman & Weekes, 2005).

In summary, the complementary patterns of spelling accuracy (double dissociation) exhibited by RG and PR constitute strong evidence that words and pseudowords are spelled by lexical and sub-lexical processes whose neural substrates are sufficiently different that they can be selectively affected by neural damage. In addition to the accuracy differences in spelling words and pseudowords, various specific attributes of the errors of these individuals provide further support for this distinction. Interestingly, the lexical/sublexical distinction seems to be present across a range of languages, regardless of the opacity or transparency of their orthography.

The Relationship between Oral and Written Spelling: JGE (Rapp & Caramazza, 1997) and JP (Kinsbourne & Warington, 1965)

In the theory being reviewed, a distinction is drawn between, on the one hand, the abstract, format-independent graphemic representations manipulated by lexical and sub-lexical systems through the level of the graphemic buffer and, on the other hand, the modality-specific representations of letter shape and letter name that are involved in written and oral spelling, respectively. An alternative possibility might be that spellings are stored in the orthographic lexicon in one modality-specific format (letter shapes or letter names) and then translated to the other. However, the organization depicted in Figure 4.1 is motivated by the observation of selective deficits to either modality of spelling output.

JGE (Rapp & Caramazza, 1997) was a right-handed man with a master's degree who worked as a high school business teacher until his retirement. At age 73 he suffered a large left occipital and posterior temporal lobe infarct (confirmed by MRI). There was also evidence of prior (unde-tected) infarcts affecting the right occipital lobe extending to the calcarine fissure as well as the supra- and peri-ventricular white matter and left thalamus. JGE's spoken language comprehension and production were excellent, and he showed no signs of visual neglect. However, he had a right visual field cut, right hemiparesis, and significant difficulties in object recognition and reading as well as in written spelling.

Although JGE used his non-dominant left hand in writing, his writing was easily legible, and his ability to copy figures with his left hand appeared to be intact (Figure 4.3). Nonetheless, he made numerous errors in written spelling, errors that were largely absent from his oral spell-ing. JGE was administered the same set of 356 words for written and oral spelling. In terms of word-level errors (semantic errors, orthographically similar word errors, or phonologically plau-sible errors), JGE produced few errors in both written and oral spelling—three phonologically plausible errors in written spelling and four in oral spelling. This rate of PPEs was within the range of normal controls and allowed us to rule out any significant deficit affecting lexical processes.

In contrast, JGE's written and oral spelling were markedly different with regard to letter-level errors (letter substitutions, additions, deletions, and transpositions). In oral spelling he produced

Spelling to dictation:
"eye" and "arrow" (left hand)

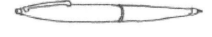

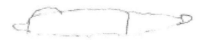

Copy (left hand)

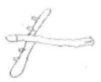

Drawing "airplane" (left hand)

Figure 4.3 Examples of JGE's drawing and writing with his non-dominant left hand.

only 17 letter errors, while in written spelling he produced 123 of these errors (Table 4.5). The highly significant difference between the two modalities reflects an impairment that arose primarily (or entirely) from a process specific to the written modality. The fact that written production was legible and that well-formed letters were always produced rules out a very peripheral locus involving motor execution. Instead, the results indicate a deficit affecting the translation of abstract graphemes to specific letter shapes at the level of the letter-shape selection process. This conclusion is consistent with the observation that in performing written spelling JGE would often produce an erroneous written response while simultaneously producing a correct oral spelling. For example, he would correctly say "t-a-b-l-e" (/ti, ei bi, ɛl, i/) while writing "F-A-P-L-E" (for other relevant cases see Anderson, Damasio, & Damasio, 1990; Baxter & Warrington, 1986; de Bastiani & Barry, 1989; Black, Behrmann, Bass, & Hacker, 1989; Friedman & Alexander, 1989; Goodman & Caramazza, 1986; Han & Bi, 2009; Kinsbourne & Rosenfield, 1974; Miozzo & de Bastiani, 2002; Patterson & Wing, 1989; Rapp & Caramazza, 1989; Rothi & Heilman, 1981; Zangwill, 1954).

Rapp and Caramazza (1997) examined JGE's written letter substitution errors to determine the nature of letter-shape representations at the level of the letter-shape selection process. Specifically, they examined whether substituted letters were similar to target letters in terms of visuospatial features or stroke features. For example, uppercase F and P were considered to be visually similar, as they have been found to be visually confusable (see Gilmore, Hersh, Caramazza, & Griffin, 1979 and van der Heijden, Malhas, & van den Roovaart, 1984), but they share only one stroke (a downward vertical). In contrast, T and L are not visually confusable, but their component strokes are highly similar (a downward vertical and a left-right horizontal). The analyses revealed that while 30 percent of JGE's written target/error pairs could be classified as being similar in terms of stroke features, only 10 percent could be classified as visually similar. Furthermore, the observed rate of visual similarity was well within the range generated by a random pairing of 1,000 target letters and errors, whereas the observed stroke similarity rate was never generated by this random process. The authors concluded that JGE's deficit originated primarily in the misselection of similar letter shapes within a system that represented letter shape in a stroke-based format.

A contrasting pattern of accuracy in oral and written spelling to that displayed by JGE was exhibited by JP (Kinsbourne & Warrington, 1965). JP was a car maintenance worker who suffered an infarct in the territory of the left middle cerebral artery. He exhibited no sensory loss or field defect. His spoken language comprehension was unimpaired, as was his single word reading; however, he had moderate difficulties in spoken language production and very specific difficulties in spelling. With regard to spelling, JP was 93 percent correct in the written spelling of three-, four-, and five-letter words that were dictated to him. However, he was only 7 percent correct in orally spelling the same set of words (also see Bub & Kertesz, 1982). Thus, JP exhibited a striking dissociation between impaired oral spelling and intact written spelling.

The combined patterns exhibited by JGE and JP create difficulties for hypotheses that propose that our knowledge of the spellings of words is represented in either a letter-name or letter-shape

Table 4.5 Frequency of JGE's Letter Errors in Written and Oral Spelling

	Written Spelling	*Oral Spelling*
Substitution	66	3
Transposition	5	3
Addition	7	3
Deletion	36	8
Other	9	0
Total	123/1899	17/1899

format. If orthographic knowledge is represented in a letter-name format, then JP's ability to write down spellings he cannot orally produce cannot be readily explained; if orthographic knowledge is represented in a letter-shape format, then JGE's ability to orally spell using letter names whose shapes have been incorrectly selected is left unaccounted for. However, both patterns are easily interpretable within the architecture depicted in Figure 4.1 that assumes that word spellings are stored in an abstract graphemic code and then given specific form by distinct (and independently lesionable) letter-shape and letter-name selection processes.

Further dissociations have been reported between different formats of letter shapes. For example, there have been a number of cases reported of individuals who have selective difficulties writing uppercase letters, without a corresponding impairment in either oral spelling or writing cursive letters (e.g., Del Grosso Desteri et al., 2000; Ingles et al., 2014; Menchielli, Rapp, & Semenza, 2008). These results suggest that the neural systems responsible for representing letter-shape information for different cases (upper vs. lower) and fonts is sufficiently distinct that certain letter-shape formats can be damaged while leaving other formats relatively unaffected.

Orthographic Working Memory Deficits: LB (Caramazza, Miceli, Villa, & Romani, 1987)

Orthographic working memory (OWM), or graphemic buffering, is assumed to be shared by lexical and sub-lexical processes, regardless of modality or format of output. The working memory process is assumed to be responsible for maintaining the activation levels of the abstract graphemic representations that have been addressed in the orthographic output lexicon or assembled by the sub-lexical phonology-to-orthography conversion system while the slower, serial processes involved in letter-shape or letter-name production are executed. Given its position within the spelling architecture, damage to OWM should result in highly similar deficits in oral and written spelling of both words and pseudowords. Furthermore, given that OWM is a limited-capacity working memory system, it is expected that longer words will place a greater burden on the orthographic working memory system than shorter words. Given this, a disruption to orthographic working memory should manifest itself in a higher error rate for longer versus shorter words. These predictions were borne out in the case of LB (Caramazza et al., 1987). LB was a 65-year-old, Italian-speaking, right-handed man who had university degrees in engineering and mathematics. He suffered a stroke that, according to CT scans, affected frontal and parietal areas in the left hemisphere. LB's language abilities were essentially normal except for reading and spelling.

Caramazza and colleagues (1987) reported LB's spelling abilities across a range of tasks with words and nonwords that were 4 to 12 letters in length (Table 4.6). First, a clear effect of length was observed for both word and nonword stimuli in both written and oral spelling. The length effect suggests a deficit at the level of a component (such as orthographic working memory) that is sensitive to word length. A length effect is not ubiquitous in dysgraphia; for example, it was not observed either in the case of RG (Beauvois & Derouesne, 1981), who had an orthographic output lexicon deficit, or in the case of JGE (Rapp & Caramazza, 1997), who suffered from damage at the level of letter-shape selection. Second, the fact that both the spelling of words and the spelling of nonwords were affected in both written and spoken output modalities suggests damage to a mechanism shared across these processes. Error rates, although not identical, were similar across word and nonword spelling and oral and written spelling. Furthermore, as indicated in Table 4.7, the distributions of error types for words and nonwords were virtually identical.

In order to account for the similarities in performance across these tasks and modalities Caramazza and colleagues (1987) proposed damage to OWM. An alternative hypothesis would require assuming fairly comparable levels of damage to both the lexical and sub-lexical systems. This hypothesis would be less parsimonious in terms of the number of damaged components it assumes.

Table 4.6 LB's Error Rate in Spelling Words and Nonwords

Length	Writing to Dictation (%)	Oral Spelling (%)	Written Naming (%)
Words			
4–5	15	25	25
6–7	34	69	42
8–9	67	81	67
10–12	90	100	91
Mean	52	69	57
Nonwords			
4–5	27	31	—
6–7	51	88	—
8–9	75	88	—
10–12	100	100	—
Mean	63	77	—

Table 4.7 LB's Distribution of Errors in Writing Words and Nonwords to Dictation

	Words (%)	Nonwords (%)
Substitutions	37	36
Insertions	8	9
Deletions	34	37
Transpositions	21	18

Furthermore, it would readily account for the length effect for words observed in LB's case but *not* in the case of individuals who exhibit the characteristics of a lexical deficit.

A number of case studies have been reported of individuals whose pattern of performance indicates an impairment to orthographic working memory (Buchwald & Rapp, 2009; Caramazza & Miceli, 1990; Cotelli, Aboutabeli, Zorzi, & Cappa, 2003; Costa et al., 2011; Jónsdottír, Shallice, & Wise, 1996; Katz, 1991; Kan, Biran, Thompson-Schill, & Chatterjee, 2006; Kay & Harley, 1994; McCloskey, Badecker, Goodman-Shulman, & Aliminosa, 1994; Miceli, Silveri, & Caramazza, 1985; Posteraro, Zinelli, & Mazzucchi, 1988; Rapp & Kane, 2002; Schiller, Greenhall, Shelton, & Caramazza, 2001; Tainturier & Rapp, 2004; Ward & Romani, 1998). While these individuals share a number of characteristics—similar patterns of performance across input and output modality for both words and nonwords, effects of word length but not of word frequency, and the absence of phonologically plausible spelling errors—there are also clear differences between some of the cases. Interestingly, individuals have been shown to differ in terms of the distribution of accuracy across letter positions, with two basic patterns having been reported. In the first pattern, errors predominate in central positions, thus yielding a bow-shaped error distribution (e.g., Buchwald & Rapp, 2009; Caramazza & Miceli, 1990; Jónsdottír, Shallice, & Wise, 1996; McCloskey et al., 1994; Tainturier & Rapp, 2004). The second pattern is characterized by errors increasing roughly monotonically from initial to final position in the written string (e.g., Katz, 1991; Schiller, et al., 2001; Miceli et al., 2004; Ward & Romani, 1998).

Costa et al. (2011) argued that these differences in error distribution suggest that the orthographic working memory system is composed of several subcomponents, each of which can be independently damaged. They specifically proposed a distinction between a set of processes that maintain the activation of the correct sequence of graphemes during the time it takes to spell the word and another set of processes that ensure that each grapheme in the sequence is represented with sufficient distinctiveness from the other graphemes held in OWM. Costa et al. argued that individuals, whose OWM impairment leaves them unable to maintain the activation of the sequence of graphemes over time, show monotonically increasing error rates, while individuals who have difficulties maintaining representational distinctiveness show bow-shaped error distributions. Research outside the area of spelling has provided considerable evidence that WM is instantiated in complex, multi-component systems, and the evidence from acquired dysgraphia supports these conclusions.

Integration of Lexical and Sub-Lexical Processes: LAT (Rapp, Epstein, & Tainturier, 2002), JJ (Hillis & Caramazza, 1991), and RCM (Hillis, Rapp, & Caramazza, 1999)

In an earlier section the empirical motivation for positing independently lesionable lexical and sub-lexical processes was discussed. However, the fact that the two processes are independent (in the sense that neither requires nor subsumes the other) does not preclude them from interacting. A number of patterns of dysgraphic performance indicate that lexical and sub-lexical systems integrate their outputs at the level of orthographic working memory (see Figure 4.1).

LAT (Rapp, Epstein, & Tainturier, 2002) was a 78-year-old, right-handed man who was diagnosed with probable Alzheimer's disease. LAT was a college graduate and retired engineer. MRI scans at the time of diagnosis showed diffuse cortical atrophy and prominent ventricles as well as increased signal intensity in the periventricular white matter. SPECT scans showed generalized cortical hypoperfusion, especially affecting both temporo-parietal regions.

LAT had no difficulty repeating each dictated stimulus before and after spelling it, and he produced written responses easily without struggling or hesitation. His ability to spell nonwords was excellent, with accuracy ranging from 90 to 98 percent correct. In contrast, he had greater difficulties in spelling words. Although he was able to provide excellent definitions for dictated words (Martyr: "a martyr is someone who will sacrifice himself for a particular concept"), his word spelling exhibited effects of word frequency and PG probability. As discussed earlier, these are characteristics of a deficit within the lexical system. Further confirmation of this was the fact that LAT's errors in word spelling were almost entirely phonologically plausible errors ("persuit" → PERSUTE; "pretty" → PRITY). Thus, LAT would correctly define a stimulus word and then produce a PPE in spelling it (e.g., Knowledge: "knowledge is the accumulation of important information K-N-O-L-E-G-E").

LAT's good nonword spelling ruled out a post-lexical deficit locus and his good word comprehension and definitions indicated intact processing through the lexical semantic system. On this basis, Rapp and colleagues concluded that LAT's deficit lay in accessing the correct spellings of words in the orthographic output lexicon.

If LAT's PPEs arose when he was unable to access the correct spelling in the orthographic output lexicon, his PPE's should reflect the functioning of the PG system. However, one thing that was striking about LAT's PPEs was that they sometimes included extremely unusual, low-probability PG mappings. For example, *bouquet* was spelled as BOUKET; *autumn* was spelled as AUTOMN. It is not surprising that the PG system would produce K for /k/ (in BOUKET) since this is the most common spelling for the phoneme /k/; however, it is somewhat surprising that the PG conversion system would yield ET as a spelling for /eI/ and MN for /m/. Although low-probability spellings such as /eI/ → ET should occur very occasionally (under the assumption that the frequency with which the PG system produces spellings corresponds to their occurrence in the English language), such low-probability spellings should not be produced often. Critically, the low-frequency mappings in LAT's PPEs were very often "lexically correct." That is, it is not just that ET is a low-probability spelling for /eɪ/, it is the spelling that is correct for the lexical target *bouquet* (but not for *delay*). Thus, Rapp and colleagues were interested in accounting for the observation that LAT's PPEs often included both highly frequent PG mappings, such as /k/ → K, as well as relatively unusual—yet lexically correct—spellings, such as /eɪ/ → ET.

One hypothesis was that the PPEs were generated entirely by the PG system but that LAT's PG system was unusual in that low-probability mappings were represented more strongly than would be expected based on their distribution in the language. Another hypothesis was that LAT's PPEs reflected integration of information from both lexical and sub-lexical systems—and that the unusual spellings originated from the lexical system. According to this hypothesis, word stimuli might activate lexical spellings sufficiently to contribute activation to their respective letters, although not sufficiently to yield a correct response. For example, under this hypothesis, in the spelling BOUKET, the PG system generated activation supporting K, the lexical system supported ET, and either or both systems might have contributed to the remaining letters.

One prediction is that if the low-probability spellings (/eɪ/ spelled as ET) actually originated in the PG systems then they should appear at comparable rates in both LAT's phonologically plausible errors to word stimuli and in his spelling of comparable nonwords. That is, according to this hypothesis a PPE in response to /boʊkeɪ/ and a plausible spelling of the nonword /loʊkeɪ/ (rhyming with *bouquet*) should be equally likely to include ET. In contrast, if the unusual spelling originated in the lexical system and reflected lexical/sub-lexical integration, then one might expect to find higher rates of low-probability, lexically correct spellings in the PPEs than in the spellings of matched pseudowords. Rapp and colleagues tested these hypotheses by administering a list of 97 word stimuli that each contained at least one low-probability PG mapping (e.g., /n/ → KN in *knowledge*) and a matched set of pseudowords that differed from each word by only one phoneme (e.g., /pɒlɪdʒ/, rhyming with knowledge, serves as its control).

The results clearly supported the hypothesis that the low-probability PG mappings originated in the lexical system and were produced as a result of lexical/sub-lexical integration. The findings were that low-probability, lexically correct PG mappings (e.g., /eɪ/→ ET) were used in 52 percent of cases in LAT's phonologically plausible errors produced in response to word stimuli, but in only 36 percent of cases in his responses to matched pseudowords. Thus, the evidence clearly supports the hypothesis of integration between lexical and sub-lexical systems.

Other patterns of dysgraphia also find explanation if lexical/sub-lexical integration is assumed. Hillis and Caramazza (1991) described the case of JJ, who made 30 to 40 percent errors in written and spoken naming to picture stimuli and comprehension of items from all semantic categories (except animals). His naming and comprehension errors were semantic errors. This pattern indicates a deficit at the level of the lexical semantic system. Interestingly, however, he produced no semantic errors in spelling to dictation.

Why should written picture naming and spelling to dictation yield such different results? If JJ relied only on the lexical system for spelling, given his semantic-level deficit, he should have produced semantic errors in both written naming and writing to dictation. Hillis and Caramazza accounted for the absence of semantic errors in JJ's spelling to dictation by assuming that JJ was able to combine the outputs of lexical and sub-lexical processes to eliminate semantic errors. For example, as a result of lexical semantic damage, the picture of a pear might generate an impoverished semantic representation (e.g., yellow, fruit) that would be consistent with, and thus lead to the activation of, multiple lexical candidates in the orthographic output lexicon (e.g., APPLE, PEAR, BANANA). In written picture naming one of these candidates would be selected for output, sometimes resulting in a semantic error—APPLE or BANANA. In writing to dictation, however, the phonological input from the stimulus (/pɛər/) would be processed by the sub-lexical system that would generate a plausible spelling such as P-A-I-R. Hillis and Caramazza argued that the sub-lexically generated output, although incorrect, would be sufficient to select among the multiple lexically generated candidates (APPLE, BANANA, PEAR) and yield the correct response (see also Hillis & Caramazza, 1995a).

Hillis and Caramazza did not describe a specific mechanism for the combination of lexical and sub-lexical information that would lead to such a result. However, lexical/sub-lexical integration at the level of the graphemic buffer in combination with feedback from letters to lexical representations would provide an account of JJ's pattern of performance (see McCloskey, Macaruso, & Rapp, 2006 for a discussion of feedback from OWM to the orthographic output lexicon). In JJ's case we must assume that in spelling to dictation the auditory stimulus /pɛər/ ("pear") results in the activation of the lexical candidate's PEAR, BANANA, and APPLE, and also that the sub-lexical system generates activation of candidate letters such as P-A-I-R. Feedback from these letters to the lexical level will increase the activation of orthographically related words such as PEAR relative to BANANA or APPLE, tipping the balance in favor of the correct response rather than a semantic error. This disambiguating input from the sub-lexical systems is not available in written picture naming where there is no auditory stimulus to drive the sub-lexical system.[1]

According to this account, the sub-lexical system plays a crucial role in eliminating semantic errors in writing to dictation. This makes very specific predictions regarding what would be expected if the sub-lexical system were unavailable or if it were unavailable and then were recovered. These predictions were tested in Hillis et al. (1999).

Hillis and colleagues described the case of RCM, an 82-year-old, right-handed woman who suffered a subacute infarct in the left frontal cortex. Spoken and written word comprehension were normal, and she exhibited only mild word-finding difficulties and somewhat reduced word fluency. Performance on oral picture naming and oral reading was excellent, with accuracy levels of 100 percent and 95 percent, respectively. Her spelling, in contrast, was considerably impaired and characterized by numerous semantic errors. On this basis her spelling deficit was localized to the orthographic output lexicon.

RCM was evaluated during two time periods. Study 1 took place in the first week after her stroke, study 2 took place two weeks later. At the time of study 1, 56 percent of RCM's errors in spelling were semantic errors (Table 4.8). Importantly, for the hypothesis under examination, her sub-lexical system was severely compromised such that no pseudowords were spelled correctly. Many of her errors in response to pseudowords bore no resemblance to the target ("besk" → TO) and others were phonologically or orthographically related words ("pon" → POWDER, "teef" → BEEF). Scoring of pseudoword spelling according to individual phonological segments (rather than the whole stimulus string) yielded 58 percent errors. Further evidence of a severely impaired sub-lexical system is the fact that no phonologically plausible errors were observed in her attempts to spell words.

Table 4.8 RCM's Error Rates and Distribution of Errors for Words and Pseudowords at Two Different Time Points for Spelling

	Study 1 (%)	*Study 2 (%)*
Error rate: words	49	37
Semantic	56	10
Ortho/phon similar	21	49
PPE	0	4
Other nonword	21	36
Other	3	1
Error rate (by segments): pseudowords	58	33

In contrast, at the time of study 2 RCM's rate of semantic errors dropped sharply to only 10 percent of her spelling errors. There were various indications that this drop was related to increased sub-lexical input. First, spelling of nonwords improved somewhat such that 3 percent of pseudowords were correctly spelled and the error rate on individual segments dropped from 58 percent in study 1 to 33 percent in study 2. Furthermore, RCM began to occasionally produce phonologically plausible responses to word stimuli. Finally, although the rate of semantic errors dropped, the rate of orthographically and phonologically similar errors (e.g., "myth" → METHOD) increased. This latter effect would be expected under an integration hypothesis. By way of the feedback connections between graphemes and the orthographic lexicon, the sub-lexically generated information would contribute to the activation of not only the target, but also of words that share the letters generated by the sub-lexical system. For example, the stimulus "myth" might yield sub-lexically generated activation of the letters M-I-T-H. Through letter-word feedback, words such as METHOD, MYTH, MATH should also receive activation. In this way, when there continues to be disruption at the level of the orthographic output lexicon, the correct response may still not be the most highly activated one, and orthographically similar words might be produced instead.

In sum, RCM's performance is consistent with very specific predictions of the hypothesis of lexical/sub-lexical integration and, in this way, provides further support for this aspect of the architecture depicted in Figure 4.1 (for other relevant papers see Beeson, 1998; Folk & Jones, 2004; Folk, Rapp, & Goldrick, 2002; Jones, Folk, & Rapp, 2009; Hillis & Caramazza, 1995b; Miceli, Capasso, & Caramazza, 1994).

Understanding the Internal Structure and Organization of Orthographic Representations

The performance of dysgraphic individuals can provide information not only regarding the basic organization of a cognitive system but also regarding detailed aspects of how our knowledge of word spellings is mentally represented. A number of studies have provided fundamental information regarding the question: *What do we know when we know the spelling of a word?* For example, what knowledge do we have and how is it organized for the spelling of a word such as FALLING? In this section we will highlight four aspects of orthographic representations revealed by the analysis of dysgraphic spelling errors: (1) morphemes, (2) consonants and vowels, (3) double letters, and (4) letter position.

The Representation of Orthographic Morphemes: Morpho-Orthography

While there have been hundreds of studies examining the representation of multi-morphemic words in spoken language processing and in reading, there have been only a handful that have considered whether, in spelling, the morphemes of a multi-morphemic word are independently represented (FALL + ING) or if, instead, the representation of the spelling consists simply of a linear string of letters (F + A + L + L + I + N + G).

Rapp and Fischer-Baum (2014) reviewed four cases that provided key information on this question. One of the cases was PW, who was an English-speaking, right-handed man who had been the manager of a meat department until he suffered a stroke that affected left parietal and posterior frontal areas (see Rapp et al., 1997 for more details). One of the striking aspects of PW's performance is that he produced morphological errors (affix deletions and substitutions) in written but not spoken production. PW was asked to produce both spoken and written sentences to describe the same pictures, and his accuracy in producing verb inflections in his spoken responses was 99 percent while in his written responses it was only 26 percent. In his written responses he produced errors such as THE MAN **SIT** ON THE BENCH while he accurately said "The man is **sitting** on the bench." Importantly, the researchers were able to show that these errors in written production did not result simply from difficulties in writing the ends of written words nor were they were whole-word substitutions of orthographic neighbors. A pattern such as this one, in which errors are concentrated on the morphological inflections in spelling but not in speaking, can be understood only if we assume that orthographic representations distinguish between the component morphemes of multi-morphemic words (see Figure 4.4). Given morpho-orthographically decomposed representations, one can imagine a deficit that disrupts access to or assembly of the morphological affixes in spelling, while the corresponding processes may be intact in speaking (for additional cases, see also Berndt & Haendiges, 2000).

A mental representation of a word's spelling such as the one depicted in Figure 4.4, in which both bound and free morphemes are distinguished, also predicts that there may be individuals with deficits specifically affecting the spelling of stems. Such an individual was reported by Badecker, Rapp, and Caramazza (1996). BH produced phonologically plausible errors on irregularly spelled stems but not on irregularly spelled affixes. For example, in spelling to dictation he spelled "surfed" as SOURPHED (not SOURPHT) and "cabooses" was spelled as CABUSES (not CABUSIZ). These cases, as well as additional evidence provided by Hillis and Caramazza (1989) and Badecker, Hillis, and Caramazza (1990), all reveal that our mental representations of the spellings of multi-morphemic words are not simply linear strings of concatenated graphemes but, instead, are internally structured according to the constituent morphemic units.

The Representation of Orthographic Consonants and Vowels

Evidence from acquired dysgraphia has also been used to argue that the brain distinguishes between *orthographic* consonants and vowels. Evidence for this claim comes from several sources. First, dysgraphic individuals have been reported with selective deficits affecting either consonants (e.g., Miceli et al., 2004) or vowels (e.g. Cubelli, 1991; Cotelli et al., 2003) in spelling. This double dissociation indicates substantial neural independence of these two types of representations, such that one category of letters can be damaged while the other stays relatively intact.

Additional evidence comes from analyzing the substitution errors of individuals with orthographic working memory deficits. For example, Caramazza and Miceli (1990) analyzed the

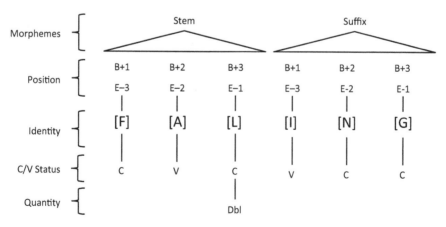

Figure 4.4 A schematic depiction of the internal structure of orthographic representations, including the representation of orthographic morphemes, consonant/vowel status, letter doubling, and letter position.

letter substitution errors produced by LB. LB's most frequent type of error was letter substitutions: on the list of 5,089 words administered to him, LB made 741 letter substitutions, with about half of the errors on consonants and half on vowels. What was striking was the fact that in 99.3 percent of the substitutions, vowels were substituted for vowels and consonants for consonants. Similar observations have been made with a number of individuals with OWM deficits (e.g., Buchwald & Rapp, 2006; Jónsdottír et al., 1996; Kay & Harley, 1994; McCloskey et al., 1994; Ward & Romani, 2000). Caramazza and Miceli (1990) proposed that this high consonant/vowel (C/V) matching rate in substitution errors is possible if we assume that letter identity information may be disrupted while information regarding C/V status may remain intact (see Figure 4.4). In other words, the orthographic representation of the word LIGHT could be disrupted such that the identity of some of the letters—including the G—may not be available. In that case, the C/V information may still be available, and if so, a response consistent with the available information may be produced, such as "light" spelled as LINHT. Buchwald and Rapp (2006) put this hypothesis to a test, demonstrating the matching of C/V status in substitution errors was specifically an orthographic and not a phonological effect.

The Representation of Double Letters

Another set of observations concerns the representation of double letters (or geminates). Caramazza and Miceli (1990) noted that LB would sometimes incorrectly produce double letters that did not belong in a word. These errors consisted of: geminate shifts ("sorella" [sister] → SOR-RELA), geminate duplications ("abisso" [abyss] → abbisso), and geminate substitutions ("marrone" [brown] → MAZZONE). These errors occurred almost exclusively in words containing a double letter. That is, it was not the case that LB would introduce double letters at random in his error responses, producing doubling errors on words without geminates. Responses such as "verita" (truth) → VETTIVA occurred on only 0.2 percent of LB's errors. It was this observation that led Caramazza and Miceli to propose that information regarding doubling is also independent from letter identity information (Figure 4.4). The double "feature" may be dissociated from its proper position and reassigned to another, leading to a geminate shift or even duplication. Furthermore, geminate substitutions can be accounted for by assuming that they occur on those occasions where information regarding identity is lost while doubling information is retained. The independent representation of doubling and identity information would also account for observations indicating that double letters behave as a unit. Examples include movement errors involving geminates, such as exchange errors ("cellula" [cell] → LECCULA) or shifts ("palazzao" [palace] → PAL-LAZO). In these errors both elements of the geminates always "traveled" together (never LECU-LULA or PALALZO). The fact that both elements of a geminate move together is hard to account for if double letters are assumed to be represented simply as a linear sequence of two consonants, comparable to the consonants within a consonant cluster The same basic patterns of results have been subsequently reported in cases in English (Jónsdóttir, Shallice, & Wise, 1996; McCloskey et al. 1994; Schiller et al., 2001; Tainturier & Caramazza, 1996) and other languages (German and Finnish: Blanken et al., 1999).

Fischer-Baum and Rapp (2014) presented evidence of a different sort for the independent representation of letter identity and doubling information. They reported the case of LSS who intruded letters into his spelling responses that did not appear in the correct spelling, but instead the intruded letters were repetitions of letters from previous responses. These errors are referred to as perseveration errors. Table 4.9 shows a sequence of LSS's target words and responses. On the error trial (referred to as E), "under" was misspelled as UNDEL, and the L is a letter intrusion. On the five trials prior to trial E (E-1 through E-5), the letter L appeared in the responses on trials E-1 (MOLDEL) and E-2 (SHOULD). Because the L-intrusion was preceded by prior responses

Table 4.9 Example of an Intrusion Error (Trial E: "under" spelled as UNDEL) produced by LSS, along with the five preceding trials (E-1, immediately preceding trial; E-5, five trials prior to the error)

Trial	Target	Response
E	UNDER	UNDEL
E-1	MOTEL	MOLDEL
E-2	SHOULD	SHOULD
E-3	VULGAR	CHEUPIVE
E-4	CHEAP	CHEAP
E-5	CERTAIN	ABSEVE

that contained an "L" it is likely that the L in UNDEL was a perseveration with a source in one of those two prior responses.

Critically, with respect to the issue of double-letter representation, Fischer-Baum and Rapp observed that in addition to intruding individual letters from previous responses, LSS made significant numbers of errors in which he intruded a double letter in the response. For example, he spelled "tragic" as TRRACE, an error in which the response contained a double letter but the target did not. Importantly these double-letter intrusions tended to occur immediately after LSS wrote words that were spelled with a double letter (e.g., EXCESS). Fischer-Baum and Rapp interpreted this pattern to mean that there is an independent double-letter feature, which occasionally perseverated from one response to the next, even though the identity of the doubled letter in the previous response did not perseverate. The error in which "tragic" was spelled as TRRACE can be explained by assuming that the double-letter feature associated with the SS in EXCESS perseverated into the subsequent response, even though the letter identity doubled in the word EXCESS (S) did not.

The Representation of Letter Position

The representation of letter position is obviously necessary to distinguish different words composed of the same letters (e.g., ACT vs. CAT). But how is letter position represented? The position of the E in the word NEST could be represented as the second letter from the beginning of the word, the letter between the N and the S, or the nucleus of the first orthographic syllable. In the first case, the position of the E is defined relative to a word-beginning reference point. In the second case, the position of the E is defined relative to the letters that precede and follow it. In the final case, the position of the E is defined by its syllabic position in the word. Each case is a viable alternative hypothesis (or *representational scheme*) for how letter position is represented in spelling.

Fischer-Baum, McCloskey, and Rapp (2010) addressed this issue through analysis of the spelling errors of two individuals who perseverated letters in spelling-to-dictation, LSS, discussed just above, and an additional individual with acquired dysgraphia, CM. When LSS and CM perseverated letters from one response to the next, the letters sometimes appeared in the same position in both the error and the prior response (referred to as the source response). For example, immediately after producing the response FRENCE, CM spelled "edge" as ERGE. Not only did the intruded R persist from the previous response, it was produced as the second letter from the beginning of the word in both the error and the source response, so it appeared in the same position according to a word-beginning-based scheme. However, according to other representational schemes, the R in ERGE and the R in FRENCE are not in the same position. By a letter-context scheme, the R in ERGE is between the E and the G, whereas the R in FRENCE is between the

F and the E. By a syllabic scheme, the R in ERGE is in a syllable coda position, while the R in FRENCE is in an onset position.

Fischer-Baum and colleagues assessed how often LSS and CM's intrusion errors appeared in the same position in the error and source response, with position defined by a range of different representational schemes. They found that for both of the individuals intrusion errors were significantly more likely to occur in the same position in the source and error when position was defined according to a **"beginning and end-based" representational scheme**. According to this scheme for representing letter position, every letter is represented in terms of its distance from *both* the beginning and end of the word (see Figure 4.4). In support of this conclusion, Fischer-Baum and colleagues (2010) found the following three types of statistically significant patterns. (1) Intruded letter/s in an error response had the same position as in the source response based on position of the letter/s counting from *either* the beginning or the end of the words. For example, "swim" was spelled as SWIP when preceded by DAMP. (2) Intruded letter/s in an error response had the same position as in the source response based on the position of the letter/s counting from the beginning of the word but not the end. For example, "edge" was spelled as ERGE when it was preceded by the response FRENCE. In this case the R was in the second position from the beginning in both source and error responses, but the R was not in the same position in source and error responses when counting from the end of the responses. (3) Intruded letter/s in an error response had the same position as in the source response based on the position of the letters counting from the end of the word but not the beginning. For example, "kitchen" was spelled as KITCHEM when it was preceded by the response SYSTEM, where the intruded M is one position from the end in both source and error responses. The observed values for these three types of perseverative letter intrusion errors that maintained beginning and/or end-based position was 78 percent and 87 percent for the two individuals. These values were significantly greater than expected by chance and were significantly greater than values obtained by any other single position representation scheme or combinations of schemes. This work provides strong support for a beginning and end-based representation of letter position in spelling (see McCloskey, Fischer-Baum, & Schubert, 2013 for evidence for similar conclusions in reading).

Summary: The Internal Structure of Orthographic Representations

The evidence that orthographic representations encode morphological structure and consonant/vowel distinctions, that doubling information is represented independently of identity information, and that letter position is represented by distance from the beginning and end of a word provide a rich characterization of what we know when we know the spelling of a word. However, these examples only begin to illustrate how much we have been able to learn about orthographic representations using data from individuals with acquired dysgraphia. Analysis of dysgraphic errors have provided insight into other aspects of orthographic representation, including such things as syllabic structure (Caramazza & Miceli, 1990; Fischer-Baum & Rapp, 2014) and the representation of digraphs, which are multi-letter units that correspond to a single sound (Fischer-Baum & Rapp, 2014; Tainturier & Rapp, 2004). These studies illustrate that careful investigations of the spelling errors produced by dysgraphic individuals have provided key insights into not only the cognitive architecture of the spelling system, but also the structure of our orthographic representations.

Conclusions

As indicated earlier, spelling is the cognitive domain in which the study of deficits has most prominently contributed to our understanding of the organization and functioning of the component mental processes. In this chapter we hope to have shown how case study research with dysgraphic individuals has been used to test specific hypotheses regarding both the organization of the system and the content of the representations that are manipulated and generated in the course of spelling. This work has revealed a highly structured cognitive system that manipulates knowledge representations with a rich internal structure.

The following chapters in this volume, by Rapcsak and Beeson and Beeson and Rapcsak, make use of this theory of the spelling process as a framework within which to discuss the neural bases of the various cognitive functions that have been posited and the manner in which deficits of spelling can be diagnosed and remediated.

Acknowledgment

Support for writing this chapter for the 2nd edition of the *Handbook* was made possible by the support of NIH grant P50-DC012283.

Note

1 That is, unless the individual him- or herself can generate a phonological representation of the picture stimulus that may serve as input to the sub-lexical process. In JJ's case this was not possible since spoken naming was equally affected by the deficit at the level of the lexical semantic system.

References

Allport, D. A., & Funnel, E. (1981). Components of the mental lexicon. *Philosophical Transactions of the Royal Society of London B, 295*, 397–410.

Anderson, S.W., Damasio, A.R., & Damasio, H. (1990). Troubled letters but not numbers: Domain specific cognitive impairments following focal damage in frontal cortex. *Brain, 113*, 749–766.

Ardila, A. (1991). Errors resembling semantic paralexias in Spanish-speaking aphasics. *Brain and Language, 41*, 437–445.

Badecker, W., Hillis, A., & Caramazza, A. (1990) Lexical morphology and its role in the writing process: Evidence from a case of acquired dysgraphia. *Cognition, 35*, 205–243.

Badecker, W., Rapp, B., & Caramazza, A. (1996). Lexical morphology and the two orthographic routes. *Cognitive Neuropsychology, 13*, 161–175.

Basso, A., Taborelli, A., & Vignolo, L.A. (1978). Dissociated disorders of speaking and writing in aphasia. *Journal of Neurology, Neurosurgery, and Psychiatry, 41*, 556–563.

Baxter, D.M., & Warrington, E.K. (1986). Ideational agraphia: A single case study. *Journal of Neurology, Neurosurgery, and Psychiatry, 49*, 369–374.

Baxter D.M., & Warrington, E.K. (1987). Transcoding sound to spelling: Single or multiple sound unit correspondences? *Cortex, 23*, 11–28.

Beauvois, M.F., & Derouesne, J. (1981). Lexical or orthographic agraphia. *Brain, 104*, 21–49.

Beeson, P.M. (1998). Problem-solving in acquired agraphia: How do you spell relief? Paper presented at the Meeting of the Academy of Aphasia. Santa Fe, NM.

Behrmann, M., & Bub, D. (1992). Surface dyslexia and dysgraphia: Dual routes, single lexicon. *Cognitive Neuropsychology, 9*, 209–251.

Berndt, R.S., & Haendiges, A.N. (2000). Grammatical class in word and sentence production: Evidence from an aphasic patient. *Journal of Memory and Language, 43*, 249–273.

Black, S. E., Behrmann, M., Bass, K., & Hacker, P. (1989). Selective writing impairment: Beyond the allographic code. *Aphasiology, 3*(3), 265–277.

Blanken, G., Schäfer, C., Tucha, O., & Lange, K.W. (1999). Serial processing in graphemic encoding: Evidence from letter exchange errors in a multilingual patient. *Journal of Neurolinguistics, 12*, 13–39.

Brown, G.D., & Loosemore, R.P. (1994). Computational approaches to normal and impaired spelling. In G.D.A. Brown & N.C. Ellis (Eds.), *Handbook of spelling: Theory, process, and intervention.* New York: Wiley.

Brown, J.W. (1972). *Aphasia, apraxia, and agnosia.* Springfield, IL: Charles C Thomas.

Bub, D., & Kertesz, A. (1982). Evidence for lexicographic processing in a patient with preserved written over oral single word naming. *Brain, 105*, 697–717.

Buchwald, A., & Rapp, B. (2006). Consonants and vowels in orthography. *Cognitive Neuropsychology, 23,* 308–337.

Buchwald, A., & Rapp, B. (2009). Distinctions between orthographic long-term memory and working memory. *Cognitive Neuropsychology, 26,* 724–751.

Caramazza, A., & Hillis, A. (1990). Where do semantic errors come from? *Cortex, 26,* 95–122.

Caramazza, A., & Miceli, G. (1990). The structure of graphemic representations. *Cognition, 37,* 243–297.

Caramazza, A., Miceli, G., Villa, G., & Romani, C. (1987). The role of the graphemic buffer in spelling: Evidence from a case of acquired dysgraphia. *Cognition, 26,* 59–85.

Coltheart, M., & Funnel, E. (1987). Reading and writing: One lexicon or two? In D.A. Allport, D. McKay, W. Prinz, & E. Scheerer (Eds.), *Language perception and production: Common processes in listening, speaking, reading, and writing.* London: Academic Press.

Costa, V., Fischer-Baum, S., Capasso, R., Miceli, G., & Rapp, B. (2011). Temporal stability and representational distinctiveness: Key functions of orthographic working memory. *Cognitive Neuropsychology, 28,* 338–362.

Cotelli, M., Abutalebi, J., Zorzi, M. & Cappa, S.F. (2003). Vowels in the buffer: A case study of acquired dysgraphia with selective vowel substitutions. *Cognitive Neuropsychology, 20,* 99–114.

Cubelli, R. (1991). A selective deficit for writing vowels in acquired dysgraphia. *Nature, 353,* 258–260.

Cuetos, F., & Labos, E. (2001). The autonomy of the orthographic pathway in a shallow language: Data from an aphasic patient. *Aphasiology, 15,* 333–342.

De Bastiani, P., & Barry, C. (1989). A cognitive analysis of an acquired dysgraphic patient with an "allographic" writing disorder. *Cognitive Neuropsychology, 6*(1), 25–41.

Del Grosso Destreri, N., Farina, E., Alberoni, M., Pomati, S., Nichelli, P., & Mariani, C. (2000). Selective uppercase dysgraphia with loss of visual imagery of letter forms: A window on the organization of graphomotor patterns. *Brain and Language, 71,* 353–372.

De Partz, M.P., Seron, X., & Van der Linden, M. (1992). Re-education of a surface dysgraphic with a visual imagery strategy. *Cognitive Neuropsychology, 9,* 369–401.

Fischer-Baum, S., McCloskey, M. & Rapp, B. (2010). Representation of letter position in spelling: Evidence from acquired dysgraphia. *Cognition, 115,* 466–490.

Fischer-Baum, S., & Rapp, B. (2014). The analysis of perseverations in acquired dysgraphia reveals the internal structure of orthographic representations. *Cognitive Neuropsychology, 31,* 237–265.

Folk, J.R., & Jones, A.C. (2004). The purpose of lexical/sublexical interaction during spelling: Further evidence from dysgraphia and articulatory suppression. *Neurocase, 10,* 65–69.

Folk, J.R., Rapp, B., & Goldrick, M. (2002). The interaction of lexical and sublexical information in spelling: What's the point? *Cognitive Neuropsychology, 19,* 653–671.

Friedman, R. B., & Alexander, M. (1989). Written spelling agraphia. *Brain and Language, 36,* 503–517.

Frith, U. (1979). Reading by eye and writing by ear. In P.A. Kolers, M. Wrolstad, & H. Bouma (Eds.), *Processing of visible language, I.* New York: Plenum Press.

Geschwind, N. (1969). Problems in the anatomical understanding of aphasia. In A.L. Benton (Ed.), *Contributions of clinical neuropsychology.* Chicago: University of Chicago Press.

Gilmore, G.C., Hersh, H., Caramazza, A., & Griffin, J. (1979). Multidimensional letter similarity derived from recognition errors. *Perception & Psychophysics,* 25(5), 425–431

Glushko, R.J. (1979). The organization and activation of orthographic knowledge in reading aloud. *Journal of Experimental Psychology: Human Perception and Performance, 5,* 674–691.

Goodman, R. A., & Caramazza, A. (1986). Aspects of the spelling process: Evidence from a case of acquired dysgraphia. *Language and Cognitive Processes, 1,* 263–296.

Goodman-Shulman, R. A., & Caramazza, A. (1987). Patterns of dysgraphia and the nonlexical spelling process. *Cortex, 23,* 143–148.

Grashey, H. (1885). On aphasia and its relations to perception (Über Aphasie und ihre Beziehungen zur Wahrnehmung). *Archiv für Psychiatire und Nervenkrankheiten, 16,* 654–688. (English version: *Cognitive Neuropsychology, 6*(1989), 515–546.)

Han, Z., & Bi, Y. (2009). Oral spelling and writing in a logographic language: Insights from a Chinese dysgraphic individual. *Brain and Language, 110,* 23–28.

Hanley, J.R., & McDonnell, V. (1997). Are reading and spelling phonologically mediated? Evidence from a patient with a speech production impairment. *Cognitive Neuropsychology, 14,* 3–33.

Hanna, P.R., Hanna, R.E., Hodges, J.S., & Rudorf Jr., E.H. (1966). *Phoneme-grapheme correspondences as cues to spelling improvement.* Washington, DC: Government Printing Office, U.S. Office of Education.

Harm, M.W., & Seidenberg, M.S. (2004). Computing the meanings of words in reading: cooperative division of labor between visual and phonological processes. *Psychological Review, 111,* 662–720.

Hatfield, F.M., & Patterson, K. E. (1983). Phonological spelling. *Quarterly Journal of Experimental Psychology, 35A*, 451–458.

Head, H. (1926). *Aphasia and kindred disorders of speech*. London: Cambridge University Press.

Hecaen, H., & Angelergues, R. (1965). *Pathologie du language, vol. 1*. Paris: Larousse.

Henry, M.L., Beeson, P.M., Stark, A.J., & Rapcsak, S.Z. (2007). The role of left perisylvian cortical regions in spelling. *Brain and Language, 100*, 44–52.

Hier, D.B., & Mohr, J.P. (1977). Incongruous oral and written naming. *Brain and Language, 4*, 115–126.

Hillis, A.E., & Caramazza, A. (1989). The graphemic buffer and attentional mechanisms. *Brain and Language, 36*, 208–235.

Hillis, A. E., & Caramazza, A. (1991). Mechanisms for accessing lexical representations for output: Evidence from a category-specific semantic deficit. *Brain and Language, 40*, 106–144.

Hillis, A. E., & Caramazza, A. (1995a). Converging evidence for the interaction of semantic and sublexical phonological information in accessing lexical representations for spoken output. *Cognitive Neuropsychology, 12*(2), 187–227.

Hillis, A. E., & Caramazza, A. (1995b). "I know it but I can't write it": Selective deficits in long- and short-term memory. In R. Campbell (Ed.), *Broken memories: Neuropsychological case studies*. London: Blackwell.

Hillis, A.E., & Rapp, B. (2004). Cognitive and neural substrates of written language comprehension and production. In, M. Gazzaniga (Ed.), *The new cognitive neurosciences* (3rd ed.). New York: W.W. Norton & Company.

Hillis, A.E., Rapp, B., & Caramazza, A. (1999). When a rose is a rose in speech but a tulip in writing. *Cortex, 35*, 337–356.

Hotopf, N. (1980). Slips of the pen. In U. Frith (Ed.), *Cognitive processes in spelling*. London: Academic Press.

Ingles, J.L., Fisk, J.D., Fleetwood, I., Burrell, S., & Darvesh, S. (2014). Peripheral dysgraphia: dissociations of lowercase from uppercase letters and of print from cursive writing. *Cognitive and Behavioral Neurology, 27*, 31–47.

Iribarren, L. C, Jarema, G., & Lecours, A.R. (2001). Two different dysgraphic syndromes in a regular orthography, Spanish. *Brain and Language, 77*, 166–175.

Jones, A.C., Folk, J.R., & Rapp, B. (2009). All letters are not equal: Subgraphemic texture in orthographic working memory. *Journal of Experimental Psychology: Learning, Memory, and Cognition, 35*, 1389.

Jónsdottír, M.K., Shallice, T., & Wise, R. (1996). Phonological mediation and the graphemic buffer disorder in spelling: Cross language differences? *Cognition, 59*, 169–197.

Kan, I.P., Biran I., Thompson-Schill S., & Chatterjee, A. (2006). Letter selection and letter assembly in acquired dysgraphia. *Cognitive and Behavioral Neurology, 19*, 225–236.

Katz, R.B. (1991). Limited retention of information in the graphemic buffer. *Cortex, 27*, 111–119.

Kay, J., & Harley, R. (1994). Peripheral spelling disorders: The role of the graphemic buffer. In G.D.A. Brown & N.C. Ellis (Eds.), *Handbook of spelling: Theory, process, and intervention*. New York: Wiley.

Kemmerer, D., Tranel, D., & Manzel, K. (2005). An exaggerated effect for proper nouns in a case of superior written over spoken word production. *Cognitive Neuropsychology, 22*, 3–27.

Kinsbourne, M., & Rosenfield, D.B. (1974). Agraphia selective for written spelling. *Brain and Language, 1*, 215–225.

Kinsbourne, M., & Warrington, E.K. (1965). A case showing selectively impaired oral spelling. *Journal of Neurology, Neurosurgery, and Psychiatry, 28*, 563–567.

Law, S.P., Wong, W., & Kong, A. (2006). Direct access from meaning to orthography in Chinese: A case study of superior written to oral naming. *Aphasiology, 20*, 565–578.

Levine, D.N., Calvanio, R., & Popovics, A. (1982). Language in the absence of inner speech. *Neuropsychologia, 4*, 391–409.

Lichtheim, L. (1885). On aphasia (Über Aphasie). *Deutsches Archiv für klinische Medizin, 36*, 204–268. (English version: *Brain, 7*, 433–485.)

Luria, A.R. (1966). *Higher cortical functions in man*. New York: Basic Books.

Luzzi, S., Bartolini, M., Coccia, M., Provinciali, L., Piccirilli, M., & Snowden, J.S. (2003). Surface dysgraphia in a regular orthography: Apostrophe use by an Italian writer. *Neurocase, 9*, 285–296.

Marcel, A.J. (1980). Surface dyslexia and beginning reading: A revised hypothesis of the pronunciation of print and its impairments. In M. Coltheart, K. E. Patterson, & J.C. Marshall (Eds.), *Deep dyslexia*. London: Routledge and Kegan Paul.

McCloskey, M., Badecker, W., Goodman-Shulman, R. A., & Aliminosa, D. (1994). The structure of graphemic representations in spelling: Evidence from a case of acquired dysgraphia. *Cognitive Neuropsychology, 2*, 341–392.

McCloskey, M., Fischer-Baum, S., & Schubert, T. (2013). Representation of letter position in single-word reading: Evidence from acquired dyslexia. *Cognitive Neuropsychology, 30*, 396–428.

McCloskey, M., Macaruso, P., & Rapp, B. (2006). Grapheme-to-lexeme feedback in the spelling system: Evidence from a dysgraphic patient. *Cognitive Neuropsychology, 23*, 278–307.

Menichelli, A., Rapp, B., & Semenza, C. (2008). Allographic agraphia: A case study. *Cortex, 44*(7), 861–868.

Miceli, G., Capasso, R., Benvegnù, B., & Caramazza, A. (2004). The categorical distinction of vowel and consonant representations: Evidence from dysgraphia. *Neurocase, 10*, 109–121.

Miceli, G., Benvegnù, B., Capasso, R., & Caramazza, A. (1997). The independence of phonological and orthographic lexical forms: Evidence from aphasia. *Cognitive Neuropsychology, 14*, 35–69.

Miceli, G., Capasso, R., & Caramazza, A. (1994). The interaction of lexical and sublexical processes in reading, writing, and repetition. *Neuropsychologia, 32*, 317–333

Miceli, G., Silveri, C., & Caramazza, A. (1985). Cognitive analysis of a case of pure dysgraphia. *Brain and Language, 25*, 187–221.

Miozzo, M., & De Bastiani, P. (2002). The organization of letter-form representations in written spelling: Evidence from acquired dysgraphia. *Brain and Language, 80*, 366–392.

Nickels, L. (1992). The autocue? Self-generated phonemic cues in the treatment of a disorder of reading and naming. *Cognitive Neuropsychology, 9*, 155–182.

Parkin, A.J. (1993). Progressive aphasia without dementia: A clinical and cognitive neuropsychological analysis. *Brain and Language, 44*, 201–220.

Patterson, K. (1986). Lexical but nonsemantic spelling? *Cognitive Neuropsychology, 3*, 341–367.

Patterson, K., & Wing, A.M. (1989). Processes in handwriting: A case for case. *Cognitive Neuropsychology, 6*(1), 1–23.

Piras, F., & Marangolo, P. (2004). Independent access to phonological and orthographic lexical representations: A replication study. *Neurocase, 10*, 300–307.

Plaut, D.C., McClelland, J.L., Seidenberg, M.S., & Patterson, K. (1996). Understanding normal and impaired word reading: Computational principles in quasi-regular domains. *Psychological Review, 103*, 56–115.

Posteraro, L., Zinelli, P., & Mazzucchi, A. (1988). Selective impairment of the graphemic buffer in acquired dysgraphia: A case study. *Brain and Language, 35*, 274–286.

Raman, I., & Weekes, B.S. (2005). Deep dysgraphia in Turkish. *Behavioural Neurology, 16*, 59–69.

Rapcsak, S.Z., & Beeson, P.M. (2004). The role of left posterior inferior temporal cortex in spelling. *Neurology, 62*, 2221–2229

Rapp, B., Benzing, L., & Caramazza, A. (1997). The autonomy of lexical orthography. *Cognitive Neuropsychology, 14*, 71–104

Rapp, B., & Caramazza, A. (1989). Letter processing in reading and spelling: Some dissociations. *Reading and Writing, 1*, 3–23.

Rapp, B., & Caramazza, A. (1997). From graphemes to abstract letter shapes: Levels of representation in written spelling. *Journal of Experimental Psychology: Human Perception and Performance, 23*, 1130–1152.

Rapp, B., Epstein, C., & Tainturier, M.J. (2002). The integration of information across lexical and sublexical processes in spelling. *Cognitive Neuropsychology, 19*, 1–29.

Rapp, B., & Fischer-Baum, S. (2014). Representation of orthographic knowledge. In M. Goldrick, V. Ferreira, & M. Miozzo (Eds.), *The Oxford handbook of language production*. New York: Oxford University Press.

Rapp, B., & Kane, A. (2002). Remediation of deficits affecting different components of the spelling process. *Aphasiology, 16*, 439–454.

Roeltgen, D.P., (1985). Agraphia. In K.M. Heilman & E. Valenstein (Eds.), *Clinical neuropsychology* (2nd ed.). New York: Oxford University Press.

Roeltgen, D.P., Rothi, L.G., & Heilman, K.M. (1986). Linguistic semantic agraphia: A dissociation of the lexical spelling system from semantics. *Brain and Language, 27*, 257–280.

Roeltgen, D.P., Sevush, S., & Heilman, K.M. (1983). Phonological agraphia: Writing by the lexical-semantic route. *Neurology, 33*, 755–765.

Rothi, L.J., & Heilman, K.M. (1981). Alexia and agraphia with spared spelling and letter recognition abilities. *Brain and Language, 12*, 1–13.

Sanders, R.J., & Caramazza, A. (1990). Operation of the phoneme-to-grapheme conversion mechanism in a brain injured patient. *Reading and Writing, 2*, 61–82.

Schiller, N.O., Greenhall, J.A., Shelton, J.R., & Caramazza, A. (2001). Serial order effects in spelling errors: Evidence from two dysgraphic patients. *Neurocase, 7*, 1–14.

Seidenberg, M., & McClelland, J.L. (1989). A distributed developmental model of word recognition and naming. *Psychological Review, 96*, 523–568.

Shallice, T. (1981). Phonological agraphia and the lexical route in writing. *Brain, 104*, 413–429.

Tainturier, M.J., & Caramazza, A. (1996). The status of double letters in graphemic representations. *Journal of Memory and Language, 35*, 53–73.

Tainturier, M.J., Moreaud, O., David, D., Leek, E.C., & Pellat, J. (2001). Superior written over spoken picture naming in a case of frontotemporal dementia. *Neurocase, 7*, 89–96.

Tainturier, M.J., & Rapp, B. (2004). Complex graphemes as functional spelling units: Evidence from acquired dysgraphia. *Neurocase, 10*, 122–131.

Van der Heijden, A. H. C., Malhas, M.S.S., & van den Roovaart, B.P. (1984). An empirical interletter confusion matrix for continuous-line capitals. *Perception and Psychophysics, 35*, 85–88.

Van Orden, G.C., Johnston, J.C., & Hale, B.L. (1988). Word identification in reading proceeds from spelling to sound to meaning. *Journal of Experimental Psychology: Learning, Memory, and Cognition, 14*, 371–386.

Ward, J., & Romani, C. (1998). Serial position effects and lexical activation in spelling: Evidence from a single case study. *Neurocase, 4*, 189–206.

Ward, J., & Romani, C. (2000). Consonant-vowel encoding and ortho-syllables in a case of acquired dysgraphia. *Cognitive Neuropsychology, 17*, 641–663.

Weekes, B., & Coltheart, M. (1996). Surface dyslexia and surface dysgraphia: Treatment studies and their theoretical implications. *Cognitive Neuropsychology, 13*, 277–315.

Weekes, B.S., Davies, R.A., Parris, B.A., & Robinson, G.A. (2003). Age of acquisition effects on spelling in surface dysgraphia. *Aphasiology, 17*, 563–584.

Wernicke, C. (1886). Neurology: Recent contributions on aphasia (Nervenheilkunde: Die neueren Arbeiten über Aphasie). *Fortschritte der Medizin, 4*, 463–482. (English version: *Cognitive Neuropsychology, 6*(6 [1989]), 547–569.)

Zangwill, O.L. (1954). Agraphia due to a left parietal glioma in a left-handed man. *Brain, 77*, 510–520.

5

NEUROANATOMICAL CORRELATES OF SPELLING AND WRITING

Steven Z. Rapcsak and Pélagie M. Beeson

It is evident that writing can be disordered by circumscribed lesions of widely different areas of the cerebral cortex, but in every case the disorder in writing will show qualitative peculiarities depending on which link is destroyed and which primary defects are responsible for the disorder of the whole functional system.
—A.R. Luria (1980)

Introduction

In setting out to explore the neural substrates of spelling and writing, a useful theoretical point of departure is to consider the development of written language from an evolutionary perspective. In this context, it is important to note that writing systems are relatively recent cultural inventions that first appeared approximately 6,000 years ago (Gelb, 1963). By contrast, the evolutionary origins of spoken language can be traced back to a much more remote era, perhaps as long as 150,000 to 200,000 years ago. The comparatively late arrival of written language on the phylogenetic time scale is mirrored by the late emergence of literacy skills in the course of ontogenetic development. Unlike mastery of spoken language that seems to develop naturally given adequate exposure, proficiency in reading and writing is only acquired as the result of explicit and prolonged instruction in school-aged children who already possess considerable speech production/comprehension, visuoperceptual, and manual motor skills. Collectively, these observations suggest that the culturally transmitted skills of reading and writing cannot be mediated by genetically specified neural circuitry and instead must utilize phylogenetically and ontogenetically older brain systems evolved for spoken language, visual form discrimination, and tool use. At the neural level, the development of written language constitutes an example of "cultural recycling" that involves remodeling evolutionarily older brain circuits to support the acquisition of new cognitive abilities (Dehaene & Cohen, 2007). These neurobiological principles have been incorporated into the "primary systems" hypothesis of written language processing, which asserts that there are no specialized brain regions dedicated to reading or writing that do not also participate in other language or cognitive functions (Henry, Beeson, Alexander, & Rapcsak, 2012; Lambon Ralph & Patterson, 2005; Patterson & Lambon Ralph, 1999). Critically, this hypothesis predicts that acquired disorders of spelling and writing (agraphia) should result from damage to a limited set of primary brain systems and that deficits in written language production will always be accompanied by evidence of impaired speech production/comprehension (aphasia), reading dysfunction (alexia), or defective motor control involving the programming and execution of skilled hand movements (apraxia). Support for the primary systems view would also be provided by functional imaging studies in normal individuals demonstrating that spelling and writing activate the same cortical regions that are engaged during tasks involving spoken language processing, reading/visual object recognition, and tool use.

In this chapter we provide an overview of what is currently known about the neuroanatomical localization of the cortical networks that support written language production. To accomplish our objective, we draw on complementary sources of scientific evidence derived from functional neuroimaging investigations of spelling and writing in normal individuals and lesion-deficit correlation studies in patients with various forms of agraphia produced by focal or degenerative brain disease. Prior to considering the neural systems involved, however, we present a cognitive model of spelling and writing that serves as the theoretical framework for our discussion.

Cognitive Systems Involved in Writing

From a neuropsychological perspective, the writing process can be subdivided into central and peripheral components (Ellis, 1988). Central components are linguistic in nature and are responsible for selecting the appropriate words for written output and for providing information about their correct spelling. Central components can also be used to generate plausible spellings for unfamiliar words or pronounceable nonwords (e.g., *dake*). According to the cognitive model of written language depicted in Figure 5.1, spelling depends on dynamic interactions between three central processing domains: phonology, orthography, and semantics. Specifically, the model postulates two major sources of input to orthography during spelling: semantic and phonological. Functionally linked central processing components involved in activating or computing orthographic representations in response to these two types of codes are referred to as the lexical-semantic and sublexical spelling routes. The lexical-semantic route relies on interactions between word-specific phonological, semantic, and orthographic memory representations. In particular, it is assumed that information about the spoken and written forms of familiar words is represented in distinct but interconnected phonological and orthographic lexicons that interface with conceptual knowledge of word meanings stored in semantic memory. The integrity of the lexical-semantic route is essential for conceptually mediated writing tasks, such as written composition and written naming, but it is also the dominant pathway normally used for spelling familiar words to dictation. The lexical-semantic route can successfully process both regular words that have predictable spelling-sound relationships (e.g., *stand*) and irregular words that contain atypical or inconsistent letter-sound or grapheme-phoneme mappings (e.g., *choir*). However, it cannot produce correct spellings for unfamiliar words or nonwords because these novel items do not have preexisting representations in lexical-semantic memory. Attempts to spell nonwords by a lexical-semantic strategy result in real word responses referred to as "lexicalization" errors (e.g., *dake* spelled as *cake*). In contrast to the whole-word retrieval strategy employed by the lexical-semantic route, the sublexical spelling route relies on the serial conversion of individual phonemes to the corresponding graphemes. The sublexical route is essential for accurate spelling of unfamiliar words or nonwords, but it can also be used to spell regular words that conform to spelling-sound conversion rules. However, attempts to spell irregular words by the sublexical procedure give rise to phonologically plausible "regularization" errors (e.g., *choir* spelled as *quire* or *kwire*). Thus, according to dual-route theory, only the lexical-semantic route can succeed in spelling irregular words, whereas only the sublexical route can render a correct response to novel nonwords. From the clinical perspective, this means that irregular word and nonword spelling scores can serve as relatively pure measures of the functional integrity of the lexical-semantic and sublexical spelling pathways in patients with acquired agraphia. On the other hand, because regular words can be spelled correctly by either pathway, performance on these items is less informative regarding the level of breakdown within the spelling process. The hypothesis that both pathways can contribute to regular word spelling receives empirical support from demonstrations that performance for these stimuli can be accurately predicted from irregular word and nonword spelling scores in individuals with agraphia (Rapcsak, Henry, Teague, Carnahan, & Beeson, 2007). In this context, it is important to emphasize that although dual-route models postulate separate lexical-semantic and sublexical pathways, this functional division need not imply that the two spelling procedures are completely independent. Instead, it is assumed that both pathways are obligatorily engaged during spelling in a parallel fashion for all types of stimuli, with cooperative and competitive interactions taking place at the orthographic output stage. Thus, the orthographic representations computed during spelling are always partly *addressed* (i.e., retrieved from lexical-semantic memory) and partly *assembled* by sublexical phoneme-grapheme conversion mechanisms. The degree of reliance or division of labor between the two spelling pathways is modulated in a context-dependent manner by task demands (e.g., spelling to dictation vs. written composition) and by stimulus type (e.g., spelling irregular word vs. nonwords).

As shown in Figure 5.1, orthographic representations generated by central spelling routes interact with the graphemic buffer—a working memory system that keeps orthographic information in an active state while graphemes are serially selected for motor output and converted into the appropriate letter shapes by the peripheral components of the writing process. Orthographic information maintained by the graphemic buffer can also be converted into letter names for oral spelling or into a sequence of keystrokes during typing, but these other peripheral output modalities will not be discussed here in detail.

Before considering the neural implementation of the cognitive processes involved in spelling and writing, we wish to point out that the functional architecture of the model shown in Figure 5.1 is consistent with the basic tenets of the primary systems hypothesis of written language

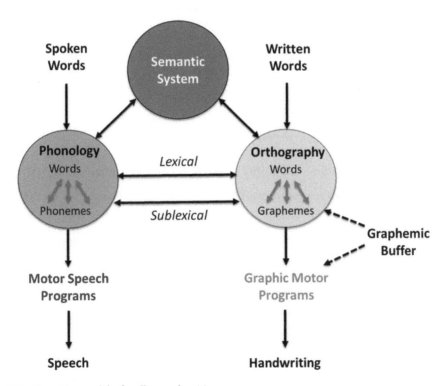

Figure 5.1 Cognitive model of spelling and writing.

processing. In particular, although spelling depends on reciprocal interactions between phonology, semantics, and orthography, these central processing domains are not specific to written language production. Phonological and semantic representations play a critical role in speech production and comprehension, and semantic representations are also involved in a variety of nonverbal conceptual tasks (e.g., recognizing objects and demonstrating their use, identifying familiar people or environmental sounds). Access to phonological and semantic representations from orthography is also required for comprehending written words and for accurate oral reading. Furthermore, orthographic processing itself is considered to emerge as the result of functional specialization within the visual system that had originally evolved for the purposes of object recognition, and it is assumed that the same orthographic lexical representations support both reading and spelling. The principle of shared neural substrates can also be extended to the working memory systems that support written spelling and to the peripheral components of the model involved in the production of handwriting movements. For instance, it has been proposed that active maintenance of orthographic information by the putative graphemic buffer is required during both reading and spelling (Caramazza, Capasso, & Miceli, 1996; Tainturier & Rapp, 2003) and, as we shall see, this functional component may play an even more general role in visuospatial attention and working memory. Similarly, the motor control of handwriting develops as a result of experience-dependent functional reorganization within cortical networks originally evolved for manipulating tools and later adapted for the purposes of picture drawing that is considered the cultural precursor of writing (Gelb, 1963).

The primary systems framework has important implications for efforts aimed at elucidating the neural correlates of written language production. In particular, due to its emphasis on shared cognitive representations and neural substrates, primary systems theory predicts that attempts to isolate distinct cortical areas specialized for spelling or writing are conceptually misguided and likely to prove futile. Instead of searching for putative "writing centers," a more sensible approach might be to identify the brain systems that mediate various aspects of the writing process while also contributing to spoken language functions, reading, visual object recognition, working memory/attention, and manual motor control. According to this view, the neurobiological substrates of writing correspond to coordinated patterns of neural activation or functional connectivity across large-scale cortical networks that participate in multiple cognitive tasks rather than reflect the activity of dedicated brain regions. With these caveats in mind, we now examine what functional imaging investigations in normal subjects and lesion-deficit correlation studies in patients with agraphia have revealed about localization of the neural systems that contribute to spelling and writing.

Functional Neuroanatomy of Written Language Production

Although neuroimaging research of language function in normal individuals has focused primarily on speech production/comprehension and reading, there have been a number of studies that attempted to identify the neural networks that support the central and peripheral components of writing (for reviews, see Planton, Jucla, Roux, & Demonet, 2013; Purcell, Turkeltaub, Eden, & Rapp, 2011). Insights gained from these investigations regarding the putative localization of the cognitive systems postulated in Figure 5.1 are briefly summarized below.

Central Components

Orthography

One of the most consistently activated brain regions in imaging studies of spelling and writing is the left-ventral occipito-temporal cortex (lvOT) corresponding to the mid-portions of the fusiform gyrus (Beeson et al., 2003; Ludersdorfer, Kronbichler, & Wimmer, 2015; Planton et al.,

2013; Purcell et al., 2011; Rapp & Lipka, 2010). The same cortical region is also reliably activated in functional imaging studies of reading and has been referred to as the "visual word form area" (VWFA)(Cohen et al., 2002; Dehaene & Cohen, 2011; McCandliss, Cohen, & Dehaene, 2003; Price & Devlin, 2011). Overlapping patterns of neural activation in the VWFA during reading and spelling confirm the central role of this region in orthographic processing and provide compelling evidence that written word recognition and production rely on shared orthographic representations with a common neural substrate (Rapp & Lipka, 2010). It has been demonstrated that neural responses in the VWFA are modulated by whole-word frequency during both reading and spelling (Bruno, Zumberge, Manis, Lu, & Goldman, 2008; Kronbichler et al., 2004; Rapp & Dufor, 2011; Rapp & Lipka, 2010). In particular, VWFA activation is negatively correlated with written word frequency (low > high), indicating that familiar orthographic patterns are processed more efficiently. The finding that the efficiency of neural computations by the VWFA is influenced by word frequency reflecting prior experience with orthographic word forms suggests that this cortical region may perform the functions ascribed to the orthographic lexicon in cognitive models of written language processing. During reading, orthographic lexical representations in the VWFA are activated in a "bottom-up" fashion by external visual input and the information is transmitted to cortical language systems involved in phonological and semantic processing. By contrast, during spelling, orthographic lexical representations in the VWFA are activated by "top-down" input from phonological and semantic networks and the information is subsequently made available to motor systems responsible for the programming of handwriting movements (Figure 5.1). Importantly, VWFA activation is also observed when reading (Kronbichler et al., 2007; Mano et al., 2013; Mechelli, Gorno-Tempini, & Price, 2003; Taylor, Rastle, & Davis, 2013) or spelling nonwords (Beeson & Rapcsak, 2003; DeMarco, Wilson, Rising, Rapcsak, & Beeson, in preparation; Ludersdorfer et al., 2015), suggesting that, in addition to its role in orthographic lexical processing, this region contributes to sublexical phoneme-grapheme conversion.

Although neuroimaging studies have consistently implicated the VWFA in the orthographic components of reading and spelling, there is considerable controversy in the literature regarding the issue of whether this cortical region is domain specific and therefore recruited only by tasks involving written word recognition and production. In particular, a number of studies have shown that the VWFA is also activated when subjects view or name pictures of objects and other complex nonorthographic visual stimuli such as faces, suggesting that this cortical area may play a more general role in visual shape processing and/or in linking visual information with higher-order phonological and semantic representations (for reviews, see Dehaene & Cohen, 2011; Behrmann & Plaut, 2013, 2014; Mano et al., 2013; Price & Devlin, 2011). Although the degree of domain-specificity within the VWFA requires further investigation, the neuroimaging findings are consistent with the contention of the primary systems hypothesis that orthographic processing emerges as the result of experience-dependent neural plasticity within cortical systems originally evolved for visual object recognition. During literacy acquisition, VWFA neurons progressively increase the selectivity of their tuning to orthographic stimuli and strengthen their functional connectivity to cortical networks involved in phonological and semantic processing. This dynamic learning process that involves both bottom-up and top-down integration of visual, phonological, and semantic information ultimately establishes the VWFA as the critical neural interface between spoken and written language.

Phonology

Written language production has been shown to be associated with activation in several perisylvian cortical areas, including posterior inferior frontal gyrus (pIFG)/operculum, precentral gyrus (PCG), insula, superior temporal gyrus/sulcus (STG/STS), and supramarginal gyrus (SMG)

(Beeson et al., 2003; DeMarco et al., in preparation; Ludersdorfer et al., 2015; Purcell et al., 2011; Rapp & Lipka, 2010). These perisylvian regions are not dedicated exclusively to spelling or writing, however, as the same cortical areas are activated during tasks involving speech production/perception, reading, phonological working memory, and phonological awareness (Acheson, Hamidi, Binder, & Postle, 2011; Buchsbaum et al., 2011; Burton, LoCasto, Krebs-Noble, & Gullapalli, 2005; Jobard, Crivello, & Tzourio-Mazoyer, 2003; Katzir, Misra, & Poldrack, 2005; Price, 2012; Vigneau et al., 2006). These observations indicate that the perisylvian language areas recruited during spelling are part of a large-scale neural system that plays a general or modality-independent role in phonological processing. In fact, it has been proposed that these functionally linked perisylvian cortical regions comprise the dorsal language pathway involved in mapping phonological information represented in STG/STS onto frontal lobe articulatory networks (pIFG/PCG/insula) for speech production (Hickok & Poeppel, 2007). During spelling, levels of activation within the phonological network are modulated by whole-word frequency (low > high), providing evidence of sensitivity to the familiarity of phonological word forms (Rapp & Dufor, 2011; Rapp & Lipka, 2010). The phonological network also shows robust activation during nonword spelling, indicating that it contributes to both whole-word and subword-level mappings between phonology and orthography (Beeson & Rapcsak, 2003; DeMarco et al., in preparation; Ludersdorfer et al., 2015). Collectively, the results of functional imaging studies suggest that lexical and sublexical phonological information used in spelling is generated, maintained, and manipulated by a distributed network of perisylvian cortical regions that plays an essential role in phonological processing during both spoken and written language tasks.

Semantic System

Functional imaging studies have provided compelling evidence that modality-independent semantic processing is mediated by a distributed network of extrasylvian brain regions that include left prefrontal cortex (PFC, especially anterior inferior frontal gyrus), anterior temporal lobe (ATL) structures (temporal pole, anterior middle/inferior temporal gyri, anterior fusiform gyrus), and temporo-parietal (TP) cortex (posterior middle/inferior temporal gyri, angular gyrus) (for reviews, see Binder, Desai, Graves, & Conant 2009; Bonner, Peelle, Cook, & Grossman, 2013; Price, 2012; Visser, Jefferies, & Lambon Ralph, 2009). The multimodal semantic network is consistently engaged during comprehension tasks involving spoken words, written words, and a variety of nonverbal stimuli (e.g., pictures of objects, famous faces, familiar environmental sounds) (Binder et al., 2009; Price, 2012; Visser et al., 2009). Semantic network activation is also reliably observed during speech production tasks requiring conceptually guided lexical retrieval (e.g., picture naming, verbal fluency, generating a spoken narrative) (Price, 2012) and during oral reading, especially for irregular words (Binder, Medler, Desai, Conant, & Liebenthal, 2005; Graves, Desai, Humphries, Seidenberg, & Binder, 2010; Jobard et al., 2003; Price, 2012; Taylor et al., 2013).

Given the central role of semantic representations in both spoken and written language processing, it might seem surprising that recent meta-analyses of the imaging literature have not revealed compelling evidence of semantic network activation during writing tasks (Planton et al., 2013; Purcell et al., 2011). These negative results, however, should not be taken to imply that semantic input is not required for written language production. Instead, the main reason for the lack of semantic network activation may be that most studies have failed to include the stimulus-type or task manipulations best suited for demonstrating engagement of semantic representations. For instance, in spelling to dictation tasks semantic activation is most likely to occur when processing irregular words because these items can only be spelled correctly by a lexical-semantic strategy. Furthermore, semantic contributions during spelling may be best revealed by direct contrasts between irregular words and nonwords, since the latter are not expected to engage semantic representations. Unfortunately, most imaging studies have not compared patterns of activation associated with spelling irregular words versus nonwords. Regarding the influence of task manipulations on semantic activation, conceptually driven writing tasks involving written composition, written verbal fluency, or written picture naming are expected to place greater demands on semantic processing than simple lexical transcoding tasks such as spelling to dictation. Consistent with this hypothesis, Brownsett and Wise (2010) observed prominent activation of the left angular gyrus (AG) using a task that required generation of written narratives. The same AG region was also activated during production of spoken narratives, confirming the central role of this cortical area in modality-independent semantic processing. Similarly, Beeson et al., (2003) documented strong left PFC activation involving anterior inferior frontal gyrus using a written verbal fluency task that placed high demands on semantically guided lexical retrieval and, in a subset of participants, this task was also associated with left AG activation. Finally, we note that the apparent lack of activation in regions implicated in semantic processing during writing tasks may also be related to technical limitations. For instance, there is broad consensus that the ATL is a critical hub within the semantic network (Patterson, Nestor, & Rogers, 2007), but this brain region has been difficult to image with fMRI due to magnetic susceptibility artifact resulting in signal dropout (Visser et al., 2009). These considerations highlight the more general point that information from functional imaging studies alone is not sufficient to draw firm conclusions about brain-behavior relationships. As we shall see, there is in fact compelling support for the role of semantic representations in writing from lesion-deficit correlation studies in neurological patients.

Graphemic Buffer

As discussed earlier, the graphemic buffer is responsible for maintaining the orthographic representations generated by central spelling routes in a high state of accessibility while they are being converted into movements of the pen by the peripheral or motor components of the writing process. Based on imaging evidence, it has been suggested that the neural correlates of this working memory system depend on functional interactions between left intraparietal sulcus/superior parietal lobule (IPS/SPL) and the caudal portions of the superior frontal sulcus (SFS) bordered by the posterior banks of the superior and middle frontal gyri (SFG/MFG) (Purcell et al., 2011; Rapp & Dufor, 2011). These cortical areas demonstrate sensitivity to word length manipulations during spelling tasks (long > short), consistent with the expectation that longer words should increase processing demands on neural systems involved in orthographic working memory (Rapp & Dufor, 2011). In line with proposals postulating a more general role for the graphemic buffer in orthographic processing (Rapp & Dufor, 2011), these frontoparietal regions, especially IPS/SPL, are also activated during reading (Binder et al., 2005; Ihnen, Petersen, & Schlaggar, 2013; Taylor et al., 2013; Valdois et al., 2006; Vogel, Miezin, Petersen, & Schlaggar, 2012). However, the functional contributions of this cortical network cannot be considered specific to written language because the same dorsal frontoparietal system is also recruited during a variety of visuospatial attention and working memory tasks that do not involve orthographic stimuli (Corbetta & Shulman, 2002; Courtney, Petit, Maisog, Ungerleider, & Haxby, 1998; Ikkai & Curtis, 2011; Nee et al., 2013; Szczepanski, Pinsk, Douglas, Kastner, & Saalmann, 2013).

Peripheral Components

Motor Programming and Neuromuscular Execution

Converging evidence from multiple imaging studies indicates that the motor control of writing is mediated by a left-hemisphere frontoparietal network that includes anterior IPS/SPL, dorsolateral premotor cortex located within the SFS and posterior SFG/MFG (sometimes referred to as Exner's writing center), supplementary motor area (SMA), and the primary sensorimotor region for the hand (Beeson et al., 2003; Sugihara, Kaminaga, & Sugishita, 2006; Roux et al., 2009; Segal & Petrides, 2011; Purcell et al., 2011; Planton et al., 2013). The parietal and frontal premotor components of the proposed neural circuit for handwriting movements partially overlap with the dorsal frontoparietal attention network that mediates the functions ascribed to the graphemic buffer (see above). These findings are consistent with the notion of a working memory system interfacing between the central and peripheral components of the writing process and illustrate the close anatomical and functional relationship between visuospatial attention and the planning and programming of spatially oriented hand movements within dorsal frontoparietal cortex. The production of handwriting is also associated with activation in several subcortical regions implicated in motor control, including basal ganglia, thalamus, and the cerebellum (Planton et al., 2013; Purcell et al., 2011). It has been proposed that these subcortical structures are functionally integrated into basal ganglia thalamocortical and cerebello-cortical motor loops that are responsible for generating concrete kinematic parameters for handwriting movements specifying stroke size, speed, duration, and force (Rapcsak & Beeson, 2002).

Consistent with the predictions of the primary systems hypothesis, the left-hemisphere frontoparietal networks involved in the visuomotor control of handwriting are also activated during performance of other types of skilled manual movements such as tool use (Choi et al., 2001; Frey, 2008; Hermsdorfer, Terlinden, Muhlau, Goldenberg, & Wohlschlager, 2007; Johnson-Frey, 2004; Johnson-Frey, Newman-Norlund, & Grafton, 2005; Moll, et al., 2000; Peigneux, et al., 2004) and drawing (Harrington, Farias, & Davis, 2009; Harrington, Farias, Davis, & Buonocore, 2007). These findings support the view that the motor control of handwriting develops as a result of functional adaptation within phylogenetically older brain circuits originally evolved for visuomotor coordination during reaching, grasping, and manipulating objects in space.

Neuropsychological Disorders of Spelling and Writing

Although imaging studies in healthy individuals can identify the neural systems recruited during written language production, they cannot confirm with certainty the functional role of different cortical areas or even prove that the activated brain regions are necessary for normal performance. Conclusive evidence that a specific cortical area is essential for spelling and writing can be obtained by lesion studies demonstrating that damage to the region produces the expected behavioral deficit. Therefore, results from functional imaging and lesion-deficit correlation studies need to be integrated and the two methodological approaches should play a complementary and synergistic role in identifying the neural correlates of written language production. In this section we review what neuropsychological investigations in patients with focal or degenerative brain disorders have revealed about the cognitive mechanisms and neural substrates of writing. In particular, we discuss distinct agraphia syndromes that result from damage to the neural systems that support the central and peripheral components of the writing process.

Central Agraphias

Disruption of the Lexical-Semantic Spelling Route: Surface Agraphia

According to the model shown in Figure 5.1, the lexical-semantic route is normally used for spelling all familiar words, but this pathway is particularly important for correct production of irregular words that contain atypical or inconsistent letter-sound mappings. Damage to the lexical-semantic route results in surface (or "lexical") agraphia characterized by disproportionate impairment in processing irregular words compared to regular words, giving rise to an increased *regularity effect* in spelling (Beauvois & Dérouesné, 1981). In addition to spelling-sound consistency/orthographic regularity, performance in surface agraphia is strongly influenced by whole-word frequency, with the spelling deficit being especially pronounced for low-frequency irregular words. By contrast, spelling of regular words and nonwords is relatively spared, presumably because these items contain predictable sound-letter relationships that can be processed accurately by relying on a rule-based sublexical phoneme-grapheme conversion strategy. Excessive reliance on the sublexical spelling route in surface agraphia is indicated by the tendency to produce phonologically plausible "regularization" errors on irregular words (e.g., *circuit* → *serkit*).

In terms of cognitive mechanisms, it has been suggested that surface agraphia may result from damage to the putative orthographic lexicon (see Rapcsak & Beeson, 2002 for a review). Neuroanatomical evidence for the proposal that surface agraphia reflects the loss or degradation of word-specific orthographic information is provided by observations that the responsible lesions frequently involve lvOT cortex centered on the VWFA (Rapcsak & Beeson, 2002, 2004; Tsapkini & Rapp, 2010; Purcell, Shea, & Rapp, 2014). The most common etiology in patients with this lesion profile is stroke in the distribution of the left posterior cerebral artery (PCA) (Rapcsak & Beeson, 2004). An orthographic basis of surface agraphia following lvOT damage is also supported by functional imaging studies in normal individuals demonstrating overlapping activations in the VWFA during reading and spelling, suggesting that this cortical region plays a central role in lexical orthographic processing (Purcell et al., 2011; Rapcsak & Beeson, 2004; Rapp & Lipka, 2010). Consistent with the notion of shared orthographic representations mediating written word recognition and production, some patients with damage to the VWFA are impaired in both reading and spelling irregular words, demonstrating a combination of surface alexia and agraphia (Bowers, Bub, & Arguin, 1996; Friedman & Hadley, 1992; Patterson & Kay, 1982; Purcell et al., 2014). It is important to bear in mind, however, that spelling is a more difficult task than reading in part because sound-to-spelling correspondences in English are much more inconsistent than spelling-to-sound mappings (Barry & Seymour, 1988). Therefore, individuals with damage to the VWFA may exhibit the typical behavioral profile of surface agraphia but experience only mild difficulty in reading irregular words (Rapcsak & Beeson, 2004; Tsapkini & Rapp, 2010). Furthermore, patients with relatively mild damage to orthographic lexical representations tend to produce visually similar real word substitution errors in reading rather than the phonologically plausible regularization errors that characterize spelling performance, indicating excessive reliance on sublexical phoneme-grapheme conversion (Rapcsak & Beeson, 2004). These observations suggest that fairly substantial degradation of orthographic lexical representations may be required to induce a switch to reading by a sublexical strategy. Finally, lvOT lesions in the vicinity of the VWFA may give rise to a combination of surface agraphia (or surface alexia/agraphia) and letter-by-letter (LBL) reading, providing evidence of both a central orthographic deficit and an additional peripheral processing impairment interfering with rapid parallel access to orthographic lexical representations from visual input (Bowers et al., 1996; Patterson & Kay, 1982; Rapcsak & Beeson, 2004; Rapcsak, Rubens & Laguna, 1990). It is likely that the peripheral/prelexical reading deficit in these patients is attributable to damage to posterior fusiform gyrus and underlying white matter that degrades or disconnects visual input to the VWFA, as typically seen in cases of pure alexia/LBL reading, whereas the central orthographic lexical impairment that affects both reading and spelling is produced by damage to the VWFA proper (Rapcsak & Beeson, 2004; Epelbaum et al., 2008; Sebastian, Gomez, Leigh, Davis, Newhart, & Hillis, 2014).

Patients with reading and spelling impairment following damage to the VWFA frequently demonstrate additional difficulties on nonorthographic visual tasks such as picture naming and face recognition, consistent with the proposal that this cortical region plays a more general role in visual shape processing and is recruited for all tasks that require fine-grained discrimination between complex visual stimuli based on high spatial frequency foveal information (for reviews, see Behrmann & Plaut, 2013, 2014; Roberts et al., 2013). However, in other individuals with similar lesion profiles the visual processing deficit appeared to be selective for orthographic stimuli (Tsapkini & Rapp, 2010; Purcell et al., 2014). The neuroanatomical basis of this variability remains to be determined and it may be that these conflicting results reflect premorbid individual differences in the cortical representation of visual categories.

Surface agraphia has also been described in association with damage to left-hemisphere extrasylvian cortical regions that show modality-independent activation in functional imaging studies of semantic processing in normal individuals, including ATL and TP cortex (Rapcsak & Beeson, 2002). Unlike the orthographic form of surface agraphia that follows damage to the VWFA, the cognitive mechanisms underlying the spelling impairment in patients with this lesion profile may reflect degraded semantic knowledge or reduced semantic input to orthography. Although the semantic form of surface agraphia may be produced by focal damage within the semantic network (Beauvois & Dérouesné, 1981; Roeltgen & Heilman, 1984; Vanier & Caplan, 1985), the spelling disorder is more often associated with neurodegenerative disorders, especially the semantic variant of primary progressive aphasia (svPPA) (Faria et al., 2013; Graham, 2014; Graham, Patterson, & Hodges, 2000; Henry et al., 2012; Shim, Hurley, Rogalski, & Mesulam, 2012) and Alzheimer's disease (AD) (Croisile et al., 1996; Croisile, Carmoi, Adeleine, & Trillet, 1995; Hughes, Graham, Patterson, & Hodges, 1997; Lambert et al., 2007; Platel et al., 1993; Rapcsak, Arthur, Bliklen, & Rubens, 1989). In fact, the highly reliable association between surface agraphia/alexia and svPPA has provided the motivation for the inclusion of these written language disorders among the clinical diagnostic criteria for this PPA subtype (Gorno-Tempini et al., 2011). Although most patients with svPPA demonstrate a combination of surface agraphia/alexia, due to the task difficulty effects alluded to above, the spelling impairment is usually more severe and may precede the onset of the reading disorder (Caine, Breen, & Patterson, 2009; Faria, et al., 2013; Graham et al., 2000; Henry et al., 2012; Patterson et al., 2006).

The semantic deficit hypothesis of surface agraphia in svPPA is supported by multiple lines of behavioral evidence. First, although the spelling disorder may be evident when semantic deficits are relatively mild, it typically appears in the context of demonstrable impairments on a variety of verbal and nonverbal semantic tasks (e.g., picture naming, verbal fluency, spoken-word/picture comprehension, object/person recognition). Second, the severity of the deficit on nonorthographic measures of semantic knowledge (e.g., picture naming, spoken-word/picture comprehension) has been shown to correlate with spelling accuracy for irregular words (Graham et al., 2000; Henry et al., 2012; Shim et al., 2012). Third, the erosion of semantic memory in svPPA creates qualitatively similar difficulties in processing unfamiliar or atypical items (as exemplified by low-frequency irregular words) not only in spelling or reading, but also in other language and nonverbal cognitive tasks (e.g., picture naming, past-tense verb generation, object decisions, drawing) (Hodges & Patterson, 2007; Patterson et al., 2006). In all these domains, errors involve over-regularizations based on preserved knowledge of more familiar or typical exemplars (e.g., naming the picture of a *zebra* as *horse*, producing the past-tense form of *give* as *gived* rather than gave). Taken together, these results provide compelling evidence that surface agraphia in svPPA is just one manifestation of a central or modality-independent semantic deficit.

A possible semantic basis of surface agraphia in patients with neurodegenerative disorders is also supported by neuroanatomical observations. Specifically, in svPPA the characteristic combination of semantic impairment and surface agraphia/alexia occurs in the setting of profound ATL atrophy/hypometabolism (Brambati, Ogar, Neuhaus, Miller, & Gorno-Tempini, 2009; Gorno-Tempini et al., 2004, 2011; Mion et al., 2010; Wilson et al., 2009). Similarly, in mixed groups of PPA patients poor irregular word spelling has been shown to correlate with atrophy involving left ATL and TP cortex, overlapping with brain regions where atrophy is associated with defective irregular word reading and impaired performance on nonorthographic semantic tasks (Brambati et al., 2009; Henry et al., 2012; Sepelyak et al., 2011; Shim et al., 2012). In some PPA case series (Shim et al., 2012) irregular word spelling scores correlated with both ventral ATL and mid-fusiform atrophy involving the VWFA, consistent with the hypothesis that semantic and orthographic processing deficits may both contribute to surface agraphia. PPA patients who predominantly produced phonologically plausible spelling errors were also found to have prominent atrophy of white matter tracts (inferior longitudinal fasciculus, inferior fronto-occipital fasciculus) connecting modality-specific posterior visual association areas, including the VWFA, to ATL and PFC regions implicated in modality-independent semantic processing (Faria et al., 2013). Structural damage to occipito-temporal and occipito-frontal white matter pathways may contribute to surface agraphia by disconnecting cortical regions responsible for mapping between semantic and orthographic lexical representations. Although the neuroanatomical basis of surface agraphia in AD has not been extensively investigated, patients with this disorder frequently manifest semantic memory impairment that correlates with atrophy/hypometabolism involving left ATL and posterior TP cortex (Ahn et al., 2011; Domoto-Reilly, Sapolsky, Brickhouse, & Dickerson, 2012; Hirini, Kivisaari, Monsch, & Taylor, 2013; Joubert et al., 2010; Zahn et al., 2004). Furthermore, in a PET study of AD patients irregular word spelling scores correlated with metabolic activity in the left AG (Penniello et al., 1995).

Surface agraphia, however, is not the only written language production deficit documented in patients with semantic impairment. Because the lexical-semantic route provides the only mechanism for incorporating meaning into writing, damage to semantic representations or reduced semantic input to orthography compromises performance on all conceptually mediated writing tasks, including written composition, written verbal fluency, and written naming. Due to defective semantically guided retrieval of orthographic word forms, written narratives have poor information content and may contain empty circumlocutions (Harnish & Neils-Strunjas, 2008). In severe cases, written output consists of vague or incoherent sentences, irrelevant intrusions, or it may be limited to a few disconnected words. Spontaneous writing and written naming may also be marred by the production of semantic errors. Reduced written verbal fluency and omission errors in written naming tasks are common. In addition, the disruption of semantic influence on writing creates difficulties in spelling homophones to dictation, a writing disorder sometimes referred to as "semantic agraphia" (see Rapcsak & Beeson, 2002 for a review). Homophones have identical sound patterns, but they are spelled differently and have different meanings (e.g., *seen* → *scene*). The correct spelling of homophonic words depends critically on semantic context (e.g., "he had *seen* that movie" vs. "he arrived at the *scene*"). Patients with semantic agraphia cannot use contextual information to disambiguate dictated homophones reliably and, therefore, frequently produce the semantically inappropriate orthographic word form. In terms of neural correlates, semantic agraphia has been documented in association with focal damage or neurodegenerative process (e.g., svPPA or AD) encroaching on the PFC, ATL, and TP components of the distributed semantic network (Harnish & Neils-Strunjas, 2008; Neils, Roeltgen, & Constantinidou, 1995; Rapcsak & Beeson, 2002; Rapcsak & Rubens, 1990; Roeltgen, Rothi, & Heilman, 1986). Thus, semantic agraphia and the other disorders of conceptually mediated written expression discussed in this section have overlapping neural substrates with surface agraphia, providing evidence that their frequent co-occurrence reflects a common underlying semantic impairment.

According to the neuroanatomical model of written language production shown in Figure 5.2, the operations of the lexical-semantic spelling route are supported by multiple parallel pathways converging on the VWFA. In particular, it is proposed that during written expression the activation of orthographic word forms within the VWFA occurs in response to combined inputs from nodes within the distributed semantic network and from phonological lexical information represented in STG/STS. Note that in terms of its neural implementation the lexical-semantic

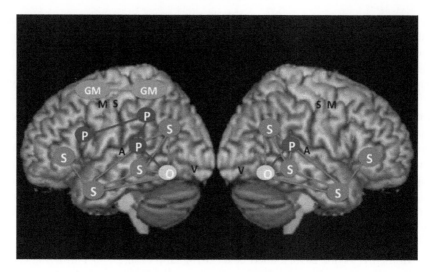

Figure 5.2 Neuroanatomical model of written language production. P = perisylvian phonological network; S = extrasylvian semantic network; O = orthographic processing/VWFA; GM = dorsal frontoparietal networks involved in attention, working memory, and graphomotor control; SM, V, and A = primary sensorimotor, visual, and auditory cortex (see text for details).

route used for generating written language overlaps with, and is parasitic upon, evolutionarily older brain systems that include the ventral language pathway implicated in bidirectional mappings between phonological and semantic representations during speech production/comprehension (Hickok & Poeppel, 2007) and the ventral visual object recognition pathway (Kravitz, Saleem, Baker, Ungerleider, & Mishkin, 2013) that allows for direct mapping between modality-specific perceptual representations of objects/faces processed in specialized regions within lvOT cortex and multimodal semantic information stored in ATL. These neuroanatomical relationships are consistent with the view that the acquisition of written language involves recycling preexisting neural systems supporting spoken language and higher-order object vision.

Although lesion-deficit correlation studies have provided compelling evidence for the central role of semantic representations in written language production, the specific contribution of different cortical regions within the extrasylvian semantic network remains to be elucidated. In this context, we note that contemporary neuropsychological models postulate two interactive functional components underpinning semantic cognition: representation and executive control (Jefferies & Lambon Ralph, 2006; Noonan, Jefferies, Visser, & Lambon Ralph, 2013). Specifically, it is assumed that multimodal semantic knowledge is represented in ATL and that executive processes regulating the activation of semantic information in a task-appropriate fashion depend on the PFC and TP components of the network. Damage to semantic representations versus executive control systems may result in qualitatively different written language production deficits. Thus, although left ATL, PFC and TP lesions may all interfere with semantically based activation of orthographic lexical representations within the VWFA (Figure 5.2), the neuropsychological mechanisms and clinical characteristics of the ensuing writing disorder may vary as a function of lesion location. For instance, damage to executive control systems may interfere with strategic lexical search and selection procedures and also with appropriate monitoring of the product of semantically guided lexical retrieval to ensure that it is consistent with the message the writer wishes to communicate (Rapcsak & Beeson, 2002). Consistent with this prediction, damage to left PFC results in a deregulation of the lexical-semantic pathway manifested by the production of semantically incoherent written narratives, impaired written naming, and difficulties with homophone spelling (Rapcsak & Rubens, 1990). The breakdown of executive control over the operations of the lexical-semantic spelling pathway may also explain reports of surface agraphia following left ventral PFC lesions (Hillis, Chang, Breese, & Heidler, 2004; Rapcsak et al., 1988) centered on the inferior frontal junction (IFJ) (the intersection of inferior frontal sulcus and pre-central sulcus, see Derrfuss, Brass, Neumann, & von Cramon, 2005). These patients did not show evidence of multimodal semantic deficit or reading impairment, suggesting that neural systems representing conceptual knowledge and orthographic information were preserved. Instead, the spelling deficit may have been caused by defective strategic control over the retrieval and selection of orthographic lexical representations, perhaps coupled with insufficient inhibition of competing information generated by the sublexical spelling route. According to this view, frontal executive systems exert context-dependent top-down control over the division of labor between the spelling pathways (i.e., depending on whether the task involves spelling real words vs. nonwords) and are responsible for detecting and resolving conflict between orthographic representations computed by lexical-semantic versus sublexical procedures. The executive demands associated with compe-tition between spelling pathways are particularly high when processing low-frequency irregular words and if unresolved, the conflict may result in the production of phonologically plausible spelling errors consistent with the profile of surface agraphia.

Additional support for the proposal that damage to different components of the distributed semantic system may give rise to qualitatively distinct written language deficits comes from Jef-feries, Rogers, Hopper, and Lambon Ralph (2010) who reported that in a spelling to dictation task svPPA patients demonstrated greater sensitivity to orthographic regularity and frequency and produced more regularization errors than patients with stroke-induced "semantic aphasia" following focal left PFC or TP lesions. Since the two groups were similar in terms of overall lev-els of semantic impairment, qualitative differences in spelling performance were likely to reflect the nature of the underlying semantic deficit. In particular, differences in spelling profiles may have been attributable to the fact that ATL atrophy in svPPA produced a genuine degradation of semantic knowledge, whereas focal damage to PFC and TC resulted in defective executive control of activation within the semantic network interfering with reliable access to otherwise preserved lexical-semantic representations.

Finally, we note that it has been proposed that in some patients surface agraphia (and surface alexia) may result from defective mapping between otherwise preserved semantic and orthographic lexical representations produced by damage to the putative "orthography-semantics interface region" that corresponds to the basal temporal language area located posterior to the temporal pole and anterior to the VWFA (Purcell et al., 2014).

Regardless of the specific cognitive mechanisms involved and the exact location of the respon-sible lesions within the lexical-semantic spelling pathway, patients with surface agraphia attempt to compensate for their deficit by relying on sublexical phoneme-grapheme conversion. These observations suggest that the neural substrates of subword-level translations between phonology and orthography must be at least partially independent from the cortical systems implicated in lexical-semantic spelling. We next examine what lesion-deficit correlation studies have revealed about the anatomical localization of the neural networks that support spelling by a sublexical strategy.

Damage to the Sublexical Spelling Route: Phonological Agraphia

As discussed earlier, spelling by the sublexical route relies on the systematic application of phoneme-grapheme conversion rules that encode knowledge about the statistical regularities of sound-letter correspondences in English. Specifically, it is assumed that during sublexical spelling phonological representations are first segmented into their component sounds, following which individual phonemes are converted into their most common graphemic equivalents and assembled into an orthographic string for written production. The sublexical pathway is critical for generating plausible spellings for unfamiliar words or novel nonwords that do not have preexisting lexical-semantic representations. The sublexical procedure can also produce correct spellings for regular words that contain predictable sound-spelling correspondences. However, the application of phoneme-grapheme conversion rules to irregular words gives rise to phonologically plausible spelling errors.

As shown in Figure 5.1, spelling information generated by the sublexical pathway is integrated with the output of the lexical-semantic spelling route at the grapheme level. In addition, the sublexical spelling system can influence lexical activation and selection via feedback connections from the grapheme level to the orthographic lexicon. Through these dynamic interactions with the lexical-semantic route, the sublexical system can aid spelling performance by reinforcing the correct lexical targets and their constituent graphemes (Folk, Rapp, & Goldrick, 2002, see also preceding chapter, this volume). Contributions from the sublexical route may be particularly important for correct spelling of stimuli that are processed relatively inefficiently by the lexical-semantic pathway, including low-frequency words and items with impoverished semantic representations (abstract words, functors, bound morphemes). Sublexical/lexical integration can also serve to strengthen the target word against interference from lexical or semantic competitors and thereby reduce the risk of form-related (*trail* → *train*) or semantic (*apple* → *pear*) spelling errors (Folk et al., 2002). Thus, although it is assumed that the lexical-semantic pathway plays a preeminent role in spelling familiar words, contributions from the sublexical route are also necessary for normal performance. The division of labor or relative balance between the two spelling procedures may be subject to individual variation in healthy persons reflecting levels of education and spelling expertise, and it can be altered in a dramatic fashion following brain injury. However, even in the damaged system the pathways continue to interact and jointly contribute to spelling performance, as indicated by the finding that the spelling errors of patients with acquired agraphia often reflect a combination of lexical-semantic and sublexical influences (for a review, see Rapp, Epstein, & Tainturier, 2002).

Damage to the sublexical route produces the syndrome of phonological agraphia characterized by a disproportionate difficulty in processing unfamiliar nonwords compared to familiar words, giving rise to an enlarged *lexicality effect* in spelling (Shallice, 1981). Spelling errors on nonwords include unrelated responses, phonologically incorrect but visually similar renditions of the target (*gope* → *glipe*), and lexicalizations (*flig* → *flag*). Although nonword spelling can be severely compromised or even abolished, real word spelling performance is relatively preserved. Several observations suggest that the residual spelling abilities of patients with phonological agraphia are mediated by the lexical-semantic pathway. For instance, patients may be unable to spell words to dictation unless they have access to their meaning (Bub & Kertesz, 1982b; Shallice, 1981). Furthermore, spelling performance is typically influenced by lexical-semantic variables, such as word frequency (high > low), imageability (concrete > abstract), and grammatical word class (nouns > verbs > functors). Spelling errors on real words are usually phonologically implausible, but they often retain visual/orthographic similarity to the target (*secret* → *securt*) indicating partial lexical knowledge (Ellis, 1982). Morphological errors (*works* → *worked*) and functor substitutions (*where* → *what*) are also commonly observed. Phonological agraphia is closely related to the syndrome of deep agraphia (Bub & Kertesz, 1982a). In particular, deep agraphia shares all the characteristic clinical features of phonological agraphia, but it is empirically distinguished from the latter by the production of frequent semantic spelling errors (e.g., *night* → *sleep*). Although phonological and deep agraphia were originally considered distinct entities, there is much evidence to suggest that the differences between these two writing disorders are quantitative rather than qualitative in nature (for a review, see Rapcsak et al., 2009). Therefore, phonological and deep agraphia are more appropriately conceptualized as points along a continuum, with the latter representing a more severe version of the former. Acknowledging this overlap, we will refer to both entities by the common term phonological agraphia throughout most of our discussion.

The proposed breakdown of the sublexical route provides an adequate explanation of the nonword spelling impairment in phonological agraphia, since this pathway is considered essential for spelling novel items not represented in lexical-semantic memory. Similarly, the real word spelling difficulties of these patients may be accounted for by assuming that sublexical support is normally required for spelling items that are relatively unfamiliar and/or have sparse semantic representations (low-frequency words, abstract words, functors, bound morphemes), and also to eliminate potential form-related and semantic spelling errors arising from interference by lexical or semantic competitors. According to this hypothesis, the characteristic spelling profile in phonological agraphia reflects the intrinsic functional limitations of the lexical-semantic spelling route when this system must operate in isolation without support from sublexical phonological inputs to orthography. Alternatively, the real word spelling impairments in phonological agraphia may be indicative of additional damage to the lexical-semantic pathway (see below).

Although descriptions of phonological agraphia have focused primarily on processing impairments apparent at the single-word level in spelling to dictation or written naming tasks, patients with this writing disorder also manifest characteristic deficits affecting written narrative production. Specifically, written compositions generated by patients with phonological agraphia are typically reduced in length and contain simplified sentence constructions, sometimes resulting in telegraphic output consisting mostly of nouns with relatively few verbs and frequent omissions of functors and bound morphemes. These production features may reflect the fact that the retrieval of orthographic representations for items with reduced semantic weight normally requires phonological inputs to orthography via the sublexical spelling route (see above). To emphasize the close functional relationship and possible common origin of single-word and sentence-level written language production deficits in patients with phonological agraphia, we have referred to this written narrative profile as "phonological text agraphia" (Beeson et al., 2012). Writing impairments in phonological agraphia may be more pronounced at the sentence level because of the increased demands on limited phonological short-term memory capacity that creates disproportionate difficulties in maintaining phonological traces for lexical items that cannot benefit from additional semantic support. However, it is conceivable that text-level writing impairments in phonological agraphia are manifestations of an underlying general syntactic deficit or agrammatism, in which case patients would be expected to show qualitatively similar difficulties in spoken narrative production.

There is compelling behavioral evidence from both single-case and group studies that the core functional deficit in phonological agraphia involves damage to central phonological representations that support both spoken and written language (Rapcsak et al., 2009). In terms of clinical presentation, the writing disorder is usually observed in aphasic patients with phonological deficits affecting speech production and perception (i.e., Broca's, conduction, and Wernicke's aphasia). Furthermore, the vast majority of patients with phonological agraphia demonstrate parallel impairments and increased lexicality effects on spoken language tasks such as oral repetition and on tests of phonological awareness that require the identification, maintenance, and manipulation of sublexical phonological information (e.g., rhyme judgments, phoneme segmentation and blending) (for reviews, see Jefferies, Sage, & Lambon Ralph, 2007; Rapcsak et al., 2009). Patients with phonological agraphia also typically show exaggerated lexicality effects in reading, consistent with the profile of phonological alexia (Crisp & Lambon Ralph, 2006; Jefferies et al., 2007; Rapcsak et al., 2009). Critically, it has been demonstrated that performance on nonorthographic tests of phonological awareness strongly correlates with, and is predictive of, both nonword and real word spelling (and reading) accuracy (Rapcsak et al., 2009). The close association between general phonological ability and written language performance has been documented both in patients with stroke-induced aphasia (Crisp & Lambon Ralph, 2006; Rapcsak et al., 2009) and in individuals with language dysfunction due to PPA (Henry et al., 2012; Shim et al., 2012). Taken together, these findings are consistent with the view that the highly correlated and qualitatively similar written and spoken language impairments in patients with phonological agraphia/alexia have a common origin and are merely different manifestations of a central phonological deficit. The proposed phonological impairment gives rise to enlarged lexicality effects across all language tasks because the unfamiliar phonological elements that make up nonwords are more difficult to process and are less stable than the familiar phonological patterns that correspond to real words, and also because in interactive language systems phonological lexical representations can receive additional top-down support from semantic representations (Figure 5.1) (Crisp & Lambon Ralph, 2006; Jefferies et al., 2007; Patterson, Suzuki, & Wydell, 1996; Rapcsak et al., 2009).

The phonological deficit hypothesis of phonological agraphia is also strongly supported by converging evidence from lesion-deficit correlation studies in neurological patients and functional imaging studies of language processing in healthy individuals. In particular, the writing disorder is reliably associated with damage to perisylvian cortical regions that show activation in imaging studies of normal subjects during a variety of written and spoken language tasks requiring phonological processing, including speech production/perception, reading, spelling, phonological awareness, and phonological short-term memory (for a review, see Henry, Beeson, Stark, & Rapcsak, 2007; Rapcsak et al., 2009). The responsible lesions are typically strokes in left middle cerebral artery (MCA) territory, involving pIFG, PCG, insula, STG/STS, and SMG in various combinations. The lesions also produce substantial damage to white matter pathways connecting these perisylvian cortical areas, including the arcuate fasciculus (AF)/superior longitudinal fasciculus (SLF) fiber tract system. Phonological impairment associated with perisylvian damage is also the likely neuropsychological mechanism of phonological agraphia documented in individuals with nonfluent or logopenic PPA (Faria et al., 2013; Graham, 2014; Henry et al., 2012; Sepelyak et al., 2011; Shim et al., 2012). Consistent with this hypothesis, patients with nfPPA and lvPPA produce phonological errors in spoken language tasks, have difficulty with repetition, and perform poorly on tests of phonological short-term memory (Ash et al., 2010; Gorno-Tempini et al., 2004, 2008; Grossman, 2012). These spoken language deficits are associated with prominent atrophy/hypometabolism involving the anterior (pIFG/PCG/insula in nfPPA) or posterior (STG/STS, SMG in lvPPA) components of the perisylvian phonological network (Gorno-Tempini et al., 2004, 2008, 2011; Grossman, 2012; Mesulam, 2013). White matter structural abnormalities have also been identified in the AF/SLF fiber tract system in these PPA variants, providing evidence of defective structural connectivity within the perisylvian language zone (Galantucci et al., 2011). Furthermore, in mixed groups of PPA patients, nonword spelling, nonword reading, and performance on nonorthographic tests of phonological awareness have been found to correlate with overlapping regions of atrophy within anterior and posterior perisylvian cortex (Brambati et al., 2009; Henry et al., 2012; Shim et al., 2012). Finally, evidence for the participation of posterior perisylvian cortical regions (STG/STS and SMG) in sublexical phoneme-grapheme conversion during spelling and reading has been provided by cortical stimulation studies in patients with brain tumors (Roux, Durand, Rehault, Reddy, & Demonet 2012; Roux et al., 2014). Thus, regardless of the nature of the underlying neurological disorder (focal vs. degenerative), the critical neural substrate of phonological agraphia is damage to perisylvian phonological networks that play an essential role in both spoken and written language processing.

Phonological agraphia is the most common spelling disorder encountered in clinical practice, reflecting the high prevalence of strokes in the distribution of the left MCA that includes the perisylvian cortical language areas. However, it is important to emphasize that the spelling profiles of individuals with perisylvian lesions are distributed along a continuum that mirrors and is determined by the severity of the underlying phonological impairment (Rapcsak et al., 2009). When the phonological deficit is relatively mild, the disproportionate reduction in nonword spelling accuracy gives rise to a large lexicality effect consistent with the profile of phonological agraphia. With more severe phonological impairment, the additional decline in real word spelling ability significantly reduces the size of the lexicality effect until the difference between real words and nonwords becomes negligible and patients demonstrate equally severe spelling deficits for both types of items, consistent with global agraphia (Beeson & Henry, 2008; Rapcsak et al., 2009). Thus, the full spectrum of spelling disorders in patients with perisylvian lesions follows a severity continuum that ranges from "pure" phonological agraphia at one end and global agraphia at the other, with deep agraphia occupying an intermediate position (Rapcsak et al., 2009). Within the framework of the cognitive model depicted in Figure 5.1, these observations suggest that mild phonological impairment caused by perisylvian lesions primarily compromises the sublexical spelling route, but more severe damage also degrades phonological lexical representations thereby disrupting both word- and subword-level phonological inputs to orthography. According to this view, the nonword and real word spelling deficits in patients with perisylvian lesions have a common underlying mechanism and reflect different degrees of phonological impairment. Consistent with this hypothesis, we found that both nonword and real word spelling scores correlated with nonorthographic measures of phonological ability in patients with perisylvian lesions (Rapcsak et al., 2009). Furthermore, spelling and phonological awareness scores both showed a correlation with the overall extent of the perisylvian network damage (as reflected by the total number of perisylvian ROIs involved) (Rapcsak et al., 2009). However, patients with severe real word spelling deficits, especially those with the clinical profile of deep or global agraphia, often have large lesions that extend outside the strict confines of the perisylvian region into extrasylvian cortical areas implicated in semantic processing. Thus, real word spelling impairments in these patients may in part be caused by semantic network disruption. The proposal that phonological and semantic impairments can both contribute to real word spelling deficits receives support from investigations that included phonological and semantic composite scores as independent nonorthographic predictors of written language performance in patients with aphasia due to stroke or PPA (Crisp & Lambon Ralph, 2006; Henry et al., 2012). These studies found that whereas nonword performance was predicted entirely by phonological scores, both phonological and semantic scores contributed to explaining variance in accuracy for real words. Thus, a complete characterization of the neuropsychological deficits underlying the phonological–deep–global agraphia continuum will require incorporating independent measures of phonological and semantic ability into the assessment and correlating spelling performance with damage to the neural systems that support these cognitive domains.

So far we have discussed the phonological agraphia continuum as writing disorders that reflect the residual output of the damaged left-hemisphere spelling system. However, the extensive destruction of left-hemisphere language areas documented in some patients raises the possibility that writing performance in these individuals may have been mediated by the intact right hemisphere (Rapcsak, Beeson, & Rubens, 1991). According to this hypothesis, the phonological–deep–global agraphia continuum reflects the intrinsic functional limitations of the normal right-hemisphere language system. Neuropsychological studies of right-hemisphere language ability in split-brain and dominant hemispherectomy patients offer some support for this view (for reviews, see Coltheart, 1980; Ogden, 1996; Rapcsak et al., 1991; Weekes, 1995; Zaidel, 1990). For instance, investigations of auditory and written word comprehension in this patient population have provided evidence that the semantic system of the right hemisphere lacks the precise functional organization of the left-hemisphere semantic network, making it susceptible to semantic errors. These studies have also revealed that the right-hemisphere lexicon is biased toward high-frequency, concrete words, and may have limited representation of low-frequency, abstract words, functors, and bound morphemes. In addition, the right hemisphere seems to have limited phonological competence and may completely lack the sublexical phonological skills necessary to perform phoneme-grapheme conversion. Perhaps most importantly, it has been demonstrated that the isolated right hemisphere is capable of generating elementary written expression, with a linguistic profile that is consistent with phonological or deep agraphia (for a review, see Rapcsak et al., 1991). Taken together, these results indicate that right-hemisphere writing remains a viable explanation of phonological/deep agraphia in patients with extensive left-hemisphere damage. However, the fact that many patients with large left-hemisphere lesions cannot produce meaningful writing at all suggests that right-hemisphere writing capacity may be subject to considerable individual variation. Based on these observations, right-hemisphere contributions to recovery from agraphia following left-hemisphere damage might be expected to range from a profile of phonological/ deep agraphia at the upper limit to global agraphia at the lower. Given the limited capacity of the right hemisphere for written expression, it appears that good functional recovery from agraphia requires the reengagement or reorganization of left-hemisphere cortical networks that originally supported spelling and writing.

In terms of our neuroanatomical model (Figure 5.2), the lesion profiles of patients with the phonological agraphia continuum suggest that the sublexical and lexical phonological codes used in spelling are generated, maintained, and manipulated by functionally linked perisylvian cortical areas that collectively constitute the dorsal language pathway involved in mapping phonological representations onto articulatory networks during speech production (Hickok & Poeppel, 2007). Critical components of the distributed phonological network include STG/STS, SMG, pIFG, PCG, and insula, along with the white matter pathways connecting these regions, primarily via the AF/SLF. According to the model, direct mapping between word and subword-level phonological and orthographic representations during spelling is mediated primarily by functional interactions between STG/STS and the VWFA, although connections between other components of the phonological network and the VWFA may also be involved. Specifically, we propose that during written language production phonological lexical representations of familiar words are retrieved from STG/STS and that the same region is involved in constructing novel sound-based representations for unfamiliar nonword targets in spelling to dictation tasks. During the spelling process, phonological representations computed within STG/STS are maintained in an active state and refreshed by articulatory rehearsal mechanisms mediated via the dorsal language pathway that constitutes a common neural substrate of phonological short-term memory and auditory-motor integration during all speech production tasks, including spontaneous speech, naming, repetition, and oral reading (Hickok & Poeppel, 2007). Processing of information within the phonological network and the efficiency of the direct phonological-to-orthographic mapping procedure is influenced by stimulus familiarity reflecting prior spelling (and reading) experience in translating between spoken and written word forms, with an advantage for high-frequency over low-frequency lexical items. Nonwords contain unfamiliar combinations of phonological elements, and spelling these novel stimuli requires the explicit identification, maintenance, and manipulation of sublexical phonological representations that can be mapped onto the corresponding orthographic units. Thus, nonword spelling places greater demands on phonological processing resources, including phonological short-term memory and phonological awareness, than spelling familiar real words. Consequently, the reduction in phonological capacity following perisylvian network damage will have a disproportionate impact on nonword processing, manifested by an increased lexicality effect in spelling. Phonological representations for familiar words are more resistant to phonological network damage and, unlike nonwords that have no meaning, they can receive additional activation from semantic representations supported by spared left-hemisphere extrasylvian cortical regions. Furthermore, some lexical items, particularly high-frequency concrete words, could potentially be spelled correctly without obligatory phonological mediation by relying on direct connections between semantic network nodes and orthographic lexical representations within the VWFA or by the successful integration of preserved semantic and degraded phonological inputs to orthography (Figures 5.1 and 5.2). Lastly, as we have seen, spelling by a lexical-semantic strategy can also be partially supported by language networks located within the intact right hemisphere (Figure 5.2). Thus, the redundant and bilateral organization of lexical-semantic networks may explain the relative sparing of real word spelling in phonological agraphia while the strong left-hemisphere lateralization of perisylvian cortical systems critical for sublexical phonological processing accounts for the disproportionate impairment of nonword spelling in these patients.

It should be readily apparent from our review of the relevant neuropsychological literature that the status of central phonological representations reflecting the integrity of perisylvian cortical regions is a key determinant of spelling performance in patients with agraphia following left-hemisphere damage. Poor phonological skills and impaired awareness of the phonological structure of spoken words are also considered core functional deficits in individuals with developmental dyslexia/dysgraphia and have been associated with structural and functional abnormalities within the same perisylvian cortical regions and white matter pathways that are implicated in acquired cases of phonological alexia/agraphia (e.g., Darki, Peyrard-Janvid, Matsson, Kere, & Klingberg, 2012; Richlan, Kronbichler, & Wimmer, 2009, 2013; Vandermosten et al., 2012). Thus, developmental abnormality or neurological damage affecting perisylvian cortical networks originally evolved for speech processing can both result in poorly structured phonological representations that cannot adequately support written language performance in general and sublexical phoneme-grapheme conversion in particular. The quality of phonological representations is also a powerful predictor of recovery from acquired agraphia and training phonological awareness skills along with regaining mastery of the alphabetic principle regarding the systematic mappings between individual sounds and letters are critical components of rehabilitation efforts in these patients (Beeson, Rising, Kim, & Rapcsak, 2010).

Agraphia Caused by Dysfunction of the Graphemic Buffer: The Role of Visuospatial Attention and Working Memory Systems in Spelling and Writing

Cognitive models of written language production postulate the existence of a graphemic buffer, conceptualized as a working memory system that maintains the orthographic representations generated by central spelling routes in a high state of accessibility while they are being converted into motor output by the peripheral components of the writing process. Damage to the buffer interferes with the processing of all activated graphemic representations, irrespective of lexical status (words vs. nonwords), lexical-semantic features (frequency, imageability, grammatical word class), or orthographic regularity. Stimulus length, however, has a strong effect on performance because each additional grapheme imposes further demands on limited orthographic working memory capacity. Dysfunction of the buffer results in the loss of information relevant to the serial order and identity of stored graphemes, leading to letter substitutions, omissions, additions, and transpositions (Caramazza, Miceli, Villa, & Romani, 1987). These grapheme-level errors give rise to phonologically inaccurate misspellings that frequently retain visual similarity to the target. The distribution of errors may be influenced by letter position. Specifically, some patients produce errors primarily on letters located at the end of the word, consistent with a serial left-to-right read-out process operating over a rapidly decaying orthographic memory trace, while in other cases, errors mostly involved letters in the middle of the word presumably because letters in internal positions are more susceptible to interference from neighboring items than letters located at either end (for reviews, see Buchwald & Rapp, 2009; Costa, Fischer-Baum, Capasso, Miceli, & Rapp, 2011). In addition to working memory capacity, the retrieval of information from the graphemic buffer may also be influenced by impairments affecting the allocation of visuospatial attention. For instance, it has been demonstrated that some patients with unilateral neglect produce more errors on the side of the word opposite their lesion, regardless of stimulus length and modality of output, and independent of whether they spell in conventional left-to-right order or in reverse (Baxter & Warrington, 1983; Caramazza & Hillis, 1990; Hillis & Caramazza, 1989, 1995). These observations are consistent with a unilateral disruption of attention over an internal orthographic representation in which the order of graphemes is spatially coded within a word-centered coordinate frame (Caramazza & Hillis, 1990).

In our neuroanatomical model, we assigned a central role to the VWFA in orthographic processing during spelling (Figure 5.2). In particular, we suggested that orthographic representations are addressed or assembled within this cortical region in response to converging input from neural networks involved in phonological and semantic processing. Thus, the VWFA serves as the critical neural interface for integrating orthographic information generated by the sublexical and lexical-semantic spelling routes (Figures 5.1 and 5.2). As we have seen, the VWFA also makes an essential contribution to orthographic processing during reading, and it is assumed that a common set of orthographic representations support both written word recognition and production. Reading also requires keeping orthographic information active in working memory while familiar letter combinations are identified and mapped onto their corresponding phonological and semantic representations. Therefore, temporary maintenance of orthographic representations computed within the VWFA is an important component of both reading and spelling, and it has been suggested that a common graphemic buffer supports both written language functions (Caramazza, et al., 1996; Tainturier & Rapp, 2003). Note, however, that reading and spelling make different demands on orthographic working memory capacity. Given the relatively slow, serial nature of written language production, orthographic representations need to be maintained in an active state longer during spelling than reading. Furthermore, whereas spelling words and nonwords both rely on serial processing, reading familiar words is normally accomplished by rapid parallel processing of multiple letter identities. As a result, only reading unfamiliar nonwords is likely to place significant demands on orthographic working memory because these items need to be decoded by a serial grapheme-phoneme conversion strategy (Tainturier & Rapp, 2003).

Functional imaging studies in normal subjects have attempted to localize the putative graphemic buffer by identifying cortical regions that showed sensitivity to word length manipulations during spelling. Specifically, Rapp and Dufor (2011) suggested that orthographic working memory was supported by a dorsal frontoparietal network composed of IPS/SPL and caudal SFS/posterior SFG/MFG. Neuropsychological observations in patients with spelling profiles indicative of damage to the graphemic buffer are consistent with this proposal, as the responsible lesions typically involved the same frontoparietal cortical areas (for reviews, see Cloutman et al., 2009; Purcell et al., 2011; Rapcsak & Beeson, 2002; Rapp & Dufor, 2011). Furthermore, consistent with the hypothesis that a common orthographic working memory system supports written word recognition and production, the dorsal frontoparietal cortical network is engaged during reading tasks, especially when processing unfamiliar nonwords or when stimuli are presented in an unusual format (vertical, rotated, or mirror-reversed) that interferes with rapid parallel word identification, forcing subjects to adopt an attention-demanding serial letter-by-letter strategy (Binder et al., 2005; Church et al., 2011; Cohen et al., 2008; Ihnen et al., 2013; Taylor et al., 2013; Valdois et al., 2006). Collectively, these results suggest that the maintenance of orthographic information during reading and spelling rely on functional interactions between the VWFA and the dorsal frontoparietal attention/working memory system. Regarding the nature of the proposed interaction, we suggest that the dorsal frontoparietal network performs the functions ascribed to the graphemic buffer by providing top-down attentional amplification and enhancement of orthographic representations computed within the VWFA during spelling and reading. The allocation of attentional resources is modulated by task difficulty, including the time required for maintaining orthographic representations in an active state during written word recognition and production. Additional contributions of the frontoparietal network to orthographic analysis include setting the size of the attentional window and thereby regulating the number of graphemes processed simultaneously, reducing interference from neighboring items, and directing attention to specific spatial locations within the graphemic string. Reduction in attentional resources following damage to the dorsal frontoparietal network can explain the characteristic clinical features of graphemic buffer agraphia, including the length-dependent loss of information about the identity and serial ordering of graphemes and also the unilateral spatial bias in spelling performance reported in some patients. Note that according to our proposal there is no independent and neuroanatomically distinct "graphemic buffer module" that receives and temporarily stores orthographic information, as implied by some cognitive models of spelling. Instead, orthographic working memory emerges from dynamic task-dependent modulations of functional connectivity between the VWFA and the dorsal frontoparietal network that provides top-down control of selective attention.

Although findings from functional imaging studies of reading/spelling in normal subjects and neuropsychological observations in patients with graphemic buffer agraphia strongly implicate dorsal frontoparietal cortex in orthographic working memory, the functions of this neural system are not specific to written language processing. Instead, the available evidence suggests that the dorsal attention network is recruited in a variety of cognitive tasks that require maintenance and manipulation of visuospatial information in working memory in preparation for movements directed toward behaviorally relevant objects and locations within external visual space (Corbetta & Shulman, 2002; Courtney et al., 1998; Ikkai & Curtis, 2011; Szczepanski et al., 2013). An example of this type of spatially oriented motor behavior is the production of handwriting movements.

Peripheral Agraphias

Peripheral agraphias reflect the breakdown of the cognitive and motor processes involved in converting orthographic information into handwriting movements. We will provide only a brief summary of these writing disorders here in order to highlight the relevant neural systems implicated. For a comprehensive review of the various peripheral agraphia syndromes and their neural correlates, see Rapcsak and Beeson (2002).

Impaired Selection, Programming, and Control of Handwriting Movements: Allographic Writing Disorders, Apraxic Agraphia, and Related Disorders of Motor Execution

Handwriting is a highly complex manual motor skill that takes several years to master. In addition to the fine motor control required for executing the stroke sequences needed to produce different letter shapes or allographs (Ellis, 1982) (uppercase vs. lowercase, print vs. script), the writing process involves visuomotor coordination and online monitoring of sensory feedback (Rapcsak & Beeson, 2002). Functional imaging studies in normal individuals have indicated that the programming and execution of writing movements are mediated by a left-lateralized dorsal frontoparietal cortical network (regardless of the hand used for writing), the key components of which include anterior IPS/SPL, caudal SFS/posterior SFG/MFG (Exner's area), SMA, and the primary sensorimotor area for the hand (for reviews, see Planton et al., 2013; Purcell et al., 2011). Handwriting also recruits subcortical structures involved in motor control, including basal ganglia, thalamus, and the cerebellum (Planton et al., 2013; Purcell et al., 2011).

As noted earlier, the IPS/SPL and caudal SFS/posterior SFG/MFG (Exner's area) components of the handwriting network have also been implicated in orthographic working memory

(Rapp & Dufor, 2011; Purcell et al., 2011). These observations underscore the intimate functional and neuroanatomical relationship between visuospatial working memory, attention, and the planning of spatially directed movements within dorsal frontoparietal cortex (Corbetta & Shulman, 2002; Courtney et al., 1998; Ikkai & Curtis, 2011; Szczepanski et al., 2013). Supported by shared neural substrates, these closely related cognitive operations are used to construct a priority map of space critical for transforming internal mental representations or behavioral goals into diverse visuomotor acts directed at objects or locations in the environment (Ikkai & Curtis, 2011). Writing can be considered a special example of this general class of visuomotor behaviors in which internally generated orthographic representations are used to guide motor actions of the hand in external space. Thus, translating orthographic representations into letter-specific motor programs, maintaining a map of external visual space suitable for motor planning and execution, and online monitoring of the evolving handwriting movement may all depend on partially overlapping or anatomically adjacent neural systems within left dorsal frontoparietal cortex. Although essential for converting orthographic information into movements of the pen, other spelling output modalities that involve spatially oriented hand movements would also be expected to engage the frontoparietal network. Consistent with this hypothesis, Purcell, Napoliello, and Eden, (2011) found that the frontoparietal cortical regions involved in the production of handwriting were also recruited during typing. By the same token, oral spelling and reading aloud should be associated with lower levels of activation within the dorsal frontoparietal network, because although these language tasks require orthographic working memory, they do not involve spatially oriented limb movements for motor execution. As noted earlier, consistent with the general role of dorsal frontoparietal cortex in the programming of visually guided limb movements, the cortical regions involved in handwriting also show robust activation during tool use and picture drawing. These observations support the view that handwriting builds on phylogenetically older neural networks originally evolved for visuomotor control of reaching/grasping and later adopted for skilled object use (cf., Segal & Petrides, 2011).

Lesion studies of patients with peripheral agraphia have confirmed the central role of left dorsal frontoparietal cortex in the programming and execution of handwriting movements. In particular, focal damage or cortical stimulation of IPS/SPL and SFG/MFG have been associated with allographic writing disorders characterized by defective activation or impaired selection of correct letter shapes for written production, implying faulty mapping between orthographic representations and letter-specific motor programs (Magrassi, Bongetta, Bianchini, Berardesca, & Arienta, 2010; Rapcsak & Beeson, 2002; Roux et al., 2009). Lesions involving dorsal frontoparietal cortex can also result in apraxic agraphia characterized by gross errors of letter morphology in written production (Alexander, Fischer, & Friedman, 1992; Rapcsak & Beeson, 2002; Sakurai et al., 2007). It has been suggested that apraxic agraphia following IPS/SPL lesions may reflect damage to graphic motor programs that contain abstract spatiotemporal information about the sequence of strokes necessary to produce different letters, whereas apraxic agraphia following damage to frontal premotor regions (Exner's area, SMA) results from an inability to translate the information contained in these programs into motor commands for neuromuscular execution (Rapcsak & Beeson, 2002). In addition to focal lesions, a progressive form of apraxic agraphia has been described in patients with neurodegenerative disorders that have a predilection for involving components of the dorsal frontoparietal motor network, including corticobasal degeneration (Heilman, Coenen, & Kluger, 2008; Passov, Gavrilova, Strand, Cerhan, & Josephs, 2011) and posterior cortical atrophy (Kas et al., 2011; Renner et al., 2004; Ross et al., 1996; Tsai, Teng, Liu, & Mendez, 2011; Whitwell et al., 2007). Finally, apraxic agraphia has been documented following damage to subcortical motor regions (thalamus, cerebellum) that are functionally integrated with dorsal frontoparietal cortex for the control of skilled limb movements (De Smet, Engelborghs, Paquier, De Deyn, & Marien, 2011; Ohno, Bando, Nagura, Ishii, & Yamanouchi, 2000). Damage to subcortical motor areas can also interfere with generating the appropriate kinematic parameters for writing movements resulting in defective control of writing force, speed, and amplitude. Examples of this type of motor writing disorder include the micrographia of patients with Parkinson's disease and the poorly coordinated writing movements produced by patients with cerebellar dysfunction (Rapcsak & Beeson, 2002). In all these peripheral agraphia syndromes oral spelling is preserved, providing evidence of the functional independence of neural systems that support the central components of written language production.

Conclusions

Learning to read and write is accompanied by experience-dependent functional reorganization within neural systems dedicated to spoken language production/comprehension, visual object recognition, and tool use. In literate adults, written language production involves both word- and subword-level translations between phonology, semantics and orthography mediated via the lexical-semantic and sublexical spelling pathways. In terms of neural substrates, evidence from functional imaging and lesion–deficit correlation studies suggests that during spelling orthographic representations are addressed or assembled within the VWFA in response to converging input from perisylvian phonological and extrasylvian semantic networks. At the clinical level, the breakdown of the lexical-semantic pathway results in the spelling profile of surface agraphia and is associated with lesions that either damage critical nodes within the distributed semantic network, degrade word-specific orthographic information within the VWFA, or disrupt the mapping between semantic and orthographic lexical representations. By contrast, damage to phonological representations supported by perisylvian cortical networks primarily interferes with the operations of the sublexical spelling pathway and gives rise to the syndrome of phonological agraphia. Orthographic representations computed within the VWFA are maintained in an active state and converted into motor commands for handwriting movements by partially overlapping neural networks within dorsal frontoparietal cortex that play a critical role in visuospatial attention, working memory, and the planning and execution of spatially oriented limb movements. Damage to these neural systems produces writing impairment attributable to reduced orthographic working memory capacity (graphemic buffer agraphia), or it may result in peripheral agraphia syndromes characterized by impaired selection and implementation of motor programs for handwriting movements (allographic writing disorders, apraxic agraphia). Defective execution of handwriting movements can also be associated with damage to subcortical motor areas that are functionally linked with the dorsal frontoparietal motor control network.

With respect to future directions, we believe that systematic comparisons of spelling performance and lesion profiles across groups of neurological patients with different disease etiologies (i.e., focal vs. degenerative) and in patients with acute (e.g., Hillis et al., 2002, 2005; Philipose et al., 2007; Sebastian et al., 2014) versus chronic stroke (e.g., Henry et al., 2007; Rapcsak & Beeson, 2004; Rapcsak et al., 2009) would be of considerable interest. We anticipate further that the combined use of high-resolution structural and functional neuroimaging techniques, both in patients with agraphia and in normal individuals, will continue to refine our understanding of the precise role of different cortical regions and white matter pathways in spelling and writing. In addition, multimodal neuroimaging methods have excellent potential for studying the dynamic reorganization of cortical networks in patients with agraphia following brain injury and can inform us about neural plasticity and also about the neurobiological correlates of behavioral change associated with various therapeutic interventions in written language rehabilitation.

Acknowledgment

This work was supported by NIH grants 2R01-DC07646 and P30AG19610.

References

Acheson, D.J., Hamidi, M., Binder, J.R., & Postle, B.R. (2011). A common neural substrate for language production and verbal working memory. *Journal of Cognitive Neuroscience, 23*(6), 1358–1367.

Ahn, H.-J., Seo, S.W., Chin, J., Suh, M.K., Lee, B.H., Kim, S.T., . . . Na, D.L. (2011). The cortical neuroanatomy of neuropsychological deficit in mild cognitive impairment and Alzheimer's disease: A surface-based morphometric analysis. *Neuropsychologia, 49*(14), 3931–3945.

Alexander, M.P., Fischer, R.S., & Friedman, R. (1992). Lesion localization in apractic agraphia. *Archives of Neurology, 49*(3), 246–251.

Ash, S., McMillan, C., Gunawardena, D., Avants, B., Morgan, B., Khan, A., . . . Grossman, M. (2010). Speech errors in progressive non-fluent aphasia. *Brain and Language, 113*(1), 13–20.

Barry, C., & Seymour, P.H.K. (1988). Lexical priming and sound-to-spelling contingency effects in nonword spelling. *Quarterly Journal of Experimental Psychology, 40*(1), 5–40.

Baxter, D.M., & Warrington, E.K. (1983). Neglect dysgraphia. *Journal of Neurology, Neurosurgery, and Psychiatry, 46*(12), 1073–1078.

Beauvois, M.F., & Dérouesné, J. (1981). Lexical or orthographic agraphia. *Brain, 104*(1), 21–49.

Beeson, P.M., & Henry, M.L. (2008). Comprehension and production of written words. In R. Chapey (Ed.), Language intervention strategies in aphasia and related neurogenic communication disorders (5th ed.) (pp. 159–165). Baltimore: Lippincott, Williams and Wilkins.

Beeson, P.M., & Rapcsak, S.Z. (2003). The neural substrates of sublexical spelling. *Journal of the International Neuropsychological Society, 9*, 304.

Beeson, P.M., Rapcsak, S.Z., Plante, E., Chargualaf, J., Chung, A., Johnson, S.C., & Trouard, T.P. (2003). The neural substrates of writing: A functional magnetic resonance imaging study. *Aphasiology, 17*(6–7), 647–665.

Beeson, P.M., Rising, K., Kim, E.S., & Rapcsak, S.Z. (2010). A treatment sequence for phonological alexia/agraphia. *Journal of Speech, Language, and Hearing Research, 53*(2), 450–468.

Beeson, P.M., Rising, K., Howard, T., Northrop, E., Wilheim, R., Wilson, S., & Rapcsak, S. (2012). The nature and treatment of phonological text agraphia. *Procedia—Social and Behavioral Sciences, 61*, 22–23.

Behrmann, M., & Plaut, D.C. (2013). Distributed circuits not circumscribed centers mediate visual recognition. *Trends in Cognitive Sciences, 17*(5), 210–219.

Behrmann, M., & Plaut, D.C. (2014). Bilateral hemispheric processing of words and faces: Evidence from word impairments in prosopagnosia and face impairments in pure alexia. *Cerebral Cortex, 24*(4) 1102–1118.

Binder, J.R., Medler, D.A., Desai, R., Conant, L.L., & Liebenthal, E. (2005). Some neurophysiological constraints on models of word naming. *NeuroImage, 27*(3), 677–693.

Binder, J.R., Desai, R.H., Graves, W.W., & Conant, L.L. (2009). Where is the semantic system? A critical review and meta-analysis of 120 functional neuroimaging studies. *Cerebral Cortex, 19*(12), 2767–2796.

Bonner, M.F., Peelle, J.E., Cook, P.A., & Grossman, M. (2013). Heteromodal conceptual processing in angular gyrus. *NeuroImage, 71*, 175–186.

Bowers, J.S., Bub, D., & Arguin, M.A. (1996). Characterization of the word superiority effect in a case of letter-by-letter surface alexia. *Cognitive Neuropsychology, 13*(3), 415–441.

Brambati, S.M., Ogar, J., Neuhaus, J., Miller, B.L., & Gorno-Tempini, M.L. (2009). Reading disorders in primary progressive aphasia: A behavioral and neuroimaging study. *Neuropsychologia, 47*(8), 1893–1900.

Brownsett, S.L.E., & Wise, R.J.S. (2010). The contribution of the parietal lobes to speaking and writing. *Cerebral Cortex, 20*(3), 517–523.

Bruno, J.L., Zumberge, A., Manis, F.R., Lu, Z.-L., Goldman, J.G. (2008). Sensitivity to orthographic familiarity in the occipito-temporal region. *NeuroImage, 39*(4), 1988–2001.

Bub, D., & Kertesz, A. (1982a). Deep agraphia. *Brain and Language, 17*(1), 146–165.

Bub, D., & Kertesz, A. (1982b). Evidence for lexicographic processing in a patient with preserved written over oral single word naming. *Brain, 105*(4), 697–717.

Buchsbaum, B.R., Baldo, J., Okada, K., Berman, K.F., Dronkers, N., D'Esposito, M., & Hickok, G. (2011). Conduction aphasia, sensory-motor integration, and phonological short-term memory—an aggregate analysis of lesion and fMRI data. *Brain and Language, 119*(3), 119–128.

Buchwald, A., & Rapp, B. (2009). Distinctions between orthographic long-term memory and working memory. *Cognitive Neuropsychology, 26*(8), 724–751.

Burton, M.W., LoCasto, P.C., Krebs-Noble, D., & Gullapalli, R.P. (2005). A systematic investigation of the functional neuroanatomy of auditory and visual phonological processing. *NeuroImage, 26*(3), 647–661.

Caine, D., Breen, N., & Patterson, K. (2009). Emergence and progression of "non-semantic" deficits in semantic dementia. *Cortex, 45*(4), 483–494.

Caramazza, A., Miceli, G., Villa, G., & Romani, C. (1987). The role of the graphemic buffer in spelling: Evidence from a case of acquired dysgraphia. *Cognition, 26*(1), 59–85.

Caramazza, A., & Hillis, A.E. (1990). Spatial representation of words in the brain implied by studies of a unilateral neglect patient. *Nature, 346*(6281), 267–269.

Caramazza, A., Capasso, R., & Miceli, G. (1996). The role of the graphemic buffer in reading. *Cognitive Neuropsychology, 13*(5), 673–698.

Choi, S.H., Na, D.L., Kang, E., Lee, K.M., Lee, S.W., & Na, D.G. (2001). Functional magnetic resonance imaging during pantomiming tool-use gestures. *Experimental Brain Research, 139*(3), 311–317.

Church, J.A., Balota, D.A., Petersen, S.E., & Schlaggar, B.L. (2011). Manipulation of length and lexicality localizes the functional neuroanatomy of phonological processing in adult readers. *Journal of Cognitive Neuroscience, 23*(6), 1475–1493.

Cloutman, L., Gingis, L., Newhart, M., Davis, C., Heidler-Gary, J., Crinion, J., & Hillis, A.E. (2009). A neural network critical for spelling. *Archives of Neurology, 66*(2), 249–253.

Cohen, L., Lehéricy, S., Chochon, F., Lemer, C., Rivaud, S., & Dehaene, S. (2002). Language-specific tuning of visual cortex? Functional properties of the Visual Word Form Area. *Brain, 125*(5), 1054–1069.

Cohen L., Dehaene S., Vinckier F., Jobrt, A., & Montavont, A. (2008). Reading normal and degraded words: Contribution of the dorsal and ventral visual pathways. *NeuroImage, 40*(1), 353–366.

Coltheart, M. (1980). Deep dyslexia: A right hemisphere hypothesis. In M. Coltheart, K. Patterson, & J. Marshall (Eds.). *Deep dyslexia* (pp. 326–380). London: Routledge & Kegan Paul.

Corbetta, M., & Shulman, G.L. (2002). Control of goal-directed and stimulus-driven attention in the brain. *Nature Reviews Neuroscience, 3*(3), 210–215.

Costa, V., Fischer-Baum, S., Capasso, R., Miceli, G., & Rapp, B. (2011). Temporal stability and representational distinctiveness: Key functions of orthographic working memory. *Cognitive Neuropsychology, 28*(5), 338–362.

Courtney, S.M., Petit, L., Maisog, J.M., Ungerleider, L.G., & Haxby, J.V. (1998). An area specialized for spatial working memory in human frontal cortex. *Science, 279*(5355), 1347–1351.

Crisp, J., & Lambon Ralph, M.A. (2006). Unlocking the nature of the phonological-deep dyslexia continuum: The keys to reading aloud are in phonology and semantics. *Journal of Cognitive Neuroscience, 18*(3), 348–362.

Croisile, B., Carmoi, T., Adeleine, P., & Trillet, M. (1995). Spelling in Alzheimer's disease. *Behavioral Neurology, 8*(3–4), 135–143.

Croisile, B., Brabant, M. J, Carmoi, T., Lepage, Y., Aimard, G., & Trillet, M. (1996). Comparison between oral and written spelling in Alzheimer's disease. *Brain and Language, 54*(3), 361–387.

Darki, F., Peyrard-Janvid, M., Matsson, H., Kere, J., & Klingberg, T. (2012). Three dyslexia susceptibility genes DYX1C1, DCDC2, and KIAA0319, affect temporo-parietal white matter structure. *Biological Psychiatry, 72*(8), 671–676.

Dehaene, S., & Cohen, L. (2007). Cultural recycling of cortical maps. *Neuron, 56*(2), 384–398.

Dehaene, S., & Cohen, L. (2011). The unique role of the visual word form area in reading. *Trends in Cognitive Sciences, 15*(6), 254–262.

DeMarco, A.T., Wilson, S.M., Rising, K., Rapcsak, S.Z., & Beeson, P.M. (in preparation). Neural substrates of sublexical processing for spelling.

Derrfuss, J., Brass, M., Neumann, J., & von Cramon, D.Y. (2005). Involvement of the inferior frontal junction in cognitive control: Meta-analysis of switching and Stroop studies. *Human Brain Mapping, 25*(1), 22–34.

De Smet, H.J., Engelborghs, S., Paquier, P.F., De Deyn, P.P., & Marien, P. (2011). Cerebellar induced apraxic agraphia: a review and three new cases. *Brain and Cognition, 76*(3), 424–434.

Domoto-Reilly, K., Sapolsky, D., Brickhouse, M., & Dickerson, B.C. (2012). Naming impairment in Alzheimer's disease is associated with left anterior temporal lobe atrophy. *NeuroImage, 63*, 348–355.

Ellis, A.W. (1982). Spelling and writing (and reading and speaking). In A.W. Ellis (Ed.), *Normality and pathology in cognitive functions*. London: Academic Press.

Ellis, A.W. (1988). Normal writing processes and peripheral acquired dysgraphias. *Language and Cognitive Processes, 3*(2), 99–127.

Epelbaum, S., Pinel, P., Gaillard, R., Delmaire, C., Perrin, M., Dupont, S., Dehaene, S., & Cohen, L. (2008). Pure alexia as a disconnection syndrome: New diffusion imaging evidence for an old concept. *Cortex, 44*, 962–974.

Faria, A.V., Crinion, J., Tsapkini, K., Newhart, M., Davis, C., Cooley, S., . . . Hillis, A.E. (2013). Patterns of dysgraphia in primary progressive aphasia compared to post-stroke aphasia. *Behavioural Neurology, 26*(1–2), 21–34.

Folk, J.R., Rapp, B., & Goldrick, M. (2002). The interaction of lexical and sublexical information in spelling: what is the point? *Cognitive Neuropsychology, 19*(7), 653–671.

Frey, S.H. (2008). Tool use, communicative gesture and cerebral asymmetries in the modern human brain. *Philosophical Transactions of the Royal Society of Biological Sciences, 363*(1499), 1951–1957.

Friedman, R.B., & Hadley, J.A. (1992). Letter-by-letter surface alexia. *Cognitive Neuropsychology, 9*(3), 185–208.

Galantucci, S., Tartaglia, M.C., Wilson, S.M., Henry, M.L., Filippi, M., Agosta, F., . . . Gorno-Tempini, M.L. (2011). White matter damage in primary progressive aphasia: A diffusion tensor tractography study. *Brain, 134*(10), 3011–3029.

Gelb, I.J. (1963). *A study of writing*. Chicago: University of Chicago Press.

Gorno-Tempini, M.L., Dronkers, N.F., Rankin, K.P., Ogar, J.M., Phengrasamy, L., Rosen, H.J., . . . Miller, B.L. (2004). Cognition and anatomy in three variants of primary progressive aphasia. *Annals of Neurology, 55*(3), 335–346.

Gorno-Tempini, M.L., Brambati, S.M., Ginex, V., Ogar, J., Dronkers, N.F., Marcone, A., . . . Miller, B.L. (2008). The logopenic/phonological variant of primary progressive aphasia. *Neurology, 71*(16), 1227–1234.

Gorno-Tempini, M.L., Hillis, A.E., Weintraub, S., Kertesz, A., Mendez, M.F., Cappa, S.F., . . . Grossman, M. (2011). Classification of primary progressive aphasia and its variants. *Neurology, 76*(11), 1006–1014.

Graham, N.L. (2014). Dysgraphia in primary progressive aphasia: Characterisation of impairments and therapy options. *Aphasiology, 28(8–9)*, 1092–1111.

Graham, N.L., Patterson, K., & Hodges, J.R. (2000). The impact of semantic memory impairment on spelling: Evidence from semantic dementia. *Neuropsychologia, 38*(2), 143–163.

Graves, W.W., Desai, R., Humphries, C., Seidenberg, M.S., & Binder, J.R. (2010). Neural systems for reading aloud: A multiparametric approach. *Cerebral Cortex, 20*(8), 1799–1815.

Grossman, M. (2012). The non-fluent/agrammatic variant of primary progressive aphasia. *Lancet Neurology, 11*(6), 545–555.

Harnish, S.M., & Neils-Strunjas, J. (2008). In search of meaning: reading and writing in Alzheimer's disease. *Seminars in Speech and Language, 29*(1), 44–59.

Harrington, G.S., Farias, D., Davis, C.H., & Buonocore, M.H. (2007). Comparison of the neural basis for imagined writing and drawing. *Human Brain Mapping, 28*(5), 450–459.

Harrington, G.S., Farias, D., & Davis, C.H. (2009). The neural basis for simulated drawing and the semantic implications. *Cortex, 45*(3), 386–393.

Heilman, K.M., Coenen, A., & Kluger, B. (2008). Progressive asymmetric apraxic agraphia. *Cognitive and Behavioral Neurology, 21*(1), 14–17.

Henry, M.L., Beeson, P.M., Stark, A.J., & Rapcsak, S.Z. (2007). The role of left perisylvian cortical regions in spelling. *Brain and Language, 100*(1), 44–52.

Henry, M.L., Beeson, P.M., Alexander, G.E., & Rapcsak, S.Z. (2012). Written language impairments in primary progressive aphasia: a reflection of damage to central semantic and phonological processes. *Journal of Cognitive Neuroscience, 24*(2), 261–275.

Hermsdorfer, J., Terlinden, G., Muhlau, M., Goldenberg, G., & Wohlschlager, A.M. (2007). Neural representations of pantomimed and actual tool use: evidence from an event-related fMRI study. *NeuroImage, 36*(2), T109–T118.

Hickok, G., & Poeppel, D. (2007). The cortical organization of speech processing. *Nature Reviews Neuroscience, 8*(5), 393–402.

Hillis, A.E., & Caramazza, A. (1989). The graphemic buffer and attentional mechanisms. *Brain and Language, 36*(2), 208–235.

Hillis, A.E., & Caramazza, A. (1995). Spatially specific deficits in processing graphemic representations in reading and writing. *Brain and Language, 48*(3), 263–308.

Hillis A.E., Kane A., Tuffiash E., Beauchamp, N.J., Barker, P.B., Jacobs, M.A., & Wityk, R.J. (2002). Neural substrates of the cognitive processes underlying spelling: Evidence from MR diffusion and perfusion imaging. *Aphasiology, 16(4–6)*, 425–438.

Hillis, A.E., Chang, S., Breese, E., & Heidler, J. (2004). The crucial role of posterior frontal regions in modality specific components of the spelling process. *Neurocase, 10*(2), 175–187.

Hillis A.E., Newhart M., Heidler J., Barker, P., Herskovits, E., & Degaonkar, M. (2005). The roles of the "visual word form area" in reading. *NeuroImage, 24(2)*. 548–559.

Hirini, D.I., Kivisaari, S.L., Monsch, A.U., & Taylor, K.I. (2013). Distinct neuroanatomical bases of episodic and semantic memory performance in Alzheimer's disease. *Neuropsychologia, 51*(5), 930–937.

Hodges J.R., & Patterson K. (2007). Semantic dementia: a unique clinicopathological syndrome. *Lancet Neurology, 6*(11), 1004–1014.

Hughes, J.C., Graham, N., Patterson, K., & Hodges, J.R. (1997). Dysgraphia in mild dementia of Alzheimer's type. *Neuropsychologia, 35*(4), 533–545.

Ihnen, S.K.Z., Petersen, S.E., & Schlaggar, B.L. (2013). Separable roles for attention control subsystems in reading tasks: A combined behavioral and fMRI study. *Cerebral Cortex*. doi:10.1093/cercor/bht313

Ikkai, A., & Curtis, C.E. (2011). Common neural mechanisms supporting spatial working memory, attention, and motor intention. *Neuropsychologia, 49*(6), 1428–1434.

Jefferies, E., & Lambon Ralph, M.A. (2006). Semantic impairment in stroke aphasia versus semantic dementia: A case series comparison. *Brain, 129*(8), 2132–2147.

Jefferies, E., Sage, K., & Lambon Ralph, M.A. (2007). Do deep dyslexia, dysphasia and dysgraphia share a common phonological impairment? *Neuropsychologia, 45*(7), 1553–1570.

Jefferies, E., Rogers, T.T., Hopper, S., & Lambon Ralph, M.A. (2010). "Pre-semantic" cognition revisited: critical differences between semantic aphasia and semantic dementia. *Neuropsychologia, 48*(1), 248–261.

Jobard, G., Crivello, F., & Tzourio-Mazoyer, N. (2003). Evaluation of the dual route theory of reading: A meta-analysis of 35 neuroimaging studies. *NeuroImage, 20*(2), 693–712.

Johnson-Frey, S.H. (2004). The neural basis of complex tool use in humans. *Trends in Cognitive Sciences, 8*(2), 71–78.

Johnson-Frey, S.H., Newman-Norlund, R., & Grafton, S.T. (2005). A distributed left hemisphere network active during planning of everyday tool use skills. *Cerebral Cortex, 15*(6), 681–695.

Joubert, S., Brambati, S.M., Ansado, J., Barbeau, E.J., Felician, O., Didic, M., . . . Kergoat, M.-J. (2010). The cognitive and neural expression of semantic memory impairment in mild cognitive impairment and early Alzheimer's disease. *Neuropsychologia, 48*(4), 978–988.

Kas, A., de Souza, L.C., Samri, D., Bartolomeo, P., Lacomblez, L., Kalafat, M., . . . Sarazin, M. (2011). Neural correlates of cognitive impairment in posterior cortical atrophy. *Brain, 134*(5), 1464–1478.

Katzir, T., Misra, M., & Poldrack, R.A. (2005). Imaging phonology without print: Assessing the neural correlates of phonemic awareness using fMRI. *NeuroImage, 27*(1), 106–115.

Kravitz, D.J., Saleem, K.S., Baker, C.I., Ungerleider, L.G., & Mishkin, M. (2013). The ventral visual pathway: An expanded neural framework for the processing of object quality. *Trends in Cognitive Sciences, 17*(1), 26–49.

Kronbichler, M., Hutzler, F., Wimmer, H., Mair, A., Staffen, W., & Ladurner, G. (2004). The visual word form area and the frequency with which words are encountered: Evidence from a parametric fMRI study. *NeuroImage, 21*(3), 946–953.

Kronbichler, M., Bergmann, J., Hutzler, F., Staffen, W., Mair, A., Ladurner, G., & Wimmer, H. (2007). Taxi vs. taksi: On orthographic word recognition in the left ventral occipitotemporal cortex. *Journal of Cognitive Neuroscience, 19*(10), 1584–1594.

Lambert, J., Giffard, B., Nore, F, de la Sayette, V., Pasquier, F., & Eustache, F. (2007). Central and peripheral agraphia in Alzheimer's disease: From the case of Auguste D. to a cognitive neuropsychology approach. *Cortex, 43*(7), 935–951.

Lambon Ralph, M.A., & Patterson, K. (2005). Acquired disorders of reading. In M.J. Snowling & C. Hulme (Eds.). *The science of reading: A handbook* (pp. 413–430). Malden, MA: Blackwell Publishing.

Ludersdorfer, P., Kronbichler, M., & Wimmer, H. (2015). Accessing orthographic representations from speech: the role of left ventral occipitotemporal cortex in spelling. *Human Brain Mapping*, in press.

Luria, A.R. (1980). *Higher cortical function in man* (2nd ed.). New York: Basic Books.

Magrassi, L., Bongetta, D., Bianchini, S., Berardesca, M., & Arienta, C. (2010). Central and peripheral components of writing depend on a defined area of the dominant superior parietal gyrus. *Brain Research, 1346*, 145–154.

Mano, Q.R., Humphries, C., Desai, R.H., Seidenberg, M.S., Osmon, D.C., Stengel, B.C., & Binder, J.R. (2013). The role of left occipitotemporal cortex in reading: Reconciling, stimulus, task, and lexicality effects. *Cerebral Cortex, 23*(4), 988–1001.

McCandliss, B.D., Cohen, L., & Dehaene, S. (2003). The visual word form area: Expertise for reading in the fusiform gyrus. *Trends in Cognitive Sciences, 7*(7), 293–299.

Mechelli, A., Gorno-Tempini, M.L., & Price, C.J. (2003). Neuroimaging studies of word and pseudo-word reading: Consistencies, inconsistencies, and limitations. *Journal of Cognitive Neuroscience, 15*(2), 260–271.

Mesulam, M.-M. (2013). Primary progressive aphasia and the language network: The 2013 H. Houston Merrit Lecture. *Neurology, 81*(5), 456–462.

Mion, M., Patterson, K., Acosta-Cabronero, J., Pengas, G., Izquierdo-Garcia, D., Hong, Y.T., . . . Nestor, P.J. (2010). What the left and right anterior fusiform gyri tell us about semantic memory. *Brain, 133*(11), 3256–3268.

Moll, J., de Oliveira-Souza, R., Passman, L.J., Cunha, F.C., Souza-Lima, F., & Andreiuolo, P.A. (2000). Functional MRI correlates of real and imagined tool-use pantomimes. *Neurology, 54*(6), 1331–1336.

Nee, D.E., Brown, J.W., Askren, M.K., Berman, M.G., Demiralp, E., Krawitz, A., & Jonides, J. (2013). A meta-analysis of executive components of working memory. *Cerebral Cortex, 23*(2), 264–282.

Neils, J., Roeltgen, D.P., & Constantinidou, F. (1995). Decline in homophone spelling associated with loss of semantic influence on spelling in Alzheimer's disease. *Brain and Language, 49*(1), 27–49.

Noonan, K.A., Jefferies, E., Visser, M., & Lambon Ralph, M.A. (2013). Going beyond inferior prefrontal involvement in semantic control: evidence for the additional contribution of dorsal angular gyrus and posterior middle temporal cortex. *Journal of Cognitive Neuroscience, 25*(11), 1824–1850.

Ogden, J.A. (1996). Phonological dyslexia and phonological dysgraphia following left and right hemispherectomy. *Neuropsychologia, 34*(9), 905–918.

Ohno, T., Bando, M., Nagura, H., Ishii, K., & Yamanouchi, H. (2000). Apraxic agraphia due to thalamic infarction. *Neurology, 54*(12), 2336–2339.

Patterson, K.E., & Kay, J. (1982). Letter-by-letter reading: Psychological descriptions of a neurological syndrome. *Quarterly Journal of Experimental Psychology, 34*(3), 411–441.

Patterson, K., Suzuki, T., & Wydell, T.N. (1996). Interpreting a case of Japanese phonological alexia: The key is in phonology. *Cognitive Neuropsychology, 13*(6), 803–822.

Patterson, K., & Lambon Ralph, M.A. (1999). Selective disorders of reading? *Current Opinion in Neurobiology, 9*(2), 235–239.

Patterson, K., Lambon Ralph, M.A., Jefferies, E., Woollams, A., Jones, R., Hodges, J.R., & Rogers, T.T. (2006). "Presemantic" cognition in semantic dementia: Six deficits in search of an explanation. *Journal of Cognitive Neuroscience, 18*(2), 169–183.

Patterson, K., Nestor, P.J., & Rogers, T.T. (2007). Where do you know what you know. *Nature Reviews Neuroscience, 8*(12), 976–987.

Passov, V., Gavrilova, R.H., Strand, E., Cerhan, J.H., & Josephs, K.A. (2011). Sporadic corticobasal syndrome with progranulin mutation presenting as progressive apraxic agraphia. *Archives of Neurology, 68*(3), 376–380.

Peigneux, P., Van der Linden, M., Garraux, G., Laureys, S., Degueldre, C., Aerts, J., Del Fiore, G., Moonen, G., Luxen, A., & Salmon, E. (2004). Imaging a cognitive model of apraxia: The neural substrate of gesture-specific cognitive processes. *Human Brain Mapping, 21*(3), 119–142.

Penniello, M.-J., Lambert, J., Eustache, F., Petit-Taboué, M.C., Barré, L., Viader, F., ... Baron, J.-C. (1995). A PET study of the functional neuroanatomy of writing impairment in Alzheimer's disease: The role of the left supramarginal and angular gyri. *Brain, 118*(3), 697–707.

Philipose L.E., Gottesman R.F., Newhart M., Kleinman, J.T., Herskovits, E.H., Pawlak, M.A., ... Hillis, A.E. (2007). Neural regions essential for reading and spelling of words and pseudowords. *Annals of Neurology, 62*(5), 481–192.

Planton, S., Jucla, M., Roux., F.E., & Demonet, J.-F. (2013). The "handwriting brain": A meta-analysis of neuroimaging studies of motor versus orthographic processes. *Cortex, 49*(10), 2772–2787.

Platel, H., Lambert, J, Eustache, F., Cadet, B., Dary, M., Viader, F., & Lechevalier, B. (1993). Characteristic evolution of writing impairment in Alzheimer's disease. *Neuropsychologia, 31*, 1147–1158.

Price, C.J. (2012). A review and synthesis of the first 20 years of PET and fMRI studies of heard speech, spoken language and reading. *NeuroImage, 62*(2), 816–847.

Price, C.J., & Devlin, J.T. (2011). The Interactive Account of ventral occipitotemporal contributions to reading. *Trends in Cognitive Sciences, 15*(6), 246–253.

Purcell, J.J., Napoliello, E.M., & Eden, G.F. (2011). A combined fMRI study of typed spelling and reading. *NeuroImage, 55*(2), 750–762.

Purcell, J.J., Turkeltaub, P.E., Eden, G.F., & Rapp, B. (2011). Examining the central and peripheral processes of written word production through meta-analysis. *Frontiers in Psychology, 2*, 239.

Purcell, J.J., Shea, J., & Rapp, B. (2014). Beyond the visual word form area: The orthography-semantics interface in spelling and reading. *Cognitive Neuropsychology* [e-pub ahead of print].

Rapcsak, S.Z., Arthur, S.A., & Rubens, A. B. (1988). Lexical agraphia from focal lesion of the left precentral gyrus. *Neurology, 38*(7), 1119.

Rapcsak, S.Z., Arthur, S. A., Bliklen, D. A., & Rubens, A.B. (1989). Lexical agraphia in Alzheimer's disease. *Archives of Neurology, 46*(1), 66–68.

Rapcsak, S.Z., & Beeson P.M. (2002). Neuroanatomical correlates of spelling and writing. In A.E. Hillis (Ed.), *Handbook of adult language disorders: Integrating cognitive neuropsychology, neurology, and rehabilitation* (pp. 71–99). Philadelphia: Psychology Press.

Rapcsak, S.Z., & Beeson, P.M. (2004). The role of left posterior inferior temporal cortex in spelling. *Neurology, 62*(12), 2221–2229.

Rapcsak, S., Beeson, P., Henry, M., Leyden, A., Kim, E., Rising, K., Andersen, S., & Cho, H. (2009). Phonological dyslexia and dysgraphia: Cognitive mechanisms and neural substrates. *Cortex, 45*(5), 575–591.

Rapcsak, S.Z., Beeson, P.M., & Rubens, A.B. (1991). Writing with the right hemisphere. *Brain and Language, 41*(4), 510–530.

Rapcsak, S.Z., & Rubens, A.B. (1990). Disruption of semantic influence on writing following a left prefrontal lesion. *Brain and Language, 38*(2), 334–344.

Rapcsak, S., Rubens, A.B., & Laguna, J. (1990). From letters to words: Procedures for word recognition in letter-by-letter reading. *Brain and Language, 38(4)*, 504–514.

Rapcsak, S.Z., Henry, M.L., Teague, S.L., Carnahan, S.D., & Beeson, P.M. (2007). Do dual-route models accurately predict reading and spelling performance in individuals with acquired alexia and agraphia? *Neuropsychologia, 45*(11), 2519–2524.

Rapp, B., Epstein, C., & Tainturier, M.J. (2002). The integration of information across lexical and sublexical processes in spelling. *Cognitive Neuropsychology, 19*(1), 1–29.

Rapp, B., & Lipka, K. (2010). The literate brain: the relationship between spelling and reading. *Journal of Cognitive Neuroscience, 23*(5), 1–18.

Rapp, B., & Dufor, O. (2011). The neurotopography of written word production: An fMRI investigation of the distribution of sensitivity to length and frequency. *Journal of Cognitive Neuroscience, 23*(12), 4067–4081.

Renner, J.A., Burns, J.M., Hou, C.E., McKeel, D.W., Storandt, M., & Morris, J.C. (2004). Progressive posterior cortical dysfunction. A clinicopathological series. *Neurology, 63*(7), 1175–1180.

Richlan, F., Kronbichler, M., & Wimmer, H. (2009). Functional abnormalities in the dyslexic brain: A quantitative meta-analysis of neuroimaging studies. *Human Brain Mapping, 30*(10), 3299–3308.

Richlan, F., Kronbichler, M., & Wimmer, H. (2013). Structural abnormalities in the dyslexic brain: A meta-analysis of voxel-based morphometry studies. *Human Brain Mapping, 34*(11), 3055–3065.

Roberts, D.J., Woollams, A.M., Kim, E., Beeson, P.M., Rapcsak, S.Z., & Lambon Ralph, M.A. (2013). Efficient visual object and word recognition relies on high spatial frequency coding in the left posterior fusiform gyrus: Evidence from a case-series of patients with ventral occipito-temporal cortex damage. *Cerebral Cortex, 23*(11), 2568–2580.

Roeltgen, D.P., & Heilman, K.M. (1984). Lexical agraphia: Further support for the two-system hypothesis of linguistic agraphia. *Brain, 107*(3), 811–827.

Roeltgen, D.P., Rothi, L.G., & Heilman, K.M. (1986). Linguistic semantic agraphia: A dissociation of the lexical spelling system from semantics. *Brain and Language, 27*(2), 257–280.

Ross, S.J.M., Graham, N., Stuart-Green, L., Prins, M., Xuereb, J., Patterson, K., & Hodges, J.R. (1996). Progressive biparietal atrophy: An atypical presentation of Alzheimer's disease. *Journal of Neurology, Neurosurgery, and Psychiatry, 61*(4), 388–395.

Roux, F.E., Dufor, O., Giussani, C., Wamain, Y., Draper, L., Longcamp, M., & Demonet, J.F. (2009). The graphemic/motor frontal area Exner's area revisited. *Annals of Neurology, 66*(4), 537–545.

Roux, F.E., Durand, J.B., Rehault, E., Reddy, M., & Demonet, J.F. (2012). Segregation of lexical and sub-lexical reading processes in left perisylvian cortex. *PLoS ONE, 7*(11), e50665. doi:10.1371/journal. pone.0050665

Roux, F.E., Durand, J.B., Rehault, E., Planton, S., Draper, L., & Demonet, J.F. (2014). The neural basis for writing from dictation in the temporoparietal cortex. *Cortex, 50*, 64–75.

Sakurai, Y., Onuma, Y., Nakazawa, G., Ugawa, Y., Momose, T., Tsuji, S., & Mannen, T. (2007). Parietal dysgraphia: characterization of abnormal writing stroke sequences, character formation and character recall. *Behavioral Neurology, 18*(2), 99–114.

Sebastian R., Gomez Y., Leigh R., Davis C., Newhart M., & Hillis A.E. (2014). The roles of occipitotemporal cortex in reading, spelling, and naming. *Cognitive Neuropsychology.* [e-pub ahead of print]

Segal, E., & Petrides, M. (2011). The anterior superior parietal lobule and its interactions with language and motor areas during writing. *European Journal of Neuroscience, 35*(2), 1–14.

Sepelyak, K., Crinion, J., Molitoris, J., Epstein-Peterson, Z., Bann, M., Davis, C., . . . Hillis, A.E. (2011). Patterns of breakdown in spelling in primary progressive aphasia. *Cortex, 47*(3), 342–352.

Shallice, T. (1981). Phonological agraphia and the lexical route in writing. *Brain, 104*(3), 413–429.

Shim, H.S., Hurley, R.S., Rogalski, E., & Mesulam, M.-M. (2012). Anatomic, clinical, and neuropsychological correlates of spelling errors in primary progressive aphasia. *Neuropsychologia, 50*(8), 1929–1935.

Szczepanski, S.M., Pinsk, M.A., Douglas, M.M., Kastner, S., & Saalmann, Y.B. (2013). Functional and structural architecture of the human dorsal frontoparietal attention network. *Proceedings of the National Academy of Science, 110*(39), 15806–15811.

Sugihara, G., Kaminaga, T., & Sugishita, M. (2006). Interindividual uniformity and variety of the "Writing center": A functional MRI study. *NeuroImage, 32*(4), 1837–1849.

Tainturier, M.J., & Rapp, B. (2003). Is a single graphemic buffer used in reading and spelling? *Aphasiology, 17*(6–7), 537–562.

Taylor, J.S.H., Rastle, K., Davis, M.H. (2013). Can cognitive models explain brain activation during word and pseudoword reading? *Psychological Bulletin, 139*(4), 766–791.

Tsai, P.H., Teng, E., Liu, C., & Mendez, M.F. (2011). Posterior cortical atrophy: Evidence for discrete syndromes of early onset Alzheimer's disease. *American Journal of Alzheimer's Disease & Other Dementias, 26*(5), 413–418.

Tsapkini K., & Rapp, B. (2010). The orthography-specific functions of the left fusiform gyrus: evidence of modality and category specificity. *Cortex, 46*(2), 185–205.

Valdois, S., Carbonell, S., Juphard, A., Baciu, M., Ans, B., Peyrin, C., & Segebarth, C. (2006). Polysyllabic pseudo-word processing in reading and lexical decision: Converging evidence from behavioral data, connectionist stimulations and functional MRI. *Brain Research, 1085*(1), 149–162.

Vandermosten, M., Boests, B., Poelmans, H., Sunaert, S., Wouters, J., & Ghesquiere, P. (2012). A tractography study of dyslexia: Neuroanatomic correlates of orthographic, phonological, and speech processing. *Brain, 135*(3), 935–948.

Vanier, M., & Caplan, D. (1985). CT correlates of surface dyslexia. In K.E. Patterson, J.C. Marshall, & M. Coltheart (Eds.). *Surface dyslexia: Neuropsychological and cognitive studies of phonological reading.* London: Lawrence Erlbaum.

Vigneau, M., Beaucousin, V., Hervé, P.Y., Duffau, H., Crivello, F., Houdé, O., Mazoyer, B., & Tzourio-Mazoyer, N. (2006). Meta-analyzing left hemisphere language areas: Phonology, semantics, and sentence processing. *NeuroImage, 30*(4), 1414–1432.

Visser, M., Jefferies, E., & Lambon Ralph, M.A. (2009). Semantic processing in the anterior temporal lobes: A meta-analysis of the functional neuroimaging literature. *Journal of Cognitive Neuroscience, 22*(6), 1083–1094.

Vogel, A., Miezin, F.N., Petersen, S.E., & Schlaggar, B.L. (2012). The putative visual word form area is functionally connected to the dorsal attention network. *Cerebral Cortex, 22*(3), 537–549.

Weekes, B. (1995). Right hemisphere writing and spelling. *Aphasiology, 9*(4), 305–319.

Whitwell, J.L., Jack, C.R., Kantarchi, K., Weigand, S.D., Boeve, B.F., Knopman, D.S., . . . Josephs, K.A. (2007). Imaging correlates of posterior cortical atrophy. *Neurobiology of Aging, 28*(7), 1051–1061.

Wilson S.M., Brambati S.M., Henry R.G., Handwerker, D.A., Agosta, F., Miller, B.L., . . . Gorno-Tempini, M.L. (2009). The neural basis of surface dyslexia in semantic dementia. *Brain, 132*(1), 71–86.

Zahn, R., Juengling, F., Bubrowski, P., Jost, E., Dykierek, P., Talazko, J., & Huell, M. (2004). Hemispheric asymmetries of hypometabolism associated with semantic memory impairment in Alzheimer's disease: A study using positron emission tomography with fluorodeoxyglucose-F18. *Psychiatry Research: Neuroimaging, 132*(2), 159–172.

Zaidel, E. (1990). Language functions in the two hemispheres following complete cerebral commissurotomy and hemispherectomy. In F. Boller & J. Grafman (Eds.). *Handbook of neuropsychology: Vol. 4.* Amsterdam: Elsevier Science Publishers.

6

CLINICAL DIAGNOSIS AND TREATMENT OF SPELLING DISORDERS

Pélagie M. Beeson and Steven Z. Rapcsak

Introduction

Daily needs for spelling range from jotting down grocery lists or "to do" lists, to composition of electronic mail messages, to carefully crafted literary prose or scholarly papers. While these activities require varying degrees of linguistic competence, they all depend on the ability to spell single words. Clearly some individuals are more dependent on the written word than others, so an acquired impairment of spelling will have varied impact in accordance with one's lifestyle. Isolated impairments of spelling or writing can result in significant reduction in one's ability to exchange information, leading to marked changes in vocational and personal activities. More often, acquired agraphia is part of a central language impairment, as is common in aphasia. In that context, the loss or impairment of written expression compounds the difficulties posed by disturbances of spoken communication.

Given that spoken language is the primary means of daily interaction for most people, it is not surprising that aphasia treatment typically is focused on spoken rather than written communication. That fact does not diminish the importance of clinical assessment and treatment of writing at the appropriate time in the rehabilitation process. In fact, in some cases of aphasia, writing may be better preserved than spoken language so that it becomes the dominant or most successful means of communication (Bub & Kertesz, 1982a; Clausen & Beeson, 2003; Ellis, Miller, & Sin, 1983; Levine, Calvanio, & Popovics, 1982). Similarly, writing may prove to be more amenable to remediation than speech in some patients (Beeson, 1999; Beeson, Rising, & Volk, 2003; Hillis Trupe, 1986; Robson, Marshall, Chiat, & Pring, 2001). Writing also may serve to facilitate spoken productions, so that it can be an important aspect of strategic compensation for impaired communication abilities (Beeson & Egnor, 2006; de Partz, 1986; Holland, 1998; Nickels, 1992). Thus, the clinical treatment of writing may be motivated by several goals: to reestablish premorbid writing skills, to serve as an adjunct or stimulant for spoken language, or to provide a substitute for spoken communication.

In this chapter, we describe clinical tasks that structure the examination of the cognitive processes necessary for writing that were detailed in chapter 5, followed by a review of evidence-based approaches to agraphia treatment. It is our premise that careful determination of the status of the component processes for writing should lead to the formulation of hypotheses regarding the locus (or loci) of impairment and an understanding of preserved processes. In turn, this information provides the rationale for the selection or development of an appropriate treatment plan. An individual's response to treatment may further clarify the nature of the impairment, and thus offer additional insight to direct rehabilitation efforts.

Clinical Evaluation of Spelling and Writing

A comprehensive evaluation of written language production should include a variety of tasks and stimulus materials designed to examine the functional status of the central and peripheral processing components identified in the previous chapter (Figure 5.1). As indicated in Table 6.1, different spelling tasks rely on specific cognitive processes and representations, so that comparative performance across several tasks helps to isolate the locus of impairment. As discussed in chapter 5, spelling can be accomplished via the lexical-semantic and sublexical spelling routes. The lexical-semantic route supports conceptually mediated spelling that is critical for spontaneous written communication and is based on the association between word meanings and the orthographic and phonological forms of familiar words. The sublexical route can be used for spelling both familiar words and unfamiliar words or nonwords, and depends on knowledge of sound-letter or phoneme-grapheme conversion rules. Orthographic information derived from lexical-semantic or sublexical procedures is maintained by a working memory system, referred to as the graphemic buffer, while graphic motor programs are activated and specific motor movements for writing are implemented. In addition to written spelling, other peripheral processes can also be used to produce oral spelling or typing (see Table 6.1).

A detailed analysis of impaired and preserved spelling processes and an examination of spelling errors should provide a clear picture of the nature of the acquired agraphia. It also should

Table 6.1 Tasks Used for Spelling Assessment (Check marks indicate processes or representations necessary to accomplish the various tasks.)

Task	Central Spelling Processes			Interface	Peripheral Processes			
	Lexical-Semantic		*Sublexical*	*Attention*	*Motor Planning & Implementation*			
	Semantic representation	*Orthographic lexicon*	*Phoneme-grapheme conversion*	*Graphemic buffer*	*Allographic conversion*	*Graphic motor programs (handwriting)*	*Hand movements (keyboard)*	*Speech (letter naming)*
Written naming	√	√		√	√	√		
Writing to dictation	√	√		√	√	√		
Writing homophones	√	√		√	√	√		
Typing	√	√		√	√ᵃ		√	
Anagram spelling	√	√		√	√ᵃ			
Oral spelling	√	√		√				√
Writing nonwords			√	√	√	√		
Delayed copy		√		√	√	√		
Direct copy		√ᵇ			√ᵇ	√		
Case conversion					√	√		

ᵃ Typing and anagram spelling could be accomplished with reliance on recognition (rather than selection) of letter shape.

ᵇ Direct copy may be accomplished without activation of orthographic lexicon, letter shape selection, or graphic motor programs if performed in a pictorial (nonlinguistic) fashion.

be possible to determine whether the patient fits the diagnostic criteria of the various agraphia syndromes reviewed in chapter 5 and summarized in Table 6.2. We acknowledge that the use of syndrome labels can be justifiably criticized for the potential oversimplification of the impairment and the fact that a given syndrome may reflect damage to different components of the spelling process; however, syndrome classifications provide the benefit of a shorthand to communicate the presence of a symptom cluster and are useful in a clinical context. As we use syndrome labels, we note their limitations and emphasize that when individual patterns of acquired agraphia fail to conform to a recognized syndrome they are best characterized by the description of the impaired and preserved processes.

Assessment of Lexical-Semantic Spelling Procedures

The lexical-semantic spelling route supports all conceptually driven writing tasks, so it is critical for most everyday writing activities. To determine the functional status of this spelling route, it is useful to obtain a sample of self-generated written communication before proceeding with a structured assessment of single-word writing. Spontaneous writing can be elicited as a descriptive narrative or as a picture description task, such as written description of standard stimuli like the "cookie theft" picture from the *Boston Diagnostic Aphasia Examination* (Goodglass & Kaplan, 1976; Goodglass, Kaplan, & Barresi, 2001) or the "picnic scene" from the *Western Aphasia Battery* (Kertesz, 1982; WAB-Revised, Kertesz, 2006). Written narratives may provide a sample of spelling errors and reveal the types of words that are spelled in error or omitted. This information provides clues regarding the nature of the spelling impairment that may be further investigated using carefully constructed word lists. Written narratives also allow for examination of lexical retrieval, syntactic structure, and other linguistic and cognitive abilities that are not the focus of this chapter but clearly are of interest in clinical and research contexts. Writing should be compared to spoken language to determine the extent to which the observed agraphia reflects impairments to semantic, phonological, or syntactic processes that are common to writing and speaking.

Written Naming

Just as written narratives and picture descriptions allow for the assessment of conceptually motivated spellings, written naming of pictured stimuli allows for examination of spellings derived from semantic representations. Relatively common, concrete nouns are typically used as picture stimuli for a written naming task. Adequate visual perception and object recognition must occur in order to activate the appropriate semantic representation for the pictured item, which should in turn activate the appropriate entry in the orthographic lexicon. It is likely that the presentation of pictured items evokes overt or subvocal spoken naming, but the written naming task can at times be accomplished without the ability to produce the spoken name. Failure to correctly write the name of a visually perceived item may reflect impairment to any of the necessary central or peripheral spelling processes indicated in Table 6.1. Clues regarding the locus of impairment may be derived from a comparison of written naming to writing to dictation. For example, if written naming is impaired relative to writing to dictation, it may reflect damage to the semantic system or a failure of the semantic system to activate the appropriate representation in the orthographic lexicon.

Writing to Dictation

Writing familiar words to dictation is typically accomplished via the lexical-semantic route. The spoken word activates the associated entry in the phonological lexicon, which addresses the

Table 6.2 Observed Effects on Spelling Accuracy Typically Associated with Impairment to Certain Spelling Processes and the Syndrome Labels Associated with the Spelling Profile

		Effects							
Locus of Damage	*Agraphia Syndrome*	*Word freq.* HF > LF	*Image* HI > LI	*Gram. Class* noun > func	*Lexicality* words > non	*Regularity* reg > irregular	*Length* short > long	*Semantic Errors*	*Homophone Errors*
Lexical-Semantic Spelling Route	*Surface agraphia*	√				√			√[a]
Sublexical Spelling Route	*Phonological/deep*[b] *Agraphia*	√	√	√	√			√Deep	
Sublexical and Lexical-Semantic Spelling Routes	*Global agraphia*	★	★	★	★			★	
Graphemic Buffer	*Graphemic buffer impairment*						√		

Key: HF > LF = high frequency > low frequency; HI > LI = high imagery > low imagery; func = functors; non = nonwords; reg = regularly spelled.

[a] Some patients with surface agraphia also produce frequent homophone errors, demonstrating features of "semantic agraphia."
[b] Deep agraphia may include damage to lexical-semantic spelling routes, as well.
★ Global agraphia may result in too few correct responses to demonstrate significant effects or to produce semantic errors.

appropriate semantic representation and the corresponding entry in the orthographic lexicon (Figure 5.1). If the phonological lexicon is damaged or fails to appropriately address the semantic system, then writing to dictation may be more impaired relative to tasks that do not depend on auditory input, such as spontaneous writing, written picture description, and written naming. Adequate processing of auditory input can be confirmed by means of spoken word-to-picture matching tasks. When written spelling to dictation is impaired, performance should be contrasted with other output modalities, such as oral spelling, typing, or spelling by the arrangement of component letters (i.e., an anagram task). A central spelling impairment will result in similar spelling errors for a given patient across modalities because they all depend upon activation of a common orthographic representation. In contrast, a peripheral agraphia may result in modality-specific errors such as the case in which poor written spelling is accompanied by preserved oral spelling.

Writing single words to dictation allows for control over orthographic features such as spelling regularity (i.e., the extent to which sounds map onto orthography in a predictable manner) and word length (number of letters). Stimuli can also be controlled on a number of lexical-semantic features that may influence spelling accuracy, such as word frequency, imageability (or concreteness), grammatical class, and morphological complexity. Several research groups have created controlled word lists to be used for testing spelling, including the *Psycholinguistic Assessments of Language Processing in Aphasia* (PALPA; Kay, Lesser, & Coltheart, 1992), *the Johns Hopkins University Dysgraphia Battery* (Goodman & Caramazza, 1986a, published in Beeson & Hillis, 2001), and the *Arizona Battery for Reading and Spelling* (Beeson et al., 2010; http://www.aphasia.arizona.edu/Aphasia_Research_Project/For_Professionals.html). Healthy, literate adults are typically familiar with the words included on such lists, so that they are spelled with relatively high accuracy and performance is not significantly affected by linguistic variables. This assumption should be supported by normative data; however, it is important to consider premorbid abilities of the individuals tested so that developmental spelling disorders are not confused with acquired impairments of writing.

In competent spellers, the effect of orthographic regularity is minimal, so when spelling accuracy is significantly better for regularly versus irregularly spelled words it is suggestive of damage to the lexical-semantic route and reliance on a sublexical spelling strategy. This regularity effect is the hallmark of **surface agraphia** (Beauvois & Dérouesné, 1981; Rapcsak & Beeson, 2004; Tsapkini & Rapp, 2010). The relatively good spelling of nonword stimuli (e.g., pseudowords like *flig*) confirms the functional integrity of the sublexical route. The characteristic profile of surface agraphia is depicted by two cases in Figure 6.1. In each case, there is a disproportionate impairment of irregularly spelled words compared to regularly spelled words and pseudowords. The example on the left (Figure 6.1a) demonstrates the orthographic form of surface agraphia following a left posterior cerebral artery stroke that damaged left ventral occipito-temporal regions (see arrows). The case on the right (Figure 6.1b) shows an individual with the semantic form of surface agraphia associated with anterior temporal lobe atrophy (greater on the left) that is consistent with the semantic variant of primary progressive aphasia (Gorno-Tempini et al., 2011; Graham, 2014; Graham, Patterson, & Hodges, 2000; Faria et al., 2013; Henry et al., 2012; Shim, Hurley, Rogalski, & Mesulam, 2012). More extensive assessment confirmed that the underlying impairment in these two individuals represents damage to different components of the lexical-semantic network: degraded memory for the spellings of words in the orthographic form of surface agraphia shown in Figure 6.1a; and disruption of the modality-independent semantic network in the individual shown in Figure 6.1b (see chapter 5 for details). Regardless of lesion etiology, or the nature of the underlying cognitive impairment (orthographic vs. semantic), individuals with surface agraphia tend to assemble spellings using knowledge of sound-to-letter correspondences (i.e., the phoneme-grapheme conversion mechanism), which often results in phonologically plausible renditions of the target word (e.g., from case examples in Figure 6.1, move → *moov;* laugh→ *laff*).

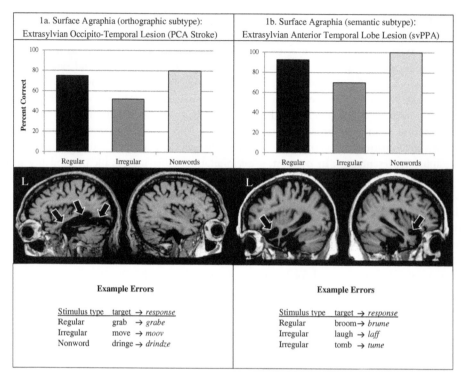

1a. Surface Agraphia (orthographic subtype): Extrasylvian Occipito-Temporal Lesion (PCA Stroke)	1b. Surface Agraphia (semantic subtype): Extrasylvian Anterior Temporal Lobe Lesion (svPPA)

Example Errors

Stimulus type	target → *response*
Regular	grab → *grabe*
Irregular	move → *moov*
Nonword	dringe → *drindze*

Example Errors

Stimulus type	target → *response*
Regular	broom → *brume*
Irregular	laugh → *laff*
Irregular	tomb → *tume*

Figure 6.1   Case examples of spelling accuracy by stimulus type and lesion location in the orthographic (1a) and semantic (1b) forms of surface agraphia.

In cases of surface agraphia attributable to reduced semantic influence on spelling, homophone errors are also observed (e.g., *suite* → *sweet*).

Assessment of Sublexical Spelling Procedures

The integrity of the sublexical spelling route can be examined in a relatively direct manner with the spelling of pronounceable pseudowords (i.e., nonwords like *prane*). If nonword spelling is good, it can be assumed that the ability to convert sounds to corresponding graphemes is intact, and the sublexical spelling route is available. When nonword spelling is notably impaired relative to real word spelling, it suggests a deficit at some level of the phoneme-grapheme conversion process (Patterson & Marcel, 1992; Rapcsak et al., 2009; Shallice, 1981). This **phonological agraphia** profile is associated with damage to left perisylvian cortical regions, so that it often accompanies perisylvian aphasias like Broca's, Wernicke's, and conduction aphasia, and those that evolve to anomic aphasia (Beeson, Rising, & Rapcsak, 2011; Henry et al., 2007; Rapcsak et al., 2009). Nonword spelling will be poor for both written and oral spelling because the tasks depend on the same phonological processes, although oral spelling may be more impaired than written spelling because it requires the additional challenge of letter naming, which is difficult for many individuals with left perisylvian damage.

The writing-to-dictation performance of three individuals with impaired phonological skills is shown in Figure 6.2. All three cases experienced damage to left perisylvian cortical regions following left middle cerebral artery stroke, and their behavioral profiles reflect different points on a continuum of phonological impairment. The case on the left (Figure 6.2a) had a relatively

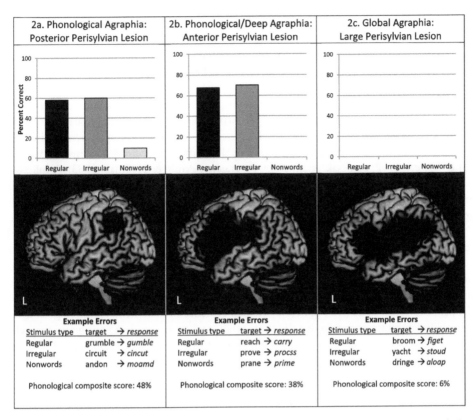

2a. Phonological Agraphia: Posterior Perisylvian Lesion	2b. Phonological/Deep Agraphia: Anterior Perisylvian Lesion	2c. Global Agraphia: Large Perisylvian Lesion

Example Errors (2a)

Stimulus type	target → *response*
Regular	grumble → *gumble*
Irregular	circuit → *cincut*
Nonwords	andon → *moamd*

Phonological composite score: 48%

Example Errors (2b)

Stimulus type	target → *response*
Regular	reach → *carry*
Irregular	prove → *procss*
Nonwords	prane → *prime*

Phonological composite score: 38%

Example Errors (2c)

Stimulus type	target → *response*
Regular	broom → *figet*
Irregular	yacht → *stoud*
Nonwords	dringe → *aloap*

Phonological composite score: 6%

Figure 6.2 Case examples of spelling accuracy by stimulus type and lesion location in patients with the phonological–deep–global agraphia continuum due to left middle cerebral artery strokes (see text for details).

circumscribed lesion affecting left supramarginal gyrus and underlying white matter that resulted in a marked impairment of nonword spelling in relation to real word spelling. The middle case (Figure 6.2b) also showed a strong lexicality effect (real words > nonwords) following extensive damage to left frontal perisylvian regions. These two cases of phonological agraphia are representative of others reported in the literature in that spelling for real words was also depressed (Baxter & Warrington, 1985; Bub & Kertesz, 1982a; Goodman-Schulman & Caramazza, 1987; Henry et al., 2007; Rapcsak et al., 2009). As shown, example errors on real words may demonstrate partial word-form knowledge (e.g., *grumble* → *gumble*), but attempts to spell the nonwords may be quite implausible (*andon* → *moamd*), or they may reflect an attempt to lexicalize the nonword (e.g., *prane* → *prime*). The individual in the center (Figure 6.2b) also made semantic errors on some real words (*reach* → *carry*), indicating a profile consistent with **deep agraphia** (Bub & Kertesz, 1982b; Marshall & Newcombe, 1966; Newcombe & Marshall, 1984; Nolan & Caramazza, 1983; Hatfield, 1985). The case on the right (Figure 6.2c) had extensive damage throughout the left perisylvian region affecting both sublexical and lexical-semantic spelling abilities so that no real words or nonwords were spelled correctly, and responses bore little resemblance to the targets. This profile is best described as **global agraphia** (Beeson & Hillis, 2001; Rapcsak et al., 2009).

When spelling is accomplished by exclusive reliance on the lexical-semantic route, performance may be influenced by variables such as word frequency (better spelling of high-frequency words like *dollar* or *sister* compared to low-frequency words like *fabric* or *bugle*; Ellis & Young, 1996; Morton, 1969; Rapcsak et al., 2009), grammatical word class (better spelling of nouns than of function words; Badecker, Hillis, & Caramazza, 1990; Baxter & Warrington, 1985; Hillis & Caramazza, 1994), and imageability/concreteness (better spelling of concrete words such as *table* than abstract words such as *wish*).

To further assess phoneme-grapheme conversion abilities, characteristic sounds for single letters may be presented orally for translation to the appropriate grapheme. Preserved phoneme-grapheme conversion for single sounds but not for words or pseudowords suggests impairment in the ability to segment words into their constituent sounds (Bolla-Wilson, Speedie, & Robinson, 1985; Patterson & Marcel, 1992; Rapcsak et al., 2009; Roeltgen, Sevush, & Heilman, 1983). A full assessment of phonological awareness and manipulation skills provides insight regarding the nature and severity of the underlying central phonological impairment in patients with phonological/deep agraphia, which can assist in treatment planning (e.g., Beeson et al., 2010; Patterson & Marcel, 1992; Rapcsak et al., 2009). For example, a central phonological impairment was evident in the three individuals shown in Figure 6.2 when evaluated on tasks that required phonological awareness and manipulation, but did not involve orthography: rhyme production, sound deletion from word/nonword, blending of sounds to produce the corresponding word/nonword, and replacement of one sound with another in a word/nonword. Individual composite scores derived from performance on those tasks (see Figure 6.2) yielded evidence of incremental phonological deficits that was in line with the assertion that the three syndromes are points on a continuum that reflect increasing degrees of central phonological impairment in the order of phonological < deep < global agraphia (Rapcsak et al., 2009).

Assessment of the Graphemic Buffer

Graphemic representations derived from either the lexical-semantic or sublexical spelling routes must be maintained in short-term memory, while peripheral writing processes are planned and implemented (Miceli, Silveri, & Caramazza, 1985; Caramazza, Miceli, Villa, & Romani, 1987; Tainturier & Rapp, 2003). The graphemic buffer serves as an interface between central and peripheral spelling processes, so impairment at this level will affect the spelling of words and nonwords in all output modalities (e.g., writing, typing, oral spelling). Given that word length is an important determinant of the amount of time an item needs to be maintained in orthographic working memory, errors are expected to be more frequent with longer words when the buffer is impaired. Word lists that are controlled for length (and balanced for other lexical-semantic features such as frequency, imagery, and grammatical class) are therefore the appropriate stimuli to test the integrity of the graphemic buffer.

The individual presented in Figure 6.3 demonstrated a marked word-length effect in his spelling accuracy following dorsal frontoparietal damage due to a middle cerebral artery stroke. As is typical of **graphemic buffer agraphia**, his spelling errors included letter substitutions (*charge* → *chargh*), deletions (*shrug* → *shug*), and transpositions (*talk* → *takl*) and combined errors (*splendid* → *splended*). There were no lexical-semantic effects (i.e., frequency, imagery, or grammatical class), and his performance was spared on the direct copy and the transcoding of letter case (uppercase to lowercase, and vice versa). As expected, errors emerged on a delayed copying task because of the demand for temporary storage of graphemic information.

Assessment of Peripheral Writing Processes

In order for abstract graphemic information to be realized as a written word, the appropriate letter shapes must be selected and the motor programs implemented to achieve the necessary

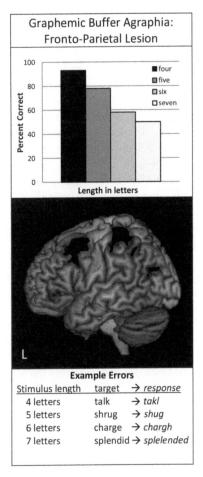

Figure 6.3 shown here with the following content:

Graphemic Buffer Agraphia: Fronto-Parietal Lesion

Percent Correct (y-axis, 0 to 100) by Length in letters (x-axis)

Legend: four, five, six, seven

L

Example Errors

Stimulus length	target	→ response
4 letters	talk	→ *takl*
5 letters	shrug	→ *shug*
6 letters	charge	→ *chargh*
7 letters	splendid	→ *splelended*

Figure 6.3 Case example of spelling accuracy by word length and lesion location in agraphia due to damage to the graphemic buffer.

movements of the pen (Ellis, 1982; Goodman & Caramazza, 1986b; Rapp & Caramazza, 1997). The allographic conversion process involves not only the determination of the appropriate letter identity but the specification of the particular physical characteristics, including case (upper vs. lower) and style (print vs. cursive). To assess the ability to select correct letter shapes, a transcoding task can be administered that requires conversion of words (or individual letters) from uppercase to lowercase letters, and vice versa. Impaired access or damage to information about letter shapes (i.e., allographs) can result in errors in letter selection and disorders of letter production that will be evident on all tasks requiring written spelling (e.g., writing words and nonwords to dictation, written naming, spontaneous written narrative, and transcoding tasks). In marked contrast, oral spelling of dictated words and nonwords will be preserved.

Direct copying tasks provide an examination of writing without demands on central spelling processes, and offer a means to examine the motor aspects of writing. Observation of copying should provide evidence as to whether it is accomplished in a lexical (whole-word), graphemic (letter-by-letter), or pictorial fashion (Ellis, 1982). Whereas lexical copying reflects activation of the orthographic lexicon via the reading system and subsequent written production of the word, graphemic copying is mediated by recognition of single letters and activation of the corresponding allographic representation. Impairments of graphomotor control will disrupt lexical or graphemic copying, so that pictorial copying of letters may be attempted in the same way that one would copy nonlinguistic visual patterns. Pictorial copying is slow and fragmented and is accomplished in a stroke-by-stroke fashion with heavy reliance on visual feedback rather than stored graphic motor programs.

As noted earlier, peripheral agraphia may be confirmed when spelling is significantly better using another output modality, such as oral spelling or anagram arrangement, that does not require written production of letters. Anagram spelling may be a particularly useful task with patients who also have letter-naming difficulty, as is common in aphasia. An assessment of typing/keyboarding or the ability to generate text messages via a mobile phone may be implemented in order to evaluate the functional impact of the writing impairment. Although there are few comparative studies of handwriting versus typing in individuals with acquired agraphia, clinical experience indicates that keyboard skills are rarely better preserved than handwriting. The exceptional cases are individuals with relatively pure apraxic agraphia who are able to type but not generate the graphomotor programs for handwriting (Alexander, Fischer, & Friedman, 1992; Hodges, 1991).

In summary, the assessment process should provide adequate information to discern the relative contribution of central and peripheral writing impairments and to guide the initial treatment plan. As noted previously, an individual's response to treatment will often clarify the nature of the deficit (e.g., Aliminosa, McCloskey, Goodman-Schulman, & Sokol, 1993; Beeson, 1999; Rapp, 2005), and improvements associated with one phase of treatment may change the profile to the extent that residual abilities are enhanced by relearned skills. Thus, clinical assessment is a dynamic process that continues throughout treatment and influences the selection of subsequent intervention strategies.

Treatment Approaches to Spelling Impairments

The clinical assessment of writing should provide information regarding impaired and preserved processes and representations that will be considered as treatment plans are devised. Writing treatment may be directed toward strengthening weakened processes (and representations) in an attempt to restore premorbid spelling procedures, and may serve to establish alternative spelling procedures or strategies that take advantage of preserved (or relearned) abilities. The rehabilitation of handwritten communication is typically the primary focus of treatment, but the need to communicate via the computer and other electronic media has increased tremendously over the past decade, so that consideration of keyboard skills and the potential value of assistive spelling devices or software warrant clinical attention (e.g., Armstrong & MacDonald, 2000; Beeson, Higginson, & Rising, 2013).

The body of literature to support evidence-based practice in the treatment of acquired agraphia has grown considerably over the past 15 years. As of this writing, there are at least 70 empirical studies examining the therapeutic effects of various treatment protocols designed to improve written language abilities in individuals with acquired agraphia. A complete list of these studies is maintained at http://aphasiatx.arizona.edu/written_writing. The majority of the research has been conducted with individuals with agraphia due to stroke, but a growing number of studies have demonstrated the value of agraphia treatment in individuals with primary progressive aphasia (Harris, Olson, & Humphreys, 2012; Raymer, Cudworth, & Haley, 2003; Rapp, 2005; Rapp & Glucroft, 2009; Tsapkini & Hillis, 2013). In this chapter, we provide a review of agraphia treatments organized according to the primary cognitive processes and procedures that are the focus of treatment. Specifically, we review approaches that target aspects of lexical-semantic spelling procedures, those that address sublexical spelling skills, and, finally, the peripheral aspects of writing.

It is important to note that some treatment outcomes serve to reinforce the dynamic interactions among the central language processing components and the attention mechanisms required for successful written communication. For example, lexical spelling treatments may also improve semantic associations for the lexical item or the individual's ability to say target words because of the repeated linking of orthography, phonology, and semantics for the targeted items (see Table 6.3). Improvements in the function of the short-term memory for orthographic information (i.e., the graphemic buffer) may also occur through repeated, structured stimulation of lexical-semantic spelling procedures.

It is clear that no one treatment approach will work for all individuals with acquired agraphia even when the impairment appears to be the same (Hillis, 1992), and the same treatment can have different effects on different individuals (Beeson et al., 2003; Rapp, 2005; Rapp & Kane, 2002). Individual variability in response to treatment conceivably reflects the unique pattern of damaged and preserved cognitive processes following brain damage, as well as differences in premorbid language abilities and the supporting neural architecture. Good clinical practice involves close monitoring of individual responses to treatment to determine whether it is effective and in what ways treatment should be adjusted to better suit the needs of the patient. Clinical management and decision making are also influenced by intrinsic and extrinsic factors that are unique to each patient, including medical, psychosocial, cultural, and contextual factors. As we proceed to discuss various treatment approaches, it is with the understanding that cognitive approaches to spelling treatment should be applied in a manner that enhances the functional communication skills of the individual patient. It should also be noted that writing treatment, like other language treatments, may include progression from one protocol to another so that individuals can take advantage of relearned or strengthened processes to further advance their progress toward maximal recovery (e.g., Beeson et al., 2010).

Table 6.3 Evidence-Based Treatment Approaches Appropriate for Various Agraphia Syndromes

Treatment Type	Example Treatment (Tx)	Semantic agraphia	Surface agraphia	Phonological agraphia	Deep agraphia	Global agraphia	Graphemic buffer agraphia	Allographic impairment
Semantic	*Semantic Elaboration Tx*	√	√		√			
	Homophone Tx	√						
Lexical	*Copy and Recall Tx (CART)*	√	√	√	√	√	√	√
Phonological	*Phonological Tx*			√	√	√		
Interactive	*Spell Check Training (including device)*		√					
Self-monitoring	*Self-Dictation*						√	
	Self-Detection/Correction		√				√	√

Lexical-Semantic Spelling Treatments

When it is evident that lexical-semantic processes are impaired, writing treatment may be directed toward strengthening semantic and/or orthographic representations or improving access to those representations. Given that the semantic system is central to all modalities of language processing, treatment to improve semantics is likely to be given high priority when clinical assessment implicates damage to that component.

Treatment to Improve Semantics and Links to Orthography

Semantic knowledge can be strengthened in the context of writing treatment with procedures that highlight the unique cluster of features that define concepts and clarify the distinctions among semantically related items. Treatment should serve to strengthen central semantic knowledge, so the benefit is not specific to written language, but spoken naming and comprehension typically improve as well (Cardell & Chenery, 1999; Hillis, 1989, 1991). Treatments that include less explicit training of semantic concepts also can serve to strengthen semantic representations for some individuals. For example, reading and writing tasks that associate the printed word to pictures (with corrective feedback) have been shown to strengthen semantic representations and reduce semantic errors (Hillis & Caramazza, 1991, 1994).

Treatment may be directed specifically toward homophones, which are problematic for individuals with surface agraphia (Behrman, 1987; Behrmann & Byng, 1992; Weekes & Coltheart, 1996). For example, Behrmann (1987) reported the value of treatment designed to improve spelling of homophonic word pairs (e.g., *main* versus *mane*) in a patient who showed impairment of the lexical-semantic spelling route with reliance on phoneme-grapheme conversion rules for spelling. The treatment focused on reestablishment of links between semantic meaning and orthography for targeted homophones using a picture-to-written-word matching task followed by written naming of each picture. Homework required the correct selection of written words to appropriately complete printed sentences, such as "After Christmas the shops have a big (sail/sale)."

De Partz, Seron, and Van der Linden (1992) used a more elaborate procedure to engage semantic processing in the retraining of irregular spellings in a French-speaking individual with surface agraphia. During treatment, they presented each target word with the challenging letters (i.e., the irregular aspect of the spelling) integrated into a drawing that was semantically related to the word. For example, because the word *pathologie* (pathology) was incorrectly spelled as *patologie* (lacking the *h*), the word was written with the letter *h* integrated into a drawing of a bed (as a hospital bed, denoting illness). This visual imagery approach proved adequate to cue the correct spelling of targeted words, and the word-specific improvement was maintained over a long period of time. In a similar manner, Schmalzl and Nickels (2006) demonstrated the value of using visual mnemonics to support spelling retraining in an individual with a semantic deficit.

Strengthening Orthographic Representations

When neural damage degrades or prevents access to the store of learned spellings, semantic and phonological representations may not successfully activate the associated orthography. The most common and direct treatment approach is to retrain individual spellings for targeted words in an item-specific manner. There are over 40 studies that have examined the value of such lexical treatments for spelling (see http://aphasiatx.arizona.edu for a complete list of references). The benefit of lexical spelling treatment has been documented across a range of individuals with impaired semantic, phonological, and/or orthographic knowledge, including those with little residual spelling ability (global agraphia), those with moderate to severe phonological or deep agraphia, and those with surface agraphia. The majority of the studies employed single-subject, multiple-baseline experimental designs, and together they provide strong, positive evidence that individuals with aphasia and acquired agraphia are typically able to relearn the spellings for targeted words. Reports of individuals who did not improve in response to treatment serve to provide guidance regarding the minimum cognitive and sensorimotor skills necessary to support single word writing for communication (Beeson, Rising, & Volk, 2003).

Lexical spelling treatments vary with regard to the exact procedures used to strengthen orthographic representations, but they share the common feature of repeated practice in the spelling of targeted words (e.g., Aliminosa et al., 1993; Beeson, 1999; Carlomagno, Iavarone, & Colombo, 1994; Hillis, 1991; Rapp & Kane, 2002; Raymer, Cudworth, & Haley, 2003; Schmalzl & Nickels, 2006). Copy and recall treatment (CART) is an example protocol for lexical spelling treatment that involves repeated copying of a targeted set of words along with subsequent trials to recall the correct spelling in the absence of a model (e.g., Beeson, 1999). Repeated copying provides stimulation of specific orthographic representations, while the recall trials place demands on the retrieval mechanism. Self-evaluation of recall trials can include reference to a written or printed model, and provides opportunities for self-correction and additional copying to further strengthen specific orthographic representations. The CART protocol varies the cognitive demands so that the initial attempt to independently generate the spelling is most challenging and is likely to evoke error responses, which should heighten attention to the correct spelling during the repeated copying from a model. The copying task tends to be relatively errorless, and the recall trial is of intermediate difficulty with errors tending to decline rapidly over the training trials. Single-subject multiple baseline designs have been useful to demonstrate the treatment effects. The typical response to CART and similar lexical treatment approaches is sequential mastery of subsets of words targeted for treatment. The number of items targeted for treatment at one time can vary, with smaller sets of about 5 items for individuals with global agraphia (e.g., Beeson et al., 2003) or larger sets of 20 to 30 items for those with less severe impairment (e.g., Rapp & Kane, 2002; Raymer et al., 2003).

It is important to note that while lexical spelling treatments focus on rebuilding orthographic representations, it is always important to reinforce links between orthography, semantics, and phonology. Spelling treatments inherently include reading, and most lexical spelling treatments include procedures that reinforce the links between written words and their meaning by the use of pictures or semantic association tasks (Beeson et al., 2003; Carlomagno et al., 1994; Hillis, 1991). Even when semantic knowledge is not specifically reinforced during treatment, it is likely to play a role in the relearning process, as demonstrated in a case reported by Kumar and Humphreys (2008). They found that high-imagery words were better maintained over time than low-imagery words in an individual with deep agraphia.

When speech production skills are adequate, a procedure like CART can be implemented with repeated spoken production of the target words, so that the spoken name is simply repeated in the course of the copying tasks. The implementation of CART plus repetition has been shown to improve lexical retrieval and speech production in individuals with aphasia (e.g., Ball, DeRiesthal, Breeding, & Mendoza, 2011; Beeson & Egnor, 2006; Hillis & Caramazza, 1994). In the case of conduction aphasia, the written word may stabilize access to phonology resulting in fewer phonemic paraphasias (Beeson & Egnor, 2006).

A variation of lexical spelling treatment includes the use of an anagram task in which the component letters of each target word are provided as part of a cueing hierarchy (e.g., Ball et al. 2011; Beeson, 1999; Hillis, 1989; Carlomagno et al., 1994). The manipulation of letters and the opportunity to judge resultant spellings provides a supportive context for relearning specific orthographic representations. The anagram task is typically paired with a copying task in order to further encode the correct spellings, so that it has been referred to as anagram and copy treatment (ACT; Beeson,

1999). Observation of the attempts to arrange letters can provide insight into the status of the orthographic representation. For example, for the target word "poker," an individual with global agraphia arranged *p_k_r* and then struggled with the decision of where the *o* and *e* should be placed. In that case, knowledge of the vowel placement improved so that the individual relearned the spelling of "poker" (Beeson, 1999).

Lexical spelling treatments that serve to strengthen orthographic representations also have been shown to reduce word-length effects thought to reflect graphemic buffer impairment (Aliminosa et al., 1993; Cardell & Chenery, 1999; Hillis, 1989; Hillis & Caramazza, 1987; Sage & Ellis, 2006). When the improvement is specific to the trained items, it suggests that strengthening orthographic representations can make them less subject to decay, and thus yielded correct spelling for trained items. In some cases, lexical spelling treatment can result in generalized improvement in spelling and reduction of the word-length effect in individuals with graphemic buffer impairment (Rapp, 2005; Raymer et al., 2003). In such cases, the treatment appeared to improve the function of attentional processes necessary to maintain information in the graphemic buffer.

Although lexical spelling treatments are most often implemented with handwritten responses, some studies have examined relearning with use of a keyboard at the computer (e.g., Katz & Nagy, 1984; Seron, Deloche, Moulard, & Rousselle, 1980) or a mobile phone keypad for text messaging (Beeson et al., 2013). The shift from handwriting to the keyboard is not trivial, and some individuals have considerable difficulty typing words. In addition to the limitations caused by hemiparesis in some agraphic individuals, the additional burden of locating letters on a keyboard should not be underestimated. Text messaging on a phone keyboard is often accomplished with one hand, so that hemiparesis may be less of an issue than keyboard typing on a personal computer. A recent case study demonstrated comparable mastery of spellings using the pullout keyboard on a cellular phone in comparison to handwriting; however, it was interesting to note that long-term follow-up testing showed stronger persistence of spellings learned using handwriting versus keyboarding (Beeson et al., 2013). The difference may relate to deeper encoding of orthographic memories by handwriting in comparison to pressing letter keys.

An obvious limitation of lexical spelling treatment is that most individuals demonstrate an item-specific treatment effect with limited generalization to untrained words. For that reason, it is important to carefully select the words to be trained. Several treatment studies included information regarding the functional benefit of item-specific treatment. For example, Hillis and Caramazza (1987) documented relearning of spellings important for the occupational demands of an individual who was able to return to work after treatment. Individuals with severely impaired spoken language skills can use single word writing as a means of everyday communication and supported conversation (e.g., Beeson, 1999; Clausen & Beeson, 2003). Another potential value of lexical spelling treatment is to establish a corpus of words that can be used as "key words" or "relay words" associated with individual sound-letter correspondences to assist individuals who proceed to treatment to strengthen sublexical spelling abilities.

Strengthening General Phonological Skills and Sublexical Spelling Procedures

The sublexical spelling route that depends upon phoneme-grapheme conversion processes typically functions in parallel with lexical-semantic spelling processes. Spelling treatment may be designed to strengthen and facilitate the use of sublexical spelling procedures and to strengthen central phonological skills. To date, nearly 20 studies have been reported that examined outcomes associated with sublexical/phonological treatment for spelling (see http://aphasiatx.arizona.edu/written_writing). Numerous case reports have documented success in retraining sound-to-letter correspondences to facilitate spelling via the sublexical route in individuals with phonological

LIVERPOOL JOHN MOORES UNIVERSITY
LEARNING SERVICES

or deep agraphia (e.g., Cardell & Cheney, 1999; Carlomagno & Parlato, 1989; Carlomagno et al., 1994; Beeson et al., 2010; Hillis Trupe, 1986; Hillis & Caramazza, 1994; Kiran, 2005; Luzzatti, Colombo, Frustaci, & Vitolo, 2000). The task of translating phonemes to graphemes for spelling requires several steps, including segmenting the word into sounds or syllables, categorizing each sound into its phoneme category, and mapping the phoneme to the corresponding grapheme. Additional training is typically required to improve phonological awareness and manipulation skills, so that sound-letter conversion skills can be applied at the word level (e.g., phonological blending treatment described in Beeson et al., 2010).

For many individuals with significant phonological impairment, the relearning of sound-letter correspondences is extremely challenging. In order to support the process, some individuals benefit from the use of "key words" that provide a means to help retrieve the sound letter correspondences (Beeson et al., 2010; Carlomagno & Parloto, 1989; Hillis & Caramazza, 1994). For example, the individual uses the key word "pie" to segment the sound /p/ and to retrieve the associated grapheme *p*. Phonological treatment may require retraining phoneme-grapheme correspondences for all consonants and vowels; however, some individuals are able to use the first letter or two to cue orthographic retrieval via the lexical route. There is also evidence that retrieval of the initial letter serves to block semantic errors in individuals with deep agraphia, demonstrating the dynamic interaction and integration of sublexical/lexical information (Folk, Rapp, & Goldrick, 2002; Hillis & Caramazza, 1994). In a few reported cases, phonological treatment has been implemented at the syllable level, wherein a corpus of preserved proper nouns served as "code words" to relearn spellings of consonant-vowel syllables (Carlomagno & Parlato, 1989).

It is apparent that spelling can be enhanced by increased reliance on and improved function of the sublexical spelling route. Beeson and colleagues (2008) demonstrated in a group study that improved phonological skills were associated with generalized improvement in the spelling of regular as well as irregularly spelled words, suggesting interactive use of sublexical and lexical knowledge (Folk et al., 2002). Generalization to untrained items is typical when treatment serves to improve the function of phonological/sublexical skills, in contrast to item-specific improvements that are typical of lexical spelling treatment. Of particular interest is the recent finding that some individuals with phonological impairment demonstrate improved writing at the text level following successful phonological treatment (Beeson et al., 2012). Specifically, individuals with relatively preserved single word spelling, but markedly impaired text-level writing (a profile that we refer to as phonological text agraphia) demonstrated significant improvement in the ability to retrieve and produce the orthography for functors and morphological markers after phonological treatment. These findings reinforce the idea that phonological/sublexical spelling skills are dynamically involved in written language processing even for familiar lexical items.

Phonological skills are highly dependent upon left perisylvian regions that are often damaged in left middle cerebral artery stroke. Although considerable improvement has been documented following phonological treatment, residual deficits are not uncommon. In such cases, individuals with phonological/deep agraphia may derive only partial orthography from phonology. Even when sound-letter transcoding skills become relatively strong, it is necessary to call upon residual lexical knowledge to correctly spell any words that do not follow fully predictable phoneme-grapheme rules. In such cases, treatment may be implemented that strives to maximize the use of partial lexical and sublexical spelling information, as described below.

Promoting Interactive Use of Lexical-Semantic and Sublexical Spelling Knowledge

It makes sense that agraphic patients should bring all available information to bear as they attempt to resolve spelling difficulties. Partial information derived from the lexical-semantic route may be supplemented by orthographic information derived from the sublexical route (Beeson, Rewega, Vail, & Rapcsak, 2000; Hillis & Caramazza, 1991; Hillis Trupe, 1986). In fact, several carefully described cases of acquired agraphia provide evidence of interaction and integration of lexical and sublexical information (Folk, Rapp, & Goldrick, 2002; Hillis & Caramazza, 1991, 1994; Rapp, Epstein, & Tainturier, 2002). Treatment can be structured to train the necessary problem-solving strategies to maximize interactive use of lexical and sublexical spelling routes (e.g., Beeson et al., 2000, 2010). Interactive spelling treatment can include the use of electronic spelling devices (or software) sensitive to plausible misspellings to assist in training self-detection and correction of spelling errors, particularly when individuals are capable of generating partial spellings or phonologically plausible spellings (Beeson et al., 2000, 2010; Hillis Trupe, 1986). Such devices or software are distinct from the typical spell-checking algorithms that are built into most word processing programs, which assume typical typing errors and a few common misspellings.

The use of a spelling device can provide compensatory support, but successful interactive treatment should result in generalized improvement in spelling abilities (Beeson et al., 2000; Beeson et al., 2010). Hillis Trupe (1986) demonstrated an additional potential benefit of this type of treatment in an individual with severe apraxia of speech who learned to type plausible spellings into a portable computer with text-to-speech capability, resulting in synthesized spoken utterances. Another individual reported that interactive treatment and use of the electronic speller allowed her to return to her hobby of writing fiction (SV; Beeson et al., 2000).

Self-Monitoring Treatments to Improve Self-Detection and Correction of Errors

It is obvious that any of the agraphia subtypes might benefit from increased attention to the selection and production of letter strings. Treatments that are specifically designed to increase self-detection and correction of errors have been implemented in individuals with surface agraphia (as described above under the heading of interactive treatment). Training to improve self-monitoring strategies also has been the specific focus of several intervention studies with individuals with graphemic buffer impairment. For example, Hillis and Caramazza (1987) trained an individual to use a search strategy to detect errors (i.e., to compare his spellings to representations in his orthographic lexicon). He also was guided to focus on the ends of words (where most of his errors occurred) and to sound out each word as it was written to call attention to phonologically implausible misspellings. This treatment successfully improved self-detection and correction of spelling errors for single words, as well as for written narratives.

Several case reports describe attempts to compensate for graphemic buffer impairment by taking advantage of relatively preserved oral spelling. The approach includes training the individual to employ self-dictation of spelling as a means to guide written spelling (Lesser, 1990; Panton & Marshall, 2008; Pound, 1996) or keyboard typing (Mortley, Enderby, & Petheram, 2001). The approach was not successful for the participant in Lesser's study, but the individuals described by Pound (1996) and Panton and Marshall (2008) responded positively to self-dictation treatment. A key feature of the self-dictation treatment is increased self-monitoring of the match (or mismatch) between orally named letters and the written production.

Treatment for Impairments to Peripheral Spelling Processes

Relatively little attention has been given to treatment that is specific to peripheral agraphias. This is not surprising given that the incidence of acquired writing impairments without significant language impairment is relatively rare. A review of 500 left-hemisphere-damaged individuals yielded only 2 who were considered to have pure agraphia (Basso, Taborelli, & Vignolo, 1978). In contrast, the co-occurrence of central and peripheral writing impairments is a far more common finding, owing to lesions that produce combined damage to neuroanatomical regions critical to lexical-semantic, sublexical, and peripheral spelling/writing processes. In cases of concomitant impairment to central and peripheral writing processes, the peripheral impairments must be overcome in order to realize the effects of treatment for central spelling processes. Fortunately, there is evidence (albeit limited) that peripheral processes may be strengthened by the repeated written productions elicited in the context of treatments for central spelling processes, such as those reviewed above. For example, the repeated copying and delayed copying of target words was associated with improved allographic conversion processes in some individuals with global agraphia (Beeson et al., 1999; Beeson et al., 2003); however, few studies have provided data to determine whether this outcome is common.

Individuals with intact central spelling processes who experience selective impairment of peripheral spelling skills may be able to circumvent their handwriting difficulty by typing/keyboarding. For example, a patient reported by Black and colleagues (Black, Behrmann, Bass, & Hacker, 1989) with a selective impairment to allographic conversion processes showed nearly normal ability to type. Similarly, individuals with damage to graphic motor programs (apraxic agraphia) may retain the ability to use a keyboard for written communication because such movements do not require the same level of skilled motor control as that needed for handwriting. In such cases, where an effective alternative to written spelling is available, rehabilitation of the peripheral writing impairment may not be a priority.

Many individuals with acquired writing impairments also have hemiparesis affecting their ability to write with the dominant hand, so they must shift to writing with the nondominant hand. Several investigators have reported on the value of various writing prostheses to support the use of the paralyzed right hand (Armstrong & MacDonald, 2000; Brown, Leader, & Blum, 1983; Leischner, 1983, 1996; Lorch, 1995a, 1995b; Whurr & Lorch, 1991). There were reports that written composition produced with the aided hemiparetic right hand can be linguistically superior to that written with the nondominant left hand; however, the mechanisms underlying this phenomenon were a matter of discussion and debate (Brown, 1995; Goldberg & Porcelli, 1995; Rothi, 1995; Lorch, 1995a, 1995b; Sasanuma, 1995; Leischner, 1996). There has been little recent research to shed additional light on the benefit of prosthetic support for the hemiparetic hand at a linguistic level, but it appears that such support can improve graphomotor control at the peripheral level for some individuals.

Conclusions

Clinical assessment of individuals with acquired agraphia should provide insight regarding the status of orthographic, semantic, phonological, and sensorimotor processes necessary for spelling and writing. The observed performance profile across a range of spelling tasks allows the formulation of hypotheses regarding the locus of the spelling impairment and the contribution from spared processes. As we have reviewed in this chapter, information derived from the assessment can subsequently guide the selection and planning of agraphia treatment directed toward specific components of central or peripheral spelling processes. This includes strengthening semantic, orthographic, and phonological lexical representations (and their links), improving the use of the sublexical spelling route, strengthening attentional control to maintain graphemic information in short-term memory, and reestablishing peripheral spelling processes.

Although the literature regarding agraphia treatment is less extensive than other areas of language rehabilitation, there is strong evidence in the form of well-controlled, single-subject experiments and some group studies to show that spelling and writing may be improved even long after the onset of agraphia. Our approach was to examine treatments directed toward specific processes and representations; however, it is apparent that the treatment tasks typically engage numerous cognitive processes, so that the stimulation provided by treatment was rarely limited to isolated processes. For that reason, it is not surprising that a given treatment approach may serve to strengthen several cognitive processes. As a result, at times it may be difficult to determine with certainty that treatment influenced a particular spelling process to the exclusion of others; however, the fact that treatment improves the function of several components of the spelling process makes for an efficacious clinical approach.

In closing, we return to the issue of the functional value of spelling and writing treatment. We assert that it is not enough to simply improve cognitive processes if such treatment has no significant impact on the functional outcome or quality of life for a given patient. Clearly the clinical treatment of writing should be influenced by patient needs and should include the necessary bridge between clinical activities and real life, and feedback regarding the functional value of treatment is important. We end this chapter with recent feedback from individuals who affirmed the value of agraphia treatment in their lives. A woman who received treatment at 10 years post stroke stated, "I thought I could never write again, but it's coming along . . . and that's really exciting." And this comment from the spouse of an individual who relearned spelling skills so that he was able to use written words to support his ability to convey information in conversation and on the phone: "It's made a world of difference!"

Acknowledgments

This work was supported by NIH grants from the National Institute on Deafness and other Communication Disorders (2R01-DC07646) and the National Institute on Aging (P30AG19610). The authors wish to thank the current and former members of the Aphasia Research Project at the University of Arizona, with particular appreciation toward Kindle Rising, Andrew DeMarco, and Reva Wilheim for their contributions to this chapter. We are also indebted to our research participants who continue to help us learn about the nature and treatment of agraphia.

References

Alexander, M.P., Fischer, R.S., & Friedman, R. (1992). Lesion localization in apractic agraphia. *Archives of Neurology, 49*(3), 246–251.

Aliminosa, D., McCloskey, M., Goodman-Schulman, R., & Sokol, S. (1993). Remediation of acquired dysgraphia as a technique for testing interpretations of deficits. *Aphasiology, 7*, 55–69.

Armstrong, L., & Macdonald, A. (2000). Aiding chronic written language expression difficulties: A case study. *Aphasiology, 14*(1), 93–108.

Badecker, W., Hillis, A., & Caramazza, A. (1990). Lexical morphology and its role in the writing process: Evidence from a case of acquired dysgraphia. *Cognition, 35*, 205–243.

Ball, A.L., de Riesthal, M., Breeding, V.E., & Mendoza, D.E. (2011). Modified ACT and CART in severe aphasia. *Aphasiology, 25*(6–7), 836–848.

Basso, A., Taborelli, A., & Vignolo, L.A. (1978). Dissociated disorders of speaking and writing in aphasia. *Journal of Neurology, Neurosurgery, & Psychiatry, 41*, 556–563.

Baxter, D.M., & Warrington, E. K. (1985). Category specific phonological dysgraphia. *Neuropsychologia, 23*, 653–666.

Beauvois, M.-F., & Dérouesné, J. (1981). Lexical or orthographic agraphia. *Brain, 104*, 21–49.

Beeson, P.M. (1999). Treating acquired writing impairment. *Aphasiology, 13*, 367–386.

Beeson, P.M., & Egnor, H. (2006). Combining treatment for written and spoken naming. *Journal of the International Neuropsychological Society, 12*(6), 816–827.

Beeson, P.M., Higginson, K., & Rising, K. (2013). Writing treatment for aphasia: A texting approach. *Journal of Speech, Language, and Hearing Research, 56*(3), 945–955.

Beeson, P.M., & Hillis, A.E. (2001). Comprehension and production of written words. In. R. Chapey (Ed.), *Language intervention strategies in adult aphasia* (4th ed.) (pp. 572–595). Baltimore: Lippincott Williams & Wilkins.

Beeson, P.M., Rewega, M., Vail, S., & Rapcsak, S.Z. (2000). Problem-solving approach to agraphia treatment: interactive use of lexical and sublexical spelling routes. *Aphasiology, 14*, 551–565.

Beeson, P.M., Rising, K., Howard, T., Northrop, E., Wilheim, R., Wilson, S., & Rapcsak, S. (2012). The nature and treatment of phonological text agraphia. *Procedia—Social and Behavioral Sciences, 61*, 22–23.

Beeson, P.M., Rising, K., Kim, E.S., & Rapcsak, S.Z. (2008). A novel method for examining response to spelling treatment. *Aphasiology, 22*(7–8), 707–717.

Beeson, P.M., Rising, K., Kim, E., & Rapcsak, S.Z. (2010). A treatment sequence for phonological alexia/agraphia. *Journal of Speech, Language, and Hearing Research, 53*, 450–468.

Beeson, P.M., Rising, K., & Rapcsak, S.Z. (2011). Acquired impairments of reading and writing. In L.L. LaPointe (Ed.), *Aphasia and related neurogenic language disorders* (4th ed., pp. 121–137). New York: Thieme Publishers.

Beeson, P.M., Rising, K., & Volk, J. (2003). Writing treatment for severe aphasia: Who benefits? *Journal of Speech, Language, and Hearing Research, 46*(5), 1038–1060.

Behrmann, M. (1987). The rites of righting writing: Homophone mediation in acquired dysgraphia. *Cognitive Neuropsychology, 4*, 365–384.

Behrmann, M., & Byng, S. (1992). A cognitive approach to the neurorehabilitation of acquired language disorders. In D.I. Margolin (Ed.), *Cognitive neuropsychology in clinical practice.* New York: Oxford University Press.

Black, S.E., Behrmann, M., Bass, K., & Hacker, P. (1989). Selective writing impairment: Beyond the allographic code. *Aphasiology, 3*, 265–277.

Bolla-Wilson, K., Speedie, L.J., & Robinson, R.G. (1985). Phonologic agraphia in a left-handed patient after a right-hemisphere lesion. *Neurology, 35*, 1778–1781.

Brown, J. (1995). What dissociation should be studied? *Aphasiology, 9*, 277–279.

Brown, J.W., Leader, B.J., & Blum, C.S. (1983). Hemiplegic writing in severe aphasia. *Brain and Language, 19*, 204–215.

Bub, D., & Kertesz, A. (1982a). Evidence for lexicographic processing in a patient with preserved written over oral single word naming. *Brain, 105*, 697–717.

Bub, D., & Kertesz, A. (1982b). Deep agraphia. *Brain and Language, 17*, 146–165.

Caramazza, A., Miceli, G., Villa, G., & Romani, C. (1987). The role of the graphemic buffer in spelling: Evidence from a case of acquired dysgraphia. *Cognition, 26*, 59–85.

Cardell, E.A., & Chenery, H.J. (1999). A cognitive neuropsychological approach to the assessment and remediation of acquired dysgraphia. *Language Testing, 16*, 353–388.

Carlomagno, S., Iavarone, A., & Colombo, A. (1994). Cognitive approaches to writing rehabilitation: From single case to group studies. In M.J. Riddoch & G.W. Humphreys (Eds.), *Cognitive neuropsychology and cognitive rehabilitation.* Hillsdale, NJ: Lawrence Erlbaum.

Carlomagno, S., & Parlato, V. (1989). Writing rehabilitation in brain damaged adult patients: A cognitive approach. In G. Deloche (Ed.), *Cognitive approaches in neuropsychological rehabilitation.* Hillsdale, NJ: Lawrence Erlbaum.

Clausen, N. & Beeson, P.M. (2003). Conversational use of writing in severe aphasia: A group treatment approach. *Aphasiology, 17*(6), 625–644.

de Partz, M.-P. (1986). Re-education of a deep dyslexic patient: Rationale of the method and results. *Cognitive Neuropsychology, 3*, 147–177.

de Partz, M.-P., Seron, X., & Van der Linden, M.V. (1992). Re-education of surface dysgraphia with a visual imagery strategy. *Cognitive Neuropsychology, 9*, 369–401.

Ellis, A.W. (1982). Spelling and writing (and reading and speaking). In A.W. Ellis (Ed.), *Normality and pathology in cognitive functions.* London: Academic Press.

Ellis, A.W., Miller, D., & Sin, G. (1983). Wernicke's aphasia and normal language processing: A case study in cognitive neuropsychology. *Cognition, 15*, 111–144.

Ellis, A.W., & Young, A.W. (1996). *Human cognitive neuropsychology: A textbook with readings.* London: Lawrence Erlbaum.

Faria, A.V., Crinion, J., Tsapkini, K., Newhart, M., Davis, C., Cooley, S., . . . Hillis, A.E. (2013). Patterns of dysgraphia in primary progressive aphasia compared to post-stroke aphasia. *Behavioural Neurology, 26*(1–2), 21–34.

Folk, J.R., Rapp, B., & Goldrick, M. (2002). The interaction of lexical and sublexical information in spelling: What is the point? *Cognitive Neuropsychology, 19*(7), 653–671.

Goldberg, G., & Porcelli, J. (1995). The functional benefits: How much and for whom? *Aphasiology, 9*, 274–277.

Goodglass, H., & Kaplan, E. (1976). *The assessment of aphasia and other disorders.* Philadelphia: Lea & Feabiger.

Goodglass, H., Kaplan, E., & Barresi, B. (2001). *The assessment of aphasia and related disorders*. Baltimore: Lippincott Williams & Wilkins.

Goodman, R. A., & Caramazza, A. (1986a). *The Johns Hopkins University dyslexia and dysgraphia batteries*. Unpublished.

Goodman, R. A., & Caramazza, A. (1986b). Aspects of the spelling process: Evidence from a case of acquired dysgraphia. *Language and Cognitive Processes, 1*, 263–296.

Goodman-Schulman, R., & Caramazza, A. (1987). Patterns of dysgraphia and the nonlexical spelling process. *Cortex, 23*, 143–148.

Gorno-Tempini, M., Hillis, A., Weintraub, S., Kertesz, A., Mendez, M., Cappa, S., . . . Grossman, M. (2011). Classification of primary progressive aphasia and its variants. *American Academy of Neurology, 76*(11), 1006–1014.

Graham, N.L. (2014). Dysgraphia in primary progressive aphasia: Characterization of impairments and therapy options. *Aphasiology*. doi:10.1080/002787038.2013.869308.

Graham, N.L., Patterson, K., & Hodges, J.R. (2000). The impact of semantic memory impairment on spelling: Evidence from semantic dementia. *Neuropsychologia, 38*(2), 143–163.

Harris, L., Olson, A., & Humphreys, G. (2012). Rehabilitation of spelling in a participant with a graphemic buffer impairment: the role of orthographic neighbourhood in remediating the serial position effect. *Neuropsychological Rehabilitation, 22*(6), 890–919.

Hatfield, F.M. (1985). Visual and phonological factors in acquired dysgraphia. *Neuropsychologia, 23*, 13–29.

Henry, M., Beeson, P., Stark, A., & Rapcsak, S. (2007). The role of left perisylvian cortical regions in spelling. *Brain and Language, 100*(1), 44–52.

Henry, M.L., Beeson, P.M., Alexander, G.E., & Rapcsak, S.Z. (2012). Written language impairments in primary progressive aphasia: A reflection of damage to central semantic and phonological processes. *Journal of Cognitive Neuroscience, 24*(2), 261–275.

Hillis, A.E. (1989). Efficacy and generalization of treatment for aphasic naming errors. *Archives of Physical Medicine and Rehabilitation, 70*, 632–636.

Hillis, A.E. (1991). Effects of separate treatments for distinct impairments within the naming process. *Clinical Aphasiology, 19*, 255–265.

Hillis, A.E. (1992). Facilitating written production. *Clinics in Communication Disorders, 2*, 19–33.

Hillis, A.E., & Caramazza, A. (1987). Model-driven treatment of dysgraphia. In R.H. Brookshire (Ed.), *Clinical aphasiology*. Minneapolis, MN: BRK Publishers.

Hillis, A.E., & Caramazza, A. (1991). Mechanisms for accessing lexical representations for output: Evidence from a category-specific semantic deficit. *Brain and Language, 40*, 106–144.

Hillis, A.E., & Caramazza, A. (1994). Theories of lexical processing and rehabilitation of lexical deficits. In M.J. Riddoch & G.W. Humphreys (Eds.), *Cognitive neuropsychology and cognitive rehabilitation*. Hillsdale, NJ: Lawrence Erlbaum.

Hillis Trupe, A.E. (1986). Effectiveness of retraining phoneme to grapheme conversion. In R.H. Brookshire (Ed.), *Clinical aphasiology*. Minneapolis, MN: BRK Publishers.

Hodges, J.R. (1991). Pure apraxic agraphia with recovery after drainage of a left frontal cyst. *Cortex, 27*(3), 469–473

Holland, A. (1998). A strategy for improving oral naming in an individual with a phonological access impairment. In N. Helm-Estabrooks & A.L. Holland (Eds.), *Approaches to the treatment of aphasia*. San Diego: Singular Press.

Katz, R.C., & Nagy, V.T. (1984). An intelligent computer-based spelling task for chronic aphasia patients. In R.H. Brookshire (Ed.), *Clinical aphasiology: Vol. 14* (pp. 159–165). Minneapolis, MN: BRK Publishers.

Kay, J., Lesser, R., & Coltheart, M. (1992). *Psycholinguistic assessments of language processing in aphasia* (PALPA). East Sussex, England: Lawrence Erlbaum.

Kertesz, A. (1982). *Western aphasia battery*. New York: Grune and Stratton.

Kertesz, A. (2006). *Western aphasia battery-revised*. New York: Pearson Publishers.

Kiran, S. (2005). Training phoneme to grapheme conversion for patients with written and oral production deficits: A model-based approach. *Aphasiology, 19*, 53–76.

Kumar, V.P., & Humphreys, G.W. (2008). The role of semantic knowledge in relearning spellings: Evidence from deep dysgraphia. *Aphasiology, 22*(5), 489–504.

Leischner, A. (1983). Side differences in writing to dictation of aphasics with agraphia: A graphic disconnection syndrome. *Brain and Language, 18*, 1–19.

Leischner, A. (1996). Word class effects upon the intrahemispheric graphic disconnection syndrome. *Aphasiology, 10*, 443–451.

Lesser, R. (1990). Superior oral to written spelling: Evidence for separate buffers? *Cognitive Neuropsychology*, 7, 347–366.

Levine, D.N., Calvanio, R., & Popovics, A. (1982). Language in the absence of inner speech. *Neuropsychologia*, 20, 391–409.

Lorch, M.P. (1995a). Laterality and rehabilitation: Differences in left and right hand productions in aphasic agraphic hemiplegics. *Aphasiology*, 9, 257–271.

Lorch, M.P. (1995b). Language and praxis in written production: A rehabilitation paradigm. *Aphasiology*, 9, 280–282.

Luzzatti, C., Colombo, C., Frustaci, M., & Vitolo, F. (2000). Rehabilitation of spelling along the sub-word-level routine. *Neuropsychological Rehabilitation*, 10, 249–278.

Marshall, J.C. & Newcombe, F. (1966). Syntactic and semantic errors in paralexia. *Neuropsychologia*, 4, 169–176.

Miceli, G., Silveri, M.C., & Caramazza, A. (1985). Cognitive analysis of a case of pure dysgraphia. *Brain and Language*, 25, 187–212.

Mortley, J., Enderby, P., & Petheram, B. (2001). Using a computer to improve functional writing in a patient with severe dysgraphia. *Aphasiology*, 15(5), 443–461.

Morton, J. (1969). Interaction of information in word recognition. *Psychological Review*, 76, 165–178.

Newcombe, F., & Marshall, J.C. (1984). Task and modality-specific aphasias. In F.C. Rose (Ed.), *Advances in neurology: Vol. 42. Progress in aphasiology*. New York: Raven Press.

Nickels, L. (1992). The autocue? Self-generated phonemic cues in the treatment of a disorder of reading and naming. *Cognitive Neuropsychology*, 9, 155–182.

Nolan, K.N., & Caramazza, A. (1983). An analysis of writing in a case of deep dyslexia. *Brain and Language*, 20, 305–328.

Panton, A., & Marshall, J. (2008). Improving spelling and everyday writing after a CVA: A single-case therapy study. *Aphasiology*, 22(2), 164–183.

Patterson, K., & Marcel, A. (1992). Phonological ALEXIA or PHONOLOGICAL Alexia? In J. Alegria, D. Holender, J. Junca de Morais, & M. Radeau (Eds.), *Analytic approaches to human cognition* (pp. 259–274). Amsterdam: Elsevier Science Publishers.

Pound, C. (1996). Writing remediation using preserved oral spelling: A case for separate output buffers. *Aphasiology*, 10, 283–296.

Rapcsak, S., & Beeson, P. (2004). The role of left posterior inferior temporal cortex in spelling. *Neurology*, 62(12), 2221–2229.

Rapcsak, S., Beeson, P., Henry, M., Leyden, A., Kim, E., Rising, K., . . . Cho, H. (2009). Phonological dyslexia and dysgraphia: Cognitive mechanisms and neural substrates. *Cortex*, 45(5), 575–591.

Rapp, B. (2005). The relationship between treatment outcomes and the underlying cognitive deficit: Evidence from the remediation of acquired dysgraphia. *Aphasiology*, 19(10–11), 994–1008.

Rapp, B., & Caramazza, A. (1997). From graphemes to abstract letter shapes: Levels of representation in written spelling. *Journal of Experimental Psychology: Human Perception and Performance*, 23, 1130–1152.

Rapp, B., Epstein, C., & Tainturier, M.J. (2002). The integration of information across lexical and sublexical processes in spelling. *Cognitive Neuropsychology*, 19(1), 1–29.

Rapp, B., & Glucroft, B. (2009). The benefits and protective effects of behavioural treatment for dysgraphia in a case of primary progressive aphasia. *Aphasiology*, 23(2), 236–265.

Rapp, B., & Kane, A. (2002). Remediation of deficits affecting different components of the spelling process. *Aphasiology*, 16, 439–454.

Raymer, A., Cudworth, C., & Haley, M. (2003). Spelling treatment for an individual with dysgraphia: Analysis of generalisation to untrained words. *Aphasiology*, 17, 607–624.

Robson, J., Marshall, J., Chiat, S., & Pring, T. (2001). Enhancing communication in jargon aphasia: A small group study of writing therapy. *International Journal of Language and Communication Disorders*, 36(4), 471–488.

Roeltgen, D.P., Sevush, S., & Heilman, K.M. (1983). Phonological agraphia: Writing by the lexical-semantic route. *Neurology*, 33, 755–765.

Rothi, L.J. (1995). Are we clarifying or contributing to the confusion? *Aphasiology*, 9, 271–273.

Sage, K., & Ellis, A. (2006). Using orthographic neighbours to treat a case of graphemic buffer disorder. *Aphasiology*, 20(9), 851–870.

Sasanuma, S. (1995). The missing data. *Aphasiology*, 9, 273–274.

Schmalzl, L., & Nickels, L. (2006). Treatment of irregular word spelling in acquired dysgraphia: Selective benefit from visual mnemonics. *Neuropsychological Rehabilitation*, 16(1), 1–37.

Seron, X., Deloche, G., Moulard, G., & Rousselle, M. (1980). A computer-based therapy for the treatment of aphasic subjects with writing disorders. *Journal of Speech and Hearing Disorders, 45*(1), 45–58.

Shallice, T. (1981). Phonological agraphia and the lexical route in writing. *Brain, 104,* 413–429.

Shim, H.S., Hurley, R.S., Rogalski, E., & Mesulam, M.-M. (2012). Anatomic, clinical, and neuropsychological correlates of spelling errors in primary progressive aphasia. *Neuropsychologia, 50*(8), 1929–1935.

Tainturier, M.J., & Rapp, B. (2003). Is a single graphemic buffer used in reading and spelling? *Aphasiology, 17*(6–7), 537–562.

Tsapkini, K., & Hillis, A.E. (2013). Spelling intervention in post-stroke aphasia and primary progressive aphasia. *Behavioural Neurology, 26,* 55–66.

Tsapkini, K., & Rapp, B. (2010). The orthography-specific functions of the left fusiform gyrus: Evidence of modality and category specificity. *Cortex, 46*(2), 185–205.

Weekes, B., & Cotheart, M. (1996). Surface dyslexia and surface dysgraphia: Treatment studies and their theoretical implications. *Cognitive Neuropsychology, 13,* 277–315.

Whurr, M., & Lorch, M. (1991). The use of a prosthesis to facilitate writing in aphasia and right hemiplegia. *Aphasiology, 5,* 411–418.

PART 3

Naming

7

THE COGNITIVE PROCESSES UNDERLYING NAMING

Donna C. Tippett and Argye E. Hillis

Verbal language is generally defined as the spoken code that relates form to meaning (Dronkers, Pinker, & Damasio, 2000). The ability to express thought, and gain access to the thoughts of others, relies on richness in language that reflects multiple levels of encoded meaning present in all languages.

Levels of language processing are typically described as assuming a hierarchy, wherein at a fundamental level lexical selections are then processed according to grammatical rules. The generated "code" enriches linguistic communication with resolution and nuance to convey meaning. Across the levels of language processing, vocabulary learning, a function that enables naming objects, is the earliest and most fundamental language activity. Correspondingly, the development of vocabulary is the language process that appears the least vulnerable to critical period effects, enabling the ability to learn new words easily across protracted periods of time. For example, delays in spoken language acquisition exert far larger effects on the development of syntax (structuring phrases and sentences) and pragmatics (contextual understanding) than on vocabulary expansion (Rice, Taylor, & Zubrick, 2008; Rice, Tomblin, Hoffman, Richman, & Marquis, 2004).

A toddler points to a dog and says, "Dog," to her parents' delight. Initially, "dog" may be used to refer only to the child's own dog, but eventually the child learns that the label is used for other dogs. In fact, the child is likely to overgeneralize, extending the name "dog" for cat, squirrels, and other nonhumans. A first encounter with horse or cow may even elicit, "Big dog!" Developmental naming patterns tell us a great deal about the relationship between meanings and names and the development of cognitive processes that support naming. Similarly, naming errors that result from focal brain injury or focal brain atrophy reveal a great deal about the cognitive processes that underlie naming. This chapter discusses some of what we have learned about the cognitive processes underlying naming by studying patterns of performance of people with aphasia. The subsequent chapters discuss the neural regions that support these processes and the diagnosis and treatment of impairments of each of these cognitive processes.

Object Recognition

Naming can be initiated with a general concept (e.g., [a furry quadruped that barks] or more plausibly a specific concept (e.g., [my furry friend who will make me feel better by wagging her tail and licking my face when I get home]). The former concept has both a meaning and a label shared by speakers of a language—"dog" in English. The latter refers to a particular instance of "dog" and has different labels assigned by different owners of dogs. Naming can also be initiated with a visual, auditory, olfactory, or tactile stimulus. We can recognize [dog] from a picture, from a bark, from a smell (perhaps), or maybe from feeling one. We can normally distinguish dogs from cats in each of these modalities of input. Dog owners can also recognize their own dog from other dogs; however, this distinction is not generally considered an act of naming, but rather one of episodic memory. As humans, we are not especially talented at recognizing our own dog from other dogs by their bark, their smell, or the texture of their coat, but that failure of episodic memory in nonvisual modalities is not considered an impairment (but might be considered an impairment in a dog).

Different Types of Impairments in Visual Recognition

Agnosias, disorders of recognition, can be specific to the visual or other sensory modalities and are distinguished as apperceptive or associative types (Bauer & Rubens, 1985; Geschwind, 1965; Vignolo, 1969). Apperceptive visual agnosia refers to impaired access to internal object representations or structural descriptions. Associative visual agnosia refers to the inability to assign meaning to a correctly perceived object (De Renzi, 2000).

Apperceptive Visual Agnosia: Impaired Access to Structural Descriptions

There are individuals with focal brain damage who, despite adequate early sensory processing, cannot recognize objects in one modality of input. For example, patients may have intact visual acuity and early visual processing (tested by simple visual matching paradigms), but cannot recognize objects visually. They can recognize an object when they hold it in their hands, hear a definition of the object, or hear its sound, but not when they see it.

There are two forms of this visual agnosia (impaired visual recognition). The first is apperceptive visual agnosia, in which the individual cannot copy an object well, recognize fragmented objects, match objects in canonical (i.e., typical or unambiguous) views to the same object from an unusual view, or distinguish real from false objects (Figure 7.1). These individuals have impaired access to fundamental component (structural) descriptions of familiar objects (Grossman, Galetta, & D'Esposito, 1997; Riddoch & Humphreys, 2003; Shelton, Bowers, Duara, & Heilman, 1994; Vecera & Gilds, 1997; Warrington & Rudge, 1995).

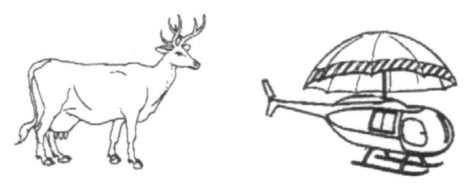

Figure 7.1 Examples of false objects. Individuals with apperceptive visual agnosia have difficulty recognizing that these figures do not depict real objects. In contrast, individuals with associative visual agnosia recognize that these figures do not depict real objects.

Associative Visual Agnosia, or "Optic Aphasia": Impaired Access to Semantics from Vision

Those with associative visual aphasia have spared access to structural descriptions, so they *can* distinguish familiar objects from false objects, match familiar objects to their appropriate color, or match an object to the same object from an unusual view. They can also, for example, match a pictured instance of cat to an identical pictured instance of cat (Figure 7.2, left), but they cannot name pictures or sort pictures into items with the same name. For example, they cannot sort pictured instances of dogs and cats into cats versus dogs (Figure 7.2, right). They have trouble associating visual input with word meaning (Charnallet, Carbonnel, David, & Moreaud, 2008; Iorio, Falanga, Fragassi, & Grossi, 1992; McCarthy & Warrington, 1986). Associative visual agnosia is also known as optic aphasia (Beauvois, 1982; Farah, 2004; Hillis & Caramazza, 1995a).

Other Modality-Specific Object Recognition Impairments

Individuals with tactile agnosia have impaired recognition specifically from the tactile modality (despite intact somatosensory skills) (Bohlhalter, Fretz, & Weder, 2002; Hömke, Amunts, Bönig, Fretz, Binkofski, Zilles, & Weder, 2009; Reed, Caselli, & Farah, 1996), while individuals with auditory agnosia have impaired recognition from the auditory modality (despite normal hearing acuity) (Buchtel & Stewart, 1989). Like associative visual agnosia or optic aphasia, there also exists individuals who recognize some auditory stimuli, but fail to associate spoken words with meaning (Auerbach, Allard, Naeser, Alexander, & Albert, 1982; Geschwind, 1965; Goldstein, 1974). This condition is known as "pure word deafness." These individuals can recognize written words, however.

Semantics

"Semantic memory" has many meanings. Here, we distinguish between general and personal knowledge of an object (everything we know about an object idiosyncratically) and

Matching Picture to Identical Picture   **Sorting Dogs Versus Cats**

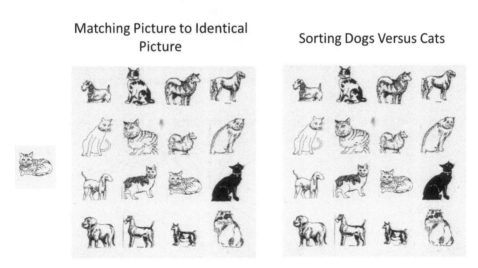

Figure 7.2 Left panel. Matching identical pictures. Individuals with apperceptive visual agnosia would have difficulty with this task; individuals with associative visual agnosia would have no difficulty with this task. Right panel. Sorting dogs versus cats. Individuals with apperceptive visual agnosia and individuals with associative visual agnosia have difficulty sorting dogs versus cats on the basis of visual information alone.

lexical-semantics—the subset of knowledge that defines a word, shared in the way the word is used by all speakers of the language. For example, we may know lots of things about dogs, only some of which are shared across cultures (e.g., <barks> <quadruped>), while other features of dogs are unique to some cultures or some instances of dogs (e.g., [used for pulling sleds], [used as police dogs], [used to help blind people], [has a black spot over one eye]). What really makes a dog a dog is its DNA. But we do not have access to the animal's DNA, so we use identifying features to identify dogs and to distinguish them from related animals. For example, we might use features like <quadruped>, <furry>, <tail>, <runs>, <barks>, and so on. Many of these features are shared with cats (except <barks>). Some are shared with wolves (except <barks>), and wolves have the feature of <nondomesticated>. These defining features serve to select a modality-independent lexical representation for output (naming).

As illustrated in Figure 7.3, shared features (e.g., <furry>, <quadruped> in our example) would activate modality-independent lexical representations for both dog and wolf. But <barks> would activate only dog. Normally, only the representation that receives activation from all of the semantic features would be selected for output. But if the lexical-semantic representation is underspecified, two or three modality-independent lexical representations (e.g., both dog and wolf) might be equally activated by the subset of semantic features.

Different Types of Semantic Impairments

Object semantics or semantic memory is the fund of general knowledge of objects. Lexical-semantics links words to meaning. Deficits in either area can result in a naming impairment.

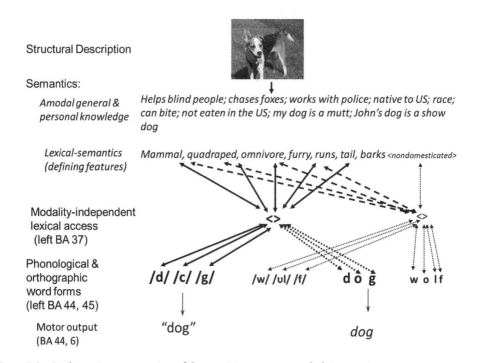

Figure 7.3 A schematic representation of the cognitive processes underlying naming.

Impaired Object Semantics

There are individuals who seem to recognize objects as familiar, and may even know which instance belongs to them, but are no longer able to link an object with general or personal knowledge. They may use the object inappropriately or respond to it inappropriately. For example, they might throw a squirrel a ball to fetch or throw the dog a diamond necklace. These patients have impaired "object semantics" or "semantic memory"; that is, they have limited general or personal knowledge of objects, usually due to semantic variant primary progressive aphasia, herpes encephalitis, or other condition that affects both the anterior/basal temporal lobes (see Sebastian & Hillis, chapter 11, this volume, for discussion). In some cases, object knowledge in particular categories of objects is affected, even when object knowledge in other categories is intact. For example, Hart, Berndt, and Caramazza (1985) reported the performance of a woman with a selective impairment of knowledge of fruits and vegetables, across a variety of language and nonlanguage tasks, following cerebral infarction. She could not judge whether drawings of fruits and vegetables were colored appropriately (e.g., a blue banana), or evaluate whether fruits and vegetables were typically eaten cooked or raw (e.g., "Is an orange typically cooked before it is eaten?). However, she showed intact performance on similar general tasks across a variety of other semantic categories, such as animals, clothing, vehicles, and tools, with items matched in frequency and familiarity.

Impaired Lexical-Semantics

Other individuals have intact general and personal knowledge about objects (and so they use objects correctly in everyday life), but appear to have impaired lexical-semantics. These individuals have trouble linking words to their meanings for both naming and word comprehension (written or spoken words). This selective impairment in lexical-semantics is manifested by the production of similar semantic errors (e.g., "cat" for dog or "fox" for dog) in oral and written naming of pictures, and in response to environmental sounds (e.g., barking), tactile stimuli (e.g., a toy dog or a real dog from tactile exploration), or when given definitions (e.g., "a furry quadruped that barks"). These individuals also make similar errors in oral and written word comprehension (e.g., confirm cat as the referent of "dog").

This characteristic pattern of errors was displayed by KE, a 52-year-old man who had a left middle cerebral artery stroke (Hillis, Rapp, Romani, & Caramazza, 1990). KE made similar semantic errors in oral reading and spelling to dictation, because he was impaired not only in lexical-semantics, but also in using phonology-to-orthography conversion and orthography-to-phonology conversion. So, when asked to write the word "chair" or write the name of a picture of a chair, KE wrote "table." When asked to read "chair," he read "bed." When asked to name aloud a pictured chair, he said "bed." His semantic errors varied across tasks and across sessions. He also sometimes produced the correct response on items that previously or later elicited a semantic error.

The fact that error rates and types of errors by KE were nearly identical across lexical tasks indicates that his deficit within the lexical system was relatively restricted to the one component common to all of these tasks. In the schematic of the cognitive processes underlying naming shown in Figure 7.3, the one component common to every lexical task is the lexical-semantic system.

Furthermore, the fact that the errors made by KE (and other patients with selective impairments in lexical-semantics) were largely coordinate semantic errors—words in the same semantic category as the target word (e.g., cat for dog)—can be explained by the hypothesis that focal brain damage may result in a selective loss of particular semantic features, leaving the individual with an underspecified lexical-semantic representation. For example, the underspecified semantic representation of dog might include features <furry> and <quadruped> and <tail>. This hypothesis leads to the prediction that individuals with lexical-semantic deficits would accept both the target object and a variety of objects in the same semantic category as the target as the referent of the name. In our example, an individual with the underspecified lexical-semantic representation of dog would accept both cat and wolf, as well as dog, as the referent of "dog," as the remaining features are consistent with all of these referents. This pattern is indeed reported in individuals with impaired lexical-semantics (Budd, Kortte, Cloutman, Newhart, Gottesman, Davis, Heidler-Gary, Seay, & Hillis, 2010; Hillis et al., 1990; Marsh & Hillis, 2005). It also predicts that they would produce the correct word and semantic coordinate errors in response to the same picture or object on separate occasions, which is also observed (Hillis & Caramazza, 1991a, 1995a).

Sometimes lexical-semantic impairments, with semantic errors in oral and written naming and spoken and written word comprehension, are specific to a given semantic category (e.g., animals, modes of transportation, body parts) (Caramazza & Hillis, 1990; Cloutman, Gottesman, Chaudhry, Davis, Kleinman, Pawlak, Herskovits, Kannan, Lee, Newhart, Heidler-Gary, & Hillis, 2009; Damasio, Tranel, Grabowski, Adolphs, & Damasio, 2004; Hillis & Caramazza, 1991b; 1995b; McKenna & Warrington, 1978; Sachett & Humphreys, 1992; Warrington & McCarthy, 1987; Warrington & Shallice, 1984). The topic of category-specific semantics, and its implications for cognitive processes involved in semantic processing, is further discussed by in chapter 10 in this volume.

Sometimes, individuals with aphasia are able to combine partial semantic information with partial phonological information to access the target phonological lexical representation for output. For example, suppose a patient has an underspecified lexical-semantic representation impairment at the level of modality-independent lexical processing that results in activation of a number of competing phonological lexical representations for output. Say, an underspecified lexical-semantic representation of dog might include <furry> <quadruped> <mammal>, and <tail>, which would activate phonological lexical phonological representations for "cat," "dog," "fox," "wolf," etc. A phonological cue, such a [dʌ] would provide additional activation of "dog," but not the competing representations, and would allow the individual to name dog. Likewise, this interaction between partial semantic information and partial phonological information may also account for correct reading of irregular words that individuals do not completely understand in some cases, as in the patient example, JJ status post a left temporal lobe lesion, described in Hillis and Caramazza (1991b).

Modality-Independent Access to Lexical Representations ("LEMMA")

One of the most common difficulties in naming is the inability to retrieve either the oral or the written name of the object despite having access to the complete semantic representation. This state of impaired word retrieval is often known as anomia. Anomia, or the "tip of the tongue" phenomenon, occurs in all of us, but occurs to a pathological degree (in terms of frequency) in dementia and after certain left hemisphere strokes. It is often the initial symptom of primary progressive aphasia, a focal neurodegenerative disease resulting from focal, progressive atrophy in the left hemisphere (Gorno-Tempini, Hillis, Weintraub, Kertesz, Mendez, Cappa, Ogar, Rohrer, Black, Boeve, Manes, Dronkers, Vandenberghe, Rascovsky, Patterson, Miller, Knopman, Hodges, Mesulam, & Grossman, 2011; Mesulam, 2001). Anomia is often the residual deficit after a variety of aphasias caused by left hemisphere stroke. But it can also occur as the only symptom of small stroke in the left posterior inferior temporal cortex (see chapter 8, this volume). Individuals with selective deficits at this level of processing make similar errors in oral and written naming, which often include semantic errors (of which they are aware; e.g., dog → "cat, well, no"), circumlocutions (e.g., dog → "my pet that fetches my paper for me"), "don't know" responses, or phonological paraphasias (e.g., dog → "doll"). Individuals with selective impairment at this level show normal performance in word comprehension tasks. For example, in Sebastian et al. (2014), a patient with a left hemisphere stroke, Dr. T. said "tie" for a picture of a shirt. He was frustrated by his errors, and very aware of them, but unable to correct them. He immediately followed his error above with, "That's not right, well, you wear it with a tie." He wrote the word "monster" for a picture of a robot. Then, he said, "something like that." He made no errors in word/picture verification with either spoken or written words. He rejected semantically related words as the names of pictures, even if he had produced the same name in response to the picture. Dr. T. used objects normally in everyday life, and was able to read aloud or spell to dictation both regular words and pseudowords. He made errors in reading and spelling irregular words. His anomia and irregular word spelling and reading were associated with poor perfusion of the left inferior temporal cortex, and improved with reperfusion of the inferior temporal cortex.

Modality-Specific Access to Lexical Representations

Detailed analyses of performance of individuals with selective impairment in naming in single-output modality (despite preserved motor output) have provided evidence that there are relatively independent orthographic and phonological lexical representations, or mechanisms for computing/accessing them, that can be independently affected by focal brain damage. To illustrate, HW and SJD both were impaired in naming verbs (actions) in a single-output modality, but had spared naming of nouns in both oral and written naming (Caramazza & Hillis, 1991). The fact that they could name nouns (objects) in both output modalities rules out a motor cause of their verb naming impairment. Rather, their highly selective deficits could best be explained by assuming impairment in (1) modality-specific access to lexical representations of verbs (phonological lexical representations for HW, orthographic lexical representations for SJD) and (2) sublexical orthography-to-phonology conversion for HW (as she could not read aloud) and sublexical phonology-to-orthography to conversion for SJD (as she could not spell the verb she said). This type of modality-specific impairment in access to lexical representations might be more prevalent than reported, because it may be difficult to detect when there is not a concomitant impairment in sublexical mechanisms for phonology-to-orthography conversion (or the opposite). That is, these sublexical mechanisms can often allow the individual to compensate for a modality-specific lexical access deficit by converting the retrieved representation from the intact modality to the impaired modality. However, in this case, the individual will make "regularization" errors in naming. For example, patient HG had severely impaired access to phonological lexical representations, but had relatively intact access to orthographic lexical representations and (following training) intact orthography-to-phonology conversion (Hillis, 1998). So, for example, when she wanted to say the word "one," she failed to access the phonological representation [wʌn], but accessed the orthographic representation, *one*. She applied orthography-to-phonology conversion and said "own" or [oʊn].

Motor Planning and Programming of Speech Articulation

Once the phonological representation is accessed (or assembled via orthography-to-phonology conversion mechanisms), the word must be articulated. Articulation requires coordinated movements of the lips, tongue, palate, jaw, vocal folds, and respiratory muscles to produce accurate phonemes. Weakness, slowness, reduced range of movement, or impaired timing of movement of any of the muscles of articulation results in consistent, predictable distortions of phonemes, known as dysarthria. In contrast, impairment in planning or programming of these movements, yielding various off-target sequences of phonemes in an attempt to produce a word, is known as apraxia of speech. Both dysarthria and apraxia of speech are pure motor speech disorders, and not strictly language disorders. They affect spoken, but not written, naming (Jordan & Hillis, 2006; Ziegler, Aichert, & Staiger, 2012).

There are other individuals who have apraxia that affects written output, but not other motor tasks performed with the limbs. This "apraxic agraphia" has been described after focal stroke (Roeltgen, 2003; Valenstein & Heilman, 1979) and even after brief, temporary lesions caused by direct electrical stimulation of Exner's area (an area posterior and superior to Broca's area), where lesions result in apraxic agraphia (Lubrano, Roux, & Démonet, 2004; Roux, Durand, Réhault, Planton, Draper, & Démonet, 2014). Because these motor deficits are only peripherally related to naming deficits, we will not consider them in detail here.

Conclusions

We have reviewed a model of the cognitive processes required to name a picture, object, or concept, schematically depicted in Figure 7.3. Many of these cognitive processes or representations are also required for other lexical tasks, so we assume these are not specifically used in the task of naming. For example, phonological lexical representations—spoken-word forms—are also accessed or assembled in reading aloud (at least irregular) words, and orthographic lexical representations—written word form—are also accessed or assembled in spelling (at least irregular) words (see chapters 1 and 4, this volume). We assume that both lexical and semantic representations are distributed representations; that is, that they are "accessed" by activating a set of components (e.g., phonemes for phonological representations, semantic features for semantic representations), and that they overlap with representations that share a subset of these components. Thus, this sort of theoretical model can be "implemented" by parallel distributed processing (PDP) sorts of computational models (see chapter 20, this volume).

References

Auerbach, S.H., Allard, T., Naeser, M., Alexander, M.P., & Albert, M.L. (1982). Pure word deafness: Analysis of a case with bilateral lesions and a defect at the prephonemic level. *Brain, 105,* 271–300.

Bauer, R.M., & Rubens, A.B. (1985). Agnosia. In: *Clinical Neuropsychology.* Second edition. Edited by K.M. Heilman and E. Valenstein. New York: Oxford University Press, pp. 187–241.

Beauvois, M.F. (1982). Optic aphasia: A process of interaction between vision and language. *Philosophical Transactions of the Royal Society Series B Biological Sciences, 298,* 35–47.

Bohlhalter, S., Fretz, C., & Weder, B. (2002). Hierarchical versus parallel processing in tactile object recognition: A behavioural-neuroanatomical study of aperceptive tactile agnosia. *Brain, 125,* 2537–2548.

Buchtel, H.A., & Stewart, J.D., (1989). Auditory agnosia: Apperceptive or associative disorder. *Brain and Language, 37,* 12–25.

Budd, M.A., Kortte, K., Cloutman, L., Newhart, M., Gottesman, R.F., Davis, C., Heidler- Gary, J., Seay, M.W., & Hillis A.E. (2010). The nature of naming errors in primary progressive aphasia versus acute post-stroke aphasia. *Neuropsychology, 24,* 581–589.

Caramazza, A., & Hillis, A.E. (1990). Where do semantic errors come from? *Cortex, 26,* 95–122.

Caramazza, A., & Hillis, A.E. (1991). Lexical organization of nouns and verbs in the brain. *Nature, 349,* 788–790.

Charnallet, A., Carbonnel, S., David, D., & Moreaud, O. (2008). Associative visual agnosia: A case study. *Behavioral Neurology, 19,* 41–44.

Cloutman, L., Gottesman, R., Chaudhry, P., Davis, C., Kleinman, J.T., Pawlak, M., Herskovits, E.H., Kannan, V., Lee, A., Newhart, M., Heidler-Gary, J., & Hillis, A.E. (2009). Where (in the brain) do semantic errors come from? *Cortex, 45,* 641–649.

Damasio, H., Tranel, D., Grabowski, T.J., Adolphs, R., & Damasio, A. (2004). Neural systems behind word and concept retrieval. *Cognition, 92,* 179–229.

De Renzi, E. (2000). Disorders of visual recognition. *Seminars in Neurology, 20,* 479–485.

Dronkers, N.F., Pinker, S., & Damasio, A. (2000). Language and the aphasias. In: *Principles of Neural Science.* Fourth edition. Edited by E.R. Kandel, J.H. Schwartz, & T.M. Jessell. New York: McGraw-Hill Companies, pp. 981–995.

Farah, M.J. (2004). *Visual Agnosia.* Second edition. Cambridge, MA: MIT Press.

Geschwind, N. (1965). Disconnexion syndromes in animals and man. Parts I and II. *Brain, 88*, 237–294, 585–644.

Goldstein, M.N. (1974). Auditory agnosia for speech (pure word deafness): Historical review with current implications. *Brain and Language, 1*, 195–204.

Gorno-Tempini, M.L., Hillis, A.E., Weintraub, S., Kertesz, A., Mendez, M., Cappa, S.F., Ogar, J.M., Rohrer, J.D., Black, S., Boeve, B.F., Manes, F., Dronkers, N.F., Vandenberghe, R., Rascovsky, K., Patterson, K., Miller, B.L., Knopman, D.S., Hodges, J.R., Mesulam, M.M., & Grossman M. (2011). Classification of primary progressive aphasia and its variants. *Neurology, 11*, 1006–1014.

Grossman, M., Galetta, S., & D'Esposito, M. (1997). Object recognition difficulty in visual apperceptive agnosia. *Brain and Cognition, 33*, 306–342.

Hart, J., Berndt, R.S., & Caramazza, A. (1985). Category-specific naming deficit following cerebral infarction. *Nature, 316*, 439–440.

Hillis, A.E. (1998). Treatment of naming disorders: New issues regarding old therapies. *Journal of the International Neuropsychological Society, 4*, 648–660.

Hillis, A.E., & Caramazza, A. (1991a). Category-specific naming and comprehension impairment: A double dissociation. *Brain, 114*, 2081–2094.

Hillis, A.E., & Caramazza, A. (1991b). Mechanisms for accessing lexical representations for output: Evidence from a category-specific semantic deficit. *Brain and Language, 40*, 106–144.

Hillis, A.E., & Caramazza, A. (1995a). Cognitive and neural mechanism underlying visual and semantic processing: Implications from optic aphasia. *Journal of Cognitive Neuroscience, 7*, 457–478.

Hillis, A.E., & Caramazza, A. (1995b). The compositionality of lexical-semantic representations: Clues from semantic errors in object naming. *Memory, 3*, 333–358.

Hillis, A.E., Rapp, B.C., Romani, C., & Caramazza, A. (1990). Selective impairment of semantics in lexical processing. *Cognitive Neuropsychology, 7*, 191–244.

Hömke, L., Amunts, K., Bönig, L., Fretz, C., Binkofski, F., Zilles, K., & Weder, B. (2009). Analysis of lesions in patients with unilateral tactile agnosia using cytoarchitectonic probabilistic maps. *Human Brain Mapping, 30*, 1444–1456.

Iorio, L., Falanga, A., Fragassi, N.A., & Grossi, D. (1992). Visual associative agnosia and optic aphasia. A single case study and a review of the syndromes. *Cortex, 28*, 23–37.

Jordan, L.C., & Hillis, A.E. (2006). Disorders of speech and language: Aphasia, apraxia and dysarthria. *Current Opinion in Neurology, 19*, 580–585.

Lubrano, V., Roux, F.E., & Démonet, J.F. (2004). Writing-specific sites in frontal areas: A cortical stimulation study. *Journal of Neurosurgery, 101*, 787–798.

Marsh, E.B., & Hillis, A.E. (2005). Cognitive and neural mechanisms underlying reading and naming: Evidence from letter-by-letter reading and optic aphasia. *Neurocase: The Neural Basis of Cognition, 11*, 325–337.

McCarthy, R.A., & Warrington, E.K. (1986). Visual associative agnosia: A clinico-anatomical study of a single case. *Journal of Neurology, Neurosurgery, and Psychiatry, 49*, 1233–1240.

McKenna, P., & Warrington, E.K. (1978). Category-specific naming preservation: A single case study. *Journal of Neurology, Neurosurgery and Psychiatry, 41*, 571–574.

Mesulam, M.M. (2001). Primary progressive aphasia. *Annals of Neurology, 49*, 425–432.

Reed, C.L., Caselli, R.J., & Farah, M.J. (1996). Tactile agnosia: Underlying impairment and implications for normal tactile object recognition. *Brain, 119*, 875–888.

Rice, M.L., Taylor, C.L., & Zubrick, S.R. (2008). Language outcomes of 7-year-old children with or without a history of late language emergence at 24 months. *Journal of Speech, Language, and Hearing Research, 51*, 394–407.

Rice, M.L., Tomblin, J.B., Hoffman, L., Richman, W.A., & Marquis, J. (2004). Grammatical tense deficits in children with SLI and nonspecific language impairment: Relationships with nonverbal IQ over time. *Journal of Speech, Language, and Hearing Research, 47*, 816–834.

Riddoch, M.J., & Humphreys, G.W. (2003). Visual agnosia. *Neurologic Clinics, 21*, 501–520.

Roeltgen, D.P. (2003). Agraphia. In: *Clinical Neuropsychology*. Edited by K.M. Heilman & E. Valenstein. New York: Oxford University Press, pp. 126–145.

Roux, F.E., Durand, J.B., Réhault, E., Planton, S., Draper, L., & Démonet, F.F. (2014). The neural basis for writing from dictation in the temporoparietal cortex. *Cortex, 50*, 64–75.

Sachett, C., & Humphreys, G.W. (1992). Calling a squirrel a squirrel but a canoe a wigwam: A category-specific deficit for artefactual objects and body parts. *Cognitive Neuropsychology, 9*, 73–86.

Sebastian, R., Gomez, Y., Leigh, R., Davis, C., Newhart, M., Hillis, A.E. (2014). The roles of occipitotemporal cortex in reading, spelling, and naming. *Cognitive Neuropsychology, 31*, 511–528.

Sebastian, R., & Hillis, A.E. (2015). Neural substrates of semantics. In: *The Handbook of Adult Language Disorders*. Edited by A.E. Hillis. New York: Psychology Press.

Shelton, P.A., Bowers, D., Duara, R., & Heilman, K.M. (1994). Apperceptive visual agnosia: A case study. *Brain and Cognition, 25*, 1–23.

Valenstein, E., & Heilman, K. (1979). Apraxic agraphia with neglect-induced paragraphia. *Archives of Neurology, 36*, 506–508.

Vecera, S. P, & Gilds, K.S. (1997). What is it like to be a patient with apperceptive agnosia? *Consciousness and Cognition, 6*, 237–266.

Vignolo, L.A. (1969). Auditory agnosia: A review and report of recent evidence. In: *Contributions to Clinical Neuropsychology*. Edited by A.L. Benton. Chicago: Aldine, pp. 172–208.

Warrington, E.K., & McCarthy, R.A. (1987). Categories of knowledge: Further fractionations and an attempted explanation. *Brain, 110*, 1273–1296.

Warrington, E.K., & Rudge, P. (1995). A comment on apperceptive agnosia. *Brain and Cognition, 28*, 173–177.

Warrington, E.K., & Shallice, T. (1984). Category specific semantic impairments. *Brain, 107*, 829–853.

Ziegler, W., Aichert, I., & Staiger, A. (2012). Apraxia of speech: Concepts and controversies. *Journal of Speech, Language, and Hearing Research, 55*, S1485–S1501.

8

THE NEURAL MECHANISMS UNDERLYING NAMING

David C. Race and Argye E. Hillis

Introduction

As described in the previous chapter, cognitive models of naming generally agree that naming takes place across two main stages—conceptual and word-form processing. The conceptual stage encompasses computation of the semantic representation of the item. The word-form stage entails linking the semantic representation to phonological representation (likely via a modality-independent lexical representation or "hidden units") and then executing the motor movements for spoken or written output. However, the task of naming often begins with recognition of a stimulus. That is, while one can certainly name a concept, naming is generally evaluated by naming stimuli, such as pictures, objects, or environmental sounds. Focal brain damage can selectively affect any of these four major stages of naming: recognition of the stimulus, the concept or meaning of the stimulus, access to the modality-independent lexical representation, or access to the spoken or written word form (see chapter 7, this volume, for further discussion). Here we will consider the lesions that selectively affect each of the cognitive processes underlying each of these stages of naming.

In naming tasks, recognition of the stimulus begins by constructing a modal structural representation that consists of features tied to the modality of stimulus presentation. For example, a picture of a horse will activate features in the visual cortex (e.g., shape, color) that combine to form a structural representation. Although modal processing is necessary for further semantic processing of the stimulus, it is not usually considered part of core semantics. Even with disruption of this level of processing in one or more modalities, speakers continue to recognize items through other modalities and verbal description and accurately describe physical and functional attributes of items when presented with its name (Beauvois, 1982; Chanoine, Ferreira, Demonet, Nespoulous, & Poncet, 1997; Coslett & Saffran, 1992; Hillis & Caramazza, 1995a; Iorio, Falanga, Fragassi, & Grossi, 1992; Lhermitte & Beauvois, 1973). As a simple illustration, a blindfolded person would not be able to recognize a picture of a horse or a real horse out in the distance, but would be able to describe aspects of horses as well as recognize a horse through sound (whinnying or galloping) or tactile input or perhaps even smell.

As the stream of processing continues, representations continue to increase in complexity, both within and across modalities, to the point of becoming amodal. As amodal representations are formed across modal inputs, accessing them is not dependent on any one modality. Damage to amodal semantic representations leads to deficits across input and output modalities. There are two levels of representation that are modality-independent: conceptual semantics (everything we know about a concept, including personal information) and lexical-semantics (the meaning of a word). Individuals with impairment of either would have difficulty with word-picture matching, as well as oral and written naming. However, only individuals with impairment of conceptual semantics would have nonlinguistic deficits related to the functional properties of items (e.g., how to use a fork and knife; see chapter 7).

Next begins the process of linking the semantic representation to a word-form. This task is rather daunting as the relationship between semantics and phonology (or orthography) is usually arbitrary. The stage of processing is sometimes called the "lemma" level of processing. For example, there is little, if any, relationship between the semantic representation of a horse and the word "horse." A horse could just as well be named a "blern." In fact the same semantic representation of a horse has many different names across the languages of the world. Although this type of flexibility is one of the main aspects that make language such a powerful tool for communication, it creates a challenge for the linking process. At minimum the linking process must be able to activate the correct phonological representation (and orthographic representation) in the midst of competitors that can overlap with the target either semantically (horse vs. zebra), phonologically/visually (cat vs. fat), or both semantically and phonologically/visually (cat vs. rat).

The word-form stage encompasses activating the phonological representation (i.e., sound structure) or orthographic representation, followed by planning and executing motor output for oral naming or written naming. Evidence that there exists a neural mechanism for computing modality-specific representations comes from brain-damaged individuals who are selectively impaired in naming in one modality (e.g., oral naming) but not the other (e.g., written naming) (Caramazza & Hillis, 1990), despite intact motor speech and writing. There are even instances where the modality-specific naming deficits are also specific to a particular grammatical category, such as nouns or verbs (Caramazza & Hillis, 1991; Hillis & Caramazza, 1995b), providing further evidence that the deficit is not a motor execution deficit.

Similar to previous stages, errors arise due to overlap between the target and competitors that overlap in composition of the representation. Successful activation (or computation) of the target involves selecting the phonemes and ordering them in the proper sequence. Phonemes are uniquely identified according to a complex combination of features related to qualities of their sound, as well as the motor movements required to make that sound. For example, in English, adduction (closure) of the vocal folds allowing vibration results in voiced phonemes as heard in the phoneme /b/, while abduction (opening) results in unvoiced sounds as heard in the phoneme /p/. Competition increases with overlap such that sounds with high overlap (/b/ vs. /p/) are in higher competition than sounds with low overlap (/b/ vs. /k/). Errors can occur when phonemes within the target word receive too much competition. For a particular target word (cat), word-form errors could either be an unrelated word (mat) or a nonword (zat). Difficulties that can arise from problems in the phonological (or motor planning) stage are highlighted in the errors made with tongue twisters.

Various types of naming tasks may also require other cognitive processes than those described above for the simple task of picture naming. For example, demanding naming tasks, such as when a verbal description initially fails to activate the target, may require the ability to use task relevant information to activate the target item and discriminate this representation from similar items. This type of activity is referred to as goal-directed processing (Badre & Wagner, 2007), which is an intricate part of semantic working memory. One of the most studied forms of goal-directed processing is controlled retrieval. Controlled retrieval is the process of using goal-related information to activate the semantic representation. The necessity of controlled retrieval increases when stimulus cues leave the target underspecified. For example, "Name the pointy objects that cowboys wear on their boots" may fail to activate the target. In this case, controlled retrieval would activate information about cowboys to help activate the target answer (spurs).

Association between Naming and Brain Regions

As should be obvious from the preceding brief overview, naming is a complex process that involves many regions interacting together to accomplish the task. The general behavioral deficit, an inability to name, can arise from impairment in any one of these processes. Therefore, it takes careful testing and observation to uncover specific behavioral deficits that manifest due to a particular process and associate it with brain regions or networks. In the following sections we provide an overview of the relationship between naming deficits and regions of the brain. It is crucial to keep in mind that there is no one-to-one correspondence between a particular aspect of the naming process and a particular region of the brain. Many regions seem to be involved across multiple aspects of naming, and also play a role in other aspects of language, such as sentence processing. As such, the structure-function relationship is discussed in relative terms with at least one region being most closely associated with a particular aspect of processing, while others may be associated but less so.

Stimulus Recognition (Input Modality-Specific Processing)

Modal processing encompasses the representation of the to-be-named object for a particular mode of input (e.g., visual, auditory, tactile) and is associated with regions such as the visual, auditory, and somatosensory cortices. Damage to these regions can lead to agnosia, in which recognition of an item is impaired although basic sensory perception is intact. Importantly, with agnosia the semantic and word-form representations are intact, such that a speaker would be able to name an item if presented in the unaffected modalities. For example, a person with visual agnosia would have difficulty naming a picture of a dog, but would be able to name dog from the sound (barking).

Visual agnosia is characterized by deficits in recognizing objects presented visually despite intact basic visual processing (e.g., normal acuity, ability to track movement) (Farah, 2004; Ffytche, Blom, & Catani, 2010; Humphreys & Riddoch, 2006). The subtypes of visual agnosia are generally divided between two broad classes: apperceptive and associative agnosia. Apperceptive agnosia is linked to difficulty with the perception of items (Grossman, Galetta, & D'Esposito, 1997). It is associated with bilateral lesions to occipital and occipital-temporal regions (Brodmann areas, or BAs, 17, 18, 19). The recognition of basic features such as color, brightness, and size are intact but difficult to combine in a manner that uniquely identifies the item. Individuals with apperceptive agnosia have difficulty copying objects. They can also have difficulty discriminating between shapes and comparing similar figures. Furthermore, they often fixate on one feature while attempting to recognize an item. This strategy may prove fruitful in some cases (e.g., correctly identifying a banana because it is yellow), but often fails. For example, one agnosic individual described the finger holes of scissors as "wheels of a big car" (Grossman, Galetta, & D'Esposito, 1997).

With associative agnosia, visual perception of items is relatively intact, but difficulty remains in linking this perception to meaning (Farah, 2004; McCarthy & Warrington, 1986). This form of agnosia is associated with bilateral lesions in the junction of the posterior inferior temporal lobe and the occipital lobe (BAs 18, 19, 37). In contrast to apperceptive agnosia, individuals are able to draw copies of items that they cannot name. Furthermore, they can discern whether two pictures match and also whether a picture depicts a real or false object (e.g., false objects constructed by combining two real objects, such as a lion's head on the body of a cow). Nevertheless, individuals with associative agnosia have difficulty in providing either the name or function of items and also have trouble sorting objects by semantic category. Errors tend to be related to visual structure rather than semantics (e.g., key named as "knife").

Optic aphasia is similar to visual associative agnosia (or is a variant of visual associative agnosia). Some authors make a distinction, such that those with optic aphasia have greater access to semantic representations of objects (Farah, 2004). Individuals with optic aphasia are able to sort items by broad semantic categories (e.g., living vs. nonliving), and their naming errors tend to be semantically related to the target (e.g., naming a goat as a "sheep") (Hillis & Caramazza, 1995a). Even when they make naming errors they often describe or gesture the correct function of the target item. Optic aphasia is associated with lesions of the left occipital cortex and the splenium, which is believed to result in a disconnection between visual processing in the right hemisphere and language processing in the left hemisphere (Freund, 1889; Hillis & Caramazza, 1995a; Marsh & Hillis, 2005).

Auditory agnosia is characterized by deficits in processing verbal or environmental sounds despite intact basic hearing (e.g., ability to hear tones within a normal range and localize sounds) (Buchtel & Stewart, 1989; Goldstein, 1974; Lewis, Wightman, Brefczynski, Phinney, Binder, & DeYoe, 2004; Saygin, Dick, Wilson, Dronkers, & Bates, 2003; Saygin, Leech, & Dick, 2010). It is associated with bilateral lesions to the middle and posterior superior temporal cortex (BAs 22, 41, 42) and to some extent the posterior middle temporal cortex (BA 21). Individuals with verbal auditory agnosia, or "pure word deafness," have difficulty comprehending speech, although reading, writing, and speech production are relatively intact. With nonverbal auditory agnosia or environmental agnosia, individuals have difficulty matching an environmental sound to its source. For example, a patient responded "cow," "baby," and "gunfire" to the sound of a sheep, a crow, and a helicopter, respectively (Saygin, Leech, & Dick, 2010).

Tactile agnosia is characterized by deficits in perceiving objects through tactile investigation despite intact basic somatosensory perception (e.g., recognition of vibration and temperature, two-point discrimination) (Bohlhalter, Fretz, & Weder, 2002; Hömke et al., 2009; Reed, Caselli, & Farah, 1996). It is associated with lesions of the somatosensory cortex (BAs 1, 2, 3, 4) and the parietal cortex (BAs 7, 39, 40). Individuals have difficulty identifying common objects through tactile investigation (e.g., calculator, bottle, combination lock), although they can describe some of their features. Individuals do retain the ability to discriminate between objects of different sizes, weights, and textures (Reed, Caselli, & Farah, 1996).

Conceptual Stage: Amodal Semantics

Amodal semantic deficits are characterized by naming errors across input and output modalities, comprehension errors, and, crucially, by nonverbal deficits (e.g., placing salad into a cup instead of a plate). Much of the data regarding the amodal representation comes from individuals with semantic dementia (now called semantic variant primary progressive aphasia, or svPPA; Gorno-Tempini et al., 2011), which is characterized by both linguistic and nonlinguistic semantic deficits in contrast to relatively normal abilities in other aspects of cognition (e.g., memory and executive functioning) and language (e.g., phonology and syntax) (Gorno-Tempini et al., 2011; Hodges, Patterson, Oxbury, & Funnell, 1992; Snowden, Goulding, & Neary, 1989).

In svPPA both linguistic and nonlinguistic processing deficits occur across all modalities (Jefferies & Lambon Ralph, 2006). In comprehension tasks, individuals with svPPA have difficulty matching an object to its spoken or written name or to a verbal description (Coccia, Bartolini, Luzzi, Provinciali, & Lambon Ralph, 2004). In production tasks, they have difficulty with spoken or written naming of an object presented in visual, auditory, or tactile form (Lambon Ralph, Graham, Ellis, & Hodges, 1998; Lambon Ralph, McClelland, Patterson, Galton, & Hodges, 2001). In addition, individuals with svPPA have trouble with nonlinguistic tasks, such as drawing a copy of an object after delay (Bozeat et al., 2003), or matching an object to the sound that it makes, its smell, or its tactile features (Bozeat, Lambon Ralph, Patterson, Garrard, & Hodges, 2000; Lambon Ralph, Graham, Patterson, & Hodges, 1999). Errors are generally semantic in nature (e.g., naming the picture of a dog as "cat"), and performance tends to be affected by item factors such as frequency, familiarity, and complexity (Bozeat et al., 2000; Funell, 1995; Jefferies & Lambon Ralph, 2006).

A point of emerging consensus is that the deficits of conceptual semantics, as seen in svPPA, generally only occur with damage to bilateral temporal cortex, including anterior temporal pole (Lambon Ralph, Cipolotti, Manes, & Patterson, 2010; Walker et al., 2011; Warren, Crinion, Lambon Ralph, & Wise, 2009; see also chapter 7, this volume). A recent study of participants with unilateral chronic lesions of the anterior temporal pole (left or right) indicated that neither unilateral anterior temporal lesion caused substantial semantic impairment; that bilateral damage was essential for the severe impairment of semantic memory seen in svPPA (Lambon Ralph, Cipolotti, Manes, & Patterson, 2010). A recent study of participants with acute unilateral left hemisphere demonstrated no association between unilateral left anterior temporal pole (BA 38) damage and amodal semantic deficits after controlling for volume of infarct (Tsapkini, Frangakis, & Hillis, 2011).

While the data from svPPA studies suggests a relationship between bilateral anterior temporal lobe (ATL) and amodal semantics, the functional imaging data provide mixed support. As a result, for models of language that incorporate the imaging data, the ATL tends to figure less prominently as a site for amodal semantics (Hickock & Poeppel, 2004; Indefrey & Levelt, 2004; Wise, 2003). Visser, Jefferies, and Lambon Ralph (2010) addressed the inconsistency within the imaging literature through a meta-analysis of functional imaging studies of language tasks to investigate the conditions in which ATL activation was reported. They found that studies were more likely to report ATL activation when (a) positron emission tomography (PET) imaging was used rather than fMRI due to the fact that the fMRI signal can become distorted in the ATL region, (b) the field of view included the whole brain rather than a smaller area that potentially did not include the ATL, (c) the ATL was included in a region of interest (ROI) analysis, which provides more statistical power towards finding significant differences when activation is relatively weak, and (d) the baseline task acted as a more stringent control for semantic processing. Although the debate is far from settled, their data indicates the possibility that the functional imaging literature may converge with the svPPA literature to a greater degree than previously thought.

Lexical-Semantic Processing (Linking Semantics and Modality Independent Representations)

Lexical semantic processing links the semantic representation of an item and its modality-independent lexical representation for both production and comprehension of words. Importantly, while lexical-semantic processing deficits affect language tasks such as naming and word-picture matching, nonlinguistic semantic processing remains intact. For example, while a patient with lexical-semantic deficits and a patient with amodal semantic deficits may have difficulty naming an object (e.g., television) or matching an object to its name or description, only the latter patient would have difficulty operating that object.

Lesions to posterior superior temporal gyrus (STG) often result in Wernicke's aphasia, which is characterized by occasions of fluent but meaningless speech, repetition, and writing, along with impaired comprehension in conversation and reading. Interestingly, individuals seem to be generally unaware of their deficits. Individuals commit a mixture of semantic errors (e.g., referring to a horse as "deer") and phonological errors (e.g., referring to a horse as "horn" or "splern"). Both acute and chronic lesions in BA 22 cause deficits in comprehension and production (Hart & Gordon, 1990; Leff et al., 2009; Lesser et al., 1986). Furthermore, in the acute setting the severity of hypoperfusion in BA 22 correlates with the severity of deficits (Hillis et al., 2001b), and restored blood flow results in improved performance (Hillis et al., 2001a; Hillis & Heidler, 2002). Functional imaging data indicates that this region is highly involved in word comprehension and production (Fridriksson & Morrow, 2005; Leff et al., 2002) along with phonological processing (Buchsbaum, Hickok, & Humphries, 2001; Okada & Hickok, 2006; Price, Wise, & Frackowiak, 1996).

Lesions to areas adjacent to BA 22, most notably the angular gyrus and posterior middle temporal gyrus (MTG) often result in transcortical sensory aphasia, which is similar to Wernicke's aphasia, except repetition is intact (Farias, Harrington, Broomand, & Seyal, 2005; Fridriksson & Morrow, 2005; Harrington, Buonocore, & Farias, 2006; Jefferies & Lambon Ralph, 2006; Kemeny et al., 2006). Functional imaging studies have revealed greater activation in these regions for picture naming and lexical-semantic tasks (e.g., semantic relative to phonological judgments) (Binder, Desai, Graves, & Conant, 2009; Mummery, Patterson, Hodges, & Price, 1998). Both regions are points of convergence across modalities, which may explain their role in linking semantics to phonology.

Modality-Independent Lexical Representations (Access to both Phonological and Orthographic Words from Lexical-Semantics)

Once an individual has computed lexical-semantic representation (the meaning of a specific word), he or she must then retrieve the word itself. (See chapter 7, this volume, for discussion of theories regarding this stage of word retrieval). Everyone has the experience of failing at this level of processing, when we know exactly what we want to say but fail to retrieve the word for it. It is on the "tip of the tongue," and one can neither say nor spell the word. This failure, known as anomia, is a modality-independent impairment in accessing lexical representations. It is the most common language deficit in all types of aphasia (and in dementia), and can be the residual deficit after recovery from nearly any large lesion in the left hemisphere.

Anomia is most commonly seen in isolation after lesion in the left posterior inferior temporal gyrus (within BA 37). Lesions to this region tend to result in semantic errors for both written and spoken output (DeLeon et al., 2007; Raymer et al., 1997). Errors arise in picture naming, naming the source of a sound, and naming from tactile input (Tranel, Grabowski, Lyon, & Damasio, 2005). Reperfusion of left BA 37 after stroke, in the acute setting, is associated with improvement in naming but not comprehension (Hillis et al., 2006).

Functional imaging studies indicate that left BA 37 is activated during oral and written naming (Emerton, Gansler, Sandberg, & Jerram, 2013; Rapcsak & Beeson, 2004) and during oral reading (Cohen et al., 2000, 2002; McCandliss et al., 2003). However, the more medial part of BA 37, in left fusiform cortex, may be more important for early written word recognition, while the lateral part of left BA 37, in inferior temporal cortex, may be important for modality-independent lexical access (Cohen, Jobert, Bihan, & Dehaene, 2004). A recent study of individuals with acute left-hemisphere ischemic stroke (Sebastian et al., 2014) supports these claims, indicating written naming and reading deficits associated with left fusiform damage and object naming deficits with lateral damage to BA 37. Furthermore, in some cases, performance improved with reperfusion to the affected area. Finally, a study of individuals with primary progressive aphasia (Race et al., 2013) revealed that atrophy of the posterior inferior temporal gyrus, which overlaps with lateral BA37, was associated with performance across a number of tasks that involved naming.

Modality-Specific Lexical Representations (Access to Word Forms)

Computation of a phonological representation (spoken-word form) can be impaired independently of computation of an orthographic representation (written word form). However, individuals with this selective deficit are relatively rare, and most have been studied after partial recovery from large lesions (Ellis, Miller, & Sin, 1983; Hillis & Caramazza, 1990; Rapp & Caramazza, 1997). However, acute lesions or atrophy in posterior frontal areas sometimes cause modality-independent output deficits in oral naming or written naming of *actions*, even when the individuals are able to speak or write names of *objects* (showing that it is not a motor deficit that limits their output) (Hillis, Wityk, Barker, & Caramazza, 2003; Hillis, Chang, & Breese, 2004; Hillis, Oh, & Ken, 2004).

Production of a spoken word also requires motor planning and execution of the muscles used for speech (i.e., the articulators). Impairment in motor planning and programming of speech articulation is most closely associated with the inferior frontal gyrus (notably Broca's area), portions of the insular gyrus, the supplementary cortex, and the premotor cortex. Damage to these regions is associated with deficits in speech praxis, or orchestration of motor plans of the lips, tongue, jaw, palate, vocal folds, and muscles of respiration to articulate speech (Ash et al., 2009; Davis et al., 2008; Hickok, Rogalsky, Chen, Herskovits, Townsley, & Hillis, 2014; Trupe et al., 2013). Note that problems with speech praxis are separate from impairment in strength, tone, rate, range, or coordination of the articulatory muscles, known as dysarthria.

Discussion

This chapter provided an overview of the relationship between cognitive processes underlying naming and regions of the brain. The to-be-named object is first processed in modality-specific regions (e.g., visual/auditory/somatosensory cortex). Next, the input activates a conceptual representation, which involves a broad region of areas in both temporal cortices that encompasses posterior and anterior regions. Anterior regions of the temporal cortex are likely involved in amodal semantic processing, while posterior regions seem more involved in linking word meanings to word forms, with lateral inferior temporal cortex portion of BA 37 being a likely candidate as the gateway for this linking process in naming. Finally, modality-specific output representations must be activated, which seems to depend on posterior inferior frontal cortex, at least for names of actions (verbs). Future studies will continue to provide more detail as to how these regions interact during naming, as well as how this network is modified in response to lesions and recovery.

References

Ash, S., Moore, P., Vesely, L., Gunawardena, D., McMillan, C., Anderson, C., et al. (2009). Non-fluent speech in frontotemporal lobar degeneration. *Journal of Neurolinguistics, 22*(4), 370–383.

Badre, D., & Wagner A.D. (2007). Left ventrolateral prefrontal cortex and the cognitive control of memory. *Neuropsychologia, 45*, 2883–2901.

Beauvois, M.F. (1982). Optic aphasia—A process of interaction between vision and language. *Philosophical Transactions of the Royal Society of London Series B-Biological Sciences, 298*(1089), 35–47.

Binder, J.R., Desai, R.H., Graves, W.W., & Conant, L.L. (2009). Where is the semantic system? A critical review and meta-analysis of 120 functional neuroimaging studies. *Cerebral Cortex, 19*, 2767–2796

Bohlhalter, S., Fretz, C., & Weder, B. (2002). Hierarchical versus parallel processing in tactile object recognition—A behavioural-neuroanatomical study of aperceptive tactile agnosia. *Brain, 125*, 2537–2548.

Bozeat, S., Lambon Ralph, M.A., Graham, K.S., Patterson, K., Wilkin, H., Rowland, J., et al. (2003). A duck with four legs: Investigating the structure of conceptual knowledge using picture drawing in semantic dementia. *Cognitive Neuropsychology, 20*(1), 27–47.

Bozeat, S., Lambon Ralph, M.A., Patterson, K., Garrard, P., & Hodges, J.R. (2000). Non-verbal semantic impairment in semantic dementia. *Neuropsychologia, 38*(9), 1207–1215.

Buchsbaum, B.R., Hickok, G., & Humphries, C. (2001). Role of left posterior superior temporal gyrus in phonological processing for speech perception and production. *Cognitive Science, 25*(5), 663–678.

Buchtel, H.A., & Stewart, J.D. (1989). Auditory agnosia—Apperceptive or associative disorder. *Brain and Language, 37*(1), 12–25.

Caramazza, A. (1997). How many levels of processing are there in lexical access? *Cognitive Neuropsychology, 14*, 177–208.

Caramazza, A., & Hillis, A.E. (1990). Levels of representation, coordinate frames, and unilateral neglect. *Cognitive Neuropsychology, 7*, 391–445.

Caramazza, A., & Hillis, A.E. (1991). Lexical organization of nouns and verbs in the brain. *Nature, 349,* 788–790.

Chanoine, V., Ferreira, C.T., Demonet, J.F., Nespoulous, J.L., & Poncet, M. (1998). Optic aphasia with pure alexia: A mild form of visual associative agnosia? A case study. *Cortex, 34*(3), 437–448.

Coccia, M., Bartolini, M., Luzzi, S., Provinciali, L., & Lambon Ralph, M.A. (2004). Semantic memory is an amodal dynamic system: Evidence from the interaction of naming and object use in semantic dementia. *Cognitive Neuropsychology, 21*(5), 513–527.

Cohen, L., Dehaene, S., Naccache, L., Lehericy, S., Dehaene-Lambertz, G., Henaff, M.A., et al. (2000). The visual word form area—Spatial and temporal characterization of an initial stage of reading in normal subjects and posterior split-brain patients. *Brain, 123,* 291–307.

Cohen, L., Jobert, A., Bihan, D.L., & Dehaene, S. (2004). Distinct unimodal and multimodal regions for word processing in the left temporal cortex. *NeuroImage, 23,* 1256–1270.

Cohen, L., Lehericy, S., Chochon, F., Lemer, C., Rivaud, S., & Dehaene, S. (2002). Language-specific tuning of visual cortex functional properties of the Visual Word Form Area. *Brain, 125,* 1054–1069.

Coslett, H.B., & Saffran, E.M. (1992). Optic aphasia and the right-hemisphere—A replication and extension. *Brain and Language, 43*(1), 148–161.

Davis, C., Kleinman, J.T., Newhart, M., Gingis, L., Pawlak, M., & Hillis, A.E. (2008). Speech and language functions that require a functioning Broca's area. *Brain and Language, 105*(1), 50–58.

DeLeon, J., Gottesman, R.F., Kleinman, J.T., Newhart, M., Davis, C., Heidler-Gary, J., et al. (2007). Neural regions essential for distinct cognitive processes underlying picture naming. *Brain, 130,* 1408–1422.

Ellis, A.W., Miller, D., & Sin, G. (1983). Wernicke's aphasia and normal language processing: A case study in cognitive neuropsychology. *Cognition, 15*(1–3), 111–144.

Emerton, B.C., Gansler, D.A., Sandberg, E.H., & Jerram, M. (2014). Functional anatomic dissociation of description and picture naming in the left temporal lobe. *Brain Imaging and Behavior, 8*(4), 570–578.

Farah, M.J., (2004). *Visual agnosia* (2nd ed.). Cambridge, MA: MIT Press.

Farias, S.T., Harrington, G., Broomand, C., & Seyal, M. (2005). Differences in functional MR imaging activation patterns associated with confrontation naming and responsive naming. *American Journal of Neuroradiology, 26*(10), 2492–2499.

Ffytche, D.H., Blom, J.D., & Catani, M. (2010). Disorders of visual perception. *Journal of Neurology Neurosurgery and Psychiatry, 81*(11), 1280–1287.

Freund, D.C. (1889). Ueber optische Aphasie un Seelenblindheit. *Archiv für Psychiatrie und Nervenkrankheiten, 20,* 371–416.

Fridriksson, J., & Morrow, L. (2005). Cortical activation and language task difficulty in aphasia. *Aphasiology, 19*(3–5), 239–250.

Funnell, E. (1995). Objects and properties: A study of the breakdown of semantic memory. *Memory, 3,* 497–518.

Goldstein, M. N. (1974). Auditory agnosia for speech (pure word deafness)—Historical review with current implications. *Brain and Language, 1*(2), 195–204.

Gorno-Tempini, M.L., Hillis, A.E., Weintraub, S., Kertesz, A., Mendez, M., Cappa, S., et al. (2011). Classification of primary progressive aphasia and its variants. *Neurology, 76*(11), 1006–1014.

Grossman, M., Galetta, S., & D'Esposito, M. (1997). Object recognition difficulty in visual apperceptive agnosia. *Brain and Cognition, 33,* 306–342.

Harrington, G.S., Buonocore, M.H., & Farias, S.T. (2006). Intrasubject reproducibility of functional MR imaging activation in language tasks. *American Journal of Neuroradiology, 27*(4), 938–944.

Hart, J., & Gordon, B. (1990). Delineation of single-word semantic comprehension deficits in aphasia, with anatomical correlation. *Annals of Neurology, 27*(3), 226–231.

Hickok, G., & Poeppel, D. (2004). Dorsal and ventral streams: A framework for understanding aspects of the functional anatomy of language. *Cognition, 92*(1–2), 67–99.

Hickok, G., Rogalsky, C., Chen, R., Herskovits, E.H., Townsley, S., & Hillis, A. (2014). Partially overlapping sensorimotor networks underlie speech praxis and verbal short-term memory: Evidence from apraxia of speech following acute stroke. *Frontiers in Human Neuroscience, 8,* 649.

Hillis, A.E., Barker, P.B., Beauchamp, N.J., Winters, B.D., Mirski, M., & Wityk, R.J. (2001a). Restoring blood pressure reperfused Wernicke's area and improved language. *Neurology, 56(5),* 670–672.

Hillis, A.E., & Caramazza, A. (1995a). The representation of grammatical categories of words in the brain. *Journal of Cognitive Neuroscience, 7,* 396–407.

Hillis, A. E., & Caramazza, A. (1995b). Cognitive and neural mechanisms underlying visual and semantic processing—Implications from optic aphasia. *Journal of Cognitive Neuroscience, 7*(4), 457–478.

Hillis, A.E., Chang, S., & Breese, E. (2004). The crucial role of posterior frontal regions in modality specific components of the spelling process. *Neurocase, 10,* 157–187.

Hillis, A.E., & Heidler, J. (2002). Mechanisms of early aphasia recovery. *Aphasiology, 16*(9), 885–895.

Hillis, A.E., Kleinman, J.T., Newhart, M., Heidler-Gary, J., Gottesman, R., Barker, P.B., et al. (2006). Restoring cerebral blood flow reveals neural regions critical for naming. *Journal of Neuroscience, 26*(31), 8069–8073.

Hillis, A.E., Oh, S., & Ken, L. (2004). Deterioration of naming nouns and verbs in primary progressive aphasia. *Annals of Neurology, 55*(2), 268–275.

Hillis, A.E., Wityk, R., Barker, P.B., & Caramazza, A. (2003). Neural regions essential for writing verbs. *Nature Neuroscience, 6*, 19–20.

Hillis, A.E., Wityk, R.J., Tuffiash, E., Beauchamp, N.J., Jacobs, M.A., Barker, P.B., et al. (2001b). Hypoperfusion of Wernicke's area predicts severity of semantic deficit in acute stroke. *Annals of Neurology, 50*(5), 561–566.

Hodges, J.R., Patterson, K., Oxbury, S., & Funnell, E. (1992). Semantic dementia: Progressive fluent aphasia with temporal-lobe atrophy. *Brain, 115*, 1783–1806.

Hömke, L., Amunts, K., Bönig, L., Fretz, C., Binkofski, F., Zilles, K., & Weder B. (2009). Analysis of lesions in patients with unilateral tactile agnosia using cytoarchitectonic probabilistic maps. *Human Brain Mapping, 30*, 1444–1456.

Humphreys, G.W., & Riddoch, M.J. (2006). Features, objects, action: The cognitive neuropsychology of visual object processing, 1984–2004. *Cognitive Neuropsychology, 23*(1), 156–183.

Indefrey, P., & Levelt, W.J.M. (2004). The spatial and temporal signatures of word production components. *Cognition, 92*(1–2), 101–144.

Iorio, L., Falanga, A., Fragassi, N.A., & Grossi, D. (1992). Visual associative agnosia and optic aphasia—A single case-study and a review of the syndromes. *Cortex, 28*(1), 23–37.

Jefferies, E., & Lambon Ralph, M.A. (2006). Semantic impairment in stroke aphasia versus semantic dementia: A case-series comparison. *Brain, 129*, 2132–2147.

Kemeny, S., Xu, J., Park, G.H., Hosey, L.A., Wettig, C.M., & Braun, A.R. (2006). Temporal dissociation of early lexical access and articulation using a delayed naming task—An fMRI study. *Cerebral Cortex, 16(4)*, 587–595.

Lambon Ralph, M.A., Cipolotti, L. Manes, F., & Patterson, K. (2010). Taking both sides: Do unilateral, anterior temporal-lobe lesions disrupt semantic memory? *Brain, 133*, 3243–3255.

Lambon Ralph, M.A., Graham K.S., Ellis A.W., & Hodges J.R. (1998). Naming in semantic dementia—What matters? *Neuropsychologia, 36*, 775–784.

Lambon Ralph, M.A., Graham K.S., Patterson K., & Hodges J.R. (1999). Is a picture worth a thousand words? Evidence from concept definitions by patients with semantic dementia. *Brain and Language, 70*, 309–335.

Lambon Ralph, M.A., McClelland J.L., Patterson K., Galton C.J., & Hodges J.R. (2001). No right to speak? The relationship between object naming and semantic impairment: Neuropsychological abstract evidence and a computational model. *Journal of Cognitive Neuroscience, 13*, 341–356.

Leff, A., Crinion, J., Scott, S., Turkheimer, F., Howard, D., & Wise, R.A. (2002). Physiological change in the homotopic cortex following left posterior temporal lobe infarction. *Annals of Neurology, 51*(5), 553–558.

Leff, A.P., Schofield, T.M., Crinion, J.T., Seghier, M.L., Grogan, A., Green, D.W., Price, C.J. (2009). The left superior temporal gyrus is a shared substrate for auditory short-term memory and speech comprehension: Evidence from 210 patients with stroke. *Brain. 132*(Pt 12), 3401–3410.

Lesser, R.P., Luders, H., Morris, H.H., Dinner, D.S., Klem, G., Hahn, J., et al. (1986). Electrical-stimulation of Wernicke's area interferes with comprehension. *Neurology, 36*(5), 658–663.

Lewis J.W., Wightman, F.L., Brefczynski, J.A., Phinney, R.E., Binder, J.R., & DeYoe, E.A. (2004). Human brain regions involved in recognizing environmental sounds. *Cerebral Cortex, 14*, 1008–1021.

Lhermitte, F., & Beauvois, M.F. (1973). Visual-speech disconnection syndrome—Report of a case with optic aphasia, agnosic alexia and color agnosia. *Brain, 96*, 695–714.

Marsh, E.B., & Hillis, A.E. (2005). Cognitive and neural mechanisms underlying reading and naming: Evidence from letter-by-letter reading and optic aphasia. *Neurocase, 11*, 325–318.

McCandliss, B.D., Cohen, L., & Dehaene, S. (2003). The visual word form area: Expertise for reading in the fusiform gyrus. *Trends in Cognitive Science, 7*(7), 293–299.

McCarthy, R.A., & Warrington, E.K. (1986). Visual associative agnosia: A clinico-anatomical study of a single case. *Journal of Neurology, Neurosurgery, and Psychiatry, 49*, 1233–1240.

Mummery, C.J., Patterson, K., Hodges, J.R., & Price, C.J. (1998). Functional neuroanatomy of the semantic system: Divisible by what? *Journal of Cognitive Neuroscience, 10*(6), 766–777.

Okada, K., & Hickok, G. (2006). Left posterior auditory-related cortices participate both in speech perception and speech production: Neural overlap revealed by fMRI. *Brain and Language, 98*(1), 112–117.

Price, C.J., Wise, R.J.S., & Frackowiak, R.S.J. (1996). Demonstrating the implicit processing of visually presented words and pseudowords. *Cerebral Cortex, 6*(1), 62–70.

Race, D.S., Tsapkini, K., Crinion, J., Newhart, M., Davis, C., Gomez, Y., et al. (2013). An area essential for linking word meanings to word forms: Evidence from primary progressive aphasia. *Brain and Language, 127*, 167–176.

Rapcsak, S.Z., & Beeson, P.M. (2004). The role of left posterior inferior temporal cortex in spelling. *Neurology, 62*(12), 2221–2229.

Raymer, A.M., Foundas, A.L., Maher, L.M., Greenwald, M.L., Morris, M., Rothi, L.J.G., et al. (1997). Cognitive neuropsychological analysis and neuroanatomic correlates in a case of acute anomia. *Brain and Language, 58*(1), 137–156.

Reed, C.L., Caselli, R.J., & Farah, M.J. (1996). Tactile agnosia: Underlying impairment and implications for normal tactile object recognition. *Brain, 119*, 875–888.

Saygin, A.P., Dick, F., Wilson, S.W., Dronkers, N.F., & Bates, E. (2003). Neural resources for processing language and environmental sounds: Evidence from aphasia. *Brain, 126*, 928–945.

Saygin, A.P., Leech, R., & Dick, F. (2010). Nonverbal auditory agnosia with lesion to Wernicke's area. *Neuropsychologia, 48*, 107–113.

Sebastian, R., Gomez, Y., Leigh, R., Davis, C., Newhart, M., & Hillis, A.E. (2014). The roles of occipitotemporal cortex in reading, spelling, and naming. *Cognitive Neuropsychology, 31*(5–6), 511–528.

Snowden J.S., Goulding P. J., & Neary, D. (1989). Semantic dementia: a form of circumscribed cerebral atrophy. *Behavioral Neurology, 2*, 167–182.

Tranel, D., Grabowski, T.J., Lyon, J., & Damasio, H. (2005). Naming the same entities from visual or from auditory stimulation engages similar regions of left inferotemporal cortices. *Journal of Cognitive Neuroscience, 17*(8), 1293–1305.

Trupe, L.A., Varma, D.D., Gomez, Y., Race, D., Leigh, R., Hillis, A. E., & Gottesman, R.F. (2013). Chronic apraxia of speech and Broca's area. *Stroke, 44*, 740–744.

Tsapkini, K., Frangakis, C., & Hillis, A.E. (2011). The function of the left anterior temporal pole: Evidence from acute stroke and infarct volume. *Brain, 134*, 3094–3105.

Visser, M., Jefferies, E., & Lambon Ralph, M.A. (2010). Semantic processing in the anterior temporal lobes: A meta-analysis of the functional neuroimaging literature. *Journal of Cognitive Neuroscience, 22*(6), 1083–1094.

Walker, G.M., Schwartz, M.F., Kimberg, D.Y., Olufunsho, F., Brecher, A., Dell, G.S., & Coslett, H.B. (2011). Support for anterior involvement in semantic error production in aphasia: New evidence from VLSM. *Brain and Language, 117*, 110–122.

Warren, J.E., Crinion, J.T., Lambon Ralph, M.A., & Wise, R.J.S. (2009). Anterior temporal lobe connectivity correlates with functional outcome after aphasic stroke. *Brain, 132*(12), 3428–3442.

Wise, R.J.S. (2003). Language systems in normal and aphasic human subjects: Functional imaging studies and inferences from animal studies. *British Medical Bulletin, 65*, 95–119.

9

CLINICAL DIAGNOSIS AND TREATMENT OF NAMING DISORDERS

Anastasia M. Raymer

Introduction

Anomia is an impairment of word retrieval that is a common symptom among individuals with neurologic diseases affecting the left cerebral hemisphere leading to aphasia. The functional impact is devastating in that word retrieval failures disrupt the ability to carry on meaningful, effective, efficient conversations. While the impact of anomia is difficulty maintaining verbal interactions in conversational speech, the clinical assessment and treatment of word retrieval impairments are most typically accomplished through the use of picture confrontation naming tasks. Thereby word retrieval impairments are often referred to as naming impairments.

As reviewed by Tippett and Hillis (see chapter 7, this volume), the process of picture naming requires not only the retrieval of the lexical phonological forms for words, but also mechanisms for visual object and semantic processing (Figure 9.1). Presumably, it is the semantic and phonological stages that are critical for the process of word retrieval in conversation, and impairments of these processes are associated with aphasia. Deficits affecting the mechanisms for visual object processing (the agnosias) may co-occur with aphasia, further complicating the picture in naming assessment and treatment.

Race and Hillis (see chapter 8, this volume) have explored the neural correlates of the complex process of picture naming distributed throughout the neural cortex. Disparate cortical regions, largely mediated by the left hemisphere, contribute different processes or types of information—visual, semantic, and phonological—to a composite outcome in picture naming. Impairments in picture naming and conversational word retrieval thereby may result from dysfunction of a number of these cortical regions associated with various neurologic diseases, such as stroke or dementia. Thus, the distributed neural architecture of word retrieval processing is compatible with a multicomponential, cognitive model of naming.

For many years now, clinical researchers have advocated the use of multicomponent models, such as the model of naming described in Figure 9.1, as a theoretical perspective to guide strategic clinical decision making in the management of individuals with acquired language disorders (Hillis, 1993; Raymer, Rothi, & Greenwald, 1995; Nickels, 2002; Raymer & Rothi, 2008). In this chapter we focus specifically on the model of naming and its implications for assessment and management of word retrieval impairments in individuals with aphasia. Although disruption of mechanisms of visual object processing may impair picture naming performance, these impairments fall into the category of sensory-specific, prelinguistic processing, which is beyond the scope of this chapter. We concentrate primarily on assessment of semantic and phonological stages of lexical processing as they undermine word retrieval functions in conversational and picture naming tasks in individuals with aphasia. We also review studies in which researchers use this framework to develop rational treatments that either target impaired naming mechanisms or take advantage of spared mechanisms to circumvent naming impairments (Raymer & Rothi, 2008).

Considerations in Assessment and Treatment

In word retrieval assessment guided by the cognitive neuropsychological perspective, the goal is to characterize the impairment of the individual with aphasia with respect to dysfunction at some stage in the naming model (Figure 9.1). In earlier work, Raymer, Rothi, and Greenwald (1995) illustrated how this approach may provide a more focused assessment of naming abilities in contrast to standardized aphasia tests alone. Two individuals with aphasia, both demonstrating comparable severity of anomia in standardized aphasia testing, had distinct differences in the mechanisms for their word retrieval impairments. One individual had an impairment in semantic activation of the output lexicons characterized by intact performance in auditory comprehension tasks and severe cross-modality anomia in all verbal and written naming tasks (Raymer, Foundas et al., 1997). The other had impairments affecting at least two stages of lexical processing: visual object activation of the semantic system, representing elements of agnosia, and semantic activation of the output lexicons, or cross-modality anomia (Raymer, Greenwald, Richardson, Rothi, & Heilman, 1997). Assessment results using this model-driven strategy led to a targeted word retrieval treatment in the second individual, as we trained word retrieval using the auditory-verbal input modality rather than the impaired visual input system, as traditionally is done in naming treatments (Greenwald, Raymer, Richardson, & Rothi, 1995).

Cross-Modality Comparisons

A key notion incorporated in the assessment geared to identify impairments in the naming system is cross-modality comparison. The naming assessment includes single word processing tasks

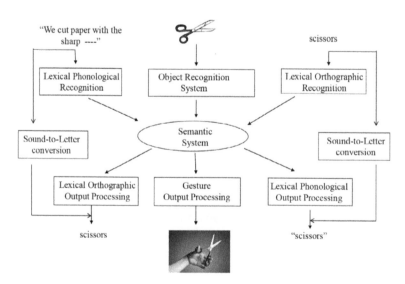

Figure 9.1   Model of lexical processing.

in which the clinician systematically varies input (written words, spoken words, viewed objects, viewed gestures) and output modalities (speech, oral and written spelling, gesture), and then analyzes patterns of performance for tasks that share modalities of processing. As shown in Table 9.1, the assessment typically includes key tasks that assess comprehension and production of single words in phonological and orthographic forms. Published psycholinguistic tests are available that allow systematic assessment of lexical processing for naming and comprehension (Psycholinguistic Assessment of Language Processing Abilities; Kay, Lesser, & Coltheart, 1992; Boston Naming Test, Kaplan, Goodglass, & Weintraub, 2001). In addition, researchers have developed experimental batteries of lexical tasks for use in their studies of naming impairments (e.g., Cambridge Semantics Battery, Adlam, Patterson, Bozeat, & Hodges, 2010; Florida Semantics Battery, Raymer & Rothi, 2008; Philadelphia Naming Test, Roach, Schwartz, Martin, Grewal, & Brecher, 1996; Northwestern Naming Battery, Thompson, Lukic, King, Mesulam, & Weintraub, 2012), some of which are accessible through online resources.

If the functioning of a lexical mechanism is disturbed by neurologic disease, modality comparisons should demonstrate impairment in all tasks dependent upon that mechanism. For example, a deficit of semantic processing will affect performance in all naming and lexical comprehension tasks (modality consistency) (Hillis, Rapp, Romani, & Caramazza, 1990; Jefferies & Lambon Ralph, 2006; Jefferies, Rogers, Hopper, & Lambon Ralph, 2010). Breese and Hillis (2004) noted that spoken-word/picture verification tasks are especially sensitive to semantic breakdown relative to other word/picture matching comprehension tasks (see Newhart et al., 2007, for a short assessment tool). Dysfunction of the phonological output lexicon will result in impairment in all verbal production tasks (e.g., oral naming of pictures, naming to definition, and oral reading of words with exceptional spellings) (Caramazza & Hillis, 1990; Schwartz, Faseyitan, Kim, & Coslett, 2012) in the presence of intact lexical comprehension (modality inconsistency). In the case of phonological output dysfunction, it is possible for performance in writing to be intact as well (modality inconsistency).

Lexical Stimuli

A second consideration in naming assessment is the selection of appropriate stimuli to use across lexical tasks. In this way, differences observed across tasks can be attributed to the modality of processing rather than differences inherent to the stimulus items. For example, we used the same set of 120 nouns across tasks when we developed the Florida Semantics Battery (Raymer & Rothi, 2008). There will be times when the clinician wants to evaluate performance for contrasting sets of words from different semantic (e.g., animals vs. tools) or grammatical categories (e.g., nouns vs. verbs). However, additional factors such as word frequency, imageability, length, familiarity, and age of acquisition (Hirsh & Ellis, 1994; Kittredge, Dell, Verkuilen, & Schwartz, 2008; Lambon Ralph, Graham, Ellis, & Hodges, 1998; Nickels & Howard, 1994, 1995) may influence naming abilities across sets. For that reason experimental tests like the Philadelphia Naming Test (Roach et al., 1996; available online at www.mrri.org/philadelphia-naming-test) are useful as the test includes a set of 175 nouns that are well characterized for psycholinguistic characteristics. When an exploration of performance across semantic categories is of interest, the Florida Semantics Battery may be a tool, as it includes 120 noun stimuli from 12 different semantic categories. Often, a comparison of nouns and verbs is at issue, in which case the standardized Object and Action Naming Battery (Druks & Masterson, 2000) may be employed. In addition, the Northwestern Naming Battery (Thompson et al., 2012) is a useful tool, as it includes subtests for both object and action naming and comprehension. To explore psycholinguistic attributes of individualized stimuli, the MRC Psycholinguistic Database can be accessed (www.psych.rl.ac.uk). Thus, clinicians can select from several tools to evaluate the influence of lexical parameters on naming failure for the individual patient.

Table 9.1 Battery of Key Tasks to Include in Lexical Assessment

Oral picture naming
Written picture naming
Oral naming to spoken definitions
Oral word reading
Writing to dictation
Auditory word-to-picture matching or verification
Written word-to-picture matching or verification

Error Patterns

The assessment of naming abilities also includes a consideration of the errors produced across lexical tasks, as patterns of errors may provide clues to the mechanism of naming failure. The same qualitative pattern of errors should be observed in all tasks that engage the suspected impaired mechanism. For example, a deficit of semantic processing may lead to semantic errors (e.g., *orange* for *apple*) in comprehension as well as naming tasks (Hillis et al., 1990; Cloutman et al., 2009). A dysfunction of phonological lexical retrieval may result in patterns of phonological errors (e.g., /apsll/ for "apple") that span verbal production tasks such as oral naming of pictures and oral reading of single words (Schwartz et al., 2012).

Examination of error type is not sufficient to distinguish the level of lexical impairment responsible for the naming error, however. Semantic errors in picture naming are a case in point (Hillis & Caramazza, 1995b; Cloutman et al., 2009). For the target picture of a carrot, semantic naming errors may include responses such as "vegetable" (superordinate), "celery" (coordinate), or "rabbit" (associated). Whereas in some individuals semantic errors represent semantic system impairment (Hillis et al., 1990; Jefferies et al., 2010; Raymer, Foundas, et al., 1997), semantic errors also can occur from impairment at the phonological retrieval stage (Caramazza & Hillis, 1990; Walker et al., 2011), or during visual-to-semantic activation (Hillis & Caramazza, 1995a; Raymer, Greenwald, et al., 1997). These observations suggest the need to analyze error patterns across lexical tasks to develop a more accurate hypothesis regarding the source of the lexical error as, for example, semantic errors do not necessarily imply semantic dysfunction (Budd et al., 2010).

Final Comments on Assessment

In addition to specifying the basis for dysfunction in lexical processing leading to naming failure, the cognitive neuropsychological approach has other advantages. Many patients with extensive neurological lesions have dysfunction affecting multiple levels in the naming process. An in-depth assessment will frequently suggest not only what mechanisms are impaired, but also what mechanisms are spared in lexical processing, information that may be beneficial as the clinician turns toward devising treatments for each individual with aphasia. Retained lexical processing in alternative mechanisms not typically part of the naming process—for example, reading and gesture mechanisms—may be implemented in compensatory methods to improve word retrieval and, thereby, communication abilities.

A clear disadvantage of this approach is the potential increased length of assessment and analysis. Although a lengthy assessment may be challenging to conduct in clinical practice, it is possible for clinicians to adapt these methods using a more circumscribed set of available materials representing a variety of semantic or grammatical categories, such as those used in Newhart et al. (2007). The systematic assessment may indeed be more cost-effective than the standard of care as clinicians characterize both their patients' impairments and retained abilities, and hence target treatments in the most efficient manner.

Application to Treatment

For several decades now, clinical researchers have expressed enthusiasm for applying a model-guided approach to aphasia treatment (Mitchum, 1992; Raymer et al., 1995; Riddoch & Humphreys, 1994; Seron & Deloche, 1989), although others have voiced some caution (Caramazza & Hillis, 1993). Naming models provide a sound basis for guiding some, though by no means all, treatment decisions. In particular, naming models are well suited to the view that the type of intervention strategy to apply should relate to the chronicity of the naming impairment. Rothi (1995) proposed that restitutive strategies, which encourage restoration of functioning in a manner compatible with normal language processing, are appropriate in early stages when neurophysiologic processes of recovery are maximal. Compensatory strategies that attempt to circumvent naming dysfunction using intact cognitive mechanisms may be beneficial during acute and chronic stages of recovery.

Semantic Impairments

Assessment

Word retrieval difficulties in some individuals may arise due to dysfunction of semantic processing. A patient with a semantic impairment will have difficulty performing any tasks that require semantic mediation (i.e., modality consistency). Therefore, of the tasks listed in Table 9.1, patients should have difficulty in comprehension of spoken words and spoken naming, not just for seen objects, but for all modalities of input (objects, spoken definitions, and so on). All modes of output will be affected as well (gesture, writing, and so on). Because sublexical letter-sound conversion mechanisms may be available for decoding or encoding written words, performance in oral word reading and writing to dictation may be less affected than naming or comprehension.

Assuming that the semantic system is structured in a similar fashion for all modalities of processing, individuals with brain damage that yields semantic system impairment should demonstrate quantitatively and qualitatively similar impairments across lexical tasks requiring semantic mediation. Researchers have described this association of impairments in some patients with vascular lesions (Hillis et al., 1990; Howard & Orchard-Lisle, 1984) and progressive neurological impairments (Hodges & Patterson, 1996; Jefferies & Lambon Ralph, 2006; Jefferies et al., 2010; Raymer & Berndt, 1996).

Semantic Tasks

In practice, it may be possible for a neurological lesion to cause extensive damage to lexical input and output stages simultaneously, leading to modality consistency of impairments that mimic semantic dysfunction. Therefore, it can be beneficial to administer additional semantic tasks that require more specific processing of semantic attributes of stimuli or that avoid the use of lexical stimuli. Individuals with semantic dysfunction should have difficulty in these types of tasks as well, whereas individuals with co-occurring input modality/output modality impairments may perform somewhat better in some of these semantic tasks that circumvent verbal disturbances. In this regard, category sorting tasks can be used in which patients sort pictures from closely related categories that require them to accomplish more fine-grained semantic processing for successful performance (e.g., fruits vs. vegetables, winter clothing vs. summer clothing). When required to sort distant semantic categories, patients may be able to accomplish the task in spite of semantic impairment by recognizing only visual characteristics or appreciating superficial semantic information.

Semantic associate tasks also can be used to assess semantic processing independent of verbal input. *Pyramids and Palm Trees* (Howard & Patterson, 1992) is a published test of this sort. In this task, participants match a target item (e.g., carrot) to a semantically related item from several choices (e.g., associate—rabbit; distractors—squirrel, duck). This type of associate task may be sensitive to subtle impairments in semantic activation (e.g., Raymer, Greenwald, et al., 1997). A more recent iteration of the semantic associate task, *Kissing and Dancing Test* (Bak & Hodges, 2003), has been developed to evaluate semantic processing for verb associate combinations. It is also possible to contrast performance in the associate task for matching spoken words and matching viewed pictures to distinguish impairments related to phonological input versus semantic stages of lexical processing. Semantic impairments are associated with difficulty whether stimuli are presented as words or pictures.

Researchers have also described individuals with aphasia whose naming and comprehension impairments fractionate, demonstrating selective preservation or impairment for specific semantic categories, such as living and nonliving things, fruits and vegetables, and animals (see review by Mahon & Caramazza, 2009). Within standard aphasia tests currently available, an astute examiner may notice either impaired or spared performance related to selective semantic categories and explore the possibility of a category-specific dysfunction with additional testing materials representing that semantic category. The Cambridge Semantics Battery (Adlam et al., 2010, available for download at www.neura.edu.au/frontier/research/test-downloads/) incorporates a comparison of living and nonliving stimuli across a series of lexical tasks. We have incorporated semantic category distinctions into the *Florida Semantics Battery*, as we test items from 12 different semantic categories (Raymer & Rothi, 2008). Results of testing that identifies selective categories of difficulty for a patient may allow the clinician to streamline efforts in rehabilitation, focusing on impaired categories and taking advantage of retained processing for other categories.

Semantic Treatments for Naming Impairments

Because semantic dysfunction may lead to naming impairments, researchers have investigated a number of treatment approaches that exploit semantic functioning in an attempt to improve naming abilities (Table 9.2). Some of the techniques tend to activate semantic processing, whereas others encourage the reconstitution of semantic representations. Although we cannot definitively state that the techniques are restorative in nature, the methods seem to encourage semantic processing according to principles that parallel what is known of normal semantic processing and thus appear to be primarily restorative.

Semantic Comprehension Treatments

Because the semantic system plays a role in both word comprehension and word selection, a number of researchers have investigated the utility of what might be termed semantic comprehension treatments to facilitate naming abilities (e.g., Howard et al., 1985; Marshall, Pound,

Table 9.2 Types of Naming Treatments That Have Been Tested

Restorative Semantic Treatments	*Restorative Phonological Treatments*
Semantic comprehension tasks	Phonological judgment tasks
Contextual priming	Phonological cueing hierarchy
Semantic feature matrix training	Oral word reading/word repetition
Typicality training	Phonological components analysis
Verb network Strengthening treatment	Errorless naming treatment
Compensatory treatments	Phoneme training
Letter-sound conversion self-cues	
Gestural facilitation	

White-Thomson, & Pring, 1990; Nickels & Best, 1996). Participants complete various semantic comprehension tasks (e.g., auditory word-picture matching, written word-picture matching, answering yes/no questions about semantic details of a picture, sort words and pictures by semantic category), and picture naming performance is evaluated. In a review of this treatment approach, Ennis (2001) reported that 17 of 20 individuals with aphasia and one group study reported improved naming for trained nouns, with little generalization to untrained nouns. Nickels (2002) noted that individuals with impairments related to either semantic or phonological dysfunction demonstrated significant improvement in naming abilities following semantic comprehension treatments.

In semantic comprehension studies, it was often mentioned that the participants also said the words during the performance of the comprehension tasks, adding a phonological component to the treatment. Two studies have contrasted treatments in which semantic comprehension tasks were performed with and without phonological production of target words to determine the role that the phonological component plays in treatment outcome (Drew & Thompson, 1999; Le Dorze, Boulay, Gaudreau, & Brassard, 1994). In both studies, participants benefited maximally during training in which comprehension tasks were paired with phonological output during training (oral reading, repetition), in keeping with the normal process of semantic-phonological activation in lexical output.

Martin and colleagues (Martin et al., 2005, 2006; Renvall et al., 2007) have implemented a modification of the comprehension paradigm called contextual priming. In this procedure, participants complete a spoken-word/picture matching task for a set of related pictures (e.g., apple, cherries, orange, banana) followed by repetition of the set of target words, thus activating both semantic and phonological information in training. The premise of this procedure is that massed repetition priming leads to spreading of activation to semantically related words. Early in the procedure some participants experienced interference in naming the set of related words, but over time, naming improvements were reported for trained words. They also indicated that the procedure worked best in individuals with retained semantic abilities.

Noting that earlier comprehension studies centered on noun retrieval, Raymer and colleagues (Raymer et al., 2007; Rodriguez et al., 2006) examined the influence of a semantic-phonologic comprehension training (answering a series of questions about semantic and phonological attributes of target verbs and nouns) for individuals with stroke-induced verb retrieval deficits. Improvements were reported for trained nouns and verbs, again with little generalization to untrained nouns and verbs. Positive outcomes for verb naming were associated with improvements appreciated in a communicative rating scale. Response to treatment was limited in individuals with severe semantic impairments.

The semantic comprehension training paradigm has been adapted for computerized presentation as part of MossTalk Words 2.0 (Fink, Brecher, Montgomery, & Schwartz, 2010) multimodality matching module in which participants complete matching tasks for spoken words/pictures, written words/pictures, and spoken words/written nouns and verbs (available for download at www.mrri.org/mosstalk-words-2). Raymer, Kohen, and Saffell (2006) showed that training with the matching module paired with practice in production of the spoken words (i.e., semantic + phonological training) led to improvements in comprehension and naming for trained nouns for individuals with both semantic and phonological anomia. The two individuals with semantic anomia in the study found the computerized training engaging and interesting, and responded with naming improvements not seen when they participated in an earlier training trial (Raymer et al., 2007).

Semantic Feature Matrix Training

Another type of naming treatment developed on the basis of cognitive theories of semantic representations incorporates semantic feature analysis (SFA). Clinicians teach individuals with aphasia to use a viewed matrix of printed cue words representing semantic features (e.g., function, properties, category, and so on) surrounding a target picture to assist in retrieving semantic information about the picture along with its name, as depicted in Figure 9.2. Although this approach can be viewed as restorative in nature, the method teaches a semantically based strategy that can be used whenever word retrieval failure occurs. A number of single participant investigations have examined the effects of SFA for individuals with various fluent and nonfluent aphasia syndromes (Boyle, 2004; Boyle & Coelho, 1995; Hashimoto & Frome, 2011; Lowell, Beeson, & Holland, 1995; Rider, Wright, Marshall, & Page, 2008; Wallace & Kimelman, 2013). Following SFA training, participants have demonstrated improved naming of trained pictures as well as generalization of the strategy to naming of some untrained pictures. Improvements in discourse measures also have been reported in some trials (Antonucci, 2009; Boyle, 2004; Rider et al., 2008; Wallace & Kimelman, 2013). Whereas most SFA studies have examined effects for noun retrieval, Wambaugh and Ferguson (2007) showed that the treatment also could be applied to verb retrieval with successful outcomes for trained words and discourse measures. None of the SFA studies has delineated the basis for word retrieval failure, although, as noted earlier, participants demonstrated a variety of aphasia syndromes.

Promoting Generalized Improvements in Semantic Training

Most studies that examined effects of semantic comprehension training demonstrated item-specific training effects, with less generalized improvements to untrained words. Kiran (2008) opined, however, that semantically based treatments should have a generalized effect to words within the same semantic category. Drawing upon perspectives in cognitive psychology that distinguish typical and atypical category members (Rosch, 1975), Kiran and colleagues (Kiran, 2007; Kiran & Johnson, 2008; Kiran, Sandberg, & Abbott, 2009; Kiran, Sandberg, & Sebastian, 2011; Kiran & Thompson, 2003) have conducted a series of naming treatment studies where they manipulated typicality of category membership of stimuli used in training. While their specific treatment approach was similar to the semantic treatments described earlier (semantic feature analysis, answering questions about semantic features of target words, sorting by categories), the nature of the training stimuli was systematically manipulated across studies to include items that were either typical for the category (e.g., vegetables: carrots; birds: robin), or atypical for the category (e.g., vegetables: artichoke; birds: penguin). Their counterintuitive findings, which have been replicated across a variety of animate and inanimate semantic categories (vegetables, birds, furniture, clothing, things at a garage sale) and in other labs (Stanczak, Waters, & Caplan, 2006), demonstrate that training of atypical category exemplars leads to improvements for untrained typical items as well, whereas training of typical exemplars does not generalize to atypical items. Kiran (2008) proposed that this effect occurs because of broader semantic activation for the variety of unique semantic features trained for atypical items compared to the more overlapping set of common core features trained across a set of typical items. Whereas the participants across these studies represent both fluent and nonfluent aphasia syndromes, the nature of word retrieval impairment for the individuals with aphasia is less clearly articulated (Kiran & Bassetto, 2008).

The studies of word retrieval training have centered on studies of patients recovering from stroke-induced aphasia and anomia. More recently, Beeson, Henry, and colleagues (Beeson et al., 2011; Henry, Beeson, & Rapcsak, 2008; Henry et al., 2013) applied semantic treatment tasks in the context of semantic category generative naming outcomes (e.g., name clothing items) for individuals with primary progressive aphasia. Treatment focused on sets of pictures from specific semantic categories wherein semantic comprehension tasks and SFA training were then implemented for that semantic category in an effort to promote semantic search strategies. Results indicated improved generation of words in trained semantic categories, as well as gains in untrained semantic categories, suggesting generalization of the search strategies.

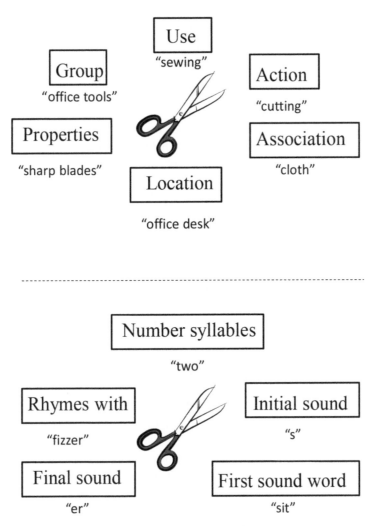

Figure 9.2 Semantic feature analysis training matrix (upper panel) and phonological components analysis training matrix (lower panel).

Whereas most studies of naming treatments for nouns and verbs have centered on picture naming outcomes, Edmonds and colleagues (Edmonds, Nadeau, & Kiran, 2009; Edmonds & Babb, 2011) have examined a semantically based treatment that connects lexical performance to sentence production—verb network strengthening training (VNeST). Participants view a written verb name (e.g., slice) and then generate multiple thematic agents (e.g., chef) and patients (e.g., carrots) associated with that verb, somewhat like SFA for verbs (Wambaugh & Ferguson, 2007). They also answer yes/no questions and make judgments about correct and semantically anomalous sentences corresponding to trained verbs, analogous to some semantic comprehension training tasks. Following this training, participants with primarily phonological forms of anomia improved production of utterances incorporating trained verbs and associated nouns, as well as some untrained verbs and nouns. Improvements in discourse measures also were reported.

Summary

A number of investigators have evaluated treatment schemes that primarily target semantic processing, recognizing aspects of the normal process of semantic activation and representation of semantic knowledge. Most semantic training protocols usually included a phonological component to the training as well. In studies examining the importance of the phonological step in semantic training, findings indicated that the phonological component was critical for optimizing treatment effects (Drew & Thompson, 1999; Le Dorze et al., 1994). Hence, training that encompasses semantic and phonological information, as in the normal process of word retrieval, appears to be particularly effective in the remediation of naming impairments. These semantic treatments have led to improved naming for individuals whose impairments arise at both semantic and phonological stages of processing, although the outcomes are limited in some studies for individuals with severe semantic impairments (Raymer et al., 2007).

Another observation among semantic training studies for naming is that, to some extent, generalization of training to untrained words may be possible. The SFA training protocol, which encourages activation of elements of semantic information, is promising in this respect. Typicality of training stimuli (i.e., training with atypical items) seems to have an important influence on potential for generalization to untrained stimuli (Kiran, 2008). With somewhat guarded optimism, we continue to recommend that clinicians plan for limited generalization to untrained words and, accordingly, select training stimuli that are functional and relevant to the individual patient's needs and interests.

Phonological Impairments

Assessment

Word retrieval difficulties in some individuals with aphasia stem from dysfunction at the level of lexical phonological output. In the case of phonological dysfunction, impairment will be evident in all verbal tasks dependent upon the integrity of stored phonological representations, including spoken naming tasks, whether to picture or definitions (Table 9.1). In addition, they may have difficulty in oral reading, particularly for words with exceptional spelling (e.g., *colonel, bread*), as sublexical processes are often insufficient to derive accurate pronunciations for those words. A variety of naming errors can be observed, representing the spectrum of impairments that may occur in the process of activating the phonological lexicon. Some individuals may produce semantic errors or no response because of difficulty accessing the phonological lexicon (Caramazza & Hillis, 1991; Le Dorze & Nespoulous, 1989; Miceli et al., 1991). Others may produce neologistic responses or phonemic paraphasias related to disturbance of the internal structure of phonological representations (Kohn et al., 1996) or postlexical phonemic processes (Ellis et al., 1992).

A key distinction that presumably is represented at the level of the phonological lexicon is grammatical category (Caramazza & Hillis, 1991). Dissociations in naming performance may be evident, as some patients with fluent aphasia and more posteriorly placed lesions may be more impaired for noun naming than verb naming. Others with nonfluent aphasia and more anterior lesions may be more impaired for verb naming than noun naming (Damasio & Tranel, 1993; Miceli, Silveri, Villa, & Caramazza, 1984; Zingeser & Berndt, 1990). Naming assessment then should incorporate tasks to explore grammatical category differences in naming. An initial step in assessing grammatical class in naming can be accomplished with the Boston Naming Test (Kaplan et al., 2001) and the Action Naming Test (Nicholas, Obler, Albert, & Goodglass, 1985). However, the Action Naming Test is not widely available and the two measures are not equated on variables such as word frequency that may influence word retrieval (Williamson, Adair, Raymer, & Heilman, 1998). An alternative resource to evaluate naming for nouns and verbs can be found in the Object and Action Naming Battery (Druks & Masterson, 2000) and the Northwestern Naming Battery (Thompson et al., 2012), which is not yet widely distributed.

Phonological Tasks

In the initial lexical assessment, tasks requiring spoken-word production will require activation of lexical phonological output. Impairment in oral naming, oral word reading, or repetition tasks in the context of good performance in auditory and reading comprehension, written naming, and writing to dictation leads one to suspect impairment of the phonological lexicon (Caramazza & Hillis, 1990). However, this dissociation between spoken and written output may arise with subsequent phonological planning impairments as well (e.g., apraxia of speech).

Although comparable impairments for spoken and written naming often represent semantic dysfunction, it is possible to develop co-occurring naming impairments from dysfunction of both the phonological and orthographic output lexicons (Miceli et al., 1991). To differentiate these deficits, however, individuals with naming impairment due to parallel dysfunctions of the phonological and orthographic output lexicons should demonstrate relatively preserved performance in comprehension tasks.

To distinguish among oral naming impairments related to phonological lexical versus subsequent phonological planning deficits, it may be necessary to administer tasks that specifically tax phonological lexical processing without motor speech. One such task is a rhyme judgment task in which participants decide whether the names of two pictures rhyme (e.g., *whale, nail*). Alternatively, a written homophone task can be implemented in which patients must verify whether two written words are pronounced the same (e.g., *pear, pair*). These tasks will prove difficult for individuals who fail to activate a full lexical representation for the pictures.

Phonological Treatments

Recognizing that word retrieval abilities depend upon the integrity of the phonological stage of naming, a number of studies have used treatment protocols incorporating phonological information in an attempt to restore naming abilities in patients with word retrieval impairments (Table 9.2). Because pictures and words usually are included in the training, presumably the treatments include activation of some semantic information as well, but these approaches emphasize phonological attributes of words during training.

Oral Reading and Repetition

In the naming model, the same phonological output representation may be activated in oral reading, word repetition, and oral picture naming. Realizing this relationship, a number of studies have required participants to practice with oral reading or repetition tasks while naming performance was monitored. Results for nouns and verb naming typically showed improvements for trained stimuli (Mason et al., 2011; Miceli, Amitrano, Capasso, & Caramazza, 1996; Mitchum & Berndt, 1994). Repetition training does not seem to have as strong or lasting of effects when compared with other treatments (Greenwald et al., 1995; Raymer & Ellsworth, 2002; Rose & Sussmilch, 2008).

Phonological Cueing Hierarchy

Other treatment studies have incorporated phonological cueing hierarchies in training to improve word retrieval impairments. In this type of protocol, patients systematically practice naming as they are given different types of phonological information as they attempt to retrieve target words (Table 9.3). A number of patients who received training with cueing hierarchies have demonstrated improvements in word retrieval for trained words, with little generalization to untrained words (Greenwald et al., 1995; Hillis, 1993, 1998; Raymer, Thompson, Jacobs, & leGrand, 1993; Wambaugh, 2003; Wambaugh et al., 1999). Several recent studies have incorporated cueing hierarchies to maximize effects by encompassing phonological, orthographic, and semantic cues in training (Henry et al., 2013; Kendall et al., 2014).

Recent studies using a combination of phonemic and orthographic cues examined factors to optimize training effects. Sage, Snell, and Ralph (2011) found that training applied in a less intensive schedule (two times per week for 5 weeks) had greater maintenance of effects over time than an intensive training schedule (five times per week for 2 weeks). Laganaro, Di Pietro, and Schnider (2006) and Snell, Sage, and Ralph (2010) compared higher and lower numbers of items incorporated in training and found no difference in proportions of words learned. Thereby training with a larger number of items had greater outcomes. Conroy, Snell, Sage, and Lambon Ralph (2012) examined cueing patterns for 22 participants from their prior studies and noted that words that responded to fewer cues at baseline were predictive of better learning and maintenance of those words after cueing treatment. Among these various phonological cueing studies, treatment was reported to be effective for individuals with either semantic or phonological word retrieval dysfunction, although improvements were more limited in some patients with semantic impairment (Hillis, 1998; Raymer et al., 1993; Snell et al., 2010).

The MossTalk Words 2.0 (Fink et al., 2010) computerized training program referred to earlier includes a cued naming training module. Given a target picture, participants with aphasia can click on buttons that provide either semantic (sentence completion) or phonological (initial phoneme and repetition) cues to the picture name. Training with the cued naming module led to improved naming of trained pictures for individuals with phonologically based naming impairments along with generalized naming improvements in some participants (Fink, Brecher, Schwartz, and Robey, 2002; Ramsberger & Marie, 2007).

Errorless Naming Training

A series of studies incorporating a cueing approach, centered primarily on phonological and orthographic cues, has evaluated the effects of error production in naming treatment (Conroy, Sage, & Lambon Ralph, 2009a; Fillingham, Hodgson, Sage, & Lambon Ralph, 2003; Fillingham, Sage, & Lambon Ralph, 2005a, 2005b, 2006; Raymer et al., 2012) for individuals with aphasia. In errorless naming treatment (ENT), the participant views a target picture and is given maximal support through repetition and oral reading to avoid production of an error during multiple opportunities to rehearse the correct name of the picture. Because the picture is present during training, activation of semantic information presumably is also a factor in training effects. One

Table 9.3 Example of a Phonological Cueing Hierarchy (after Raymer et al., 1993)

At each step, patient attempts to retrieve the target word. If correct, the patient moves to the next picture after rehearsing the correct word multiple times. If incorrect, the patient is given the next cue.

1. Patient attempts to name target picture (e.g., table).
2. Initial phoneme cue: "It starts with /t/."
3. Rhyme cue: "It sounds like fable."
4. Oral reading cue: Present word for oral reading.
5. Repetition cue: "Say table."

perspective underlying this approach is the Hebbian learning principle that 'neurons that fire together wire together.' That is, each time a response is produced, whether correct or error, the chance of that response occurring again in the future is potentially increased (Fillingham et al., 2006). Therefore, it would be important to avoid error production in training, as is typically the case in the error-driven cueing hierarchy training described earlier.

In their review of the aphasia word retrieval treatment literature, Fillingham et al. (2003) found that studies employing error-reducing (somewhat errorless) methods were as effective as errorful treatments for improving word retrieval in individuals with aphasia. They noted that treatment effects were best in individuals with 'expressive' impairments and more limited in those with 'expressive-receptive' impairments, suggesting a semantically based anomia. In their subsequent series of investigations, Fillingham and colleagues (Fillingham et al., 2005a, 2005b, 2006) found no clear difference between errorful and errorless training methods for individuals with aphasia. Both methods led to positive training effects when naming trained words with little generalized improvement for untrained words. Similar findings were evident when Conroy, Sage, and Ralph (2009a,b) compared cueing training effects in contrasting order relative to potency of cue, increasing (errorful) or decreasing (errorless). In their study, Raymer et al. (2012) reported positive effects of errorless training for individuals with both phonological and mild semantic naming impairments. Their participants often expressed preference for the errorless approach, which is inherently less frustrating during the training experience.

Phonological Judgment Treatment

Some studies have used a different type of phonological training scheme that paralleled the procedures described earlier for semantic comprehension treatment (Fisher, Wilshire, & Ponsford, 2009; Robson, Marshall, Pring, & Chiat, 1998). In these methods, participants complete tasks requiring word discrimination or judgments about phonological information for words, such as the number of syllables and the initial phoneme of words, to encourage activation of phonological output representations. Individuals with naming impairment arising at a phonological stage of lexical processing demonstrated improvement in naming pictures trained with this strategy and showed some generalization of the process in naming untrained pictures as well. Like the semantic comprehension tasks noted earlier, the phonological judgment training tasks are not as successful unless paired with spoken output of the words during training (Jacquemot, Dupoux, Robotham, & Bachoud-Levi, 2012).

Phonological Components Analysis

Knowing the successful findings reported for semantic feature analysis training, Leonard, Rochon, and Laird (2008) developed a corollary approach for phonological feature training. As shown in Figure 9.2, in the phonological components approach (PCA), a target picture is surrounded by five key properties to retrieve pertaining to phonological characteristics of the target word: rhyming word, initial phoneme, final phoneme, number of syllables, and word with same initial phoneme. If unsuccessful when retrieving the desired component, options were given for selection of an appropriate response. Repetition of the target word was also emphasized in PCA. Seven of 10 participants, all with phonological anomia, improved picture naming for trained words, with limited generalization to untrained words for 3 individuals. There was a negative correlation indicating a tendency to have poorer naming outcomes in those with more severe semantic impairment. Bose (2013) subsequently reported improvements for trained words associated with PCA in a patient with severe jargon aphasia. Together these studies provide preliminary evidence for the positive effects of the PCA approach for word retrieval in aphasia.

Phoneme-Based Treatment of Naming

All the approaches reviewed above involve training in the context of words and pictures. Thereby, the approaches engage a number of lexical mechanisms beyond the phonological system alone. Kendall and colleagues (2008) applied a focused phonemic training paradigm for individuals with aphasia, relatively devoid of lexical and semantic information. In this intensively delivered (96 total hours) phoneme training modeled after a published reading program (Lindemood & Lindemood, 2011), participants focus on phonemic awareness activities, syllable segmentation, and mapping of phonemes to articulatory postures. Although words and pictures were not incorporated in training, participants with aphasia improved picture naming following participation in this protocol. The source of naming failure was not well characterized in this study, however.

Summary

A number of researchers have investigated treatment protocols encompassing phonological aspects of words to improve naming abilities. Preliminary data suggest that the use of a phonological cueing hierarchy is more effective than simple repetition practice in remediating word retrieval impairments (Greenwald et al., 1995). These phonological treatments appear to be effective in patients with impairments related to either phonological or semantic stages of naming; however, effects may be reduced in individuals with pronounced semantic impairment (Raymer et al., 1993; Snell et al., 2008). However, a cueing hierarchy may not be as effective as an alternative semantic treatment in individuals with semantically based naming impairments (Hillis, 1998). Finally, generalization of treatment effects to untrained stimuli were much more limited in the phonological training investigations than in semantic training protocols, suggesting the need to select stimuli carefully for functional relevance to the individual patients prior to instituting these phonological treatments.

Naming Treatments: Remaining Issues

Compensatory Naming Treatments

An alternative approach to rehabilitation of naming impairments to which lexical models may contribute is the development of compensatory treatments that either circumvent an impaired lexical mechanism or vicariatively mediate word retrieval using other cognitive mechanisms. For example, the use of semantic circumlocution to describe a concept when a naming failure occurs is a compensatory semantic strategy to circumvent failure at the subsequent stage of phonological lexical retrieval. Some treatment studies have evaluated the effects of methods to vicariatively activate word retrieval using alternative cognitive mechanisms.

Orthographic Mechanisms

Hillis (1998) described an extraordinary patient who spontaneously used retained reading abilities (print-to-sound conversion abilities, access to orthographic representations) to support her failed attempts at oral naming. She often mispronounced words using regularized pronunciations (e.g., "breed" for bread). To circumvent this maladaptive strategy, Hillis taught her to pronounce words by memorizing regularized spellings of common words with exceptional spellings (e.g., *kwire* for *choir*), which she in turn used in oral naming of the same words.

Some individuals with naming impairments arising at the level of phonological lexical output may be able to access all or part of the word's spelling through retained orthographic lexical output mechanisms. In turn, print-to-sound conversion processes can be used to generate a phonemic self-cue or computerized phonemic cue to facilitate production of the intended word (Bastiannse,

Bosje, & Franssen, 1996; Bruce & Howard, 1987; DeDe, Parris, & Waters, 2002; Nickels, 1992). Holland (1998) found that the writing self-cue strategy only generalized to conversational speech when the technique was rehearsed in a generative semantic category naming task (e.g., writing words in a particular category such as animals). Many individuals with aphasia are impaired for both spelling and oral naming; however, Beeson and Egnor (2006) demonstrated that spelling training with a copy and recall treatment method can lead to improved word retrieval when spelling and spoken production of target words are paired during training.

Gesture

Cognitive models that recognize the interactive nature of verbal and gestural output processing (Rothi, Ochipa, & Heilman, 1997) suggest a means for gesture to facilitate activation of lexical retrieval. Alternatively, training with gestural pantomimes may provide a compensatory means of communication for individuals with severe aphasia who often also have profound limb apraxia that may undermine gesture use. A number of investigators have applied a verbal + gestural pantomime training paradigm, such as the one represented in Table 9.4, to facilitate recovery of word retrieval in individuals with aphasia (e.g., Pashek, 1998; Raymer & Thompson, 1991; Rose & Douglas, 2008; Rose, Douglas, & Matyas, 2002; Raymer et al., 2007; Raymer et al., 2012). Most gestural training studies have centered on effects for noun retrieval. However, Druks (2002) noted a tighter link between gestures and verbs than nouns. Positive gesture + verbal training effects have been reported for verbs as well, with no clear advantage evident for verbs over nouns (Boo & Rose, 2011; Pashek, 1998; Raymer et al., 2006; Rose & Sussmilch, 2008).

A systematic review of the gesture training literature conducted by Rose, Raymer, Lanyon, and Attard (2013) reported that gesture + verbal training led to improvements in picture naming for nouns and verbs for more than 50% of the 134 participants across the studies. Effects were largely training specific with little generalization to untrained words. Studies that compared gesture + verbal training to other verbal training methods did not show any clear advantage for the use of gesture, although training with gesture in isolation was not sufficient to improve naming. Response to gesture + verbal training has typically been best in individuals with more retained semantic abilities (Boo & Rose, 2011; Kroenke, Kraft, Regenbrecht, & Obrig, 2013; Raymer et al., 2007). A desirable outgrowth of gesture + verbal pantomime training is that participants with aphasia who often also present with limb apraxia improved their use of recognizable gestures, providing a potential alternative communication mode when verbal improvements do not develop in individuals with severe semantic anomia (Rodriguez et al., 2006).

Recent investigations have also evaluated effects of training with intentional gestures (i.e., nonmeaningful limb movements) paired with spoken production for naming (Crosson, 2008; Crosson et al., 2007; Richards et al., 2002). The premise of intentional gesture training is to use complex reaching and turning limb movements to activate frontal regions critical for initiation

Table 9.4 Gestural Facilitation Training for Word Retrieval

Present a pictured object (e.g., hammer, banana) or action (e.g., pounding, cutting).

1. Clinician provides model of gesture and corresponding word for imitation by patient.
2. Patient then rehearses only the pantomime, with clinician providing hands-on manipulation of limb as needed.
3. Patient rehearses spoken-word production, with clinician assistance as needed.
4. Patient pairs pantomime with spoken word and repeats three times.
5. After a short delay, clinician probes and patient once again provides target pantomime plus word production.

of movements, including limb and speech movements. Crosson and colleagues (2007) reported improvements in picture naming for trained words for their two groups with aphasia, along with generalized increases for untrained pictures in a group with moderately severe naming deficits. In a small trial that compared effects of intentional training and gestural pantomime training (both paired with verbal production), Ferguson, Evans, and Raymer (2012) found greater improvements for trained picture naming following intention training, and greater improvements for gesture production following pantomime training. These findings suggest that intentional training may be most applicable in individuals with mild-moderate anomia, whereas pantomime training is especially useful in individuals with severe anomia where participants may need gestures as a compensatory communication modality. The basis for naming failure was not well characterized in these studies, however.

Summary

Intact orthographic and gestural mechanisms of the lexical system may be used to support communication attempts in individuals with naming impairments. Some compensatory treatments may over time act vicariatively to improve spoken naming. At other times, the compensatory strategy remains the primary means of communication, as naming improvement is not forthcoming. It is crucial that clinicians evaluate the potential for alternative communication modes as a means to circumvent lexical impairments, particularly in individuals in more chronic stages of recovery from neurological injury.

Closing Issues

A fairly broad literature has now demonstrated the effectiveness of a variety of treatments for naming impairments. The question remains whether one treatment approach has advantages over another, particularly with respect to the nature of word retrieval failure, semantic versus phonological. Among studies that have evaluated response to contrasting semantic and phonological treatments across participants with aphasia, results favored the semantic treatment in some studies (Howard et al., 1985; Wambaugh et al., 1999) and the phonological treatment in others (Raymer & Ellsworth, 2002). In one of the only randomized controlled trials of naming treatment, Doesborgh et al. (2004) reported that both semantic and phonological treatments led to gains in their groups with semantic + phonological naming impairments, with no significant difference between treatments. Abel, Willmes, and Huber (2007) reported a similar pattern in their case series. Lorenz and Ziegler (2009) described a case series in which some participants initially responded better to phonological cues, yet the tendency was toward a more stable response to the semantic treatment over time. They also noted that there was little direct relationship between type of naming impairment (semantic or phonological) and most effective treatment, which further confirms the proposal espoused by Hillis (1993) long ago. In an extensive meta-analysis of the naming treatment literature, Wisenburn and Mahoney (2009) found that while semantic treatments led to positive outcomes in picture naming, stronger effects were associated with the phonological training studies. They also found that naming training effects were largely item specific to trained items, with some minimal generalization noted for semantic training. The source of naming impairments, whether semantic or phonological, was not considered in the meta-analysis.

Either semantic or phonological treatment seems to improve naming in individuals with either semantic or phonological impairment, although the treatment may be effective for different reasons in the two cases. For example, providing a phonological cue to a patient with a semantic deficit may help to activate the target phonological representation among many competing phonological representations activated by the damaged semantic representation. In contrast, providing a phonological cue to a patient with a deficit at the level of the phonological lexicon may provide the additional activation needed to the target lexical representation (which would have received full activation from the semantic system, but still did not quite reach threshold for selection due to damage at this level), such that the target is activated just above its threshold. In fact, the direction of treatments over time has been to combine semantic and phonological steps in training, in keeping with the normal process of lexical retrieval (Drew & Thompson, 1999; Kendall et al., in press; Raymer et al., 2007; Wambaugh et al., 2002).

One critical area for which further investigation is warranted in studies of naming treatments is the functional outcomes for patients in daily communication activities. The primary dependent variable in treatment studies for lexical impairments in aphasia has been percent improvement in the trained lexical task, typically picture naming. Fewer studies have investigated the generalization of lexical improvements to functional communication tasks and settings. Those that have examined discourse outcomes have reported modest changes in lexical use and efficiency measures for nouns and verbs following naming training, most often semantic training (Antonucci, 2009; Boyle, 2004; Cameron, Wambaugh, Wright, & Nessler, 2006; Conroy et al., 2009b; Del Toro et al., 2008; Edmonds & Babb, 2011). Likewise, some studies have reported positive changes on communication ratings scales associated with lexical treatments (Boyle & Coelho, 1995; Raymer et al., 2007). Overall, however, the functional consequences of treatments using a model-guided approach have not been well studied.

Knowledge gained from studies of the cognitive neuropsychological bases for word retrieval impairments certainly have influenced clinical practice in positive ways. A number of innovative treatment strategies have been developed on the basis of normal models of lexical and semantic processing. Although the model-guided approach to assessment and treatment can require an investment of time and energy in the clinical process, patients may anticipate maximum benefits as a result. Certainly cognitive models do not provide a sufficient basis upon which to base our clinical practice, as a number of medical, social, and experiential factors (Hillis, 1993; McClung, Rothi, & Nadeau, 2010), as well as principles of neuroplasticity (Kleim & Jones, 2008; Raymer et al., 2008), must be considered in the clinical decision-making process. However, this approach has the potential to guide and influence clinical practice in practical ways as we continue to study methods and determine who, what, and how to assess and treat naming impairments in aphasia.

Acknowledgment

Preparation of this chapter was supported in part by NIH grant R15 DC009690.

References

Abel, S., Willmes, K, & Huber, W. (2007). Model-oriented naming therapy: Testing predictions of a connectionist model. *Aphasiology, 21*(5), 411–447.

Adlam, A.L., Patterson, K., Bozeat, S., & Hodges, J.R. (2010). The Cambridge Semantic Memory Test Battery: Detection of semantic deficits in semantic dementia and Alzheimer's disease. *Neurocase, 16*, 193–207.

Antonucci, S. M. (2009). Use of semantic feature analysis in group aphasia treatment. *Aphasiology, 23*, 854–866.

Bak, T., & Hodges J.R. (2003). Kissing and dancing—a test to distinguish the lexical and conceptual contributions to noun/verb and action/object dissociation. Preliminary results in patients with frontotemporal dementia. *Journal of Neurolinguistics, 16*, 169–181.

Bastiaanse, R., Bosje, M., & Franssen, M. (1996). Deficit-oriented treatment of word-finding problems: Another replication. *Aphasiology, 10*, 363–383.

Beeson, P.M., & Egnor, H. (2006). Combining treatment for written and spoken naming. *Journal of the International Neuropsychological Society, 12*, 816–827.

Beeson, P.M., King R.M., Bonakdarpour, B., Henry, M.L., Cho, H., & Rapcsak, S.Z. (2011). Positive effects of language treatment for the logpenic variant of primary progressive aphasia. *Journal of Molecular Neuroscience, 45*, 724–736.

Boo, M., & Rose, M.L. (2011). The efficacy of repetition, semantic, and gesture treatments for verb retrieval and use in Broca's aphasia. *Aphasiology, 25*, 154–175.

Bose, A. (2013). Phonological therapy in jargon aphasia: Effects on naming and neologisms. *International Journal of Language and Communication Disorders, 48*, 482–495.

Boyle, M. (2004). Semantic feature analysis treatment for anomia in two fluent aphasia syndromes. *American Journal of Speech-Language Pathology, 13*, 236–249.

Boyle, M., & Coelho, C.A. (1995). Application of semantic feature analysis as a treatment for aphasic dysnomia. *American Journal of Speech-Language Pathology, 4*, 94–98.

Breese, E.L., & Hillis, A.E. (2004). Auditory comprehension: Is multiple choice really good enough. *Brain and Language, 89*, 3–8.

Bruce, C., & Howard, D. (1987). Computer-generated phonemic cues: An effective aid for naming in aphasia. *British Journal of Disorders of Communication, 22*, 191–201.

Budd, M.A., Kortte, K., Cloutman, L., Newhart, M., Gottesman, R.F., Davis, C., Heidler-Gary, J., Seay, M.W., & Hillis, A.E. (2010). The nature of naming errors in primary progressive aphasia versus acute post-stroke aphasia. *Neuropsychology, 24*, 581–589.

Cameron, R.M., Wambaugh, J.L., Wright, S.M., & Nessler, C.L. (2006). Effects of combined semantic/phonologic cueing treatment on word retrieval in discourse. *Aphasiology, 20*, 269–285.

Caramazza, A., & Hillis, A.E. (1990). Where do semantic errors come from? *Cortex, 26*, 95–122.

Caramazza, A., & Hillis, A.E. (1991). Lexical organization of nouns and verbs in the brain. *Nature, 349*, 788–790.

Caramazza, A., & Hillis, A. (1993). For a theory of remediation of cognitive deficits. *Neuropsychological Rehabilitation, 3*, 217–234.

Cloutman, L., Gottesman, R., Chaudhry, P., Davis, C., Kleinman, J.T., Pawlak, M., Herskovits, E.H., Kannan, V., Lee, A., Newhart, M., Heidler-Gary, J., & Hillis, A.E. (2009). Where (in the brain) do semantic errors come from? *Cortex, 45*, 641–649.

Conroy, P., Sage, K., & Ralph, M.L. (2009a). Improved vocabulary production after naming therapy in aphasia: can gains in picture naming generalise to connected speech? *International Journal of Language and Communication Disorders, 44*(6), 1036–1062.

Conroy, P., Sage, K., & Lambon Ralph, M.A. (2009b). The effects of decreasing and increasing cue therapy on improving naming speed and accuracy for verbs and nouns in aphasia. *Aphasiology, 23*(6)707–730.

Conroy, P., Snell, C., Sage, K.E., & Lambon Ralph, M.A. (2012). Using phonemic cueing of spontaneous naming to predict item responsiveness to therapy for anomia in aphasia. *Archives of Physical Medicine & Rehabilitation, 93* (Suppl. 1), S53–S60.

Crosson, B. (2008). An intention manipulation to change lateralization of word production in nonfluent aphasia: Current status. *Seminars in Speech and Language, 29*, 188–200.

Crosson, B., Fabrizio, K.S., Singletary, F., Cato, M.A., Wierenga, C.E., Parkinson, R.B., Sherod, M.E., Moore, A.B., Ciampitti, M., Holiway, B., Leon, S., Rodriguez, A., Kendall, D.L., Levy, K.F., & Rothi, L.J.G. (2007). Treatment of naming in nonfluent aphasia through manipulation of intention and attention: A phase 1 comparison of two novel treatments. *Journal of the International Neuropsychologial Society, 13*, 582–594.

Damasio, A.R., & Tranel, D. (1993). Nouns and verbs are retrieved with differently distributed neural systems. *Proceedings of the National Academy of Sciences, USA, 90*, 4957–4960.

DeDe, G., Parris, D., & Waters, G. (2003). Teaching self-cues: A treatment approach for verbal naming. *Aphasiology, 17*, 465–480.

Del Toro, C.M., Raymer, A.M., Leon, S., Blonder, L.X., Rothi, L.J.G., & Altmann, L. (2008). Changes in aphasic discourse after contrasting treatments for anomia. *Aphasiology, 22*, 881–892.

Doesborgh, S.J., van de Sandt-Koenderman, M.W., Dippel, D.W., van Harskamp, F., Koudstaal, P.J., & Visch-Brink, E.G. (2004). Effects of semantic treatment on verbal communication and linguistic processing in aphasia after stroke: A randomized controlled trial. *Stroke, 35*, 141–146.

Drew, R.L., & Thompson, C.K. (1999). Model-based semantic treatment for naming deficits in aphasia. *Journal of Speech, Language, and Hearing Research, 42*, 972–989.

Druks, J. (2002). Verbs and nouns-A review of the literature. *Journal of Neurolinguistics, 15*, 289–319.

Druks, J., & Masterson, J. (2000). *Object and Action Naming Battery*. Hove: Psychology Press.

Edmonds, L., & Babb, M. (2011). Effects of verb network strengthening treatment in moderate-to-severe aphasia. *American Journal of Speech-Language Pathology, 20*, 131–145.

Edmonds, L., Nadeau, S., & Kiran, S. (2009). Effect of verb network strengthening treatment (VNeST) on lexical retrieval of content words in sentences in persons with aphasia. *Aphasiology, 23*, 402–424.

Ellis, A.W., Kay, J., & Franklin, S. (1992). Anomia: Differentiating between semantic and phonological deficits. In D.I. Margolin (Ed.), *Cognitive neuropsychology in clinical practice*. New York: Oxford University Press.

Ennis, M.R. (2001). Comprehension approaches for word retrieval training in aphasia. *ASHA Special Interest Division 2: Neurophysiology and Neurogenic Speech and Language Disorders, 11*(2), 18–22.

Ferguson, N.F., Evans, K., & Raymer, A.M. (2012). A comparison of intention and pantomime gesture treatment for noun retrieval in people with aphasia. *American Journal of Speech-Language Pathology, 21*, 126–139.

Fillingham, J.K., Hodgson, C., Sage, K., & Lambon Ralph, M.A. (2003). The application of errorless learning to aphasic disorders: A review of theory and practice. *Neuropsychological Rehabilitation, 13*, 337–363.

Fillingham, J.K., Sage, K., & Lambon Ralph, M.A. (2005a). Further explorations and an overview of errorless and errorful therapy for aphasic word-finding difficulties: The number of naming attempts during therapy affects outcomes. *Aphasiology, 19*, 597–614.

Fillingham, J.K., Sage, K., & Lambon Ralph, M. (2006). The treatment of anomia using errorless learning. *Neuropsychological Rehabilitation, 16*, 129–154.

Fillingham, J.K., Sage, K., & Lambon Ralph, M.A. (2005b). Treatment of anomia using errorless versus errorful learning: Are frontal executive skills and feedback important? *International Journal of Language & Communication Disorders, 40*, 505–523.

Fink, R.B., Brecher, A., Schwartz, M.F., & Robey, R.R. (2002). A computer-implemented protocol for treatment of naming disorders: Evaluation of clinician-guided and partially self-guided instruction. *Aphasiology, 16*, 1061–1086.

Fink, R.B., Brecher, A., Montgomery, M., & Schwartz, M.S. (2010). *MossTalk Words 2.0*. Philadelphia: Moss Rehabilitation Research Institute. Available at www.mrri.org/mosstalk-words-2.

Fisher, C., Wilshire, C., & Ponsford, J. (2009). Word discrimination therapy: A new technique for the treatment of a phonologically based word-finding impairment. *Aphasiology, 23*, 676–693.

Greenwald, M.L., Raymer, A.M., Richardson, M. E., & Rothi, L.J.G. (1995). Contrasting treatments for severe impairments of picture naming. *Neuropsychological Rehabilitation, 5*, 17–49.

Hashimoto, N., & Frome, A. (2011). The use of a modified semantic features analysis approach. *Journal of Communication Disorder, 44*, 459–469.

Henry, M.L., Beeson, P.M., & Rapcsak, S.Z. (2008). Treatment for lexical retrieval in progressive aphasia. *Aphasiology, 22*, 826–838.

Henry, M.L., Rising, K., Demarco, A.T., Miller, B.L., Gorno-Tempini, M.L., & Beeson, P.M. (2013). Examining the value of lexical retrieval treatment in primary progressive aphasia: Two positive cases. *Brain and Language, 127*, 145–156.

Hillis, A.E. (1993). The role of models of language processing in rehabilitation of language impairments. *Aphasiology, 7*, 5–26.

Hillis, A.E. (1998). Treatment of naming disorders: New issues regarding old therapies. *Journal of the International Neuropsychological Society, 4*, 648–660.

Hillis, A.E., & Caramazza, A. (1995a). Cognitive and neural mechanisms underlying visual and semantic processing: Implications from "optic aphasia." *Journal of Cognitive Neuroscience, 7*, 457–478.

Hillis, A.E., & Caramazza, A. (1995b). The compositionality of lexical semantic representations: Clues from semantic errors in object naming. *Memory, 3*, 333–358.

Hillis, A.E., Rapp, B., Romani, C., & Caramazza, A. (1990). Selective impairment of semantics in lexical processing. *Cognitive Neuropsychology, 7*, 191–243.

Hirsh, K.W., & Ellis, A.W. (1994). Age of acquisition and lexical processing in aphasia: A case study. *Cognitive Neuropsychology, 11*, 435–458.

Hodges, J.R., & Patterson, K. (1996). Nonfluent progressive aphasia and semantic dementia: A comparative neuropsychological study. *Journal of the International Neuropsychological Society, 2*, 511–524.

Holland, A.L. (1998). A strategy for improving oral naming in an individual with a phonological access impairment. In N. Helm-Estabrooks & A.L. Holland (Eds.), *Approaches to the treatment of aphasia*. San Diego: Singular Publishing.

Howard, D., & Orchard-Lisle, V. (1984). On the origin of semantic errors in naming: Evidence from the case of a global aphasic. *Cognitive Neuropsychology, 1*, 163–190.

Howard, D., & Patterson, K. (1992). *Pyramids and palm trees*. Bury St. Edmunds: Thames Valley Publishing.

Howard, D., Patterson, K., Franklin, S., Orchard-Lisle V., & Morton, J. (1985). Treatment of word retrieval deficits in aphasia. *Brain, 108*, 817–829.

Jacquemot, C., Dupoux, E., Robotham, L., & Bachoud-Levi, A. C. (2012). Specificity in rehabilitation of word production: A meta-analysis and a case study. *Behavioral Neurology, 25*, 73–101.

Jefferies, E., & Lambon Ralph, M.A. (2006). Semantic impairment in stroke aphasia versus semantic dementia: A case-series comparison. *Brain, 129,* 2132–2147.

Jefferies, E., Rogers, T.T., Hopper, S., & Lambon Ralph, M.A. (2010). "Pre-semantic" cognition revisited: Critical differences between semantic aphasia and semantic dementia. *Neuropsychologia, 48,* 248–261.

Kaplan, E., Goodglass, H., & Weintraub, S. (2001). *The Boston naming test.* Baltimore: Lippincott Williams & Wilkins.

Kay, J., Lesser, R., & Coltheart, M. (1992). *PALPA: Psycholinguistic assessments of language processing in aphasia.* East Sussex, England: Lawrence Erlbaum.

Kendall, D., Raymer, A., Rose, M., Gilbert, J., & Rothi, L.J.G. (2014). Anomia treatment platform as a behavioral engine for use in research on physiological adjuvants to neurorehabilitation. *Journal of Rehabilitation Research & Development, 51,* 391–400.

Kendall, D.L., Rosenbek, J.C., Heilman, K.M., Conway, T., Klenberg, K., Rothi, L.J.G., & Nadeau, S.E. (2008). Phoneme-based rehabilitation of anomia in aphasia. *Brain and Language, 105,* 1–17.

Kiran, S. (2007). Complexity in the treatment of naming deficits. *American Journal of Speech-Language Pathology, 16,* 18–29.

Kiran, S. (2008). Evaluating the effectiveness of semantic-based treatment for naming deficits in aphasia: What works? *Seminars in Speech and Language, 29,* 71–82.

Kiran, S., & Bassetto, G. (2008). Evaluating the effectiveness of semantic-based treatment for naming deficits in aphasia: What works? *Seminars in Speech and Language, 29,* 71–82.

Kiran, S., & Johnson, L. (2008). Semantic complexity in treatment of naming deficits in aphasia: Evidence from well-defined categories. *American Journal of Speech-Language Pathology, 17,* 389–400.

Kiran, S., Sandberg, C., & Abbott, K. (2009). Treatment for lexical retrieval using abstract and concrete words in persons with aphasia: Effect of complexity. *Aphasiology, 23,* 835–853.

Kiran, S., Sandberg, C., & Sebastian, R. (2011). Treatment of category generation and retrieval in aphasia: Effect of typicality of category items. *Journal of Speech, Language, & Hearing Research, 54,* 1101–1117.

Kiran, S., & Thompson, C.K. (2003). The role of semantic complexity in treatment of naming deficits: Training semantic categories in fluent aphasia by controlling examplar typicality. *Journal of Speech, Language, & Hearing Research, 46,* 773–787.

Kittredge, A.K., Dell, G.S., Verkuilen, J., & Schwartz, M.F. (2008). Where is the effect of frequency in word production? Insights from aphasic picture naming error. *Cognitive Neuropsychology, 25,* 463–492.

Kleim, J.A., & Jones, T.A. (2008). Principles of experience-dependent neural plasticity: Implications for rehabilitation after brain damage. *Journal of Speech-Language-Hearing Research, 51,* S225–S239.

Kohn, S.E., Smith, K.L., & Alexander, M.P. (1996). Differential recovery from impairment to the phonological lexicon. *Brain and Language, 52,* 129–149.

Kroenke, K.M., Kraft, I., Regenbrecht, F., & Obrig, H. (2013). Lexical learning in mild aphasia: Gesture benefit depends on patholinguistic profile and lesion pattern. *Cortex, 49,* 2637–2649.

Laganaro, M., Di Pietro, M., & Schnider, A. (2006). Computerised treatment of anomia in acute aphasia: Treatment intensity and training size. *Neuropsychological Rehabilitation, 16,* 630–640.

Lambon Ralph, M.A., Graham, K.S., Ellis, A.W., & Hodges, J.R. (1998). Naming in semantic dementia: What matters? *Neuropsychologia, 36,* 775–784.

LeDorze, G., Boulay, N., Gaudreau, J., & Brassard, C. (1994). The contrasting effects of a semantic versus a formal-semantic technique for the facilitation of naming in a case of anomia. *Aphasiology, 8,* 127–141.

LeDorze, G., & Nespoulous, J.-L. (1989). Anomia in moderate aphasia: Problems in accessing the lexical representation. *Brain and Language, 37,* 381–400.

Leonard, C., Rochon, E., & Laird, L. (2008). Treating naming impairments in aphasia: Findings from a phonological components analysis treatment. *Aphasiology, 22,* 923–947.

Lindemood, P., & Lindemood, P. (2011). *Lindemood phoneme sequencing program for reading, spelling, and speech* (4th ed.). Austin, TX: ProEd.

Lorenz, A., & Ziegler, W. (2009). Semantic vs. word-form specific techniques in anomia treatment: A multiple single-case study. *Journal of Neurolinguistics, 22,* 515–537.

Lowell, S., Beeson, P.M., & Holland, A.L. (1995). The efficacy of a semantic cueing procedure on naming performance of adults with aphasia. *American Journal of Speech-Language Pathology, 4,* 109–114.

Mahon, B.Z., & Caramazza, A. (2009). Concepts and categories: A cognitive neuropsychological perspective. *Annual Review of Psychology, 60,* 27–51.

Marshall, J., Pound, C, White-Thomson, M., & Pring, T. (1990). The use of picture/word matching tasks to assist word retrieval in aphasic patients. *Aphasiology, 4,* 167–184.

Martin, N., Renvall, K., & Laine, M. (2005). Contextual priming in semantic anomia: A case study. *Brain and Language, 95,* 327–341.

Martin, N., Fink, R.B., Renvall, K., & Laine, M. (2006). Effectiveness of contextual repetition priming treatments for anomia depends on intact semantics. *Journal of the International Neuropsychological Society, 12*, 853–866.

Mason, C., Nickels, L., McDonald, B., Moses, M., Makin, K., & Taylor, C. (2011). Treatment of word retrieval impairments in aphasia: Evaluation of a self-administered home programme using personally chosen words. *Aphasiology, 25*(2), 245–268.

McClung, J.S., Rothi, L.J.G., & Nadeau, S.E. (2010). Ambient experience in restitutive treatment of aphasia. *Frontiers in Human Neuroscience, 4*(183), 1–19.

Miceli, G., Amitrano, A., Capasso, R., & Caramazza, A. (1996). The treatment of anomia resulting from output lexical damage: Analysis of two cases. *Brain and Language, 52*, 150–174.

Miceli, G., Giustollisi, L., & Caramazza, A. (1991). The interaction of lexical and non-lexical processing mechanisms: Evidence from anomia. *Cortex, 27*, 57–80.

Miceli, G., Silveri, M.C., Villa, G., & Caramazza, A. (1984). On the basis for the agrammatic's difficulty in producing main verbs. *Cortex, 20*, 207–220.

Mitchum, C.C. (1992). Treatment generalization and the application of cognitive neuropsychological models in aphasia therapy. In NIH Publication no. 93–3424: *Aphasia treatment: Current approaches and research opportunities*.

Mitchum, C.C., & Berndt, R.S. (1994). Verb retrieval and sentence construction: Effects of targeted intervention. In M.J. Riddoch & G. Humphreys (Eds.), *Cognitive neuropsychology and cognitive rehabilitation*. Hove: Erlbaum.

Newhart, M., Ken, L., Kleinman, J.T., Heidler,-Gary, J., & Hillis, A.E. (2007). Neural networks essential for naming and word comprehension. *Cognitive & Behavioral Neurology, 20*, 25–30.

Nicholas, M., Obler, L., Albert, M., & Goodglass, H. (1985). Lexical retrieval in healthy aging. *Cortex, 21*, 595–606.

Nickels, L. (2002). Therapy for naming disorders: revisiting, revising, and reviewing. *Aphasiology, 16*, 935–979.

Nickels, L. (1992). The autocue? Self-generated phonemic cues in the treatment of a disorder of reading and naming. *Cognitive Neuropsychology, 9*, 155–182.

Nickels, L., & Best, W. (1996). Therapy for naming disorders (part II): Specifics, surprises, and suggestions. *Aphasiology, 10*, 109–136.

Nickels, L., & Howard, D. (1994). A frequent occurrence: Factors affecting the production of semantic errors in aphasic naming. *Cognitive Neuropsychology, 11*, 289–320.

Nickels, L., & Howard, D. (1995). Aphasic naming: What matters? *Neuropsychologia, 33*, 1281–1303.

Pashek, G.V. (1998). Gestural facilitation of noun and verb retrieval in aphasia: A case study. *Brain and Language, 65*, 177–180.

Ramsberger, G., & Marie, B. (2007). Self-administered cued naming therapy: A single-participant investigation of a computer-based therapy program replicated in four cases. *American Journal of Speech-Language Pathology, 16*, 343–358.

Raymer, A.M., Beeson, P., Holland, A., Kendall, D., Maher, L.M., Martin, N., Murray, L., Rose, M., Thompson, C. K., Turkstra, L., Altmann, L., Boyle, M., Conway, T., Hula, W., Kearns, K., Rapp, B., Simmons-Mackie, N., & Rothi, L.J.G. (2008). Translational research in aphasia: From neuroscience to neurorehabilitation. *Journal of Speech- Language-Hearing Research, 51*, S259–S275.

Raymer, A.M., & Berndt, R.S. (1996). Reading lexically without semantics: Evidence from patients with probable Alzheimer's disease. *Journal of the International Neuropsychological Society, 2*, 340–349.

Raymer, A.M., Ciampitti, M., Holliway, B., Singletary, F., Blonder, L. X., Ketterson, T., Heilman, K.M., & Rothi, L.J.G. (2007). Lexical-semantic treatment for noun and verb retrieval impairments in aphasia. *Neuropsychological Rehabilitation, 17*, 244–270.

Raymer, A.M., & Ellsworth, T.A. (2002). Response to contrasting verb retrieval treatments: A case study. *Aphasiology, 16*, 1031–1045.

Raymer, A.M., Foundas, A.L., Maher, L.M., Greenwald, M.L., Morris, M., Rothi, L.J.G., & Heilman, K.M. (1997). Cognitive neuropsychological analysis and neuroanatomic correlates in a case of acute anomia. *Brain and Language, 58*, 137–156.

Raymer, A.M., Greenwald, M.L., Richardson, M.E., Rothi, L.J.G., & Heilman, K.M. (1997). Optic aphasia and optic apraxia: Case analysis and theoretical implications. *Neurocase, 3*, 173–183.

Raymer, A.M., Kohen, F., Blonder, L.X., Douglas, E., Sembrat, J.L., & Rothi, L.J.G. (2007). Effects of gesture and semantic-phonologic treatments for noun retrieval in aphasia. *Brain and Language, 103*, 219–220.

Raymer, A.M., Kohen, F.P., & Saffell, D. (2006). Computerised training for impairments of word comprehension and retrieval in aphasia. *Aphasiology, 20*, 257–268.

Raymer, A.M., McHose, B., Graham, K., Ambrose, A., & Casselton, C. (2012). Contrasting effects of errorless naming treatment and gestural facilitation for word retrieval in aphasia. *Neuropsychological Rehabilitation, 22*, 235–266.

Raymer, A.M., & Rothi, L.J.G. (2008). Cognitive neuropsychological approaches to assessment and treatment: Impairments of lexical comprehension and production. In R. Chapey (Ed.), *Language intervention strategies in adult aphasia* (pp. 607–631). Baltimore: Lippincott Williams & Wilkins.

Raymer, A.M., Rothi, L.J.G., & Greenwald, M.L. (1995). The role of cognitive models in language rehabilitation. *NeuroRehabilitation, 5*, 183–193.

Raymer, A.M., Singletary, F., Rodriguez, A., Ciampitti, M., Heilman, K.M., & Rothi, L.J.G. (2006). Effects of gesture + verbal treatment for noun and verb retrieval in aphasia. *Journal of the International Neuropsychological Society*, 867–882.

Raymer, A. M., & Thompson, C.K. (1991). Effects of verbal plus gestural treatment in a patient with aphasia and severe apraxia of speech. In T.E. Prescott (Ed.), *Clinical aphasiology, Vol. 12*. Austin, TX: Pro-Ed.

Raymer, A.M., Thompson, C.K., Jacobs, B., & leGrand, H.R. (1993). Phonologic treatment of naming deficits in aphasia: Model-based generalization analysis. *Aphasiology, 7*, 27–53.

Renvall, K., Laine, M., & Martin, N. (2007). Treatment of anomia with contextual priming: Exploration of a modified procedure with additional semantic and phonological tasks. *Aphasiology, 21*, 499–527.

Richards, K., Singletary, F., Rothi, L.J.G., Koehler, S., & Crosson, B. (2002). Activation of intentional mechanisms through utilization of nonsymbolic movements in aphasia rehabilitation. *Journal of Rehabilitation Research & Development, 39*, 445–454.

Riddoch, M.J., & Humphreys, G.W. (1994). Cognitive neuropsychology and cognitive rehabilitation: A marriage of equal partners? In M.J. Riddoch & G.W. Humphreys (Eds.), *Cognitive neuropsychology and cognitive rehabilitation*. London: Lawrence Erlbaum.

Rider, J.D., Wright, H.H., Marshall, R.C., & Page, J.L. (2008). Using semantic feature analysis to improve contextual discourse in adults with aphasia. *American Journal of Speech-Language Pathology, 17*, 161–172.

Roach, A., Schwartz, M.F., Martin, N., Grewal, R.S., & Brecher, A. (1996). The Philadelphia Naming Test: Scoring and rationale. *Clinical Aphasiology, 24*, 121–133.

Robson, J., Marshall, J., Pring, T., & Chiat, S. (1998). Phonologic naming therapy in jargon aphasia: Positive but paradoxical effects. *Journal of the International Neuropsychological Society, 4*, 675–686.

Rodriguez, A.M., Raymer, A.M., & Rothi, L.J.G. (2006). Effects of gesture + verbal and semantic-phonologic treatments for verb retrieval in aphasia. *Aphasiology, 20*, 286–297.

Rosch, E. (1975). The nature of mental codes for color categories. *Journal of Experimental Psychology: Human Perception & Performance, 1*, 303–322.

Rose, M., & Douglas, J. (2008). Treatment of semantic word production deficit in aphasia with verbal and gesture methods. *Aphasiology, 22*, 20–41.

Rose, M., Douglas, J., & Matyas, T. (2002). The comparative effectiveness of gesture and verbal treatments for specific phonologic naming impairment. *Aphasiology, 16*, 1001–1030.

Rose, M.L., Raymer, A.M., Lanyon, L.E., & Attard, M.C. (2013). A systematic review of gesture treatments for post-stroke aphasia. *Aphasiology, 27*, 1090–1127.

Rose, M. & Sussmilch, G. (2008). The effects of semantic and gesture treatments on verb retrieval and verb use in aphasia. *Aphasiology, 22*, 691–706.

Rothi, L.J.G. (1995). Behavioral compensation in the case of treatment of acquired language disorders resulting from brain damage. In R.A. Dixon & L. Mackman (Eds.), *Compensating for psychological deficits and declines: Managing losses and promoting gains*. Mahwah, NJ: Lawrence Erlbaum.

Rothi, L.J.G., Ochipa, C., & Heilman, K.M. (1997). A cognitive neuropsychological model of limb praxis and apraxia. In L.J.G. Rothi & K.M. Heilman (Eds.), *Apraxia: The neuropsychology of action*. East Sussex, England: Psychology Press.

Sage, K., Snell, C., & Lambon Ralph, M.A. (2011). How intensive does anomia therapy for people with aphasia need to be? *Neuropsychological Rehabilitation, 21*, 26–41.

Schwartz, M.F., Faseyitan, O., Kim, J., & Coslett, H.B. (2012). The dorsal stream contribution to phonological retrieval in object naming. *Brain, 135*, 3799–3814.

Seron, X., & Deloche, G. (Eds.). (1989). *Cognitive approaches in neuropsychological rehabilitation*. Hillsdale, NJ: Lawrence Erlbaum.

Snell, C., Sage, K., & Lambon Ralph, M.A. (2010). How many words should we provide in anomia therapy? A meta-analysis and a case series study. *Aphasiology, 24*, 1064–1094.

Stanczak, L., Waters, G., & Caplan, D. (2006). Typicality-based learning and generalization in aphasia: Two case studies of anomia treatment. *Aphasiology, 20*, 374–383.

Thompson, C., Lukic, S., King, M.C., Mesulam, M.M., & Weintraub, S. (2012). Verb and noun deficits in stroke-induced and primary progressive aphasia: The Northwestern Naming Battery. *Aphasiology, 26*, 632–655.

Walker, G.M., Schwartz, M.F., Kimberg, D.Y., Faseyitan, O., Brecher, A., Dell, G.S., & Coslett, H.B. (2011). Support for anterior temporal involvement in semantic error production in aphasia: New evidence from VLSM. *Brain and Language, 117*, 110–122.

Wallace, S.E., & Kimelman, M.D. (2013). Generalization of word retrieval following semantic feature treatment. *NeuroRehabilitation, 32*, 899–913.

Wambaugh, J.L., Doyle, P.J., Linebaugh, C.W., Spencer, K. A., & Kalinyak-Fliszar, M. (1999). Effects of deficit-oriented treatments on lexical retrieval in a patient with semantic and phonological deficits. *Brain and Language, 69*, 446–450.

Wambaugh, J.L., Doyle, P.J., Martinez, A.L., & Kalinyak-Fliszar, M. (2002). Effects of two lexical retrieval cueing treatments on action naming in aphasia. *Journal of Rehabilitation Research and Development, 39*, 455–466.

Wambaugh, J.L., & Ferguson, M.S. (2007). Application of semantic feature analysis to retrieval of action names in aphasia. *Journal of Rehabilitation Research and Development, 44*, 381–394.

Wambaugh, J.L. (2003). A comparison of the relative effects of phonologic and semantic cueing treatments. *Aphasiology, 17*, 433–441.

Williamson, D.J.G., Adair, J. C, Raymer, A.M., & Heilman, K.M. (1998). Object and action naming in Alzheimer's disease. *Cortex, 34*, 601–610.

Wisenburn, B., & Mahoney, K. (2009). A meta-analysis of word-finding treatments for aphasia. *Aphasiology, 23*, 1338–1352.

Zingeser, L.B., & Berndt, R.S. (1990). Retrieval of nouns and verbs in agrammatism and anomia. *Brain and Language, 39*, 14–32.

PART 4

Semantics

10

SEMANTIC MEMORY

Elaine Funnell and Bonnie Breining

Introduction

Standard definitions of semantic memory refer to factual knowledge shared by members of a community—the sort of information that would be found in an encyclopedia or dictionary. Encyclopedias do not include personal experience and, in this respect, they observe the distinction, first drawn by Tulving (1972), between semantic knowledge for facts and episodic knowledge of personal events. As Tulving makes clear, this distinction is intended to be a useful guideline, and not necessarily to reflect differences in memory storage for the two types of knowledge. Nevertheless, the study of semantic memory has concentrated on encyclopedic knowledge, most commonly of single entities, such as objects. On the whole, theories of semantic memory and episodic memory have evolved separately.

Squeezed between episodic memory and semantic memory, and almost forgotten, is a memory for factual knowledge concerning common events—such as going to a restaurant or visiting the dentist (Schank & Abelson, 1977; Schank, 1982). This knowledge is also generally not considered to be part of semantic memory, despite the fact that it is shared by those who belong to the same culture and, in this respect, fits the standard definition of semantic memory. Kintsch (1980) has argued forcibly that knowledge of entities and events is not distinct, but forms the end points on a continuum of meaning from the least to the most context bound. The separation of semantic memory from context will be one aspect that will be discussed in this chapter.

The scientific investigation of the organization of semantic memory has been driven in recent years by the study of semantic disorders following brain damage. Double dissociations have been reported between the processing of different types of material (pictures and words), different input modalities (visual, auditory, tactile), different types of words (concrete and abstract; nouns and verbs), different categories of objects, and different types of semantic features (visual and functional). Such findings have raised a series of questions about the organization of semantic memory that mainly revolve around one issue: is there one semantic system or many? Separable semantic systems have been proposed for processing different types of material, different input modalities, and different types of content. The main goal of this chapter will be to review the evidence that has given rise to these claims. The chapter will close with a model of semantic memory that attempts to integrate the representation of isolated entities with that of context into a continuum of levels of meaning.

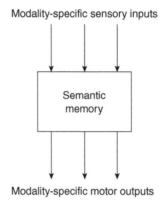

Modality-specific sensory inputs

Semantic memory

Modality-specific motor outputs

Figure 10.1

Separable Semantic Systems?

Let us start with the simplest theory possible about semantic memory, illustrated in Figure 10.1. It is a parsimonious model consisting of a single semantic system that can be accessed by all types of incoming information; for example, by words, pictures, and environmental sounds. It can activate responses in the form of linguistic output, drawing, and physical actions relating to object use. The model predicts that a disorder that affects semantic memory should disrupt the ability to comprehend all types of input and to express understanding in all types of output.

The case for a single semantic system has had serious challenges. In a seminal paper, Warrington (1975) investigated the residual semantic knowledge of two patients (AB and EM) who had a specific loss of semantic memory. Both patients defined spoken words to a similar level, but when the same items were presented visually as pictures for naming AB was relatively impaired while EM achieved significantly superior scores.[1] To account for these differences in performance given either visual or verbal materials, Warrington argued that semantic knowledge must be represented in partially separable semantic systems: a visual system specialized for pictorial material and a verbal system for written and spoken words.

Methods Used for Identifying Semantic Memory Deficits

Warrington and Shallice (1984) argued that if the semantic representation for a particular object is damaged, then there should be errors each time the defective information is accessed. Likewise, if the semantic representation for a particular object is intact, a correct response should be expected each time that representation is accessed. Using this logic, they examined the consistency of responses across repeated tests using either pictorial or verbal material in two patients (JBR and SBY) who had semantic knowledge deficits. JBE and SBY showed consistent, item-specific effects across tests using visually presented objects, and SBY also showed consistent effects across tests using spoken object names. But neither patient showed a consistent relationship when responses made to visual and verbal material were compared. Instead, different items were affected in the two tests. From this, Warrington and Shallice argued that the semantic information accessed from pictorial material and spoken words must be distinct.

Some methodological aspects of Warrington and Shallice's study undermine the conclusions (see Rapp & Caramazza, 1993; Riddoch, Humphreys, Coltheart, & Funnell, 1988). First, JBR was not given repeated tests using spoken words. Thus, his consistency within the auditory domain was assumed rather than demonstrated.[2] Second, in one of four comparisons, SBY produced a consistent performance across tests. Furthermore, Rapp and Caramazza (1993) questioned the assumption that damage to conceptual representations must necessarily produce consistent responses to the same items across tests. They argue that if damage affects a subset of semantic features, the remaining features might activate a set of related responses that include the correct response. In this case the correct response might be produced on some occasions and a related error response on others, and so produce inconsistent responses across tests (see also Chertkow & Bub, 1990).

Response consistency is just one of a set of five characteristics that have been argued to signify damage to stored representations (Shallice, 1988a). The remaining characteristics are a strong effect of word frequency, a lack of response to priming, better access to shared properties than to specific properties of objects, and no effect of presentation rate on performance. However, as Rapp and Caramazza (1993) point out, few patients have been fully examined on all the characteristics and, even when fully tested, do not always show patterns of performance that support clear distinctions between deficits of access and storage. For each characteristic proposed to reflect semantic damage, Rapp and Caramazza propose plausible alternative frameworks in which the assumption that performance patterns reflect damage to stored representations do not hold.

Theoretical Accounts of Separable Material-Specific Semantic Systems

The distinction between visual and verbal systems has been defended by Shallice (1988a, 1988b) on the basis that the systems process different types of information. Visual semantic representations process visual scenes and scenarios, while verbal semantic representations are involved in interpreting sentences by identifying propositions and determining the sense of the words. At the level of object recognition and single object names, Shallice argues that some semantic properties of objects, such as their function, might be accessed frequently from both verbal and visual input, and for these properties the distinction between visual and verbal semantic systems is more difficult to sustain. He suggests, instead, that semantic knowledge of these properties might be represented in a network in which specific regions form subsystems specialized for different types of processing. Such subsystems may be determined by the connections that each region has to process concerned with intention and action (see Allport, 1985).

Caramazza, Hillis, Rapp, and Romani (1990, p. 162) organize previous arguments and claims into a set of four hypotheses concerning the organization of separable semantic systems for visual pictorial material and verbal material.

The *modality-specific format hypothesis* is concerned with the form in which the semantic information is stored in the separable semantic systems. Visual information is stored in a "visual/imagistic code," while verbal information is stored in symbolic or propositional form (see also Paivio, 1978). This theory, however, lacks theoretical motivation and empirical evidence.

The *modality-specific input hypothesis* proposes that the visual and verbal semantic systems contain the same material. According to this hypothesis, "visual" and "verbal" capture differences in the nature of the input material rather than semantic distinctions (see also Riddoch et al., 1988). Caramazza and colleagues argued that this hypothesis could not account for data from neurologically impaired subjects who made identical types and rates of semantic errors across all input modalities. For example, their patient KE made errors of the type, dog → cat, in oral reading, oral naming, writing to dictation, written naming, spoken-word comprehension, and written word comprehension. These comprised 25 to 30 percent of his responses, and virtually all of his errors, in all of these tasks. The only way to account for this pattern of errors within a model that proposes separate semantic systems for each input modality is to assume that KE had identical damage to each of these semantic systems (Hillis, Rapp, Romani, & Caramazza, 1990).

The *modality-specific content hypothesis* distinguishes between different types of content for the visual and verbal systems. The visual system contains the visually specified attributes (e.g., object shape) and associations between objects seen together. The verbal system contains information about abstract relations (e.g., class membership) expressed through language. Both systems also include information derived in the context of the object. Caramazza and colleagues conclude that the modality-specific content hypothesis might account for data that "suggest that it is possible to access part of a semantic representation (e.g., 'visual' semantics) without necessarily having access to other parts of the semantic representation of a term (e.g., 'verbal' semantics)" (p. 174). But they also propose that the same data might be explained within an organized unitary content hypothesis (OUCH), in which a single semantic memory system has privileged access from particular inputs to particular types of semantic information.

The *hypothesis of content organization within a single semantic system*, such as OUCH, represents meaning as a set of semantic predicates in amodal form (see Figure 10.2). In OUCH, semantic predicates are linked together, and those that are more highly associated have stronger links than others. The full set of semantic information associated with an object can be accessed as a complete unit from both words and pictures. However, pictures also have "privileged" access to the semantic predicates that represent the perceptual attributes of an object. For example, the tines of a visually presented fork will access the semantic feature "tines" or "for spearing" directly, whereas the word *fork* will access the feature "tines" or "for spearing" only indirectly as a component of the complete semantic representation of fork. The authors argue that if semantic damage affects a random set of semantic predicates, access to the complete semantic description will be compromised given either pictorial or verbal input. However, since pictures also have privileged access to semantic perceptual predicates, an advantage for visual pictorial input might be expected when the task requires access to only partial semantic information (such as gesture, which might be formed on the basis of the feature "for spearing" alone).

OUCH, as Shallice (1993) points out, shares many characteristics with the account of visual and verbal semantic subsystems put forward earlier (Shallice, 1988a), in which the semantic system can be viewed as an interconnected system in which subregions are more specialized for particular types of input procedure. Theoretical differences may depend upon the nature of the connections between different types of input and different "regions" within an integrated semantic memory system, rather than separations between connections linking different sorts of semantic content.

In conclusion, the strong form of the visual-verbal semantic distinction has not stood up well. First, the evidence for a distinction between semantic knowledge systems for pictorial and verbal

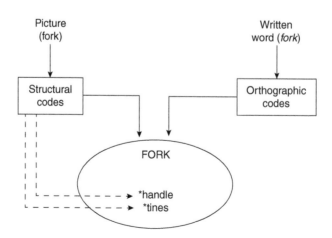

Figure 10.2

material is weak. Second, the theory of partial separation between visual and verbal semantics is not sufficiently well defined to be testable. As Caramazza and colleagues have shown, an account based on a single semantic system with additional privileged links to perceptual units from pictured inputs could provide a viable alternative. Nevertheless, the proposal of separable semantic systems is not settled. Each of the last three hypotheses regarding this issue, with evidence from more recent studies, are further discussed in the following sections.

Modality-Specific Input Hypothesis

The main source of evidence for proposing separate semantic systems distinguished by modality of input comes from optic aphasia, a rare disorder that particularly affects the naming of objects presented in the visual modality. Objects are named significantly more successfully when presented in other modalities, such as by a spoken description of the object or by holding and manipulating the object with eyes closed. Surprisingly, patients can usually demonstrate some knowledge of the visually presented object that they are unable to name. For example, they may be able to gesture the object's use, or show knowledge of the category to which the object belongs, or its function. The fact that objects that can be identified but not named from vision can, in other modalities, be both identified *and* named provides a challenge to current unitary models of semantic memory. Three different theories of optic aphasia have been put forward. These are discussed in turn.

Disconnection between Verbal Semantics and Visual Semantics

Beauvois (1982) and Beauvois and Saillant (1985) suggested that optic aphasia occurs when the links between visual and verbal semantics are impaired. This theory was based initially on findings from a patient, MP, who had an optic aphasia for color due to a stroke affecting the posterior cerebral artery resulting in damage to the left occipital pole and medial area of the left temporal lobe. The patient, a well-educated woman, had good color discrimination, but her ability to name colors and point to colors named for her was very poor.

A series of tests showed that MP's difficulty with colors emerged when the tasks involved *both* visual and verbal processing. She could provide associated names in verbal tasks (e.g., she was able to give the alternative name *jambon blanc* for *jambon de Paris*), and in purely visual tests she could point to the correctly colored version of visually presented objects. However, in visual-verbal tasks, she made errors when asked to point to a picture colored according to the color name associated with the object (e.g., a "very orange" orange rather than a more appropriate shade). She also made errors when naming the color of objects such as a gherkin that are not automatically associated with a color name and are argued to require visual imagery for the color to be identified. The authors argued that MP had suffered a disconnection between visual semantics, which contained information about the color of objects, and verbal semantics, which contained conceptual and linguistic attributes.

Optic Aphasia and Right Hemisphere Semantics

A second patient with an optic aphasia for colors, reported by Coslett and Saffran (1989), did not fit Beauvois's theory. Like MP, this patient was unable to name colors or point to the correct color given the spoken name, but he was able to name to a high level the color of named objects argued by Beauvois (1982) to require visualization (e.g., "What color is a lime?"). Thus, he could carry out tasks that involved both verbal and visual domains. Investigations suggested that his disorder could not be put down to impairments to early visual processes or semantic access. For example, he was able to distinguish between correctly drawn objects (e.g., a turtle) and incorrectly drawn objects composed of parts taken from two objects belonging to the same semantic category (e.g., a turtle with a chicken's head). He could sort pictures perfectly into categories of animals and objects, and pair together pictures of different objects sharing either the same function (e.g., a zipper and a button) or an associated function (e.g., pen and paper). To account for these findings, Coslett and Saffran (1989) proposed that optic aphasia arises from a disconnection between a visual semantic system located in the right cerebral hemisphere and the speech processing system located in the left hemisphere.[3]

Optic Aphasia and a Unitary Semantic System

The remaining theoretical account explains optic aphasia within a single semantic memory system. There are a variety of forms of this theory: the dual route theory (Ratcliff & Newcombe, 1982); the semantic access theory (Riddoch & Humphreys, 1987); and the superadditive deficit theory (Campbell & Manning, 1996; Farah, 1990). All theories have in common a specialized set of structural descriptions for object recognition that enables an object to be identified as a familiar sensory form but does not provide associated information such as knowledge of object function. These structural systems have the same function as the visual knowledge attribute systems (Coltheart et al., 1998) referred to earlier. Thus, there are sets of structural descriptions for visually processed components of objects, tactile components, and auditory components of environmental sounds associated with objects. Each set of structural descriptions has access to the central, unimodal semantic system, from whence the spoken name of the object can be retrieved (see Figure 10.3).

The Dual-Route Theory

This theory (Ratcliffe & Newcombe, 1982) proposes that each sensory input has access to a further, nonsemantic pathway from structural descriptions to naming that provides a more precise

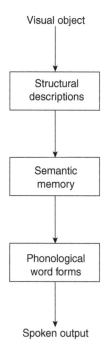

Visual object

Structural
descriptions

Semantic
memory

Phonological
word forms

Spoken output

Figure 10.3

access to the name than the semantic pathway, which is prone to error. However, Coslett and Saffran (1989) argued that their patient's performance could not be accounted for by the dual-coding theory because he could name the same objects correctly from verbal descriptions, indicating that intact semantic processing can alone support accurate naming.

The Semantic Access Theory

This theory (Riddoch & Humphreys, 1987) proposes that optic aphasia arises from a deficit to a single pathway that accesses the semantic system from the visual structural descriptions. This theory was based upon a patient, JB, who suffered damage to the left parietal/occipital region as a result of a road traffic accident. He had marked difficulties when naming common objects by vision alone, although he was able to gesture the use of many of them. He was considerably more successful at naming the same items from touch and from auditory definition.

Tests indicated that the visual processes leading up to and including the visual structural descriptions were intact: for example, he copied objects well and matched objects successfully across different views. He also demonstrated well-preserved semantic knowledge when accessed through the auditory modality. His problems arose when he was required to access the semantic system from vision, particularly when objects from semantic categories containing many structurally similar neighbors were presented. Riddoch and Humphreys (1987) argued that JB's naming problem for objects belonging to categories containing many structurally similar objects indicated an impairment to the access mechanisms to semantic information from vision. They suggested that the effects of this impairment could be explained within an interactive system in which processing at an earlier stage affects later processing stages. Supporting this view, Arguin, Bub, and Dudek (1996) have shown that in visual agnosia structural similarity is a problem only if the structurally similar items belong to the same semantic category. A simulation of optic aphasia, in which the connections linking visual with semantic information were damaged, produced errors to items that were visually and visually and semantically similar to the targets (Plaut & Shallice, 1993a). These authors proposed that a visual-semantic access account could explain optic aphasia. For additional evidence favoring this account, see DeRenzi and Saetti (1997) and Hillis and Caramazza (1995).

The Superadditivity Theory

Farah (1990) doubted that a disorder affecting visual access only could explain optic aphasia and suggested instead that "superadditivity" between two mild disorders, one affecting visual input and the other affecting spoken output, was necessary. Neither disorder would be great enough to cause problems on its own, but when combined would disrupt processing in tasks involving both sets of processes.

An optic aphasic patient, AG, provides some support for the superadditivity theory (Campbell & Manning, 1996). AG showed a mild visual impairment in tasks that required access to information about the visual characteristics of objects when these were obscured in a picture. In addition, a naming impairment was revealed in verbal fluency tests, in which object names belonging to a category must be recalled, although his naming of objects presented in domains other than vision was good. From these results, Campbell and Manning argued that superadditive effects of mild disorders to visual access and naming output could account for AG's optic aphasia. They pointed out, however, that the data would also fit the single visual access theory of Riddoch and Humphreys. Other patients, such as DHY, reported by Hillis and Caramazza (1995), have had normal verbal naming and fluency.

Perhaps the most important conclusion to be drawn from the studies by Riddoch and Humphreys and Campbell and Manning is that deficits of visual access to semantics have been demonstrated when, hitherto, it has been argued that visual to semantic processing in optic apha-sia is unimpaired. In the case of AG, the visual-to-semantic deficit was mild, revealing itself only in visual tasks in which the information was degraded. In JB, the deficits appeared when spe-cific information was sought or when decisions concerning the functional relationships between objects were made difficult by the addition of a semantically (but not functionally related) distrac-tor. Previous studies have not used such demanding tasks. It is possible, therefore, that all cases of optic aphasia might reveal deficits in visual-semantic processing if the tests given are sufficiently stringent.

Modality-Specific Content Hypothesis

Saffran and Schwartz (1994) argue forcefully that the data from neuropsychology require dis-tinctions between sensory information and conceptual representations, and suggest that the neu-ral substrates of object concepts differ according to the modality in which the information was acquired. As Saffran and Schwartz observe, there is plenty of evidence in the neuropsychological literature to indicate that different perceptual systems, such as those used for color and movement, can break down independently, indicating functionally separable systems.

Allport (1985) and Coltheart, Inglis, Cupples, et al. (1998) suggest that each perceptual domain—visual, auditory, olfactory, tactile—has a dedicated knowledge base containing the per-ceptual properties of objects. Each knowledge base functions both as a recognition device and as a store of perceptual information. For example, a visual attribute domain is used for recognizing visually presented objects and for retrieving visual attribute knowledge.[4] Damage to any sensory attribute domain gives rise to attribute-specific semantic impairments. For example, damage to the visual knowledge base will give rise to failure to recognize visually presented objects and to loss of knowledge pertaining to specific visual attributes. Allport argues that perceptual domains link together to form a distributed parallel processing system that links perceptual information with knowledge of action and lexical knowledge. Coltheart suggests that perceptual attribute domains are not linked directly. Instead, each perceptual domain accesses an additional store of nonper-ceptual knowledge organized according to functional properties, such as "dangerous." The visual domain also accesses a system dedicated to knowledge about actions (see Figure 10.4).

Coltheart et al. (1998) provided evidence for a specific visual semantic attribute system from a patient, AC, who had a left hemisphere stroke affecting the area of the left middle cerebral artery. CT scans also revealed small lesions in the white matter throughout the cerebral hemispheres. Assessments indicated that AC's early visual processes were intact. Nevertheless, he had difficulty accessing structural descriptions of animals from vision. Given pictures of real animals and non-sense animals, created by recombining heads and bodies of real animals, his performance in distin-guishing between the two was close to chance, while performance on the same test using objects was within the normal range.

AC was profoundly anomic and unable to read or write. Testing of his semantic memory for animals and objects therefore used spoken questions that probed specific semantic attributes. He was unable to respond above chance level to questions such as "Does a worm have legs?" "Does a bicycle have wheels?" "Is a bubble round?" "Is a crow colored or not?" In contrast, he answered, above chance, olfactory and auditory questions, such as "Does coffee have a characteristic smell?" "Does a star make a noise?" He was also able to answer nonperceptual questions to a high level, such as "Is a snake dangerous or not?" "Is an elephant Australian?" "Does an oyster live in water?" "Do people usually eat eagles?" On the basis of these results, Coltheart and colleagues argued that AC had an attribute-specific semantic deficit in the visual domain.[5]

In one important aspect, AC's performance does not fit the theory. The theory states that the same set of information is responsible for visual object recognition *and* visual-conceptual

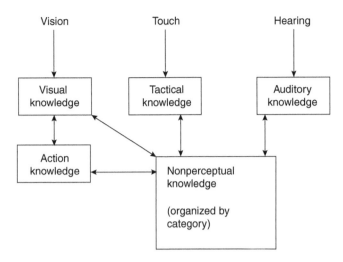

Figure 10.4

knowledge. Thus, AC's spared visual recognition for object classes other than animals predicts that he should be able to answer visual attribute questions for these spared object classes. The fact that he was unable to do so indicates that his difficulty with answering visual attribute questions arises not in the visual recognition system, but elsewhere. Within Coltheart and colleagues' model, this could arise from a problem with accessing the visual structural descriptions from the nonperceptual knowledge system. In this case, it would not be surprising if only visual attribute knowledge was affected.

Content Organization within the Semantic System

We now turn the organization of the content within the semantic system. We will discuss a set of theories that propose that the semantic system is organized according to the content of the information. The first of these theories separates information associated with different categories of objects; the second separates concrete from abstract word meanings; and the third separates object knowledge from action knowledge. The fourth proposal is that semantic information of objects and actions is embodied within the neural representations that carry out perception and actions (e.g., the representation of "kick" is embodied within the neural network responsible for orchestrating kicking). These theories will be examined in turn.

Category-Specific Disorders for Objects

Disorders affecting particular categories of objects have been widely reported. Two contrasting cases, JBR and VER, reported by Warrington (1981), began the flowering of interest in the theoretical bases of these disorders. One of these patients, JBR (referred to earlier), appeared to have a particularly marked problem with objects in the realm of living things (see also Warrington & Shallice, 1984). He named one of a set of pictures of animals and plants, but named over half of a set of manmade objects. His definitions of living things were generally empty of detailed information (e.g., daffodil → "plant"; ostrich → "unusual"), while definitions of manmade objects were well informed (e.g., tent → "temporary outhouse"; torch → "handheld light"). In contrast, the second patient (VER) had more difficulty with the processing of manmade objects (see also Warrington & McCarthy, 1983). VER had a severe aphasia, resulting from a stroke to the left frontoparietal cortex, and was virtually unable to name objects. For this reason, her knowledge of objects was tested using spoken word-picture matching tasks.[6] In a series of repeated tests, VER matched small sets of flower and animal names to pairs of pictures more successfully than names of manmade objects.[7]

As further studies made clear, the distinction between performance on living and nonliving things is not always absolute. JBR was later shown by Warrington and Shallice (1984) to perform well with body parts (a member of the living things category on which he should do badly) and badly on musical instruments (manmade objects on which he should do well). Likewise, a further patient, YOT (Warrington & McCarthy, 1987), with a deficit to manmade objects similar to VER, found some manmade objects more difficult than others. In a spoken-to-written word matching task, YOT had more problems with categories of objects that are small enough to handle (specifically furniture and kitchen utensils) compared with categories of nonmanipulable objects (such a buildings and vehicles).[8] However, this distinction was not fully consistent, for her responses to clothing, a manipulable category, were equivalent to responses to vehicles, a nonmanipulable category.

Hillis and Caramazza (1991) argued that brain damage can affect individual categories of objects. JJ, who had a stroke affecting the left temporal lobe and the left basal ganglia, had superior oral naming for pictures of land and water animals and birds, although his naming of fruit, foods, body parts, clothing, and furniture was close to zero. His performance contrasted sharply with a second patient, PS, given the same materials under the same conditions. PS had lesions resulting from a head injury that affected the left temporal lobe and smaller areas in the right temporal and frontal lobes. PS had virtually intact naming of the categories at which JJ failed, namely manmade objects, body parts, and fruit, but was clearly impaired at naming land and water animals and birds, categories at which JJ excelled. Differences in personal familiarity with animals and birds did not appear to account for these contrasting patterns in the performance of JJ and PS, since it was PS, who had a specific interest in birds and animals, who was impaired with these categories. Nevertheless, there is some evidence that personal familiarity can spare categories that might otherwise be expected to be impaired. For example, CW, an accomplished musician with a deficit for living things, did not show the usual accompanying deficit for musical instruments (Wilson & Wearing, 1995), presumably because for him these were highly familiar objects.

Differences in personal familiarity are difficult to assess, but when measures of the general familiarity of objects within a population have been collected, living things turn out to be generally less familiar than manmade objects (Funnell & Sheridan, 1992). Early studies of category-specific performance that were unaware of the importance of familiarity differences failed to control for this factor. Subsequently, some studies have shown that category-specific deficits, reported using uncontrolled materials, disappear once concept familiarity is controlled (Funnell & Sheridan, 1992; Sartori, Coltheart, Miozzo, & Job, 1994, cases 1 and 2; Stewart, Parkin, & Hunkin, 1992). In other studies, the category effect has remained, but at a considerably reduced level and confined to items of low familiarity (Funnell & De Mornay Davies, 1996; Gainotti & Silveri, 1996; Sartori, Coltheart, Miozzo, & Job, 1994 case 3; Sartori, Job, Miozzo, Zago, & Marchiori, 1993). Thus, uncontrolled differences in familiarity clearly contribute to the category-specific deficit for living things, but do not account for it entirely in all cases (see also Jefferies, Rogers, & Lambon Ralph, 2011).

Category-specific disorders are assumed to be semantic in origin (McCarthy & Warrington, 1988), yet there is good evidence that the visual properties of objects can also affect the recognition of objects in particular categories. Using a standard set of object drawings, Gaffan and Heywood (1993) found that five normal control subjects made significantly more errors when naming living things than manmade objects (when all drawings were presented at short exposure and low contrast). Moreover, within the manmade object domain, the controls made significantly more errors with musical instruments than tools. Thus, normal subjects produce a pattern similar to JBR when the materials are presented in visually degraded form.

The fact that visual degradation can effect category-specific naming in normal subjects suggests that patients with early visual processing problems might also show category-specific errors of visual identification. This was demonstrated in a patient (NA) with an apperceptive agnosia, affecting the visual processes that precede access to the structural descriptions (Funnell 2000a). Categories with very close structural similarity, such as insects, produced visual coordinate errors. Objects with few distinctive features (such as fruit and vegetables) produced visual coordinate errors (e.g., pear → apple) but also unrelated visual errors (e.g., potato → footprint). Unrelated visual errors were also typical of body parts (e.g., hair → onion) and manmade objects that were prone to visual segmentation of their parts (e.g., whip → spring). There was no effect of concept familiarity on her performance, and her understanding of object names was not impaired.

Category-specific impairments can also be found in visual associative agnosia. For example, Humphreys, Riddoch, and Quinlan (1988) reported that HJA, who was thought to have damage to the processes that link structural descriptions with the semantic system, had particular problems with objects from categories with many structurally similar objects (e.g., animals, birds, and insects). Structurally dissimilar categories (such as body parts and manmade objects) created few difficulties. His performance showed strong effects of concept familiarity and a slightly different pattern of category-specific disorders from NA (reported above), suggesting that category-specific disorders can vary according to the nature of the visual input problem.

In summary, what is clear from these studies is that a simple dichotomy between disorders affecting either living or nonliving things will not suffice. Disorders affecting living things are often associated with disorders affecting particular categories of manmade objects, such as musical instruments, while body parts, a category of living things, is usually spared. Moreover, categories themselves show further fractionations: animals and birds may be spared independently of fruit and vegetables (Hillis & Caramazza, 1991), and large, nonmanipulable objects may be spared relative to small, usable objects (Warrington & McCarthy, 1987). When semantic memory is unimpaired, early visual processing deficits, and deficits to the links between visual structural descriptions and semantics, can also show category-specific effects. Theories of the structural organization of categories based upon category-specific disorders need to take the role of visual processing factors into account. All of the theories that are supported by empirical evidence assume that semantic representations are composed of features and that either the semantic representation in its entirety or its component features is stored or processed in separate brain regions. The proposals differ as to whether the organization is based on the properties that distinguish items in a category (e.g., visual versus functional features), or on the modality (e.g., visual versus linguistic) in which the semantic representation or features are first encountered or learned, or on evolutionary pressures.

Imageable, Concrete, and Abstract Words: Processing Advantage for Imageable and Concrete Words

Concrete words are processed more readily than abstract words in a variety of laboratory tasks using unrelated words, including free recall, recognition memory, short-term memory, paired associate learning, and oral reading (see Paivio, 1991; Paivio, Yuille, & Madigan, 1968). Paivio and colleagues (1968) collected ratings on imagery (the capacity of the word to arouse sensory images) and concreteness (the capacity of the word to refer to objects, materials, or people) for a large set of nouns, and found that the two scales were closely related. A further measure of "meaningfulness" (m), based on the number of associated words produced to the target word in 1 minute, tended to be high for both abstract words and concrete/imageable words. On the basis of these results, Paivio and colleagues (1968) argued that abstract words obtain meaning largely from verbal experience (measured by m), while concrete/imageable words obtain meaning from both sensory and verbal experience.

Paivio (1978) proposed that all word meanings are represented in a verbal system specialized for processing linguistic information, but concrete and imageable words have access to a non-verbal system that stores representations of the perceptual properties of objects and events (see Figure 10.5). The two systems are independent, but richly interconnected. Connections are most direct between concrete/imageable words and become more indirect as words become more abstract.

In the neurological literature, concrete words show a marked advantage in a variety of disorders, most notably in deep dyslexia (Coltheart, Patterson, & Marshall, 1980). Within Paivio's model, the advantage to concrete/imageable words found in deep dyslexia could arise from their representation in more than one system. However, Jones (1985) suggested that concreteness and imageability ratings reflect differences in the quantity of semantic predicates (e.g., "has legs," "is old") in the underlying representation, rather than qualitative differences. Based on ratings of the ease with which subjects judged they could generate predicates, Jones proposed that abstract words contain fewer predicates than concrete/imageable words and thus are more vulnerable to brain damage.

Plaut and Shallice (1993b) used ease of predication to simulate the advantage for concrete words found in deep dyslexia. Concrete words in this computer model were assigned more than twice as many features as the abstract words. A few concrete words mapped onto some abstract features, but no abstract words shared concrete features. When the pathway from orthography to meaning was impaired, the phonological output for abstract words was more disturbed than for concrete words. Thus the greater density of semantic features for concrete words gave them an advantage when the semantic pathway was compromised.

Jones's ease of predication measure was based upon judgments rather than the actual production of predicates. When subjects were asked to produce predicates, De Mornay Davies and

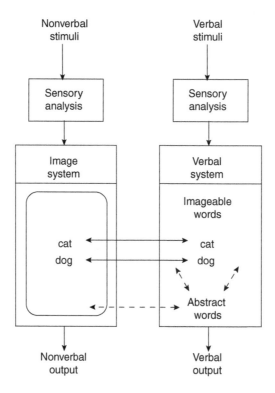

Figure 10.5

Funnell (2000) found that, in line with Jones's findings, more predicates were produced overall for concrete than for abstract words, and the numbers correlated highly with Jones's ease of predication ratings for the same words. However, when the sets of concrete and abstract words were considered separately, ease of predication ratings did not correlate significantly with the number of predicates produced, despite the fact that the number of predicates varied quite widely within each word set. Instead, ease of predication completely split the word groups into those with high ratings—all concrete words—and those with low ratings—all abstract words. From this, De Mornay Davies and Funnell argued that ease of predication reflects differences in the nature of the semantic representations rather than the number of associated predicates.

In general, the advantage for concrete/imageable words in deep dyslexia is assumed to reflect semantic processing or semantic access problems. But Newton and Barry (1997) found no evidence of deficits for comprehending abstract words in a study of a young woman (LW) who had developed deep dyslexia as a result of a left hemisphere subarachnoid hemorrhage. Despite equivalent levels of comprehension for concrete and abstract words, LW showed a marked advantage for concrete words in oral reading. Newton and Barry suggested that concrete concepts are more likely to specify a precise word form than abstract concepts, which are more likely to activate a set of related names (e.g., idea, concept, notion, thought, hypothesis, and so on), none of which may have a level of activation high enough to trigger a response. Some support for this view is provided by Funnell and Allport (1987), who found that ratings of "concept independence," defined as the ability of a word "to evoke a direct image that can be represented in isolation," correlated highly with the oral reading of two deep dyslexic subjects. Concrete/imageable words were more likely to have high-concept independence than were abstract words. Other patients with deep dyslexia, deep dysgraphia, or deep dysphasia have been shown to have *no* semantic deficit, and yet show better performance on concrete words (Hanley & Kay, in press; Hillis, Rapp, & Caramazza, 1999). Hillis and colleagues attributed the advantage for concrete words to the fact that for concrete words there are fewer items that share the majority of features with the target. On the assumption that the features of the semantic representation activate lexical representations to which they correspond, there may be numerous closely semantically related, competing words activated in the lexicon, particularly for abstract words. For example, the semantic representation of a concrete concept like *train* shares a majority of its semantic features with only a few items (van, bus, subway/underground, trolley), whereas the semantic features of an abstract word, say *faith*, shares a majority of its semantic features with many other abstract concepts (belief, credence, creed, tenet, confidence, denomination, hope, reliance, religion, trust, certainty, conviction, doctrine, dogma, persuasion, sect) in various contexts. Consequently, an impairment in accessing the target lexical representation of the word *faith* might result in activation of a large number of competing lexical representations, some of which might have higher activation than the target response (leading to an error in production).

Breedin, Saffran, and Coslett (1994) have proposed that concreteness effects in word processing arise from the activity of brain areas involved in object recognition, and Funnell (2000b) has suggested that the concrete word advantage arises in deep disorders because spoken output is restricted, abnormally, to a system used normally for nominal reference (i.e., naming things). Abstract words do not refer to nameable objects in the world and are therefore not called up by naming tasks. Thus, restricted access to a perceptually based lexical system, similar to that described by Paivio (1978), could explain the results.

In summary, deep disorders, such as deep dyslexia, demonstrate a marked advantage for the processing of concrete/imageable words, found to a lesser extent in normal behavior. Attempts to explain this advantage have suggested that concrete words benefit from (1) additional representation in a perceptually based lexical system (Paivio, 1978); (2) from possessing more semantic predicates than abstract words (Jones, 1985); (3) from specifying words with more precision than abstract words (Newton & Barry, 1997); and (4) fewer closely semantically related words in the output lexicon (Hillis et al., 1999). Finally, it has been suggested that the concrete word advantage reflects the properties of a (possibly perceptually based) output system normally used for nominal reference (Funnell, 2000b).

Reverse Concreteness Effect

Although concrete words generally show an advantage in single word processing tasks, this advantage has been reported to disappear, and even to reverse, in some pathological cases. Warrington (1975, 1981) found that AB (the patient with semantic dementia referred to earlier) had a marked deficit for defining concrete words when compared to abstract words, and a similar finding was reported by Warrington and Shallice (1984) for SBY (a patient impaired by herpes simplex encephalitis). The examples provided in these studies show a striking disparity in favor of abstract words (e.g., AB: *pact* → "friendly agreement"; *needle* → "I've forgotten"; SBY: *malice* → "To show bad will against somebody"; *frog* → "An animal—not trained"). Warrington (1981) argued that abstract and concrete words are organized by category, each category having different neural substrates. Abstract words are defined in terms of similarity (in the form of synonyms) and in terms of contrast (in the form of antonyms). Concrete words are defined in terms of superordinate category and distinguishing features.

Breedin, Saffran, and Coslett (1994) reported a second patient, DM (a patient with a progressive loss of memory for word meanings), who also showed a reverse concreteness effect. Brain imaging revealed a decrease in perfusion in the inferior temporal lobes bilaterally, consistent with a diagnosis of semantic dementia. DM's definitions generally lacked perceptual information. To explain the reverse concreteness effect, Breedin and colleagues suggested that the linguistic elements of language that support the processing of abstract words were better preserved than the perceptual attribute domains that support the processing of concrete words. They rejected the idea that concrete words benefit from a larger number of semantic features (e.g., Jones, 1985; Plaut & Shallice, 1993b) because damage to semantic features should always favor concrete words. They also rejected Paivio's dual-coding model because concrete and abstract words should benefit equally from access to verbal codes, following perceptual loss. They argued that the representations for concrete and abstract words are fundamentally different. Concrete word concepts have their basis in information acquired through the five senses, while abstract words have their basis in associations with other concepts—even concrete ones—experienced in the context of language.

Marshall, Pring, Chiat, and Robson (1995/6a) also concluded that concrete words lose their advantage when access to perceptual properties is impaired. They report the case of RG, an elderly man who suffered a left hemisphere stroke and whose speech was affected by semantic jargon. In semantic jargon, a type of expressive aphasia in which anomalous words replace appropriate words in spontaneous speech, there is usually a preponderance of abstract words. For example, RG described a picture of a woman showing a boy a signpost as "The mother is showing the . . . vision aid area to her son who doesn't really know where to go." Tests showed that RG found concrete words more difficult than abstract words. Given pictures of concrete objects (e.g., a man riding a donkey with a carrot hanging from a stick), he selected spoken abstract words (e.g., *encouragement*) to describe the picture, significantly more successfully than concrete words (e.g., *donkey*). He also named objects (e.g., *castle*) more successfully when given abstract definitions (e.g., "A fortified historic building"), than from concrete definitions (e.g., "A building with turrets and a drawbridge"). Marshall and colleagues argued that EG had well-preserved processing of abstract concepts but had an impaired ability to process the visual aspects of meaning required for concrete concepts. However, they noted that concrete *words* appear to have access to descriptions expressed in both concrete and abstract terms. This differs from a categorical account (e.g., Warrington, 1975) in which concrete and abstract words map onto different neural substrates. They suggested that RG's performance fits an account in which individual words have their meaning distributed over a variety of processing domains, in accord with Allport's theory of semantic representations (Allport, 1985).

Actions and Objects

Action names are more likely to be impaired than object names in aphasia (Thompson, Lukic, King, Mesulam, & Weintraub, 2012), but here we will consider first three case reports of patients who show the reverse pattern, and the possible implications of this dissociation for the organization of the semantic system. First, AG (one of the patients with optic aphasia reported earlier) had better preserved naming of pictured actions than objects (Campbell & Manning, 1996). For example, he named correctly only one-quarter of a set of objects pictured without actions. In contrast, he named correctly all actions pictured without objects (e.g., three men sitting without a visible seat). AG's naming of objects increased significantly when the objects were presented in pictures demonstrating object use. His object naming also improved when he was asked "What would you need to do that?" to pictures of *objectless* actions. Thus, RG was actually better at naming objects when given only relevant pictured actions than when given only pictured objects. However, while pictured actions facilitated the naming of objects, the reverse was not true: pictured objects failed to facilitate the naming of actions. The second patient, DM, reported above (Breedin et al., 1994), was able to spot, almost perfectly, the odd word out in triplets of written verbs (e.g., *to allow, to encourage, to permit*), but was significantly impaired at spotting the odd word out given triplets of written nouns (e.g., *automobile, train, car*). Finally, RG (the patient with semantic jargon aphasia reported earlier) made fewer errors when producing verbs than nouns in spontaneous speech (Marshall, Chiat, Robson, & Pring, 1995/6a, 1995/6b). He also named pictures of actions significantly more successfully than nouns, matched for word frequency.

Campbell and Manning (1996) propose three speculative accounts for AG's better naming of actions compared with objects. First, they suggest that objects possess unique, defining, perceptual characteristics that might make them more vulnerable to visual access deficits than actions, which are argued to possess more general characteristics. Second, they speculate that there may exist multiple routes from vision to semantics, with a route dedicated to actions spared in optic aphasia. Finally, they suggest that perceived actions may have a variety of resources for accessing names.

Jackendoff (1987) points out that subtle perceptual differences are required to distinguish between some structurally similar categorically related objects, such as goose, duck, and swan, and between physical actions, such as run, jog, and lope. Both Breedin and colleagues (1994) and Marshall, Chiat, and colleagues (1995/6a, 1995/6b) report differences in performance within verb sets according to their possession of perceptual properties. For example, DM (Breedin et al., 1994) was slower, and significantly less accurate, at selecting triplets of verbs of manner (e.g., *to gnaw, to gobble, to gulp*), for which knowledge of subtle differences in perceptual properties are required, than triplets of relational verbs (e.g., *to remind, to remember, to recall*) that do not possess perceptual properties. Likewise, RG was impressively good at distinguishing thematic verbs (e.g., *buy* and *sell, give* and *take*), which specify the relationship between role players, but had difficulty distinguishing between action verbs (e.g., *slide, crawl, swim*). Both studies conclude that distinctions in the meaning of action verbs are dependent upon perceptual information, while knowledge of the thematic roles of verbs is represented in a nonperceptual domain concerned with abstract verb structures. In the cases of DM and RG, the perceptual aspects of action verbs appear to have been lost, but the relational aspects of verbs, which capture psychological events represented in their functional argument structure, have been retained. The advantage of actions compared to nouns arises from the fact that some actions do not possess perceptual features.

Breedin, Saffran, and Schwartz (1998) argue that verbs with complex semantic representations are retrieved most successfully in aphasia. Thus "heavy" verbs (such as *run, grab*), which address information about the manner of the action, were retrieved more successfully than "light" verbs (such as *go, get*), which, although more frequent, are less complex. They suggest that a heavy verb is more constrained by context, and so more likely to activate one meaning, than is a light verb, which may generate a number of meanings, making selection of the most appropriate meaning for the context more difficult. However, Breedin and colleagues note also that heavy verbs may be facilitated by the presence of perceptual features.

Black and Chiat (2000) argue that differences in the processing of nouns and verbs cannot be explained entirely either in terms of differences in perceptibility or in terms of the degree to which words specify particular meanings. Even when objects and actions are both well-endowed with perceptual features, and have clearly specified meanings, a difference in naming can be observed. For example, Byng (1988; Byng, Nickels, & Black, 1994) asked a group of aphasic patients—this time with more difficulty producing action than object names—to name pictured concrete objects (e.g., *iron*) and pictured actions (e.g., *to iron*) that were associated with the objects and shared the same root morpheme. Despite the high perceptual content of both objects and actions, the objects were named significantly more successfully than the actions. Black and Chiat (2000) suggested that other aspects of meaning, besides concreteness, must account for the discrepancy between action and object naming in these patients. They observed that while nouns refer to entities, verbs specify relationships between entities: they implicitly refer to "scene schemas." Relationships may not be more difficult to process than entities; rather, there may be different mechanisms involved.

Other cases of dissociations between nouns and verbs in naming do not occur at the level of semantics, but at the level of the phonological or orthographic output lexicon (Caramazza & Hillis, 1991; Hillis, Oh, & Ken, 2004; Hillis, Wityk, Barker, & Caramazza, 2003; Thompson et al., 2012).

Embodiment

In recent years, much of the debate regarding the organization of semantic memory has centered on the hypothesis of embodiment. How does conceptual information relate to sensory and motor information? According to a strong embodiment view, conceptualization relies on the same modality-specific systems as perception (Allport, 1985; Gallese & Lakoff, 2005; Martin, 2007). Comprehending an object can be reduced to simulation in the same sensory and motor systems that are used to see, hear, smell, taste, touch, and otherwise interact with that object. For example, when interpreting the sentence "The girl watched the clouds," the same neurons that are part of visual feature maps created by past experience seeing clouds would fire to reenact earlier visual experiences with clouds. This reenactment constitutes understanding of the word "cloud" (Barsalou et al., 2003). To retrieve sensory and motor information is to retrieve the concept.

The neural plausibility of the embodiment hypothesis has been bolstered by the discovery of mirror neuron systems in nonhuman primates. Single-cell recordings in macaque premotor cortex indicate that the same neurons fire when a monkey observes another individual perform an action as when it performs that same action itself (DiPellegrino et al., 1992). Much research attention has been focused on finding a corresponding mirror neuron system in humans (e.g., Gallese et al., 1996; Rizzolati & Craighero, 2004; Rizzolatti et al., 1996; Rizzolatti et al., 2001; Rizzolatti & Luppino, 2001). Such as a system could provide a basis for embodied cognition in humans. More direct evidence bearing on the embodiment hypothesis in humans is drawn from functional neuroimaging. Numerous studies have found that conceptual processing and language comprehension activate the same modality-specific sensory and motor systems used to actually perceive stimuli (for review, see Barsalou et al., 2003; Binder & Desai, 2011; Boulenger et al., 2006; Gallese & Lakoff, 2005; Mahon & Caramazza, 2008; Martin, 2007; Martin & Chao, 2001; Pulvermüller, 2005).

Critics of strong embodiment views point out that these demonstrations of co-activation in healthy individuals do not show that activation of perceptual systems during conceptual processing is either necessary or sufficient. Evidence is equally consistent with spreading of activation from conceptual systems to perceptual systems (Mahon & Caramazza, 2008). The strong embodiment hypothesis is also inconsistent with evidence for amodal representations within the semantic system (see earlier discussion in this chapter). Furthermore, it is important to note the limited domain of the embodiment hypothesis. For the most part, the embodiment hypothesis has focused on explaining the representations of concrete objects and actions that have perceptual correspondences; it is less clear how it could be used to explain abstract concepts like truth, beauty, and justice that do not have consistently associated sensory and motor information (Mahon & Caramazza, 2008).

One recent study illustrated the limitations of evidence presented in favor of the embodiment hypothesis (de Zubicaray, Arciuli, & McMahon, 2013). The investigators showed in an fMRI study that names of manual actions evoked greater activation in motor strip compared to names of nouns not related to body parts, and the activation overlapped with that evoked by execution or observation of hand movements (the sort of result interpreted as support for embodiment). However, they also showed that pseudowords with endings associated with verb status (e.g., -eve) also evoked greater activation in the identical motor area, compared with pseudowords with endings associated with noun status (e.g., -age). These results indicate that motor cortex activation can reflect implicit processing statistical regularities that distinguish a word's grammatical class rather than conceptual content or its simulation.

On the other end of the spectrum, a strong disembodiment view suggests that concepts are symbolic and abstract. According to this view, amodal representations are completely separate from sensory and motor systems (for discussion, see Binder & Desai, 2011). Here, conceptual representations must be able to interface with sensory and motor systems, but they are completely separate (Mahon & Caramazza, 2008). For example, seeing a spoon or hearing its name would activate the abstract, symbolic concept of a spoon, which is not made up of sensory or motor information. If an individual wants to demonstrate the use of the spoon, the conceptual representation must then make contact with the motor system to perform the appropriate action. This interface between the systems is not automatic but is carried out to attain specific goals. An individual who is physically unable to perform the action due to damage to the motor system could still have an intact concept of a spoon. Evidence supporting this view comes from studies individuals with apraxia, who are able to recognize the same objects that they cannot manipulate (e.g., Gonzalez Rothi et al., 1991; Johnson-Frey, 2004; Mahon et al., 2007; Negri et al., 2007; Rosci et al., 2003). However, the neuroimaging evidence used to support the embodiment hypothesis is inconsistent with the strong form of the disembodiment hypothesis. Automatic activation of sensory and motor systems during conceptual processing suggests that the systems are not entirely separate, regardless of whether this activation is necessary or sufficient for accessing of conceptual information.

Neuropsychological evidence argues against both strong embodiment and strong disembodiment views. For individuals with damage to the motor system due to a variety of etiologies, including Parkinson's disease (Boulenger et al., 2008), progressive supranuclear palsy (Bak et al., 2006), stroke (Arévalo et al., 2012; Buxbaum & Saffran, 2002; Neininger & Pulvermüller, 2003), and motor neuron disease (Bak & Hodges, 2004; Bak et al., 2001; Grossman et al., 2008), subtle impairments to comprehension of action words are found (see Binder & Desai, 2011 for review). Similarly, healthy individuals who have transient lesions of the motor system induced by transcranial magnetic stimulation have deficits for action verb comprehension (Buccino et al., 2005; Glenberg et al., 2008; Ishibashi et al., 2011; Oliveri et al., 2004; Pobric et al., 2010; Pulvermüller et al., 2005). Such findings are inconsistent with the strong disembodiment view since the motor system does seem to contribute necessary information to the conceptual processing of action verbs. However, the subtle nature of the deficits in addition to the findings that damage to areas that are not part of the motor system also contribute to deficits for action verbs are inconsistent with the strong embodiment hypothesis since the information external to the motor and perceptual systems seems to contribute to conceptual processing. That is, motor system information plays a necessary but not sufficient role in conceptual processing of action verbs.

Given the current state of evidence on embodiment, many current hypotheses are positioned between strong embodiment and strong disembodiment views (e.g., Reilly, Harnish, Garcia, Hung, Rodriguez, & Crosson, 2014). There is general agreement that sensory and motor systems enrich conceptual representations but that modality-specific systems alone do not provide the entirety of conceptual representations' content. However, hypotheses differ as to whether conceptual representations are amodal or multimodal (Barsalou, 1999; see Binder & Desai, 2011 for review).

According to an embodied abstraction view (Binder & Desai, 2011; see also Dove, 2011; Taylor & Zwaan, 2009), there are multiple levels of abstraction from sensory and motor input that constitute multimodal representations. The level of abstraction that is accessed depends on current task demands. Higher-level schematic representations may suffice in familiar contexts, while sensory and motor systems may make more direct contributions in novel contexts that require more specific perceptual information or deeper processing.

On the other hand, according to the grounding by interaction view, conceptual representations are amodal. These abstract, symbolic representations derive their content from interactions with sensory and motor systems (Mahon & Caramazza, 2008). Sensory and motor systems are activated so that the concept can be instantiated in a particular context. In this sort of model, amodal representations are needed to bind information from the different modalities so it can be accessed efficiently (for one example, see Damasio, 1989).

Semantic Hub Hypothesis. One influential model that posits abstract, amodal representations that interact with modality-specific sensory and motor information is the distributed-plus-hub view (see Patterson, Nestor, & Rogers, 2007). In contrast with a distributed view according to which the entire semantic network is made up of separate, modality-specific sensory and motor systems as well as the connections between them, the distributed-plus-hub view adds a shared, amodal area (a "hub") that processes activation from all of the distributed modality-specific representations and forms associations between different attributes. This common hub integrates representations from many modalities into a unified representation for each concept that allows for higher-order generalizations within and between concepts. While the hub is typically claimed to exist in the anterior temporal lobe (see chapter 11 of this volume for further discussion), claims about the neuroanatomical location are tangential to the theoretical model of the semantic system this view presents. Neuropsychological evidence provides some support for the distributed-plus-hub view. According to this view, damage to distributed components should lead to category-specific, feature-specific, or modality-specific deficits, like those which have been observed in individuals after strokes or herpes simplex encephalitis (see earlier discussion in this chapter). Damage to the hub should lead to generalized semantic impairment following focal brain damage affecting all modalities of input. Such a deficit is found in semantic variant primary progressive aphasia (formerly known as semantic dementia), a neurodegenerative disorder in which individuals progressively lose both productive and receptive vocabulary and experience difficulty accessing knowledge about objects and people across all categories (Patterson, Nestor, & Rogers, 2007; Gorno-Tempini et al, 2011; Warrington, 1975).

In summary, while the debate on embodiment is still open, current evidence suggests that sensory and motor systems play a necessary but not sufficient role in conceptual processing. Understanding what they contribute as well as the nature of more abstract multimodal or amodal representations that coordinate information from modality-specific systems is an important direction of investigation into the functional organization of semantics.

Semantic Memory and Event Scripts

Scene schemas, and the role of actions in constructing the representations of events, tend to be viewed as aspects of meaning lying outside the domain of semantic memory, as episodic knowledge (Tulving, 1972) or as general event scripts (Schank, 1982; Schank & Abelson, 1977). However, Kintsch (1980) has argued that episodic knowledge and semantic knowledge form a continuum of knowledge, while Allport (1985) suggests that semantic knowledge is embedded within episodic knowledge. Recent studies of semantic dementia have indicated that the processing of current personal events plays a central role in the composition, updating, and maintenance of semantic memory, making it difficult to disconnect semantic memory entirely from wider sources of meaning.

Snowden, Griffiths, and Neary (1994) claimed that episodic memory supported the semantic processing in four patients with semantic dementia who had better preserved knowledge for personally known people and places in current experience than people and places personally known to them in their past. Further study of one of these patients showed that her recognition and use of objects was also better preserved for her own possessions than someone else's objects of the same type. In addition, her own objects were recognized more reliably when placed in their usual location in her home than when located out of context. The familiar physical properties of personal possessions and their familiar physical location appear to provide important clues to the recognition of object identity and use in these patients. Having a goal also appears to provide a context for the identification and use of objects. A patient (EP), with a well-preserved memory for the use of objects in the context of daily routines, was able to use objects appropriately as part of a goal-related task—for example, she used a needle appropriately when she was asked to sew a button on a shirt—but she was unable to demonstrate reliably the use of objects presented out of context (Funnell, 2001).

Goals, and the physical properties and location of objects, are proposed to be essential components of physical scripts that connect knowledge of physical properties of the environment with memories of the purposeful activities in which objects are used (Schank, 1982; Schank & Abelson, 1977). Scripts—and there are also personal and social scripts—form the basic level of a dynamic memory system that learns from personal experience. They are organized by structures operating at higher levels of processing, containing increasingly generalizable levels of information. In semantic dementia, it appears that these higher processing levels of information, which would enable the processing of concepts out of context, deteriorate to such an extent that information becomes progressively tied to scripts based in current experience.

Allport (1985) describes a dynamic distributed processing model that combines real-world, episodic information with object concepts. In this model, semantic memory is extracted automatically as a by-product of the encoding of many related, episodic experiences. Object concepts are stored in the episodes in which they are experienced, but also emerge from these episodes as prototypical patterns of the most common sensory and motor features experienced across episodes. These object concepts also contain scripts that encode common interactions with objects. The model predicts that semantic memory should not be lost without a corresponding loss of episodic memory entailing these semantic memories. Yet, in semantic dementia, this is what appears to occur: patients can demonstrate knowledge of the function of objects in everyday situations that they are unable to identify in semantic memory tasks.

Levels of Meaning

According to script theory, meaning is represented at different levels: as decontextualized meaning, as meaning embedded in generalizable contexts, and as meaning embedded in specific physical scripts. Figure 10.6 depicts an attempt to model these different levels of meaning (Funnell, 2001) using evidence from semantic memory and the development of object concepts. The first level, specific event knowledge, represents information regarding specific but recurring events, entailing the physical properties of the particular objects, people, and actions occurring in a particular place and time (e.g., breakfast time at home). This is the level most likely to drive personal physical and linguistic routines carried out during, or in reference to, familiar events. The second level, general event knowledge, abstracts from the physical properties of specific scenes, and now the representation reflects the typical properties and activities associated with an activity. It is likely that this is the level at which associated concepts can be accessed. At the third level, concepts (or referential level), information is represented as isolated concepts stripped of context. This is the level, captured by most current models of semantic memory, that enables isolated objects and object names to be processed out of context. Here, different categories of concepts are represented, differentiated according to the degree of specificity. Clinical tests of referential meaning, such as object naming and word-object matching, are likely to be processed at this level of meaning.

Words, pictorial materials, and other sensory information can call up meanings at each level. Names and pictures of isolated objects and actions will call up meanings at the referential level. Names and visual depictions of actions (e.g., *push, buy*) and abstract words (e.g., *steal, deny*) that capture relationships between objects, locations, and role players, will call up meaning at the level of general events, while names and pictures specifying particular objects, people, and places will call up specific scripts. In semantic dementia, the ability to recall and understand words appears to become increasingly tied to this level of specific event scripts.

The levels of meaning model can provide preliminary accounts for the phenomena reported in this chapter. Optic aphasia might arise from impaired access from visual input to the referential level of meaning, but retained access to associated aspects of meaning (including the ability to gesture object use) and frequently access to knowledge of actions represented at the general event level. Advantages for concrete/imageable words are presumed to arise at the referential level, which represents, in particular, concepts of concrete/imageable nouns. Their representation at this level may depend upon the fact that the physical properties that are confined to these items allows them to be abstracted from their context. Thus, it may be their abstractability rather than their sensory properties per se that is special. Brain damage that restricts processing to the referential level, perhaps by sparing access to names at this level, would be expected to produce concreteness effects for both nouns and verbs. In contrast, reverse concreteness effects could be argued to arise when processing at the referential level is impaired. Abstract nouns and thematic properties of verbs that capture relationships would benefit (relative to entities) from processing at the level of general event representations.

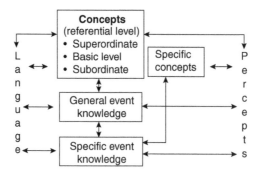

Figure 10.6

Concluding Remarks

Most current models of semantic memory are constrained by the need to account for all aspects of meaning within a single memory system that captures the encyclopedic properties of word meanings. As Kintsch (1980, p. 506) has pointed out, this type of information is just one end of "a continuum reaching from completely context-dependent episodes to truly general knowledge." Kintsch bemoaned the fact that a concentration upon sentence verification tasks had seriously limited the development and scope of semantic memory. The same might be said of the current concentration on semantic tasks that seek to isolate concepts from context.

Notes

1 AB and EM both obtained higher scores on the pictorial version of the test when the total sum of scores across all the test questions is compared. As Riddoch, Humphreys, Coltheart, and Funnell (1988) point out, this result is hard to reconcile with the claim that AB has a specific loss of visually accessed semantic information.

2 JBR has subsequently demonstrated consistent responses across tests of visual object naming and spoken name definitions (Funnell & de Mornay Davies, 1996).

3 Although naming via a right hemisphere semantic system appears to solve the problem of optic aphasia in Coslett and Saffran's patient (and also the reading pattern found in deep dyslexia; Coltheart, Patterson, & Marshall, 1980), the possibility of separable right and left hemisphere semantic systems complicates the study of semantic memory. At present, knowledge of the properties of each semantic system is rudimentary. Any complete semantic model will require a better understanding of the nature and function of each system and their interrelationship.

4 Coltheart, Inglis, Cupples, and colleagues (1998) refer to the sensory attribute domains as semantic, rather than perceptual.

5 The visual questions asked by Coltheart, Inglis, Cupples, and colleagues (1998) about ownership of legs, or wheels appear to be more specific than the more general questions asked about objects, such as "Does it make a noise?" "Does it have a smell?" Equivalent general questions in the visual domain might have been "Does it move?" Specific questions in the auditory and olfactory domains might be "Does it make a high sound?" "Does it have a sweet smell?" General questions were asked about color—"Is it colored or not?"—and were answered at chance level. This test requires a distinction between black/white and color. However, it is not clear that contrast and brightness might not have contributed to decisions about animals, such as frog, parrot, panda, and crow, in the examples provided.

6 VEE's performance was affected by the length of the interval between her pointing response and the next stimulus. At intervals of 2 seconds her performance was significantly inferior to that given longer intervals of 10 seconds or more. Warrington and McCarthy (1983) argue that this indicates a deficit in semantic access from vision. It could also reflect an interaction between visual attention and the sensory properties of the multiple stimulus arrays.

7 A significant effect of category was reported using chi square, but the use of combined data from repeated tests violates the assumptions of the chi square test (Siegel, 1956).

8 YOT's category-specific deficit was reported only at fast response interval rates of 2 seconds (see note 6).

References

Allport, D. A. (1985). Distributed memory, modular systems and dysphasia. In S.K. Newman & R. Epstein (Eds.), *Current perspectives in dysphasia*. Edinburgh: Churchill Livingstone.

Arévalo, A.L., Baldo, J.V, & Dronkers, N.F. (2012). What do brain lesions tell us about theories of embodied semantics and the human mirror neuron system? *Cortex, 48*, 242–254.

Arguin, M., Bub, D., & Dudek, G. (1996). Shape integration for visual object recognition and its implication in category-specific visual agnosia. *Visual Cognition, 3*, 193–220.

Bak, T.H., & Hodges, J.R. (2004). The effects of motor neurone disease on language: Further evidence. *Brain and Language, 89*, 354–361.

Bak, T.H., O'Donovan, D.G., Xuereb, J.H., Boniface, S., & Hodges, J.R. (2001). Selective impairment of verb processing associated with pathological changes in Brodmann areas 44 and 45 in the motor neurone disease-dementia-aphasia syndrome. *Brain, 124*, 103–120.

Bak, T.H., Yancopoulou, D., Nestor, P.J., Xuereb, J.H., Spillantini, M.G., Pulvermüller, F., & Hodges, J.R. (2006). Clinical, imaging and pathological correlates of a hereditary deficit in verb and action processing. *Brain, 129*, 321–332.

Barsalou, L.W. (1999). Perceptions of perceptual symbols. *Behavioral and Brain Sciences, 22*, 637–660.

Barsalou, L.W., Kyle Simmons, W., Barbey, A.K., & Wilson, C.D. (2003). Grounding conceptual knowledge in modality-specific systems. *Trends in Cognitive Sciences, 7*, 84–91.

Beauvois, M.F. (1982). Optic aphasia: A process of interaction between vision and language. *Philosophical Transactions of the Royal Society of London, B, 298*, 35–47.

Beauvois, M.F., & Saillant, B. (1985). Optic aphasia for colors and color agnosia: A distinction between visual and visuo-verbal impairments in the processing of colors. *Cognitive Neuropsychology, 2*, 1–48.

Binder, J.R., & Desai, R.H. (2011). The neurobiology of semantic memory. *Trends in Cognitive Sciences, 15*, 527–536.

Black, M., & Chiat, S. (2000). Putting thoughts into verbs: Developmental and acquired impairments. In W. Best, K. Bryan, & J. Maxim (Eds.), *Semantic processing: Theory and practice*. London: Whurr Publishers.

Boulenger, V., Mechtouff, L., Thobois, S., Broussolle, E., Jeannerod, M., & Nazir, T.A. (2008). Word processing in Parkinson's disease is impaired for action verbs but not for concrete nouns. *Neuropsychologia, 46*, 743–56.

Boulenger, V., Roy, A.C., Paulignan, Y., Deprez, V., Jeannerod, M., & Nazir, T. A. (2006). Cross-talk between language processes and overt motor behavior in the first 200 msec of processing. *Journal of Cognitive Neuroscience, 18*, 1607–1615.

Breedin, S.D., Saffran, E.M., & Coslett, H.B. (1994). Reversal of the concreteness effect in a patient with semantic dementia. *Cognitive Neuropsychology, 11*, 617–660.

Breedin, S.D., Saffran, E.M., & Schwartz, M.F. (1998). Semantic factors in verb retrieval: An effect of complexity. *Brain and Language, 63*, 1–31.

Buccino, G., Riggio, L., Melli, G., Binkofski, F., Gallese, V., & Rizzolatti, G. (2005). Listening to action-related sentences modulates the activity of the motor system: A combined TMS and behavioral study. *Brain Research. Cognitive Brain Research, 24*, 355–363.

Buxbaum, L.J., & Saffran, E.M. (2002). Knowledge of object manipulation and object function: Dissociations in apraxic and nonapraxic subjects. *Brain and Language, 82*, 179–199.

Byng, S. (1988). Sentence processing deficits: Theory and therapy. *Cognitive Neuropsychology, 5*, 629–676.

Byng, S., Nickels, L., & Black, M. (1994). Replicating therapy for mapping deficits in agrammatism: Remapping the deficit? *Aphasiology, 8*, 315–341.

Campbell, R., & Manning, L. (1996). Optic aphasia: A case with spared action naming and associated disorders. *Brain and Language, 53*, 183–221.

Caramazza, A., & Hillis, A.E. (1991). Lexical organization of nouns and verbs in the brain. *Nature, 349*, 788–790.

Caramazza, A., Hillis, A.E., Rapp, B. C., & Romani, C. (1990). The multiple semantics hypothesis: Multiple confusions? *Cognitive Neuropsychology, 7*, 161–190.

Chertkow, H., & Bub, D. (1990). Semantic memory loss in dementia of the Alzheimer type: What do various measures mean? *Brain, 113*, 397–417.

Coltheart, M., Inglis, L., Cupples, L., Michie, P., Bates, A., & Budd, B. (1998). A semantic subsystem of visual attributes. *Neurocase, 4*, 353–370.

Coltheart, M., Patterson, K., & Marshall, J.C. (1980). *Deep dyslexia*. London: Routledge and Kegan Paul.

Coslett, H.B., & Saffran, E.M. (1989). Preserved object recognition and reading comprehension in optic aphasia. *Brain, 112*, 1091–1110.

Damasio, A.R. (1989). Time-locked multiregional retroactivation: A systems-level proposal for the neural substrates of recall and recognition. *Cognition, 33*, 25–62.

De Mornay Davies, P., & Funnell, E. (2000). Semantic representation and ease of predication. *Brain and Language, 73*, 92–119.

DeRenzi, E., & Saetti, M.C. (1997). Associative agnosia and optic aphasia: Qualitative or quantitative difference? *Cortex, 33*, 115–130.

de Zubicaray G., Arciuli J., & McMahon, K. (2013). Putting an "end" to the motor cortex representations of action words. *Cognitive Neuroscience, 25*, 1957–1974.

Di Pellegrino, G., Fadiga, L., Fogassi, L., Gallese, V., & Rizzolatti, G. (1992). Understanding motor events: A neurophysiological study. *Experimental Brain Research, 91*, 176–180.

Dove, G. (2011). On the need for embodied and dis-embodied cognition. *Frontiers in Psychology, 1*, 129–139.

Farah, M.J. (1990). *Visual agnosia*. Cambridge, MA: MIT Press.

Funnell, E. (2000a). Apperceptive agnosia and the visual recognition of object categories in dementia of the Alzheimer type. *Neurocase, 6*, 451–463.

Funnell, E. (2000b). Deep dyslexia. In E. Funnell (Ed.), *Case studies in the neuropsychology of reading*. Hove, England: Psychology Press.

Funnell, E. (2001). Evidence for scripts in semantic dementia: Implications for theories of semantic memory. *Cognitive Neuropsychology, 18*, 323–341.

Funnell, E., & Allport, D.A. (1987). Non-linguistic cognition and word meanings: Neuropsychological exploration of common mechanisms. In A. Allport, D. MacKay, W. Printz, & E. Scheerer (Eds.), *Language perception and production: Relationships between listening, speaking, reading, and writing*. London: Academic Press.

Funnell, E., & De Mornay Davies, P. (1996). JBR: A reassessment of concept familiarity and a category-specific disorder for living things. *Neurocase, 2*, 461–474.

Funnell, E., & Sheridan, J. (1992). Categories of knowledge? Unfamiliar aspects of living and nonliving things. *Cognitive Neuropsychology, 9*, 135–153.

Gaffan, D., & Heywood, C.A. (1993). A spurious category-specific visual agnosia for living things in normal human and nonhuman primates. *Journal of Cognitive Neuroscience, 5*, 118–128.

Gainotti, G., & Silveri, M.C. (1996). Cognitive and anatomical locus of lesion in a patient with a category-specific semantic impairment for living beings. *Cognitive Neuropsychology, 13*, 357–390.

Gallese, V., Fadiga, L., Fogassi, L., & Rizzolatti, G. (1996). Action recognition in the premotor cortex. *Brain, 119*, 593–609.

Gallese, V., & Lakoff, G. (2005). The brain's concepts: The role of the sensory-motor system in conceptual knowledge. *Cognitive Neuropsychology, 22*(3), 455–479.

Glenberg, A.M., Sato, M., Cattaneo, L., Riggio, L., Palumbo, D., & Buccino, G. (2008). Processing abstract language modulates motor system activity. *Quarterly Journal of Experimental Psychology, 61*, 905–919.

Gonzalez Rothi, L.J., Ochipa, C., & Heilman, K.M. (1991). A cognitive neuropsychological model of limb praxis. *Cognitive Neuropsychology, 8*, 443–458.

Gorno-Tempini, M. L., Hillis, A. E., Weintraub, S., Kertesz, A., Mendez, M., Cappa, S.F., Ogar, J.M., et al. (2011). Classification of primary progressive aphasia and its variants. *Neurology, 76*, 1006–14.

Grossman, M., Anderson, C., Khan, A, Avants, B., Elman, L., & McCluskey, L. (2008). Impaired action knowledge in amyotrophic lateral sclerosis. *Neurology, 71*, 1396–1401.

Hanley, J.R., & Kay, J. (In press). Imageability effects and phonological errors: Implications for models of auditory repetition. *Cognitive Neuropsychology*.

Hillis, A., & Caramazza, A. (1991). Category-specific naming and comprehension impairment: A double dissociation. *Brain, 114*, 2081–2094.

Hillis, A.E., & Caramazza, A. (1995). Cognitive and neural mechanisms underlying visual and semantic processing. *Journal of Cognitive Neuroscience, 7*, 457–478.

Hillis, A.E., Oh, S., & Ken, L. (2004). Deterioration of naming nouns versus verbs in primary progressive aphasia. *Annals of Neurology, 55*, 268–275.

Hillis, A.E., Rapp, B.C., & Caramazza, A. (1999). When a rose is a rose in speaking but a tulip in writing. *Cortex, 35*, 337–356.

Hillis, A.E., Rapp, B. C., Romani, C., & Caramazza, A. (1990). Selective impairment of semantics in lexical processing. *Cognitive Neuropsychology, 7*, 191–244.

Hillis, A.E., Wityk, R., Barker, P.B., & Caramazza, A. (2003). Neural regions essential for writing verbs. *Nature Neuroscience, 6*, 19–20.

Humphreys, G.W., Riddoch, M.J., & Quinlan, P.T. (1988). Cascade processes in picture identification. *Cognitive Neuropsychology, 5*, 67–104.

Ishibashi, R., Lambon Ralph, M. A, Saito, S., & Pobric, G. (2011). Different roles of lateral anterior temporal lobe and inferior parietal lobule in coding function and manipulation tool knowledge: Evidence from an rTMS study. *Neuropsychologia, 49*, 1128–1135.

Jackendoff, R. (1987). On beyond the zebra: The relation of linguistic and visual information. *Cognition, 26*, 89–114.

Jefferies, E., Rogers, T.T., & Lambon Ralph, M.A. (2011). Premorbid expertise produces category-specific impairment in a domain-general semantic disorder. *Neuropsychologia, 49*, 3213–3223.

Johnson-Frey, S.H. (2004). The neural bases of complex tool use in humans. *Trends in Cognitive Sciences, 8*, 71–78.

Jones, G.V. (1985). Deep dyslexia, imageability, and ease of predication. *Brain and Language, 24*, 1–19.

Kintsch, W. (1980). Semantic memory: A tutorial. In R.S. Nickerson (Ed.), *Attention and performance VIII*. Cambridge, MA: Bolt Beranek and Newman.

McCarthy, R., & Warrington, E. K. (1988). Evidence for modality-specific meaning systems in the brain. *Nature, 207*, 142–175.

Mahon, B.Z., & Caramazza, A. (2008). A critical look at the embodied cognition hypothesis and a new proposal for grounding conceptual content. *Journal of Physiology, Paris, 102*, 59–70.

Mahon, B.Z., Milleville, S.C., Negri, G.A.L., Rumiati, R.I., Caramazza, A., & Martin, A. (2007). Action-related properties shape object representations in the ventral stream. *Neuron, 55*, 507–520.

Marshall, J., Pring, T, Chiat, S., & Robson, J. (1995/6a). Calling a salad a federation: An investigation of semantic jargon. Part 1: Nouns. *Journal of Neurolinguistics, 9*, 237–250.

Marshall, J., Chiat, S., Robson, J., & Pring, T. (1995/6b). Calling a salad a federation: An investigation of semantic jargon. Part 2: Verbs. *Journal of Neurolinguistics, 4*, 251–260.

Martin, A. (2007). The representation of object concepts in the brain. *Annual Review of Psychology, 58*, 25–45.

Martin, A., & Chao, L.L. (2001). Semantic memory and the brain: Structure and processes. *Current Opinion in Neurobiology, 11*, 194–201.

Negri, G.A.L., Rumiati, R.I., Zadini, A., Ukmar, M., Mahon, B.Z., & Caramazza, A. (2007). What is the role of motor simulation in action and object recognition? Evidence from apraxia. *Cognitive Neuropsychology, 24*, 795–816.

Neininger, B., & Pulvermüller, F. (2003). Word-category specific deficits after lesions in the right hemisphere. *Neuropsychologia, 41*, 53–70.

Newton, P.K., & Barry, C. (1997). Concreteness effects in word production but not word comprehension in deep dyslexia. *Cognitive Neuropsychology, 14*, 481–509.

Oliveri, M., Finocchiaro, C., Shapiro, K., Gangitano, M., Caramazza, A., & Pascual-Leone, A. (2004). All talk and no action: A transcranial magnetic stimulation study of motor cortex activation during action word production. *Journal of Cognitive Neuroscience, 16*, 374–381.

Paivio, A. (1978). The relationship between verbal and perceptual codes. In E.C. Carterette & M.P. Friedman (Eds.), *Handbook of perception, Vol. 8. Perceptual coding*. London: Academic Press.

Paivio, A. (1991). Dual coding theory: Retrospect and current status. *Canadian Journal of Psychology, 45*, 255–287.

Paivio, A., Yuille, J.C., & Madigan, S.A. (1968). Concreteness, imagery, and meaningfulness values for 925 nouns. *Journal of Experimental Psychology Monograph Supplement, 76*, 1–25.

Patterson, K., Nestor, P.J., & Rogers, T.T. (2007). Where do you know what you know? The representation of semantic knowledge in the human brain. *Nature Reviews Neuroscience, 8*, 976–987.

Plaut, D., & Shallice, T. (1993a). Perseverative and semantic influences on visual object naming errors in optic aphasia: A semantic access account. *Journal of Cognitive Neuroscience, 5*, 89–117.

Plaut, D., & Shallice, T. (1993b). Deep dyslexia: A case study of connectionist neuropsychology. *Cognitive Neuropsychology, 10*, 377–500.

Pobric, G., Jefferies, E., & Lambon Ralph, M.A. (2010). Category-specific versus category-general semantic impairment induced by transcranial magnetic stimulation. *Current Biology, 20*, 964–968.

Pulvermüller, F., Hauk, O., Nikulin, V.V., & Ilmoniemi, R.J. (2005). Functional links between motor and language systems. *The European Journal of Neuroscience, 21*, 793–797.

Rapp, B.C., & Caramazza, A. (1993). The role of representations in cognitive theory: More on multiple semantics and the agnosia. *Cognitive Neuropsychology, 10*, 235–250.

Ratcliff, G., & Newcombe, F. (1982). Object recognition: Some deductions from the clinical evidence. In A.E. Ellis (Ed.), *Normality and pathology in cognitive functions*. London: Academic Press.

Reilly, J., Harnish, S., Garcia, A., Hung, J., Rodriguez, A.D., & Crosson, B. (2014). Lesion symptom mapping of manipulable object naming in nonfluent aphasia: Can a brain be both embodied and disembodied? *Cognitive Neuropsychology, 31*, 287–312.

Riddoch, M.J., & Humphreys, G.W. (1987). Visual object processing in optic aphasia: A case of semantic access agnosia. *Cognitive Neuropsychology, 4*, 131–185.

Riddoch, M.J., Humphreys, G.W., Coltheart, M., & Funneil, E. (1988). Semantic systems or system? Neuropsychological evidence re-examined. *Cognitive Neuropsychology, 5*, 3–26.

Rizzolatti, G., & Craighero, L. (2004). The mirror-neuron system. *Annual Review of Neuroscience, 27*, 169–192.

Rizzolatti, G., Fadiga, L., & Matelli, M. (1996). Localization of grasp representations in humans by PET: 1. Observation versus execution. *Experimental Brain Research, 111*, 246–252.

Rizzolatti, G., Fogassi, L., & Gallese, V. (2001). Neurophysiological mechanisms underlying the understanding and imitation of action. *Nature Reviews Neuroscience, 2*, 1–10.

Rizzolatti, G., & Luppino, G. (2001). The cortical motor system. *Neuron, 31*, 889–901.

Rosci, C., Chiesa, V., Laiacona, M., & Capitani, E. (2003). Apraxia is not associated to a disproportionate naming impairment for manipulable objects. *Brain and Cognition, 53*, 412–415.

Saffran, E., & Schwartz, M. (1994). Of cabbages and things: Semantic memory from neuropsychological perspective: A tutorial review. In C. Umilta & M. Moscovitch (Eds.), *Attention and performance XV*. Cambridge MA: MIT Books.

Sartori, G., Coltheart, M., Miozzo, M., & Job, R. (1994). Category specificity in neuropsychological impairment of semantic memory. In C. Umilta & M. Moscovitch (Eds.), *Attention and performance XV: Conscious and nonconscious information processing.* Cambridge, MA: MIT Press.

Sartori, G., Job, R., Miozzo, M., Zago, S., & Marchiori, G. (1993). Category-specific form-knowledge deficit in a patient with herpes simplex virus encephalitis. *Journal of Clinical and Experimental Neuropsychology, 15,* 280–299.

Schank, R.C. (1982). *Dynamic memory.* Cambridge: Cambridge University Press.

Schank, R.C., & Abelson, R. (1977). *Scripts, plans, goals, and understanding.* Hillsdale, NJ: Lawrence Erlbaum.

Siegel, S. (1956). *Nonparametric statistics for the behavioural sciences.* Tokyo: McGraw-Hill.

Shallice, T. (1988a). *From neuropsychology to mental structure.* Cambridge: Cambridge University Press.

Shallice, T. (1988b). Specialisation within the semantic system. *Cognitive Neuropsychology, 5,* 133–142.

Shallice, T. (1993). Multiple semantics: Whose confusions? *Cognitive Neuropsychology, 10,* 251–262.

Snowden, J., Griffiths, H., & Neary, D. (1994). Semantic dementia: Autobiographical contribution to preservation of meaning. *Cognitive Neuropsychology, 11,* 265–288.

Stewart, F., Parkin, A.J., & Hunkin, N. M. (1992). Naming impairments following recovery from herpes simplex encephalitis: Category-specific? *Quarterly Journal of Experimental Psychology, 44A,* 261–284.

Taylor, L.J., & Zwaan, R.A. (2009). Action in cognition: The case of language. *Language and Cognition, 1,* 45–58.

Thompson, C.K., Lukic, S., King, M.C., Mesulam, M.M., & Weintraub, S. (2012). Verb and noun deficits in stroke-induced and primary progressive aphasia: The Northwestern Naming Battery. *Aphasiology, 26,* 632–655.

Tulving, E. (1972). Episodic and semantic memory. In E. Tulving & W. Donaldson (Eds.), *Organization of memory.* New York: Academic Press.

Warrington, E.K. (1975). The selective impairment of semantic memory. *Quarterly Journal of Experimental Psychology, 27,* 635–657.

Warrington, E.K. (1981). Neuropsychological studies of verbal semantic systems. *Philosophical Transactions of the Royal Society of London, B295,* 411–423.

Warrington, E.K., & McCarthy, R. (1983). Category specific access dysphasia. *Brain, 106,* 859–878.

Warrington, E.K., & McCarthy, R. (1987). Categories of knowledge: Further fractionations and an attempted integration. *Brain, 110,* 1273–1296.

Warrington, E.K., & Shallice, T. (1984). Category specific semantic impairments. *Brain, 107,* 829–854.

Wilson, B.A., & Wearing, D. (1995). Prisoner of consciousness: A state of just awakening from herpes simplex encephalitis. In R. Campbell & M.A. Conway (Eds.), *Broken memories.* Hove, England: Lawrence Erlbaum.

11

NEURAL SUBSTRATES OF SEMANTICS

Rajani Sebastian and Argye E. Hillis

Semantic processing refers to the cognitive act of accessing stored knowledge about words. Understanding the neural basis of semantics has been fraught with numerous difficulties, including various definitions of "semantics" and several models of the functional organization of semantics. One main question in the field of cognitive neuroscience is: "How does the brain code and process semantic information?" Some historical and contemporary theories emphasize that conceptualization stems from the joint action of modality-specific association cortices: the "distributed" view (Allport, 1985; Martin, 2007; for a review, see Patterson, Nestor, & Rogers, 2007), reflecting our accumulated verbal, motor, and sensory experiences. An alternative position is that, in addition to the modality-specific regions and connections, the various different surface representations connect to, and communicate through, a shared, amodal "hub" in the anterior temporal lobes: this is the "distributed-plus-hub view" (Patterson et al., 2007). Please see chapter 10 regarding different models of the functional organization of semantics.

The advent of functional neuroimaging has allowed tremendous advances in our understanding of the neural basis of semantics. In this chapter we will mostly focus our attempts to explain the neural basis of semantics at the "single-unit" (word, object) level, as words are the basic units upon which more complex semantic structures (e.g., sentences, paragraphs) likely rely. It should be noted that in addition to brain networks supporting semantic processing in general, particular regions may be relatively specialized for processing specific object categories, attributes, or types of knowledge (e.g., abstract/concrete, etc.). We refer the reader to recent reviews regarding brain regions supporting specific object categories or attributes and the controversies that surround this topic (Gainotti, 2005; Mahon & Caramazza, 2009; see also chapter 8, this volume).

In the following sections we will discuss the various brain areas found to be involved in semantics, which we will define as meaning—what defines a word, object, action, or other entity and distinguishes it from similar entities. In discussing the neurobiological basis of semantics, relevant imaging and lesion studies will be reviewed. We will also consider evidence from cortical stimulation studies and transcranial magnetic stimulation, as they also provide an important means of discerning the functional role of each of these neural structures in semantic processing. We have organized this review into four main divisions that reflect parallel but (interacting) lines of inquiry into the neural basis of semantics.

Functional Imaging Studies

In this section we will summarize a subset of recent data from functional neuroimaging that provides evidence regarding the brain regions that are involved in accessing meaning of words, sentences, objects, and actions. The literature is very extensive, and so we will only discuss selective studies that clearly illustrate key findings from this massive set of data. Researchers have adopted a variety of experimental paradigms to examine the neural basis of semantics. The tasks include word reading, word listening, categorizing (deciding whether a presented stimulus depicts a living or nonliving creature, a natural or manufactured object, a word or not), word generation (generating a verb/noun semantically related to a visual or auditory word or picture), semantic retrieval (e.g., retrieving an object property), semantic priming, sentence comprehension, etc. It is not clear that all of these tasks require meaning. For example, lexical decision might be accomplished on the basis of access to lexical representations without access to word meaning, although it is assumed that words "automatically" activate word meaning. Similarly, categorization tasks, property tasks, and so on require access to only a subset of semantic features of entities. Tasks that require access to more complete semantic representations (e.g., selecting a word or picture that is most closely related to a target from two related words or pictures) have been used less commonly (Hillis & Caramazza, 1995). All "semantic" tasks require not only access to meaning (to lesser or greater degree), but also other cognitive functions, such as searching semantic memory, visualization, selection between competitors, and so on. The location and degree of activation varies widely across paradigms, depending on these other cognitive components and the level of difficulty of the task.

Nevertheless, functional imaging studies in healthy individuals generally reveal that an extensive left-lateralized network is engaged in each of these semantic tasks. Two regions within the left hemisphere have been regularly reported as playing a major role in semantic processing: the left temporal cortex and the left inferior frontal cortex (for reviews, see Binder, Desai, Graves, & Conant, 2009; Bookheimer, 2002; Price, 2010, 2012; Vigneau et al., 2006). However, it seems clear that that the inferior frontal cortex does not have a role in representing meaning per se, but in other aspects of "cognitive control" required to accomplish semantic processing tasks (Bookheimer, 2002; Novick, Trueswell, & Thompson-Schill, 2005; Snyder, Feigenson, & Thompson-Schill, 2007). Other regions, including the angular gyrus (BA 39), supramarginal gyrus (BA 40), cingulate gyrus, and right hemisphere regions, are also engaged in semantic processing tasks.

Temporal Cortex

The superior temporal gyrus (STG; BA 22) has long been considered to play a central role in language comprehension (e.g., Geschwind 1970, 1972; Goodglass, 1993; Wernicke, 1874), but evidence using functional imaging suggests that its role is limited to early (auditory) stages of the sound-to-meaning transformation (e.g., Binder et al., 2009; Hickok & Poeppel, 2007; Turkeltaub & Coslett, 2010). A wealth of data from functional imaging studies suggests a role for left middle temporal gyrus (MTG; BA 21) in the storage and access of lexical information. Several neuroimaging studies have found reliable activation in this region during a wide range of semantic tasks whatever the modality of presentation of the stimulus (for reviews, see Binder et al., 2009; Indefrey & Levelt, 2004; Price, 2012; Vigneau et al., 2006).

Apart from left MTG, other parts of left temporal cortex have been linked to semantic processing, including more anterior and inferior temporal cortex (ITG; for reviews, see Binder et al., 2009; Price, 2012; Vigneau et al., 2006). Activation in the inferior temporal area has been reported in many studies examining lexical retrieval during naming, semantic categorization/association, or reading (e.g., Adams & Janata, 2002; Binder et al., 2003; Bookheimer, Zeffiro, Blaxton, Gaillard, & Theodore, 1995; Bright, Moss, & Tyler, 2004; Damasio, Grabowski, Tranel, Hichwa, & Damasio, 1996; Dien, Brian, Molfese, & Gold, 2013; Moore & Price, 1999; Sevostianove et al., 2002; Vingerhoets et al., 2003). A study by Whitney and colleagues (2011) shows that distinct regions in left temporal lobe (posterior MTG, mid-ITG) react differently to increased demands on semantic control and the number of meanings being retrieved. Words with multiple meanings like "bank" served as targets (in a double-prime paradigm, in which multiple meaning activation and maximal executive demands loaded onto different priming conditions). Anterior ITG was sensitive to the number of meanings that were retrieved, suggesting a role for this region in semantic representation, while posterior MTG and inferior frontal cortex showed greater activation in conditions that maximized executive demands. This study identified a double dissociation between processes related to semantic control and representation in posterior and inferior aspects of temporal cortex. Based on the results the authors propose that the left inferior temporal cortex is involved in storage of meaning, and that more posterior structures in MTG worked in concert with left inferior frontal gyrus and inferior parietal lobe to support aspects of semantic control during meaning retrieval. Although the proposal that the semantic control network extends into left posterior temporal lobe regions is controversial, other neuroimaging studies that have manipulated semantic control demands also show similar activation patterns (Bedny, McGill, & Thompson-Schill, 2008; Gennari, MacDonald, Postle, & Seidenberg, 2007; Rodd, Davis, & Johnsrude, 2005; Snijders et al., 2009; Zempleni, Renken, Hoeks, Hoogduin, & Stowe, 2007).

The anterior temporal lobes (ATL) bilaterally have been linked to semantic processing based on lesion data; however, fMRI data have produced inconsistent findings and are not in complete agreement with lesion studies. For example, many fMRI studies report activation within prefrontal and temporo-parietal areas during semantic tasks but do not observe activation within the ATLs (for a review, see Visser, Jefferies, & Lambon Ralph, 2010). A meta-analysis by Visser et al. (2010) of fMRI studies on semantic processing in ATL revealed four factors that influenced the likelihood of finding ATL activation: (1) the use of PET versus fMRI, reflecting the fact that fMRI but not PET is sensitive to distortion artifacts caused by large variations in magnetic susceptibility in the area of the ATL; (2) a field of view (FOV) of more than 15 cm, thereby ensuring whole-brain coverage; (3) the use of a high-level or active baseline task to prevent subtraction of otherwise uncontrolled semantic activation; and (4) the inclusion of the ATL as a region of interest (ROI). A recent fMRI study using enhanced protocols, including large FOV and the use of spin echo, revealed activation in bilateral ATL during semantic tasks (Binney, Embleton, Jefferies, Parker, & Lambon Ralph, 2010). Similarly, Binder et al. (2011) found activation in the ATL using an active attention-demanding control task. Together, fMRI results suggest that bilateral ATL are important in semantic processing and may serve as the "semantic hub," critical for representation of semantic entities and/or combinatorial semantic processes (Visser & Lambon Ralph, 2011).

Frontal Cortex

The inferior cortex of the left frontal lobe is another region that is critically involved in semantic processing tasks. Although this region had been initially associated with speech production, it is now well documented that this region is active during a wide range of language tasks, including those that do not involve overt production of speech. Petersen and colleagues (Petersen, Fox, Posner, Mintun, & Raichle, 1988, 1989) were among the first to suggest that regions within the left frontal lobe contribute to semantic processing, on the basis of a comparison between two speech production tasks. Since this report, a large number of studies using a variety of experimental paradigms have implicated the left inferior frontal gyrus (IFG; BA 44, 45, 47) in semantic processing (e.g., Adams & Janata, 2002; Badre & Wagner, 2002; Binder et al., 2003; Chee, Hon, Caplan, Lee, & Goh, 2002; Devlin, Matthews, & Rushworth, 2003; Gabrieli, Poldrack, & Desmond, 1998; Homae, Hashimoto, Nakajima, Miyashita, & Sakai, 2002; Kapur et al., 1994; Noppeney & Price, 2002; Nyberg et al., 2003; Poldrack et al., 1999; Thompson-Schill, D'Esposito, Aguirre, & Farah, 1997; Vingerhoets et al., 2003; Wagner, Paré-Blagoev, Clark, & Poldrack, 2001). For reviews of left frontal cortex and semantics, see Badre and Wagner (2007), Bookheimer (2002), Costafreda et al. (2006), Fiez (1997), and Thompson-Schill (2003).

Numerous experiments indicate that the left IFG is involved in the effortful retrieval, maintenance, and/or control of semantic information, whereas long-term storage of the conceptual and semantic knowledge is dependent on posterior cortical (temporal and perhaps parietal) regions (Badre, 2008; Bookheimer, 2002; Noppeney, Phillips, & Price, 2004; Thompson-Schill et al., 1997; Wagner et al., 2001; Ye & Zhou, 2009). Activation in the left IFG has been linked to task difficulty. Increased activation in the left IFG during semantic tasks may also be due to increased working memory or phonological processing demands in some studies (e.g., Adler et al., 2001; Binder, Medler, Desai, Conant, & Liebenthal, 2005; Braver et al., 1997; Braver, Barch, Gray, Molfese, & Snyder, 2001; Desai, Conant, Waldron, & Binder, 2006; Jonides et al., 1997). Some authors suggest that there is a degree of functional specialization within the left IFG, with semantic selection and controlled retrieval relying on different substructures (e.g., Badre, Poldrack, Paré-Blagoev, Insler, & Wagner, 2005; Gold et al., 2006). According to this view, dorsal aspects of left IFG (BA 45) were linked to tasks that require the selection of a subset of information competing semantic alternatives and ventral portions of left IFG (BA 47) were engaged during the controlled retrieval of semantic knowledge.

Badre et al. (2005) examined the functional and neuroanatomical relation between selection and controlled retrieval by manipulating the task requirements and the nature of the stimuli. In all trials, subjects selected a target based on its relation to the cue. First, selection demands were manipulated by varying the specificity of the semantic judgment, with participants making either a global relatedness judgment (i.e., which of the targets is most globally related to the cue) or a feature similarity judgment (i.e., which of the targets is most similar to the cue with respect to a particular feature, such as color). fMRI revealed that performance of feature (high-selection) versus relatedness (low-selection) judgments elicited greater activation in left dorsal IFG (posterior/mid ventrolateral prefrontal cortex, or VLPFC), whereas this manipulation did not affect activation levels in left ventral IFG (anterior VLPFC) and left middle temporal cortex. Within the feature similarity judgment task, selection demands were further taxed by varying the congruency. A trial was congruent if the correct target was also a pre-experimental associate of the cue and incongruent if the correct target was not the pre-experimental associate. fMRI revealed that incongruent versus congruent trials elicited greater activation in left dorsal IFG, whereas again there was no effect in left ventral IFG nor in middle temporal cortex. Thus, different parts of IFG may have different roles in semantic selection.

Parietal Cortex

The inferior parietal lobe, comprising the angular gyrus (AG, BA 39) and supramarginal gyrus (SMG, BA 40), may also play an important role in semantic processing. Activity in the left AG has been associated with semantic processing in numerous imaging studies across different tasks and modalities (e.g., Adams & Janata, 2002; Binder et al., 2003; Bookheimer et al., 1995; Giesbrecht, Camblin, & Swaab, 2004; Graves et al., 2010; Hoenig & Scheef, 2009; Ischebeck et al., 2004; Kotz et al., 2002; Mummery, Patterson, Hodges, & Price, 1998; Noppeney, Josephs, Hocking, Price, & Friston, 2008; Raettig & Kotz, 2008; Scott, Leff, & Wise, 2003; Sharp et al., 2010). A large-scale meta-analysis study conducted by Binder et al. (2009) found that the most consistent activation across 120 neuroimaging studies of tasks broadly considered to be "semantic" was located within the left AG and adjacent SMG. They described the AG as a heteromodal association area. Other meta-analysis reviews also indicate that the AG is involved in semantic processing (for reviews, see Cabeza & Nyberg, 2000; Vigneau et al., 2006).

Binder and colleagues (Binder et al., 2009) propose that the AG is specialized for conceptual integration and controlling fluent conceptual combination, such as sentence comprehension, discourse, problem solving, and planning. For example, a study by Humphries, Binder, Medler, and

Liebenthal (2006) highlights the role of the left angular gyrus in sentence-level semantic processing. Using an auditory comprehension task involving sentences and randomly ordered list of words, they found greater activation to sentences than to word lists in the left anterior superior temporal sulcus and left angular gyrus. They also found greater activation to semantically congruent stimuli than either incongruent or pseudoword stimuli in widespread, bilateral temporal lobe areas and the angular gyrus. Of the two regions that responded to syntactic structure (left anterior superior temporal sulcus and left angular gyrus), the angular gyrus showed a greater response to semantic structure, consistent with its role in combinatorial processing.

In a recent study, Seghier, Fagan, and Price (2010) used a range of different semantic tasks and stimuli to systematically subdivide semantic activations in AG according to their response properties. They collected data on 94 healthy human subjects during fixation and eight goal-directed tasks that involved semantic matching, perceptual matching, or speech production in response to familiar or unfamiliar stimuli presented in either verbal (letter) or nonverbal (picture) formats. Their results segregated three different left AG regions that were all activated by semantic relative to perceptual matching: (1) a mid-region (mAG) that was *deactivated* during all tasks relative to fixation; (2) a dorsomesial region (dAG) that was *activated* by all tasks relative to fixation; and (3) a ventrolateral region (vAG) that was activated specifically in association with semantic matching tasks. On the basis of the effects of task and stimuli in each AG subdivision, they propose that mAG is involved in a variety of semantic associations; dAG is involved in semantic search when stimulus meaning is being retrieved; and vAG is involved in later stages of conceptual identification of visual words and pictures.

Cingulate Cortex

The role of the cingulate cortex in higher cognition has received a great deal of attention in recent years. Activation in the anterior cingulate cortex has been linked to a variety of cognitive functions, including conflict monitoring, error detection, motivation, emotion, pain, and reward processing (e.g., Barch et al., 2001; Bechara, Damasio, & Damasio, 2000; Botvinick, Cohen, & Carter, 2004; Britton et al., 2006; Drevets et al., 1997; Kerns et al., 2004; Kiehl, Liddle, & Hopfinger, 2000; Liddle, Kiehl, & Smith, 2001; Mayberg et al., 1999; Noppeney et al., 2004; Phan, Wager, Taylor, & Liberzon, 2002). The anterior cingulate has been thought to play a role in semantic processing in studies examining activation associated with category judgment, ambiguity resolution, word generation, stem-completion, verbal fluency, and sentence/story comprehension (e.g., Barch, Braver, Sabb, & Noll, 2000; de Zubicaray, Zelaya, Andrew, Williams, & Bullmore, 2000; de Zubicaray, McMahon, Eastburn, & Pringle, 2006; Fu et al., 2002; Peelle, McMillan, Moore, Grossman, & Wingfield, 2004; Rossell, Bullmore, Williams, & David, 2001; Thompson-Schill et al., 1997; Whitney et al., 2009). For example, in a lexical decision priming study with short and long delays (evaluating automatic and controlled semantic priming, respectively), Rossell et al. (2001) reported different parts of anterior cingulate showed activation in response to automatic versus controlled semantic priming but did not respond differently to semantically related versus unrelated prime–target pairs. Similarly, Barch et al. (2000) found that the anterior cingulate cortex was activated during a verb-generation task when there was competition among alternative responses. In another fMRI study, Fu et al. (2002) examined the effect of manipulating task demands on activation during verbal fluency by using "easy" and "hard" letters. The hard condition was associated with greater dorsal anterior cingulate activation than the easy condition. Increased activation seen during the hard condition was thought to reflect the greater demands, particularly in terms of arousal responses with increased task difficulty and the monitoring of potential response errors. Thus, it seems that anterior cingulate, like IFG, has a role in semantic tasks with particular processing demands, rather than representation of semantics (meaning) per se.

Right Hemisphere Regions

The presence of consistent right hemisphere (RH) activation during language tasks supports the view that RH regions are involved in normal language processing. It is well recognized that the RH plays a crucial role in paralinguistic processes such as the processing of emotional prosodic information (e.g., Beaucousin et al., 2007) and the integration of context to construct a complete representation of meaning and intent (for reviews, see Bookheimer, 2002 and Lindell, 2006; see also chapter 24, this volume). Several, if not all, fMRI studies examining semantic processing have shown activation in various right hemisphere regions during semantic tasks (e.g., Adams & Janata, 2002; Booth et al., 2002; Bright et al., 2004; Dräger et al., 2004; Fiez, Balota, Raichle, & Petersen, 1999; Graves et al., 2010; Gurd et al., 2002; Hagoort et al., 1999; Ischebeck et al., 2004; McDermott, Petersen, Watson, & Ojemann, 2003; Perani et al., 1998; Petersen et al., 1989; Rogalsky & Hickok, 2009; Vingerhoets et al., 2003).

A meta-analysis done by Vigneau et al. (2011) examined the contribution of right hemisphere to phonology, semantics, and syntax. The study showed greatest activation, within the RH, in IFG, precentral gyrus, and superior temporal gyrus during tasks involving semantic association, semantic categorization, semantic retrieval, and selection (see Vigneau et al., 2011 for details).

Lesion Studies

The functional neuroimaging literature and neuropsychological studies of semantic processing mostly overlap in the areas identified as important for semantic processing. However, the results from the two methodologies have yet to be fully integrated. Lesion studies and functional neuroimaging studies answer different types of questions regarding the relationship between brain areas and cognitive processes. The main question asked in lesion studies is whether a brain area is *necessary* for a certain type of processing. If damage to a particular area consistently results in inability to perform the particular type of semantic processing, it is assumed that that area is *necessary* for that particular aspect of semantics (at least before other areas of the brain "take over" the function of the damaged part). In contrast, when areas show activation correlated with a particular aspect of semantic processing in functional neuroimaging studies in normal subjects, it can be concluded that these areas are *engaged* in that aspect of semantic processing, but it cannot be concluded that these areas are all *necessary* for that aspect of semantics. For example, some significant right hemisphere activation is observed during nearly all language tasks, but lesions to areas that are activated do not cause language impairments, indicating that they were not necessary for language. Thus, these methods provide complementary evidence about structure-function relationships, as previously argued (Fellows et al., 2005).

Studies of brain-damaged patients with semantic impairment have revealed a great deal about how semantic information is organized in the brain. Impaired semantic processing is mostly commonly associated with stroke, viral infection (e.g., herpes simplex virus encephalitis, HSvE), and two forms of neurodegenerative disease: Alzheimer's disease (AD) and semantic variant primary progressive aphasia (svPPA, previously known as semantic dementia). Lesion studies mostly implicate the role of the left temporal lobe in semantic processing, specifically the posterior and middle temporal gyrus. Another region in the temporal cortex, the anterior temporal lobe (ATL) bilaterally, has also been implicated in semantic processing, as noted earlier.

Herpes Simplex Virus Encephalitis

HSvE is the most common viral encephalitis in humans (Kennedy & Chaudhuri, 2002). The temporal lobe, including anterior MTG, ITG, and fusiform gyrus, is frequently damaged (usually bilaterally) in herpes simplex encephalitis, often resulting in profound semantic deficits (Kapur et al., 1994; Lambon Ralph, Lowe, & Rogers, 2007; Noppeney et al., 2007; Warrington & Shallice, 1984). The semantic deficit in HSvE is often category specific, with relatively well-preserved knowledge of manmade things but impaired knowledge of living things. Noppeney et al. (2007) used voxel-based morphometry to compare the pattern of brain damage in patients with semantic dementia (now svPPA) and HSvE. They found that patients with HSvE showed extensive grey matter loss, predominantly in the medial parts of the anterior temporal cortices bilaterally. The authors hypothesize that the antero-medial temporal cortex may be important for differentiating between concepts that are "tightly packed" in semantic space, such as living things. A similar proposal was made by Lambon Ralph et al. (2007) based on a computational account of neuropsychological evidence.

Stroke and Aphasia

The stroke aphasia literature similarly emphasizes the critical involvement of posterior regions (temporal and parietal) in language comprehension and semantic processing (Goodglass & Wingfield, 1997; Hart & Gordon, 1990; Hillis et al., 2001, 2002; Kertesz, Sheppard, & MacKenzie, 1982; Schwartz et al., 2009; Turken & Dronkers, 2011).

In a series of studies with acute ischemic stroke patients, Hillis and colleagues provide evidence for left posterior superior temporal cortex (BA 22) involvement in semantic processing. For example, in patients without infarct in left BA 22, severity of hypoperfusion of left BA 22 on perfusion-weighted imaging was linearly related to the severity of word comprehension deficits (Hillis et al., 2001). Furthermore, restored tissue function (via reperfusion) in this area resulted in recovery of both comprehension and naming, consistent with restored lexical-semantics (Hillis et al., 2001; Hillis et al., 2002; Hillis & Heidler, 2002). In another study, they confirmed that the severity of tissue dysfunction in left BA 22 had the greatest contribution (among all regions examined) in predicting the error rate in word/picture verification, a measure of the severity of lexical-semantic impairment (DeLeon et al., 2007). In a follow-up study, they investigated whether semantic errors result from the disruption of access either to semantics or to lexical representations (Cloutman et al., 2009). Hypoperfusion and/or infarct of left BA 22 predicted semantic errors in both naming and comprehension in acute stroke, indicating that this region is critical for linking words to their meanings. Tissue dysfunction in left BA 37 (posterior middle and inferior temporal/fusiform gyrus) predicted production of semantic errors in naming only, with spared word comprehension, indicating that this area is critical for accessing lexical representations for output.

A study by Schwartz et al. (2009) examined the role of anterior temporal lobe in word retrieval in patients with chronic aphasia. Whole-brain voxel-based lesion-symptom mapping revealed that the strongest associations between semantic errors in naming and chronic lesion were in the left anterior to mid middle temporal gyrus. The difference in localization of semantic errors in naming in acute versus chronic aphasia could be due to compensation or reorganization in the chronic stage, differences in lesion volume (larger strokes in chronic patients, as patients with small strokes recover completely), and/or the fact that the acute studies evaluated areas of hypoperfusion as well as infarct associated with errors.

Damage to specific parts of temporal and parietal cortex can also produce category-specific patterns of impairment (Gainotti, 2000; Hillis & Caramazza, 1991; Warrington & Mccarthy, 1987, 1994; Warrington & Shallice, 1984). One account of these category-specific deficits is that specific cortical fields within these regions represent particular sensory and motor features of objects (e.g., Martin, 2007; but see also Mahon & Caramazza, 2009 for an alternative account; see chapter 10, this volume, for further discussion of category-specific semantics).

Although the stroke literature traditionally implicates posterior cortical regions in decoding semantic information, there have been reports of semantic deficits following frontal lesions (Berthier, 2000, 2001). Berthier (2001) reports of a series of patients with transcortical sensory aphasia with deficits in auditory comprehension in the absence of damage to the posterior temporal cortex. All patients had frontal damage. One explanation is that the patients may have had dysfunction of posterior regions due to diaschisis or hypoperfusion. A second account is that the patients may have not had semantic deficits per se, but rather impaired response selection in semantic tasks. This latter account is in line with findings from the functional neuroimaging literature that report activation in the frontal cortex during a variety of semantic processing tasks (see Binder et al., 2009), as the hypothesized role of the frontal cortex in semantic tasks is in semantic search or selection (Bookheimer, 2002).

Semantic Variant Primary Progressive Aphasia

SvPPA is characterized by fluent and well-articulated speech with little content and with pronounced word comprehension deficits. SvPPA is commonly associated with severe naming as well as comprehension deficits (Binney et al., 2010; Bozeat, Lambon Ralph, Patterson, Garrard, & Hodges, 2000; Gorno-Tempini et al., 2004, 2011; Jefferies, Patterson, Jones, & Lambon Ralph, 2009; Jefferies & Lambon Ralph, 2006). Unlike patients with HSvE, patients with svPPA typically do not have a category-specific impairment (Lambon Ralph et al., 2003), except that they have more difficulty naming and understanding objects than actions (Hillis, Oh, & Ken, 2004).

Patients with svPPA have difficulty naming due to deterioration of the meaning of objects and their names, affecting both naming and comprehension tasks. Because impairment of the meaning of the word or concept may affect naming most profoundly, naming is often severely impaired in svPPA even relatively early in the course. This variant is associated with bilateral (left greater than right) anterior and inferior temporal atrophy (Gorno-Tempini et al., 2004, 2011; Knibb, Xuereb, Patterson, & Hodges, 2006; Nestor, Fryer, & Hodges, 2006). In part due to the profound impairment in naming and comprehension of objects associated with bilateral anterior temporal atrophy in svPPA, both anterior temporal lobes have been implicated in amodal semantic processing (Binney et al., 2010; Corbett, Jefferies, Ehsan, & Lambon Ralph, 2009; Jefferies & Lambon Ralph, 2006; Patterson et al., 2007). However, decline in object semantics is more strongly associated with atrophy in left temporal lobe than atrophy in right temporal lobe in svPPA (Breining et al., 2015).

Alzheimer's Disease

The earliest and most prominent symptom in Alzheimer's disease (AD) is a profound impairment in the ability to acquire and remember new information whether tested by recall or recognition (e.g., Grady et al., 1988; Greene et al., 1996; Grossman et al., 2003; Hodges & Patterson, 1995). Brain imaging in patients with AD reveals hypometabolism not only in the bilateral medial temporal lobes, but also in the thalamus, the posterior cingulate gyrus, and other parts of the limbic system (Nestor, Fryer, Smielwwski, & Hodges, 2003). Patients with AD exhibit notable deficits in semantic performance, even at the early stage of the disorder (Ahmed, Arnold, Thompson, Graham, & Hodges, 2008; Hodges, Erzinçlioğlu, & Patterson, 2006; Hodges, & Patterson, 1995).

Although there is a vast literature examining semantic impairment in AD, there is no clear consensus regarding the nature of the deficit. A recent study examined the nature of semantic impairment at mild and severe stages of AD (Corbett, Jefferies, Burns, & Lambon Ralph, 2012).

Both mild and severe AD patients performed below the normal level across a range of executive, semantic, naming, and category fluency tasks. When patients at mild and more severe stages of the disease were contrasted directly, however, qualitative differences in the nature of their semantic impairments emerged. The authors hypothesize that semantic deficits in the early stage of the disease are due to a failure of control processes that lead to semantic deregulation (assessed using executive/semantic tasks). In the later stages of the disease, semantic deficits are due to degradation of semantic representation (assessed using naming and category fluency tasks). These findings suggest that the evolution of AD pathology over the course of the disease affects separate components of semantic cognition at different stages.

Analyses of lesion studies indicate that all the four groups of patients (HSvE, stroke, svPPA, and AD) have semantic impairments, but there is a difference in the nature of semantic impairment across the groups. There are also differences in the nature of semantic impairments within groups: strokes in frontal versus temporal cortex cause different types of impairment on semantic tasks, and deficits in early and late AD appear to be quite distinct. These differences offer key insights into the cognitive and neural organization of semantic processing. For example, although both stroke and svPPA result in semantic impairment, there is a qualitative difference in the patterns of errors across tasks in patients with comprehension deficits due to the two etiologies, in part because svPPA affects both anterior temporal lobes (even though the atrophy generally asymmetric). The findings from the lesion studies indicate that there are at least the following interacting components that support semantic processing: (1) bilateral anterior temporal lobes, which together form a "hub" for semantic representations distributed across the temporal cortices; (2) left posterior superior temporal cortex, which links semantic representations to phonological representations; (3) left posterior inferior parietal cortex, which links "lexical-semantics" to semantic information in other modalities; and (4) left posterior inferior frontal cortex, which is critical for controlled selection of responses in semantic tasks. Functional neuroimaging studies of normal participants performing semantic tasks also point to a broadly similar neural network subserving the semantic system.

Transcranial Magnetic Stimulation

Transcranial magnetic stimulation (TMS) is another methodology that has been utilized to explore the neural substrates of semantics. Magnetic pulses are applied over a specific brain region in healthy participants, leading to relatively focal, temporary disruption or facilitation of neural activity (depending on the frequency of the pulses). Inhibitory repetitive TMS (rTMS) results in performance deficits in tasks that are underpinned by the targeted brain area (i.e., a "virtual lesion") (Pascual-Leone et al., 2000; Walsh & Rushworth, 1999; Walsh & Cowey, 2000).

Although most rTMS research to date has focused on sensory/motor systems, rTMS has also been to explore the neural basis of language and semantic memory (for a review, see Devlin & Watkins, 2007). Studies done by the Lambon Ralph's group using rTMS suggest that the ATL are a critical substrate for semantic representation (e.g., Pobric, Jefferies, & Lambon Ralph, 2007; Lambon Ralph, Pobric, & Jefferies, 2009). In the first study, Pobric et al. (2007) used rTMS over the ATL in healthy participants and demonstrated that the behavioral patterns of somewhat similar to semantic dementia can be mirrored in neurologically intact participants. Specifically, they showed that temporal disruption to neural processing in the ATL produces a selective semantic impairment leading to significant slowing in both picture naming and word comprehension.

A follow-up study by same group (Lambon Ralph et al., 2009) investigated the contribution of the right and left temporal poles in supporting verbal conceptual knowledge. The authors used rTMS to investigate the role of left and right ATL during synonym judgment (semantic task) and number matching (nonsemantic task). Stimulation of right and left temporal pole affected semantic decision times but not number judgment, indicating that both ATL are critically important in the representation and activation of semantic memory.

To further understand the role of a wider neural network underpinning semantic control, Whitney, Kirk, O'Sullivan, Ralph, and Jefferies (2011) used rTMS to produce virtual lesions within two sites, left inferior frontal gyrus and left posterior middle temporal gyrus, in healthy participants. Stimulation of both sites selectively disrupted executively demanding semantic judgments: semantic decisions based on strong automatic associations were unaffected. Performance was also unchanged in nonsemantic tasks—irrespective of their executive demands—and following stimulation of a control site. These results reveal that these frontal and posterior temporal regions are among the areas that are critical for controlled selection from semantic memory or other processes involved in executively demanding semantic judgments.

Cortical Stimulation

Direct cortical stimulation (also called electrical stimulation mapping, or ESM) is another technique that has been used to study neural correlates of semantic representation. Cortical stimulation provides a different perspective regarding the cortical organization of language by causing focal temporary brain "lesions" by stimulating electrodes implanted on subdural grids (placed to identify the appropriate area to resect in patients who have tumors or chronic epilepsy). Although the exact mechanism of cortical stimulation remains unknown, the view is that cortical stimulation transiently interacts locally with a small cortical or axonal site, as well as nonlocally, as the focal perturbation will indeed disrupt the whole or sub network sustaining a given function (Mandonnet, Winkler, & Duffau, 2010). Therefore, cortical stimulation can be used to identify with a great accuracy and reproducibility, in vivo in humans, the structures that are crucial for cognitive functions, especially language, in an individual both at cortical and subcortical (white matter and deep grey nuclei) levels (Duffau, Mortiz-Gasser, & Mandonnet, 2013). Limitations of this methodology include the fact that it is only done in patients who have chronic epilepsy or lesions that require surgery, so the individuals may have already undergone reorganization of structure-function relationships.

Results from cortical stimulation studies generally implicate both the frontal and temporal areas in semantic processing (Boatman et al., 2000; Duffau et al., 2002, 2005; Gatignol, Capelle, Bihan, & Du, 2004; Hamberger, Seidel, Goodman, Perrine, & McKhann, 2003; Ojemann, Ojemann, Lettice, & Berger, 1989; Sanai, Mirzadeh, & Berger, 2008; Schaffler, Liiders, Dinner, Lesser, & Chelune, 1993; Schaffler, Luders, & Beck, 1996). One cortical stimulation mapping study (Ojemann et al., 1989) during awake neurosurgical procedures emphasized that essential language areas vary across individuals; within the frontal lobe, they found areas specialized for semantic processing and phonology as well as articulation for some individuals. Similarly, Schäffler et al. (1993, 1996) found that transient deficits in language comprehension were elicited as frequently in Broca's areas as in Wernicke's area. As noted, however, all individuals who have ESM are patients with brain tumors or chronic epilepsy, who may have already undergone extensive reorganization of structure-function relationships because of their neurological disease.

Duffau and colleagues (Duffau et al., 2002, 2005, 2008; Mandonnet et al., 2007) used the method of intraoperative ESM to investigate the neural correlates of semantic processing both at cortical and subcortical levels. They were specifically interested in anatomo-functional connectivity underlying the semantic system. Their results indicate a functional role of the inferior occipito-frontal fasciculus in semantic processing (Duffau et al., 2005). They demonstrated that direct electrostimulation of this pathway induces semantic paraphasias with a high reproducibility, whatever the part of the bundles stimulated (namely occipito-temporal, sub-insular, or frontal part).

Although ESM has revealed some individual variability and some new insights regarding the role of certain white matter tracts, the results of cortical stimulation studies are generally in line with functional neuroimaging and lesion studies regarding brain regions underlying semantics (e.g., Binder et al., 2009; Bookheimer, 2002; Price, 2012; Vigneau et al., 2006). Further, the language disturbance induced by cortical stimulation supports the existence of a dual-stream model for auditory language processing: a ventral stream would be involved in mapping sound to meaning and a dorsal stream in mapping sound to articulation (Hickok & Poeppel, 2007; Saur et al., 2008).

Conclusions

Processing of word, object, and sentence meaning is supported by a widely distributed network of brain regions (Table 11.1). Meaning itself depends primarily on temporal regions, with left temporal regions critical for associating word meaning to phonological representations. Bilateral ATL perhaps serves as a hub for distributed multimodal meaning of objects. Left angular gyrus appears to have a critical role in combining multiple meanings. Left posterior frontal cortex, particularly IFG and anterior cingulate, appear to be critical for selection among competitors in semantic tasks, although different regions within IFG and anterior cingulate may have different roles in supporting performance on semantic tasks, including short-term memory, manipulating representations in "working memory," searching or weighing alternatives, and so on. Right hemisphere homologs to these areas also are engaged in semantic tasks, depending on the level of difficulty and the nature of the task (see also chapter 23, this volume). Lesion studies and functional imaging studies have provided complementary evidence for the complex networks of brain regions that support semantic processing, and emerging variations of these studies (including direct cortical recording, direct cortical stimulation) will continue to shed light on our understanding of this topic in the coming decades.

Table 11.1 Cognitive Processes Underlying Semantic Tasks and Their Hypothesized Neural Correlates

Cognitive Process Underlying Semantic Tasks	*Area of Brain Associated with Cognitive Process*	*Type of Study that Supports Association*
Representation of meaning of words and objects	Bilateral inferior and middle temporal cortex (perhaps ATL as "hub")	Functional imaging svPPA Herpes encephalitis Alzheimer's disease (late)
Linking word meaning to phonology (spoken-word comprehension, naming)	Left superior temporal cortex	Functional imaging Lesion studies (stroke) Cortical stimulation
Combining multiple meanings (e.g., to form semantic or syntactic structure)	Left angular gyrus	Functional imaging Lesion studies (stroke)
Retrieving meaning from written words and other visual stimuli	Left angular gyrus	Functional imaging Lesion studies (stroke)
Semantic search, selection among competitors, working memory, other executive functions	Bilateral inferior frontal gyrus, anterior cingulate cortex, inferior parietal cortex	Functional imaging Transcranial magnetic stimulation Alzheimer's disease (early)

ATL = Anterior temporal lobe

Acknowledgment

The authors and their work on this chapter were supported by NIDCD R01 DC 5375. We gratefully acknowledge this support.

References

Adams, R.B., & Janata, P. (2002). A comparison of neural circuits underlying auditory and visual object categorization. *NeuroImage, 16*(2), 361–77. doi:10.1006/nimg.2002.1088

Adler, C.M., Sax, K.W., Holland, S.K., Schmithorst, V., Rosenberg, L., & Strakowski, S.M. (2001). Changes in neuronal activation with increasing attention demand in healthy volunteers: An fMRI study. *Synapse, 42*(4), 266–72. doi:10.1002/syn.1112

Ahmed, S., Arnold, R., Thompson, S.A., Graham, K.S., & Hodges, J.R. (2008). Naming of objects, faces and buildings in mild cognitive impairment. *Cortex, 44*(6), 746–52. doi:10.1016/j.cortex.2007.02.002

Allport, D.A. (1985). Distributed memory, modular subsystems and dysphasia. In S. P. Newman & Ruth Epstein (Eds.), *Current perspectives in dysphasia* (pp. 32–60). New York: Churchill Livingstone.

Badre, D. (2008). Cognitive control, hierarchy, and the rostro-caudal organization of the frontal lobes. *Trends in Cognitive Sciences, 12*(5), 193–200. doi:10.1016/j.tics.2008.02.004

Badre, D., Poldrack, R.A., Paré-Blagoev, E.J., Insler, R.Z., & Wagner, A.D. (2005). Dissociable controlled retrieval and generalized selection mechanisms in ventrolateral prefrontal cortex. *Neuron, 47*(6), 907–18. doi:10.1016/j.neuron.2005.07.023

Badre, D., & Wagner, A. D. (2002). Semantic retrieval, mnemonic control, and prefrontal cortex. *Behavioral and Cognitive Neuroscience Reviews, 1*(3), 206–18. doi:10.1177/1534582302001003002

Badre, D., & Wagner, A.D. (2007). Left ventrolateral prefrontal cortex and the cognitive control of memory. *Neuropsychologia, 45*(13), 2883–901. doi:10.1016/j.neuropsychologia.2007.06.015

Barch, D.M., Braver, T.S., Sabb, F.W., & Noll, D.C. (2000). Anterior cingulate and the monitoring of response conflict: Evidence from an fMRI study of overt verb generation. *Journal of Cognitive Neuroscience, 12*(2), 298–309.

Barch, D.M., Braver, T.S., Akbudak, E., Conturo, T., Ollinger, J., & Snyder, A. (2001). Anterior cingulate cortex and response conflict: Effects of response modality and processing domain. *Cerebral Cortex, 11*(9), 837–48. Retrieved from http://www.ncbi.nlm.nih.gov/pubmed/11532889

Beaucousin, V., Lacheret, A., Turbelin, M.-R., Morel, M., Mazoyer, B., & Tzourio-Mazoyer, N. (2007). fMRI study of emotional speech comprehension. *Cerebral Cortex, 17*(2), 339–52. doi:10.1093/cercor/bhj151

Bechara, A., Damasio, H., & Damasio, A.R. (2000). Emotion, decision making and the orbitofrontal cortex. *Cerebral Cortex, 10*(3), 295–307. Retrieved from http://www.ncbi.nlm.nih.gov/pubmed/10731224

Bedny, M., McGill, M., & Thompson-Schill, S.L. (2008). Semantic adaptation and competition during word comprehension. *Cerebral Cortex, 18*(11), 2574–85. doi:10.1093/cercor/bhn018

Berthier, M.L. (2000). Transcortical aphasias. In S. Gilman, G.W. Goldstein, & S.G. Waxman (Eds.), *Neurobase* (3rd ed.). San Diego: Arbor Publishing.

Berthier, M.L. (2001). Unexpected brain-language relationships in aphasia: Evidence from transcortical sensory aphasia associated with frontal lobe lesions. *Aphasiology, 15*(2), 99–130. doi:10.1080/02687040042000179

Binder, J.R., McKiernan, K.A., Parsons, M.E., Westbury, C.F., Possing, E.T., Kaufman, J.N., & Buchanan, L. (2003). Neural correlates of lexical access during visual word recognition. *Journal of Cognitive Neuroscience, 15*(3), 372–93. doi:10.1162/089892903321593108

Binder, J.R., Desai, R.H., Graves, W.W., & Conant, L.L. (2009). Where is the semantic system? A critical review and meta-analysis of 120 functional neuroimaging studies. *Cerebral Cortex, 19*(12), 2767–96. doi:10.1093/cercor/bhp055

Binder, J.R., Medler, D.A., Desai, R., Conant, L.L., & Liebenthal, E. (2005). Some neurophysiological constraints on models of word naming. *NeuroImage, 27*(3), 677–93. doi:10.1016/j.neuroimage.2005.04.029

Binder, J.R., Gross, W.L., Allendorfer, J.B., Bonilha, L., Chapin, J., Edwards, J.C., . . . Weaver, K.E. (2011). Mapping anterior temporal lobe language areas with fMRI: A multicenter normative study. *NeuroImage, 54*(2), 1465–75. doi:10.1016/j.neuroimage.2010.09.048

Binney, R.J., Embleton, K. V, Jefferies, E., Parker, G.J.M., & Lambon Ralph, M.A. (2010). The ventral and inferolateral aspects of the anterior temporal lobe are crucial in semantic memory: Evidence from a novel direct comparison of distortion-corrected fMRI, rTMS, and semantic dementia. *Cerebral Cortex, 20*(11), 2728–38. doi:10.1093/cercor/bhq019

Boatman, D., Gordon, B., Hart, J., Selnes, O., Miglioretti, D., & Lenz, F. (2000). Transcortical sensory aphasia: Revisited and revised. *Brain, 123*(8), 1634–42. Retrieved from http://www.ncbi.nlm.nih.gov/pubmed/10908193

Bookheimer, S. (2002). Functional MRI of language: New approaches to understanding the cortical organization of semantic processing. *Annual Review of Neuroscience, 25*, 151–88. doi:10.1146/annurev.neuro.25.112701.142946

Bookheimer, S.Y., Zeffiro, T.A., Blaxton, T., Gaillard, W., & Theodore, W. (1995). Regional cerebral blood flow during object naming and word reading. *Human Brain Mapping, 3*(2), 93–106. doi:10.1002/hbm.460030206

Booth, J.R., Burman, D.D., Meyer, J.R., Gitelman, D.R., Parrish, T.B., & Mesulam, M.M. (2002). Modality independence of word comprehension. *Human Brain Mapping, 16*(4), 251–61. doi:10.1002/hbm.10054

Botvinick, M.M., Cohen, J.D., & Carter, C.S. (2004). Conflict monitoring and anterior cingulate cortex: An update. *Trends in Cognitive Sciences, 8*(12), 539–46. doi:10.1016/j.tics.2004.10.003

Bozeat, S., Lambon Ralph, M. A., Patterson, K., Garrard, P., & Hodges, J.R. (2000). Non-verbal semantic impairment in semantic dementia. *Neuropsychologia, 38*(9), 1207–15. Retrieved from http://www.ncbi.nlm.nih.gov/pubmed/10865096

Braver, T.S., Barch, D.M., Gray, J.R., Molfese, D.L., & Snyder, A. (2001). Anterior cingulate cortex and response conflict: Effects of frequency, inhibition and errors. *Cerebral Cortex, 11*(9), 825–36. Retrieved from http://www.ncbi.nlm.nih.gov/pubmed/11532888

Braver, T.S., Cohen, J.D., Nystrom, L.E., Jonides, J., Smith, E.E., & Noll, D.C. (1997). A parametric study of prefrontal cortex involvement in human working memory. *NeuroImage, 5*(1), 49–62. doi:10.1006/nimg.1996.0247

Breining, B.L., Lala, T., Cuitiño, M.M., Manes, F., Peristeri, E., Tsapkini, K., Faria, A.V., & Hillis, A.E. (2015). A brief assessment of object semantics in primary progressive aphasia. *Aphasiology, 29*, 488–505.

Bright, P., Moss, H., & Tyler, L.K. (2004). Unitary vs multiple semantics: PET studies of word and picture processing. *Brain and Language, 89*(3), 417–32. doi:10.1016/j.bandl.2004.01.010

Britton, J.C., Phan, K.L., Taylor, S.F., Welsh, R.C., Berridge, K.C., & Liberzon, I. (2006). Neural correlates of social and nonsocial emotions: An fMRI study. *NeuroImage, 31*(1), 397–409. doi:10.1016/j.neuroimage.2005.11.027

Cabeza, R., & Nyberg, L. (2000). Imaging cognition II: An empirical review of 275 PET and fMRI studies. *Journal of Cognitive Neuroscience, 12*(1), 1–47. Retrieved from http://www.ncbi.nlm.nih.gov/pubmed/10769304

Chee, M.W.L., Hon, N.H.H., Caplan, D., Lee, H.L., & Goh, J. (2002). Frequency of concrete words modulates prefrontal activation during semantic judgments. *NeuroImage, 16*(1), 259–68. doi:10.1006/nimg.2002.1061

Cloutman, L., Gottesman, R., Chaudhry, P., Davis, C., Kleinman, J.T., Pawlak, M., ... Hillis, A.E. (2009). Where (in the brain) do semantic errors come from? *Cortex, 45*(5), 641–9. doi:10.1016/j.cortex.2008.05.013

Corbett, F., Jefferies, E., Burns, A., & Lambon Ralph, M.A. (2012). Unpicking the semantic impairment in Alzheimer's disease: Qualitative changes with disease severity. *Behavioural Neurology, 25*(1), 23–34. doi:10.3233/BEN-2012-0346

Corbett, F., Jefferies, E., Ehsan, S., & Lambon Ralph, M.A. (2009). Different impairments of semantic cognition in semantic dementia and semantic aphasia: Evidence from the non-verbal domain. *Brain, 132*(Pt 9), 2593–608. doi:10.1093/brain/awp146

Costafreda, S.G., Fu, C.H.Y., Lee, L., Everitt, B., Brammer, M.J., & David, A.S. (2006). A systematic review and quantitative appraisal of fMRI studies of verbal fluency: Role of the left inferior frontal gyrus. *Human Brain Mapping, 27*(10), 799–810. doi:10.1002/hbm.20221

Damasio, H., Grabowski, T.J., Tranel, D., Hichwa, R.D., & Damasio, A.R. (1996). A neural basis for lexical retrieval. *Nature, 380*, 499–505.

De Zubicaray, G.I., Zelaya, F.O., Andrew, C., Williams, S.C., & Bullmore, E.T. (2000). Cerebral regions associated with verbal response initiation, suppression and strategy use. *Neuropsychologia, 38*(9), 1292–304. Retrieved from http://www.ncbi.nlm.nih.gov/pubmed/10865105

De Zubicaray, G., McMahon, K., Eastburn, M., & Pringle, A. (2006). Top-down influences on lexical selection during spoken word production: A 4T fMRI investigation of refractory effects in picture naming. *Human Brain Mapping, 27*(11), 864–73. doi:10.1002/hbm.20227

DeLeon, J., Gottesman, R.F., Kleinman, J.T., Newhart, M., Davis, C., Heidler-Gary, J., ... Hillis, A.E. (2007). Neural regions essential for distinct cognitive processes underlying picture naming. *Brain, 130*(5), 1408–22. doi:10.1093/brain/awm011

Desai, R., Conant, L.L., Waldron, E., & Binder, J.R. (2006). fMRI of past tense processing: The effects of phonological complexity and task difficulty. *Journal of Cognitive Neuroscience, 18*(2), 278–97.

Devlin, J.T., Matthews, P.M., & Rushworth, M.F.S. (2003). Semantic processing in the left inferior prefrontal cortex: A combined functional magnetic resonance imaging and transcranial magnetic stimulation study. *Journal of Cognitive Neuroscience, 15*(1), 71–84. doi:10.1162/089892903321107837

Devlin, J.T., & Watkins, K.E. (2007). Stimulating language: insights from TMS. *Brain, 130*(3), 610–22. doi:10.1093/brain/awl331

Dien, J., Brian, E.S., Molfese, D.L., & Gold, B.T. (2013). Combined ERP/fMRI evidence for early word recognition effects in the posterior inferior temporal gyrus. *Cortex, 49*(9), 2307–21. doi:10.1016/j.cortex.2013.03.008

Dräger, B., Jansen, A., Bruchmann, S., Förster, A.F., Pleger, B., Zwitserlood, P., & Knecht, S. (2004). How does the brain accommodate to increased task difficulty in word finding? A functional MRI study. *NeuroImage, 23*(3), 1152–60. doi:10.1016/j.neuroimage.2004.07.005

Drevets, W.C., Price, J.L., Simpson, J.R., Todd, R.D., Reich, R., Michael, V., & Raichle, M.E. (1997). Subgenual prefrontal cortex abnormalities in mood disorders. *Nature, 386*(6627), 824–7.

Duffau, H., Capelle, L., Sichez, N., Denvil, D., Lopes, M., Sichez, J-P., . . . Fohanno, D. (2002). Intraoperative mapping of the subcortical language pathways using direct stimulations. An anatomo-functional study. *Brain, 125*(1), 199–214. Retrieved from http://www.ncbi.nlm.nih.gov/pubmed/11834604

Duffau, H., Gatignol, P., Mandonnet, E., Peruzzi, P., Tzourio-Mazoyer, N., & Capelle, L. (2005). New insights into the anatomo-functional connectivity of the semantic system: A study using cortico-subcortical electrostimulations. *Brain, 128*(4), 797–810. doi:10.1093/brain/awh423

Duffau, H., Moritz-Gasser, S., & Mandonnet, E. (2013). A re-examination of neural basis of language processing: Proposal of a dynamic hodotopical model from data provided by brain stimulation mapping during picture naming. *Brain and Language, 131*, 1–10. doi:10.1016/j.bandl.2013.05.011

Duffau, H., Peggy Gatignol, S.T., Mandonnet, E., Capelle, L., & Taillandier, L. (2008). Intraoperative subcortical stimulation mapping of language pathways in a consecutive series of 115 patients with Grade II glioma in the left dominant hemisphere. *Journal of Neurosurgery, 109*(3), 461–71. doi:10.3171/JNS/2008/109/9/0461

Fellows, L.K., Heberlein, A.S., Morales, D. a, Shivde, G., Waller, S., & Wu, D.H. (2005). Method matters: An empirical study of impact in cognitive neuroscience. *Journal of Cognitive Neuroscience, 17*(6), 850–8. doi:10.1162/0898929054021139

Fiez, J.A. (1997). Phonology, semantics, and the role of the left inferior prefrontal cortex. *Human Brain Mapping, 5*(2), 79–83. Retrieved from http://www.ncbi.nlm.nih.gov/pubmed/10096412

Fiez, J.A., Balota, D.A., Raichle, M.E., & Petersen, S.E. (1999). Effects of lexicality, frequency, and spelling-to-sound consistency on the functional anatomy of reading. *Neuron, 24*(1), 205–18. Retrieved from http://www.ncbi.nlm.nih.gov/pubmed/10677038

Fu, C.H.Y., Morgan, K., Suckling, J., Williams, S.C.R., Andrew, C., Vythelingum, G.N., & McGuire, P.K. (2002). A functional magnetic resonance imaging study of overt letter verbal fluency using a clustered acquisition sequence: Greater anterior cingulate activation with increased task demand. *NeuroImage, 17*(2), 871–9. doi:10.1006/nimg.2002.1189

Gabrieli, J.D., Poldrack, R.A., & Desmond, J.E. (1998). The role of left prefrontal cortex in language and memory. *Proceedings of the National Academy of Sciences of the United States of America, 95*(3), 906–13. Retrieved from http://www.pubmedcentral.nih.gov/articlerender.fcgi?artid=33815&tool=pmcentrez&rendertype=abstract

Gainotti, G. (2000). What the locus of brain lesion tells us about the nature of the cognitive defect underlying category-specific disorders: A review. *Cortex, 36*(4), 539–59. Retrieved from http://www.ncbi.nlm.nih.gov/pubmed/11059454

Gainotti, G. (2005). The influence of gender and lesion location on naming disorders for animals, plants and artefacts. *Neuropsychologia, 43*(11), 1633–44.

Gatignol, P., Capelle, L., Bihan, R. Le, & Du, H. (2004). Double dissociation between picture naming and comprehension: An electrostimulation study. *NeuroReport, 15*(1), 191–5 doi:10.1097/01.wnr.0000099474.09597

Gennari, S.P., MacDonald, M.C., Postle, B.R., & Seidenberg, M.S. (2007). Context-dependent interpretation of words: Evidence for interactive neural processes. *NeuroImage, 35*(3), 1278–86. doi:10.1016/j.neuroimage.2007.01.015

Geschwind, N. (1970). The organization of language and the brain. *Science, 170*(3961), 940–4. Retrieved from http://www.ncbi.nlm.nih.gov/pubmed/5475022

Geschwind, N. (1972). Language and the brain. *Scientific American, 226*(4), 76–83.

Giesbrecht, B., Camblin, C.C., & Swaab, T.Y. (2004). Separable effects of semantic priming and imageability on word processing in human cortex. *Cerebral Cortex, 14*(5), 521–9. doi:10.1093/cercor/bhh014

Goodglass, H. (1993). *Understanding aphasia*. San Diego, CA: Academic Press.

Goodglass, H., & Wingfield, A. (Eds.). (1997). *Anomia: Neuroanatomical and cognitive correlates*. San Diego, CA: Academic Press.

Gold, B.T., Balota, D.A., Jones, S.J., Powell, D.K., Smith, C.D., & Andersen, A.H. (2006). Dissociation of automatic and strategic lexical-semantics: Functional magnetic resonance imaging evidence for differing roles of multiple frontotemporal regions. *The Journal of Neuroscience, 26*(24), 6523–32. doi:10.1523/JNEUROSCI.0808–06.2006

Gorno-Tempini, M.L., Dronkers, N.F., Rankin, K.P., Ogar, J.M., Phengrasamy, L., Rosen, H. J., . . . Miller, B.L. (2004). Cognition and anatomy in three variants of primary progressive aphasia. *Annals of Neurology, 55*(3), 335–346.

Gorno-Tempini, M.L., Hillis, A.E., Weintraub, S., Kertesz, A., Mendez, M., Cappa, S.F., . . . Grossman, M. (2011). Classification of primary progressive aphasia and its variants. *Neurology, 76*(11), 1006–14. doi:10.1212/WNL.0b013e31821103e6

Grady, C.L., Haxby, J.V., Horwitz, B., Sundaram, M., Berg, G., Schapiro, M., . . . & Rapoport, S.I. (1988). Longitudinal study of the early neuropsychological and cerebral metabolic changes in dementia of the Alzheimer type. *Journal of Clinical and Experimental Neuropsychology, 10*(5), 576–96.

Graves, W.W., Desai, R., Humphries, C., Seidenberg, M.S., & Binder, J.R. (2010). Neural systems for reading aloud: A multiparametric approach. *Cerebral Cortex, 20*(8), 1799–815. doi:10.1093/cercor/bhp245

Greene, J.D.W., Baddeley, A.D., & Hodges, J.R. (1996). Analysis of the episodic memory deficit in early Alzheimer's disease: Evidence from the doors and people test. *Neuropsychologia, 34*(6), 537–551. doi:10.1016/0028-3932(95)00151-4

Grossman, M., Koenig, P., Glosser, G., DeVita, C., Moore, P., Rhee, J., . . . Gee, J. (2003). Neural basis for semantic memory difficulty in Alzheimer's disease: An fMRI study. *Brain, 126*(2), 292–311.

Gurd, J.M., Amunts, K., Weiss, P.H., Zafiris, O., Zilles, K., Marshall, J.C., & Fink, G.R. (2002). Posterior parietal cortex is implicated in continuous switching between verbal fluency tasks: An fMRI study with clinical implications. *Brain, 125*(5), 1024–38. Retrieved from http://www.ncbi.nlm.nih.gov/pubmed/11960893

Hagoort, P., Indefrey, P., Brown, C., Herzog, H., Steinmetz, H., & Seitz, R.J. (1999). The neural circuitry involved in the reading of German words and pseudowords: A PET study. *Journal of Cognitive Neuroscience, 11*(4), 383–98. Retrieved from http://www.ncbi.nlm.nih.gov/pubmed/10471847

Hamberger, M.J., Seidel, W.T., Goodman, R.R., Perrine, K., & McKhann, G.M. (2003). Temporal lobe stimulation reveals anatomic distinction between auditory naming processes. *Neurology, 60*(9), 1478–83. doi:10.1212/01.WNL.0000061489.25675.3E

Hart, J., & Gordon, B. (1990). Delineation of single word semantic comprehension deficits in aphasia, with anatomical correlation. *Annals of Neurology, 27*(3), 226–31.

Hickok, G., & Poeppel, D. (2007). The cortical organization of speech processing. *Nature Reviews Neuroscience, 8*(5), 393–402.

Hillis, A.E., Barker, P.B., Beauchamp, N.J., Winters, B.D., Mirski, M., & Wityk, R.J. (2001). Restoring blood pressure reperfused Wernicke's area and improved language. *Neurology, 56*(5), 670–2. doi:10.1212/WNL.56.5.670

Hillis, A.E., & Caramazza, A. (1991). Category-specific naming and comprehension impairment: A double dissociation. *Brain, 114 (5)*, 2081–94. Retrieved from http://www.ncbi.nlm.nih.gov/pubmed/1933235

Hillis, A.E., & Caramazza, A. (1995). Representation of grammatical categories of words in the brain. *Journal of Cognitive Neuroscience, 7*(3), 396–407. doi:10.1162/jocn.1995.7.3.396

Hillis, A.E., & Heidler, J. (2002). Mechanisms of early aphasia recovery. *Aphasiology, 16*(9), 885–95. doi:10.1080/0268703

Hillis, A.E., Oh, S., & Ken, L. (2004). Deterioration of naming nouns versus verbs in primary progressive aphasia. *Annals of Neurology, 55*(2), 268–75. doi:10.1002/ana.10812

Hillis, A.E., Tuffiash, E., Wityk, R.J., & Barker, P.B. (2002). Regions of neural dysfunction associated with impaired naming of actions and objects in acute stroke. *Cognitive Neuropsychology, 19*(6), 523–34. doi:10.1080/02643290244000077

Hodges, J.R., Erzinçlioğlu, S., & Patterson, K. (2006). Evolution of cognitive deficits and conversion to dementia in patients with mild cognitive impairment: A very-long-term follow-up study. *Dementia and Geriatric Cognitive Disorders, 21*(5–6), 380–91. doi:10.1159/000092534

Hodges, J.R., & Patterson, K. (1995). Is semantic memory consistently impaired early in the course of Alzheimer's disease? Neuroanatomical and diagnostic implications. *Neuropsychologia, 33*(4), 441–59.

Hoenig, K., & Scheef, L. (2009). Neural correlates of semantic ambiguity processing during context verification. *NeuroImage, 45*(3), 1009–19. doi:10.1016/j.neuroimage.2008.12.044

Homae, F., Hashimoto, R., Nakajima, K., Miyashita, Y., & Sakai, K.L. (2002). From perception to sentence comprehension: The convergence of auditory and visual information of language in the left inferior frontal cortex. *NeuroImage, 16*(4), 883–900. doi:10.1006/nimg.2002.1138

Humphries, C., Binder, J.R., Medler, D.A., & Liebenthal, E. (2006). Syntactic and semantic modulation of neural activity during auditory sentence comprehension. *Journal of Cognitive Neuroscience, 18*(4), 665–79. doi:10.1162/jocn.2006.18.4.665

Indefrey, P., & Levelt, W.J.M. (2004). The spatial and temporal signatures of word production components. *Cognition, 92*(1–2), 101–44. doi:10.1016/j.cognition.2002.06.001

Ischebeck, A., Indefrey, P., Usui, N., Nose, I., Hellwig, F., & Taira, M. (2004). Reading in a regular orthography: An FMRI study investigating the role of visual familiarity. *Journal of Cognitive Neuroscience, 16*(5), 727–41. doi:10.1162/089892904970708

Jefferies, E., & Lambon Ralph, M.A. (2006). Semantic impairment in stroke aphasia versus semantic dementia: A case-series comparison. *Brain*, 129(8), 2132–47. doi:10.1093/brain/awl153

Jefferies, E., Patterson, K., Jones, R.W., & Lambon Ralph, M.A. (2009). Comprehension of concrete and abstract words in semantic dementia. *Neuropsychology, 23*(4), 492–9. doi:10.1037/a0015452.

Jonides, J., Schumacher, E.H., Smith, E.E., Lauber, E.J., Awh, E., Minoshima, S., & Koeppe, R.A. (1997). Verbal working memory load affects regional brain activation as measured by PET. *Journal of Cognitive Neuroscience, 9*(4), 462–75. doi:10.1162/jocn.1997.9.4.462

Kapur, N., Barker, S., Burrows, E.H., Ellison, D., Brice, J., Illis, L.S., . . . Loates, M. (1994). Herpes simplex encephalitis: Long term magnetic resonance imaging and neuropsychological profile. *Journal of Neurology, Neurosurgery, and Psychiatry, 57*(11), 1334–42. Retrieved from http://www.pubmedcentral.nih.gov/articlerender.fcgi?artid=1073183&tool=pmcentrez&rendertype=abstract

Kapur, S., Rose, R., Liddle, P.F., Zipursky, R.B., Brown, G.M., Stuss, D., Houle, S., & Tulving, E. (1994). The role of the left prefrontal cortex in verbal processing: Semantic processing or willed action? *NeuroReport, 5*, 2193–6.

Kennedy, P.G.E., & Chaudhuri, A. (2002). Herpes simplex encephalitis. *Journal of Neurology, Neurosurgery, and Psychiatry, 73*(3), 237–8. Retrieved from http://www.pubmedcentral.nih.gov/articlerender.fcgi?artid=1738005&tool=pmcentrez&rendertype=abstract

Kerns, J.G., Cohen, J.D., MacDonald, A.W., Cho, R.Y., Stenger, V.A., & Carter, C.S. (2004). Anterior cingulate conflict monitoring and adjustments in control. *Science, 303*(5660), 1023–6. doi:10.1126/science.1089910

Kertesz, A., Sheppard, A., & Mackenzie, R. (1982). Localization in transcortical sensory aphasia. *Archives of Neurology, 39*(8), 475–8.

Kiehl, K.A., Liddle, P.F., & Hopfinger, J.B. (2000). Error processing and the rostral anterior cingulate: An event-related fMRI study. *Psychophysiology, 37*(2), 216–23. Retrieved from http://www.ncbi.nlm.nih.gov/pubmed/10731771

Knibb, J.A., Xuereb, J.H., Patterson, K., & Hodges, J.R. (2006). Clinical and pathological characterization of progressive aphasia. *Annals of Neurology, 59*(1), 156–65. doi:10.1002/ana.20700

Kotz, S. (2002). Modulation of the lexical–semantic network by auditory semantic priming: An event-related functional MRI study. *NeuroImage, 17*(4), 1761–72. doi:10.1006/nimg.2002.1316

Lambo Ralph, M.A., Patterson, K., Garrard, P., & Hodges, J.R. (2003). Semantic dementia with category specificity: A comparative case-series study. *Cognitive Neuropsychology, 20*(3), 307–26. doi:10.1080/02643290244000301

Lambon Ralph, M.A., Lowe, C., & Rogers, T.T. (2007). Neural basis of category-specific semantic deficits for living things: Evidence from semantic dementia, HSVE and a neural network model. *Brain: A Journal of Neurology, 130*(Pt 4), 1127–37. doi:10.1093/brain/awm025

Lambon Ralph, M.A., Pobric, G., & Jefferies, E. (2009). Conceptual knowledge is underpinned by the temporal pole bilaterally: Convergent evidence from rTMS. *Cerebral Cortex, 19*(4), 832–8. doi:10.1093/cercor/bhn131

Liddle, P.F., Kiehl, K.A., & Smith, A.M. (2001). Event-related fMRI study of response inhibition. *Human Brain Mapping, 12*(2), 100–9. Retrieved from http://www.ncbi.nlm.nih.gov/pubmed/11169874

Lindell, A.K. (2006). In your right mind: Right hemisphere contributions to language processing and production. *Neuropsychology Review, 16*(3), 131–48. doi:10.1007/s11065-006-9011-9

Mahon, B.Z., & Caramazza, A. (2009). Concepts and categories: A cognitive neuropsychological perspective. *Annual Review of Psychology, 60*, 27–51. doi:10.1146/annurev.psych.60.110707.163532

Mandonnet, E., Nouet, A., Gatignol, P., Capelle, L., & Duffau, H. (2007). Does the left inferior longitudinal fasciculus play a role in language? A brain stimulation study. *Brain, 130*(3), 623–9. doi:10.1093/brain/awl361

Mandonnet, E., Winkler, P.A., & Duffau, H. (2010). Direct electrical stimulation as an input gate into brain functional networks: Principles, advantages and limitations. *Acta Neurochirurgica, 152*(2), 185–93. doi:10.1007/s00701–009–0469–0

Martin, A. (2007). The representation of object concepts in the brain. *Annual Review of Psychology, 58*, 25–45. doi:10.1146/annurev.psych.57.102904.190143

Mayberg, H.S., Liotti, M., Brannan, S.K., McGinnis, S., Mahurin, R.K., Jerabek, P.A., . . . Fox, P.T. (1999). Reciprocal limbic-cortical function and negative mood: Converging PET findings in depression and normal sadness. *American Journal of Psychiatry, 156*(5), 675–82. Retrieved from http://www.ncbi.nlm.nih.gov/pubmed/10327898

McDermott, K.B., Petersen, S.E., Watson, J.M., & Ojemann, J.G. (2003). A procedure for identifying regions preferentially activated by attention to semantic and phonological relations using functional magnetic resonance imaging. *Neuropsychologia, 41*(3), 293–303. Retrieved from http://www.ncbi.nlm.nih.gov/pubmed/12457755

Moore, C.J., & Price, C.J. (1999). A functional neuroimaging study of the variables that generate category-specific object processing differences. *Brain, 122*, 943–62. Retrieved from http://www.ncbi.nlm.nih.gov/pubmed/10355678

Mummery, C.J., Patterson, K., Hodges, J.R., & Price, C.J. (1998). Functional neuroanatomy of the semantic system: Divisible by what? *Journal of Cognitive Neuroscience, 10*(6), 766–77. Retrieved from http://www.ncbi.nlm.nih.gov/pubmed/9831743

Nestor, P.J., Fryer, T.D., & Hodges, J.R. (2006). Declarative memory impairments in Alzheimer's disease and semantic dementia. *NeuroImage*, 30(3), 1010–20. doi:10.1016/j.neuroimage.2005.10.008

Nestor, P.J., Fryer, T.D., Smielewski, P., & Hodges, J.R. (2003). Limbic hypometabolism in Alzheimer's disease and mild cognitive impairment. *Annals of Neurology, 54*(3), 343–51. doi:10.1002/ana.10669Noppeney, U., Josephs, O., Hocking, J., Price, C.J., & Friston, K.J. (2008). The effect of prior visual information on recognition of speech and sounds. *Cerebral Cortex, 18*(3), 598–609. doi:10.1093/cercor/bhm091

Noppeney, U., Patterson, K., Tyler, L.K., Moss, H., Stamatakis, E.A., Bright, P., . . . Price, C.J. (2007). Temporal lobe lesions and semantic impairment: A comparison of herpes simplex virus encephalitis and semantic dementia. *Brain, 130*(4), 1138–47. doi:10.1093/brain/awl344

Noppeney, U., Phillips, J., & Price, C. (2004). The neural areas that control the retrieval and selection of semantics. *Neuropsychologia, 42*(9), 1269–80. doi:10.1016/j.neuropsychologia.2003.12.014

Noppeney, U., & Price, C.J. (2002). A PET study of stimulus- and task-induced semantic processing. *Neuro-Image, 15*(4), 927–35. doi:10.1006/nimg.2001.1015

Novick, J.M., Trueswell, J.C., & Thompson-Schill, S.L. (2005). Cognitive control and parsing: Reexamining the role of Broca's area in sentence comprehension. *Cognitive, Affective, & Behavioral Neuroscience, 5*(3), 263–81. doi:10.3758/CABN.5.3.263

Nyberg, L., Marklund, P., Persson, J., Cabeza, R., Forkstam, C., Petersson, K.M., & Ingvar, M. (2003). Common prefrontal activations during working memory, episodic memory, and semantic memory. *Neuropsychologia, 41*(3), 371–7. Retrieved from http://www.ncbi.nlm.nih.gov/pubmed/12457761

Ojemann, G., Ojemann, J., Lettich, E., & Berger, M. (1989). Cortical language localization in left, dominant hemisphere. An electrical stimulation mapping investigation in 117 patients. *Journal of Neurosurgery, 71*(3), 316–326.

Pascual-Leone, A., Walsh, V., & Rothwell, J. (2000). Transcranial magnetic stimulation in cognitive neuroscience—virtual lesion, chronometry, and functional connectivity. *Current Opinion in Neurobiology, 10*(2), 232–7. Retrieved from http://www.ncbi.nlm.nih.gov/pubmed/10753803

Patterson, K., Nestor, P.J., & Rogers, T.T. (2007). Where do you know what you know? The representation of semantic knowledge in the human brain. *Nature Reviews Neuroscience, 8*(12), 976–87. doi:10.1038/nrn2277

Peelle, J.E., McMillan, C., Moore, P., Grossman, M., & Wingfield, A. (2004). Dissociable patterns of brain activity during comprehension of rapid and syntactically complex speech: Evidence from fMRI. *Brain and Language, 91*(3), 315–25. doi:10.1016/j.bandl.2004.05.007

Perani, D., Paulesu, E., Galles, N.S., Dupoux, E., Dehaene, S., Bettinardi, V., . . . Mehler, J. (1998). The bilingual brain. Proficiency and age of acquisition of the second language. *Brain: A Journal of Neurology, 121*(Pt 1), 1841–52. Retrieved from http://www.ncbi.nlm.nih.gov/pubmed/9798741

Petersen, S.E., Fox, P.T., Posner, M.I., Mintun, M., & Raichle, M.E. (1988). Positron emission tomographic studies of cortical anatomy of single-word processing. *Nature, 331*(6257), 585–9.

Petersen, S.E., Fox, P.T., Posner, M.I., Mintun, M., & Raichle, M.E. (1989). Positron emission tomographic studies of the processing of singe words. *Journal of Cognitive Neuroscience, 1*(2), 153–70. doi:10.1162/jocn.1989.1.2.153

Phan, K.L., Wager, T., Taylor, S.F., & Liberzon, I. (2002). Functional neuroanatomy of emotion: A meta-analysis of emotion activation studies in PET and fMRI. *NeuroImage, 16*(2), 331–48. doi:10.1006/nimg.2002.1087

Pobric, G., Jefferies, E., & Lambon Ralph, M.A. (2007). Anterior temporal lobes mediate semantic representation: mimicking semantic dementia by using rTMS in normal participants. *Proceedings of the National Academy of Sciences of the United States of America, 104*(50), 20137–41. doi:10.1073/pnas.0707383104

Poldrack, R.A., Wagner, A.D., Prull, M.W., Desmond, J.E., Glover, G.H., & Gabrieli, J.D. (1999). Functional specialization for semantic and phonological processing in the left inferior prefrontal cortex. *NeuroImage, 10*(1), 15–35. doi:10.1006/nimg.1999.0441

Price, C.J. (2010). The anatomy of language: A review of 100 fMRI studies published in 2009. *Annals of the New York Academy of Sciences, 1191*, 62–88. doi:10.1111/j.1749–6632.2010.05444.x

Price, C.J. (2012). A review and synthesis of the first 20 years of PET and fMRI studies of heard speech, spoken language and reading. *NeuroImage, 62*(2), 816–47. doi:10.1016/j.neuroimage.2012.04.062

Raettig, T., & Kotz, S.A. (2008). Auditory processing of different types of pseudo-words: an event-related fMRI study. *NeuroImage, 39*(3), 1420–8. doi:10.1016/j.neuroimage.2007.09.030

Rodd, J.M., Davis, M.H., & Johnsrude, I.S. (2005). The neural mechanisms of speech comprehension: fMRI studies of semantic ambiguity. *Cerebral Cortex, 15*(8), 1261–9. doi:10.1093/cercor/bhi009

Rogalsky, C., & Hickok, G. (2009). Selective attention to semantic and syntactic features modulates sentence processing networks in anterior temporal cortex. *Cerebral Cortex, 19*(4), 786–96. doi:10.1093/cercor/bhn126

Rossell, S.A., Bullmore, E.T., Williams, S.C., & David, A.S. (2001). Brain activation during automatic and controlled processing of semantic relations: A priming experiment using lexical-decision. *Neuropsychologia, 39*(11), 1167–76. Retrieved from http://www.ncbi.nlm.nih.gov/pubmed/11527554

Sanai, N., Mirzadeh, Z., & Berger, M.S. (2008). Functional outcome after language mapping for glioma resection. *The New England Journal of Medicine, 358*(1), 18–27. doi:10.1056/NEJMoa067819

Saur, D., Kreher, B.W., Schnell, S., Kümmerer, D., Kellmeyer, P., Vry, M.-S., . . . Weiller, C. (2008). Ventral and dorsal pathways for language. *Proceedings of the National Academy of Sciences of the United States of America, 105*(46), 18035–40. doi:10.1073/pnas.0805234105

Schaffler, L., Lüders, H.O., Dinner, D.S., Lesser, R.P., & Chelune, G.J. (1993). Comprehension deficits elicited by electrical stimulation of Broca's area. *Brain, 116*, 695–715.

Schaffler, L., Luders, H.O., & Beck, G.J. (1996). Quantitative comparison of language deficits produced by extraoperative electrical stimulation of Broca's, Wernicke's, and basal temporal language areas. *Epilepsia, 37*(5), 463–75. doi:10.1111/j.1528–1157.1996.tb00593.x

Schwartz, M.F., Kimberg, D.Y., Walker, G.M., Faseyitan, O., Brecher, A., Dell, G.S., & Coslett, H.B. (2009). Anterior temporal involvement in semantic word retrieval: Voxel-based lesion-symptom mapping evidence from aphasia. *Brain, 132*(12), 3411–27. doi:10.1093/brain/awp284

Scott, S.K., Leff, A.P., & Wise, R.J. (2003). Going beyond the information given: A neural system supporting semantic interpretation. *NeuroImage, 19*(3), 870–876. doi:10.1016/S1053–8119(03)00083–1

Seghier, M.L., Fagan, E., & Price, C.J. (2010). Functional subdivisions in the left angular gyrus where the semantic system meets and diverges from the default network. *The Journal of Neuroscience, 30*(50), 16809–17. doi:10.1523/JNEUROSCI.3377–10.2010

Sevostianov, A., Horwitz, B., Nechaev, V., Williams, R., Fromm, S., & Braun, A.R. (2002). fMRI study comparing names versus pictures of objects. *Human Brain Mapping, 16*(3), 168–75. doi:10.1002/hbm.10037

Sharp, D.J., Awad, M., Warren, J.E., Wise, R.J.S., Vigliocco, G., & Scott, S.K. (2010). The neural response to changing semantic and perceptual complexity during language processing. *Human Brain Mapping, 31*(3), 365–77. doi:10.1002/hbm.20871

Snijders, T.M., Vosse, T., Kempen, G., Van Berkum, J.J.A., Petersson, K.M., & Hagoort, P. (2009). Retrieval and unification of syntactic structure in sentence comprehension: An fMRI study using word-category ambiguity. *Cerebral Cortex, 19*(7), 1493–503. doi:10.1093/cercor/bhn187

Snyder, H.R., Feigenson, K., & Thompson-Schill, S.L. (2007). Prefrontal cortical response to conflict during semantic and phonological tasks prefrontal cortical response to conflict during semantic and phonological tasks. *Journal of Cognitive Neuroscience, 19*(5), 761–75.

Thompson-Schill, S.L. (2003). Neuroimaging studies of semantic memory: Inferring "how" from "where." *Neuropsychologia, 41*(3), 280–92. Retrieved from http://www.ncbi.nlm.nih.gov/pubmed/12457754

Thompson-Schill, S.L., D'Esposito, M., Aguirre, G.K., & Farah, M.J. (1997). Role of left inferior prefrontal cortex in retrieval of semantic knowledge: A reevaluation. *Proceedings of the National Academy of Sciences of the United States of America, 94*(26), 14792–7. Retrieved from http://www.pubmedcentral.nih.gov/articlerender.fcgi?artid=25116&tool=pmcentrez&rendertype=abstract

Turken, A.U., & Dronkers, N.F. (2011). The neural architecture of the language comprehension network: Converging evidence from lesion and connectivity analyses. *Frontiers in Systems Neuroscience, 5*(2), 1. doi:10.3389/fnsys.2011.00001

Turkeltaub, P.E., & Coslett, H.B. (2010). Localization of sublexical speech perception components. *Brain and Language, 114*(1), 1–15. doi:10.1016/j.bandl.2010.03.008

Vigneau, M., Beaucousin, V., Hervé, P.Y., Duffau, H., Crivello, F., Houdé, O., . . . Tzourio-Mazoyer, N. (2006). Meta-analyzing left hemisphere language areas: Phonology, semantics, and sentence processing. *NeuroImage, 30*(4), 1414–32. doi:10.1016/j.neuroimage.2005.11.002

Vigneau, M., Beaucousin, V., Hervé, P.-Y., Jobard, G., Petit, L., Crivello, F., . . . Tzourio-Mazoyer, N. (2011). What is right-hemisphere contribution to phonological, lexico-semantic, and sentence processing? Insights from a meta-analysis. *NeuroImage, 54*(1), 577–93. doi:10.1016/j.neuroimage.2010.07.036

Vingerhoets, G., Borsel, J.V., Tesink, C., Noort, M.V.D., Deblaere, K., Seurinck, R., . . . Achten, E. (2003). Multilingualism: An fMRI study. *NeuroImage, 20*(4), 2181–96. doi:10.1016/j.neuroimage.2003.07.029no

Visser, M., Jefferies, E., & Lambon Ralph, M.A. (2010). Semantic processing in the anterior temporal lobes: A meta-analysis of the functional neuroimaging literature. *Journal of Cognitive Neuroscience, 22*(6), 1083–94. doi:10.1162/jocn.2009.21309

Visser, M., & Lambon Ralph, M.A. (2011). Differential contributions of bilateral ventral anterior temporal lobe and left anterior superior temporal gyrus to semantic processes. *Journal of Cognitive Neuroscience, 23*(10), 3121–31. doi:10.1162/jocn_a_00007

Wagner, A. D., Paré-Blagoev, E.J., Clark, J., & Poldrack, R.A. (2001). Recovering meaning: Left prefrontal cortex guides controlled semantic retrieval. *Neuron, 31*(2), 329–38. Retrieved from http://www.ncbi.nlm.nih.gov/pubmed/11502262

Walsh, V., & Cowey, A. (2000). Transcranial magnetic stimulation and cognitive neuroscience. *Nature Reviews Neuroscience, 1*(1), 73–9. doi:10.1038/35036239

Walsh, V., & Rushworth, M. (1999). A primer of magnetic stimulation as a tool for neuropsychology. *Neuropsychologia, 37*(2), 125–35. Retrieved from http://www.ncbi.nlm.nih.gov/pubmed/10080370

Warrington, E.K., & McCarthy, R.A. (1987). Categories of knowledge. *Brain, 110*(5), 1273–96. doi:10.1093/brain/110.5.1273

Warrington, E.K., & McCarthy, R.A. (1994). Multiple meaning systems in the brain: A case for visual semantics. *Neuropsychologia, 32*(12), 1465–73.

Warrington, E.K., & Shallice, T. (1984). Category specific semantic impairments. *Brain, 107*, 829–53.

Wernicke, C. (1874). *Der Aphasische Symptomen Komplex.* Breslau: Cohn & Weigart.

Whitney, C., Huber, W., Klann, J., Weis, S., Krach, S., & Kircher, T. (2009). Neural correlates of narrative shifts during auditory story comprehension. *NeuroImage, 47*(1), 360–6. doi:10.1016/j.neuroimage.2009.04.037

Whitney, C., Jefferies, E., & Kircher, T. (2011). Heterogeneity of the left temporal lobe in semantic representation and control: Priming multiple versus single meanings of ambiguous words. *Cerebral Cortex, 21*(4), 831–44. doi:10.1093/cercor/bhq148

Whitney, C., Kirk, M., O'Sullivan, J., Ralph, M.A.L., & Jefferies, E. (2011). Executive semantic processing is underpinned by a large-scale neural network: Revealing the contribution of left prefrontal, posterior temporal, and parietal cortex to controlled retrieval and selection using TMS. *Journal of Cognitive Neuroscience, 24*(1), 133–47.

Ye, Z., & Zhou, X. (2009). Conflict control during sentence comprehension: fMRI evidence. *NeuroImage, 48*(1), 280–90. doi:10.1016/j.neuroimage.2009.06.032

Zempleni, M.-Z., Renken, R., Hoeks, J.C.J., Hoogduin, J.M., & Stowe, L.A. (2007). Semantic ambiguity processing in sentence context: Evidence from event-related fMRI. *NeuroImage, 34*(3), 1270–9. doi:10.1016/j.neuroimage.2006.09.048

12

DIAGNOSIS AND TREATMENT OF SEMANTIC IMPAIRMENTS

Sofia Vallila-Rohter and Swathi Kiran

Introduction

Much progress has been made in our understanding of language processing, with many theories emerging specifically related to semantic processing. Such theories are important in the interpretation and understanding of semantic deficits that arise in aphasia. In addition, research in aphasia has led to the observation that multiple distinct and specific patterns arise in semantic deficits. An understanding of the specific deficits that arise in semantic aphasia is therefore critical for appropriate diagnosis and treatment. Clinicians must learn to observe patterns of errors and word finding difficulties as they surface in individual patients. Available theories can then help clinicians understand how to interpret these errors within the semantic system as a whole in order to select appropriate evidence-based therapies.

In this chapter, we will outline methods of diagnosing semantic deficits within the context of available semantic processing theories. We will review currently researched treatment methods and discuss strengths and limitations of these treatments.

Assessment of Semantic Deficits

Model Constructs Guiding Assessment

Two broad views of the semantic system are most often discussed in the research literature: a modality-specific view and an amodal view. Theories that support the modality-specific view suggest that we have multiple semantic systems: a visual semantic system, a tactile semantic system, a verbal semantic system, etc. (McCarthy & Warrington, 1988; Shallice, 1988). The conceptual store of information into each of these semantic systems depends upon the modality of input and will also influence the modality of output. Words encountered through reading, for example, will be stored in an orthographic semantic system, with the most direct output form being a written word. Words experienced auditorily will be stored in the verbal semantic system, leading most directly to spoken-word output (see Figure 12.1). Under these types of modal accounts of semantic organization, information in each system can be accessed via multiple modalities, but access from alternate modalities is indirect, and therefore potentially incomplete.

In contrast, amodal views of semantic organization propose that we have one unified conceptual store, and that the semantic system is therefore the same regardless of the input modality or desired output modality (Caramazza, Hillis, Rapp, & Romani, 1990; Caramazza & Mahon,

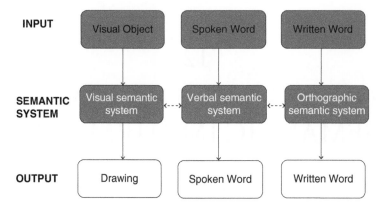

INPUT — Visual Object, Spoken Word, Written Word

SEMANTIC SYSTEM — Visual semantic system, Verbal semantic system, Orthographic semantic system

OUTPUT — Drawing, Spoken Word, Written Word

Figure 12.1 Representation of a modal view of the semantic system in which input modality influences the modality of output. Although this is one instantiation of a modality-specific semantics account, other possibilities exist, and it is not clear that any authors have clearly proposed this particular account (Caramazza et al., 1990; see also chapter 10, this volume).

2003; Humphreys & Forde, 2001; Lambon Ralph, McClelland, Patterson, Galton, & Hodges, 2001; McClelland & Rogers, 2003; Rogers & McClelland, 2008; Taylor, Devereux, & Tyler, 2011; Tyler & Moss, 2001). Amodal accounts are often based on connectionist principles or correlated structure principles (see Capitani et al., 2003). Correlated experience leads to differential weighting of perceptual characteristics among items and categories (McClelland & Rogers, 2003; Tyler & Moss, 2001). Concepts are therefore gradually organized into feature lists or semantic descriptions that are distributed across perceptual networks regardless of the modality of initial input (Barsalou, Kyle Simmons, Barbey, & Wilson, 2003). The result is a single semantic system that contains several organizational attributes (see Figure 12.2).

Among the organizing principles of the semantic system are concept category (Kolinsky et al., 2002; Tyler & Moss, 2001), object properties and features (Garrard, Ralph, Hodges, & Patterson, 2001; Warrington & McCarthy, 1987), typicality (Garrard et al., 2001; Kiran & Thompson, 2003a; Rosch & Mervis, 1975), frequency (Kittredge, Dell, Verkuilen, & Schwartz, 2008; Nozari, Kittredge, Dell, & Schwartz, 2010), imageability (Nickels & Howard, 1995), and part of speech (Bird, Howard, & Franklin, 2000). Each of the organizational properties of the semantic system is susceptible to damage, therefore each is important to characterize in the assessment of semantic impairment in aphasia.

Assessing the Modality of Deficits

Several studies have examined semantic impairments under specific modality access conditions. For instance, studies have assessed nonverbal comprehension using tasks such as selecting the appropriate color for objects (De Renzi, Faglioni, Scotti, & Spinnler, 1972; Miceli et al., 2001), demonstrating appropriate object use (Bozeat, Lambon Ralph, Patterson, & Hodges, 2002), matching environmental sounds to pictures (Caramazza & Shelton, 1998; Saygin, Dick, Wilson, Dronkers, & Bates, 2003; Spinnler & Vignolo, 1966; Varney, 1980), and matching gestures to pictures (Gainotti & Lemmo, 1976). Such tests examine the integrity of concept knowledge and access to and from the semantic system when written language or spoken speech are neither the input nor output modalities (see Table 12.1).

In addition to examining concept knowledge from multiple modalities, many studies have designed semantic batteries that specifically examine whether dissociations arise between modalities

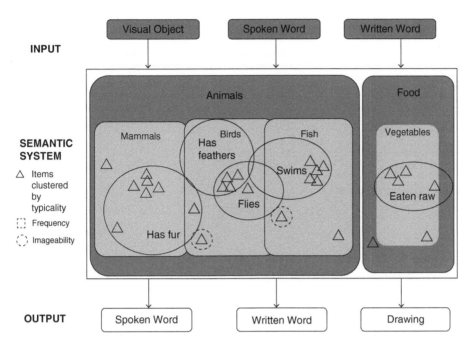

INPUT

SEMANTIC
SYSTEM

△ Items
clustered
by
typicality

⟦⟧ Frequency

⟨⟩ Imageability

OUTPUT

Figure 12.2 Representation of an amodal view of the semantic system that specifies a unified conceptual store organized in terms of attributes such as categories, features, frequency, typicality, imageability, and part of speech. Note that most architectures specify a number of additional cognitive processes that must be computed between modality-specific input and the semantic system, and between the semantic system and modality-specific output (not shown here, as the emphasis is on the semantic system; see chapter 7, this volume, for models of naming).

Table 12.1 Assessments of Specific Modalities

Input Modality	Output Modality/Task	References
Nonverbal comprehension		
Environmental sounds and pictures	Matching task	Bozeat et al., 2002; Garrard & Carroll, 2006; Saygin et al., 2003; Spinnler & Vignolo, 1966; Varney, 1980
Gestures and pictures	Matching task	Gainotti & Lemmo, 1976
Colors and objects	Matching task	De Renzi et al., 1972; Garrard & Carroll, 2006; Miceli et al., 2001
Familiar objects	Drawing objects from memory	Gainotti, Silveri, Villa, & Caltagirone, 1983
Familiar objects	Object use	Bozeat et al., 2002
Performed actions and pictured actions	Matching task	Bozeat et al., 2002
Object pictures and function pictures	Matching task	Bozeat et al., 2002
Tool pictures and recipient pictures (e.g., garlic press with garlic, onion, pepper or cheese)	Matching task	Bozeat et al., 2002

(Continued)

Table 12.1   (Continued)

Input Modality	Output Modality/Task	References
Verbal comprehension		
Spoken words and pictures	Matching task	Levin et al., 2005
Written words and pictures	Matching task	Bozeat et al., 2002; Jefferies & Lambon Ralph, 2006; Levin et al., 2005
Sounds and written words	Matching task	Bozeat et al., 2002
Spoken words and pictures	Matching task	Bozeat et al., 2002
Naming to distinct modalities		
Pictures	Spoken naming	Caramazza & Shelton, 1998; Hart & Gordon, 1992; Levin et al., 2005; Sartori & Job, 1988
Familiar objects	Spoken naming	Bozeat et al., 2002; Hart & Gordon, 1992; Levin et al., 2005
Auditory stimuli/sounds	Spoken naming	Levin et al., 2005
Definitions	Spoken naming	Levin et al., 2005; Sartori & Job, 1988
Additional output modalities		
Pictures	Written naming	Hillis & Caramazza, 1991
Familiar objects	Written naming	Levin et al., 2005
Normed assessments/ item lists		
Pyramids and Palm Trees Test (PPT)	Test of semantic association: Picture and written word versions	Howard & Patterson, 1992
Camel and Cactus Test (CCT)	Test of semantic association: Picture and written word versions	Bozeat et al., 2000
Psycholinguistic Assessment of Language (PAL)	Spoken and written word-picture matching, spoken and written sentence-picture matching, written picture naming subtests	Caplan & Bub, 1990
Psycholinguistic Assessment of Language Processing in Aphasia (PALPA)	Picture naming, picture matching subtests	Kay et al., 1992
Boston Diagnostic Aphasia Exam (BDAE)	Spoken word to picture matching, spoken and written picture naming, picture-word match	Goodglass et al., 2000
Boston Naming Test (BNT)	Picture naming	Kaplan, Goodglass, & Weintraub, 1983
Northwestern Naming Battery (NNB)	Picture naming, spoken word recognition	Thompson, Lukic, King, Mesulam, & Weintraub, 2012
Western Aphasia Battery (WAB)	Spoken and written word to picture matching, spoken and written word to object matching, object naming	Kertesz, 1982
260-item picture list (black-and-white line drawings)	Picture naming	Snodgrass & Vanderwart, 1980

(Bozeat et al., 2002; Jefferies & Lambon Ralph, 2006; Levin, Ben-Hur, Biran, & Wertman, 2005; Warrington & Crutch, 2007). Jefferies and Lambon Ralph (2006) for example, described a semantic battery of tests designed to provide a comparison of semantic performance based on input and output modality. Specifically, researchers included three versions of an environmental sounds test: word-picture matching, sound-picture matching, and sound-word matching. Target items were identical across conditions so that researchers could directly compare performance across modalities. Similarly, performance was compared on picture and word versions of the Pyramids and Palm Trees (PPT) test (D. Howard & Patterson, 1992) and the Camel and Cactus test (CCT; Bozeat et al., 2002). Both of these are normed assessments that present participants with a target item accompanied by two (PPT) to four (CCT) additional items. Participants are instructed to select the item that is most closely associated with the target. Assessments are administered in two forms: a picture form and a written word form. Items are matched across forms to allow for comparisons between linguistic and nonlinguistic versions of the task. Such comparisons provide insights into a patient's representational system for words and for pictures.

Experiments examining the dissociation between modalities have compared performance between tasks in which input modality is held constant but output modality is varied, such as oral naming and written naming (Hillis & Caramazza, 1991; Levin et al., 2005) or object naming versus object use (Bozeat et al., 2002). Studies have also held output modality constant while varying input modality, comparing performance on tasks such as written versus spoken-word comprehension (Warrington & Crutch, 2007) or naming to auditory stimuli compared with naming of tactile objects and naming to definition (Levin et al., 2005).

Identifying Category-Specific Deficits

In addition to the modality-specific deficits that can arise in aphasia, many studies have demonstrated the presence of category-specific deficits (Bunn, Tyler, & Moss, 1998; Capitani, Laiacona, Mahon, & Caramazza, 2003; Farah, McMullen, & Meyer, 1991; Hart & Gordon, 1992; Laiacona, Capitani, & Barbarotto, 1997; Warrington & Shallice, 1984). Naming deficits are more often seen among categories of living things over nonliving things. Categories of artifacts such as tools are less frequently impacted (Bunn, et al., 1998; Capitani, et al., 2003; Farah et al., 1991; Hart & Gordon, 1992; Laiacona, Barbarotto, & Capitani, 1993; Sartori & Job, 1988; Warrington & Shallice, 1984).

Category-specific deficits are often thought to arise because categories differentially depend on individual modalities or semantic features. Categories of living things, for example, contain items often referred to via visually descriptive features that likely lead to a robust visual semantic representation. In contrast, nonliving things such as manipulable artifacts are more likely to be described by their function and will have more robust functional associations and representations (see Capitani et al., 2003 for a review). Consequently, researchers hypothesize that impairments impacting visual-sensory modalities or sensory properties will have a greater likelihood of impairing naming for living than for nonliving things, thus leading to the higher incidence of naming deficits for living things.

Naming tasks are frequently used to assess naming ability for categories of living and nonliving things (Bi et al., 2011; Caramazza & Shelton, 1998; Crutch, Randlesome, & Warrington, 2007; De Renzi & Lucchelli, 1994; Farah & Wallace, 1992; Hart, Berndt, & Caramazza, 1985; Hart & Gordon, 1992; Samson & Pillon, 2003; Sartori & Job, 1988; Snodgrass & Vanderwart, 1980). Additional tasks have also been proposed as effective means of isolating category-specific deficits (see Table 12.2). Sorting tasks in which participants are instructed to sort pictures by category (Bunn et al., 1998; Kelter, Cohen, Engel, List, & Strohner, 1977; Whitehouse, Caramazza, & Zurif, 1978) or tasks requiring a yes/no response (Devlin et al., 2000) can be an effective means of assessing category-specific deficits under conditions that pose light linguistic demands on patients.

Table 12.2 Assessments of Specific Categories

Naming of Living Things

Animal naming/word-picture matching (land animals, water animals, birds, insects); food naming/word-picture matching (fruits, vegetables); flower/plant naming; body part naming/body part identification	Bi et al., 2011; Caramazza & Shelton, 1998; Crutch et al., 2007; De Renzi & Lucchelli, 1994; Farah & Wallace, 1992; Hart & Gordon, 1992; Samson & Pillon, 2003; Sartori & Job, 1988; Snodgrass & Vanderwart, 1980

Naming of Nonliving Things

Musical instrument naming; tool naming; vehicle/transportation naming; kitchenware naming; furniture naming; weapon naming; clothing naming; occupation naming; color naming; country naming/place-name verification	Bi et al., 2011; Caramazza & Shelton, 1998; Crutch et al., 2007; Hart & Gordon, 1992; Samson & Pillon, 2003; Snodgrass & Vanderwart, 1980

Additional Tasks: Verbal Output

Generative naming by category	Jefferies & Lambon Ralph, 2006
Definition generation by category	Funnell & Sheridan, 1992

Additional Tasks: Comprehension

Category-sorting tasks: sorting and classifying pictures	Bunn et al., 1998; Kelter et al., 1977; Whitehouse et al., 1978
Category-sorting tasks organized by defining and characteristic features (identifying typicality effects)	Hampton, 1995
Category odd-one-out judgments	Crutch, Connell, & Warrington, 2009; Bi et al., 2011
Category verification tasks	Kiran & Thompson, 2003b
Semantic categorization task: multiple cue words presented sequentially. Participants make a speeded decision about whether an additional word belongs to the same or different category.	Devlin et al., 2000
Word comprehension by category	Crutch et al., 2007; Laiacona et al., 1993
Face recognition; Boston Famous Faces Task	Caramazza & Shelton, 1998

Normed Assessments/Item Lists

Pyramids and Palm Trees Test (PPT)	Howard & Patterson, 1992
Boston Diagnostic Aphasia Exam (BDAE): Colors, letters, numbers, body parts, tools, foods, animals, places,	Goodglass et al., 2000
Northwestern Naming Battery (NNB): Animals, fruits, vegetables, tools, clothing	Thompson et al., 2012

Assessing Superordinate and Subordinate Categories: Coordinate and Associative Items

In the evaluation of category-specific deficits, it is not only important to consider overall categories that are named correctly or incorrectly, but to analyze the error patterns produced in naming. Research has shown that individuals with aphasia often make semantic errors that can be characterized as *coordinate semantic errors* (Jefferies & Lambon Ralph, 2006). A coordinate semantic error is a within-category naming substitution, such as the verbalization of *cat* in response to target item *dog*.

Similarly, *associative errors* such as verbalizing *bone* in response to target *dog* also commonly arise in aphasia (Jefferies & Lambon Ralph, 2006; Nickels & Howard, 1995). Researchers have posited that coordinate and associative semantic errors commonly arise in patients who have underspecified semantic representations or impaired access to semantic representations (Cloutman et al., 2009; Hillis & Caramazza, 1995; Marsh & Hillis, 2005; chapter 7, this volume). Patients who produce coordinate and associative semantic errors may have preserved access to superordinate information, but impaired storage of basic-level attributes, making access at the basic level difficult (Humphreys & Forde, 2005; Shallice, 1988).

Associative and coordinate deficits can be identified through error analyses and response patterns on tasks such as naming or category sorting. Normed associative match tasks such as the PPT (Howard & Patterson, 1992) and the CCT (Bozeat et al., 2002) provide useful insight into the integrity of an individual's superordinate and subordinate categories. However, the norms may be specific to the UK, where these tests were developed and normed, as some items or associations may not be familiar to individuals in other cultures. Therefore, a shortened form of the PPT has been developed that has been normed across cultures and identifies individuals with semantic deficits (Breining et al., submitted). Finally, the synonym judgment subtest of the Psycholinguistic Assessment of Language Processing in Aphasia (PALPA; (Kay, Lesser, & Coltheart, 1992) also provides information about integrity of category coordinates and associations. See Table 12.3 for a list of additional tasks.

Table 12.3 Assessments of Superordinate and Subordinate Categories: Coordinate and Associative Items

Nonstandardized Assessments

Category sorting	Bunn et al., 1998; Kelter et al., 1977; Whitehouse et al., 1978
Assessments of attribute knowledge arranged by superordinate attributes, subordinate attributes, associative functional features, and associative contextual features	Caramazza & Shelton, 1998; Laiacona et al., 1997
Associative match tasks: Target associated with one of two probe pictures	Caramazza & Shelton, 1998
Associative versus similarity-based odd-one-out tasks	Bi et al., 2011; Crutch et al., 2009
Judgments of association/similarity	Crutch & Warrington, 2007
Reading accuracy following semantic associative priming	Crutch & Warrington, 2007
Word synonym tasks	Warrington, McKenna, & Orpwood, 1998
Coordinate verification tasks	
Category verification tasks: Superordinate and subordinate items	Kiran & Thompson, 2003a

Normed assessments

Pyramids and Palm Trees Test (PPT)	Howard & Patterson, 1992
Camel and Cactus Test (CCT)	Bozeat et al., 2000
Psycholinguistic Assessment of Language Processing in Aphasia (PALPA): Synonym judgment subtest	Kay et al., 1992

Assessing Feature and Attribute Knowledge Related to Categories

As described in the section *model constructs guiding assessments*, many models of semantic organization propose that concepts are organized into feature lists or semantic descriptions. With experience and increased within- and between-category differentiation, feature lists are thought to cluster together in an organized manner. Distributed network accounts of semantic organization such as the Organized Unitary Content Hypothesis (OUCH; Caramazza et al., 1990) propose that objects that share many properties tend to form conceptual clusters based on the frequency with which descriptive properties co-occur. Accounts such as these suggest that brain damage affects concept clusters because they are stored in adjacent neural areas or because damage affects conceptual properties, and thus entire category clusters (Caramazza & Mahon, 2003). Assessments of feature knowledge, therefore, can help identify whether predominant deficits arise in one type of feature or another and may help explain observed category- or modality-specific deficits.

Table 12.4 Assessments of Feature and Attribute Knowledge

Attribute Knowledge Tasks

Target attribute matching (e.g., which item has a tail?)	Caramazza & Shelton, 1998
Visual attribute correspondence (e.g., select appropriately colored animals)	Hart & Gordon, 1992
Forced choice attribute knowledge (e.g., do bears like honey? Is this artifact real?)	Bi et al., 2011; Caramazza & Shelton, 1998; Laiacona et al., 1993; Moss et al., 1997; Samson et al., 1998
Verbalization of attribute knowledge (e.g., what color is an elephant?)	Hart & Gordon, 1992
Part decision task: Identify which of four pictured body parts corresponds to an incomplete target animal	Caramazza & Shelton, 1998; De Renzi & Lucchelli, 1994; Sartori & Job, 1988
Naming to definition	Gainotti, Miceli, & Caltagirone, 1979; Kelter et al., 1976; Semenza, Denes, Lucchese, & Bisiacchi, 1980
Feature Reality Test (FRT): Participant presented with pairs of pictures that differ along a single feature dimension	Garrard & Carroll, 2006
Identify semantic associations with pictured concepts	Cohen, Kelter, & Woll, 1980; Semenza et al., 1980; Gainotti et al., 1979

Feature Matching Tasks

Feature matching of sensory properties, functional attributes, perceptual characteristics, and thematic relationships	Bisiacchi, Denes, & Semenza, 1976

Sorting Tasks

Sorting of items with strong functional associations vs. sorting of items with strong sensory associations	Bunn et al., 1998

Normed Assessments

Psycholinguistic Assessment of Language (PAL): Spoken and written forced-choice attribute verification subtest	Caplan & Bub, 1990
Boston Diagnostic Aphasia Exam (BDAE): Semantic probe feature verification task	Goodglass et al., 2000

Research has described several attribute knowledge tasks that probe individuals' knowledge about item attributes through open-ended questions about attributes, yes/no questions, verification of attributes of pictorial stimuli, and naming to definition (Bi et al., 2011; Caramazza & Shelton, 1998; Hart & Gordon, 1992; Laiacona et al., 1993; Moss, Tyler, & Jennings, 1997; Samson, Pillon, & De Wilde, 1998). See Table 12.4 for a list of assessment tasks. Sorting tasks and feature matching tasks are also effective ways of assessing attribute knowledge. The Psycholinguistic Assessment of Language (PAL; Caplan & Bub, 1990) contains spoken and written attribute verification subtests. Similarly, the Boston Diagnostic Aphasia Exam (BDAE; Goodglass, Kaplan, & Barresi, 2000) contains a semantic probe feature verification task.

Within these task structures, researchers have proposed that secondary analyses can investigate whether differential results arise in the sorting and feature matching abilities of items heavily described by sensory or functional associations. Similarly, differences might also be observed between the sorting, feature matching, or naming abilities of typical versus atypical category items.

Assessing Semantic Ability with Respect to the Imageability of Items

Imageability, an indication of how easily a word produces a mental image (Bird, et al., 2000), presents another attribute often observed to impact the semantic ability of both patients with aphasia and nonaphasic individuals (Nickels & Howard, 1995; Strain, Patterson, & Seidenberg, 1995). Researchers have observed patterns that suggest that items that are less imageable are harder to access, as demonstrated through longer access times or greater incidences of word finding difficulty. In contrast, highly imageable words are accessed more quickly and more consistently (Bird et al., 2000).

Imageability effects are often observed among concrete and abstract word forms, and these word forms are therefore included in semantic assessment batteries (see Table 12.5). Concrete words have been described as more imageable than abstract words, as concrete concepts are experienced by multiple senses. In their Normal Isolated Centrally Expressed (NICE) model, Newton and Barry (1997) propose that the high imageability of concrete words leads to a high degree of specificity. High degrees of specificity facilitate lexical retrieval since conceptual activation is strong and specific. In contrast, abstract words are less imageable and are loosely associated with multiple concepts. Diffuse representations are thought to lead to a spread of activation that hinders lexical retrieval.

Table 12.5 Assessments Related to the Imageability of Items

Tests Probing Concrete/Abstract Words	
Concrete and abstract word reading	Crutch & Warrington, 2007; Newton & Barry, 1997
Odd-one-out tasks for concrete and abstract words	Crutch et al., 2009
Spoken definition-to-printed word matching task including concrete and abstract words	Newton & Barry, 1997

Normed and Standardized Assessments Probing Concrete/Abstract Words	
Psycholinguistic Assessment of Language Processing in Aphasia (PALPA): Semantic association of abstract words subtest	Kay et al., 1992
Psycholinguistic Assessment of Language (PAL): Spoken and written relatedness judgment for affixed words, spoken and written relatedness judgment for abstract words subtests	Caplan & Bub, 1990

Assessing Differential Impairments in Nouns and Verbs

Differential impairments have also been observed in aphasia between noun and verb naming (Bird et al., 2000; Orpwood & Warrington, 1995; Zingeser & Berndt, 1990). Some accounts suggest that dissociations arise due to distinct levels of imageability between nouns and verbs (Bird et al., 2000; Crepaldi et al., 2006; Luzzatti & Chierchia, 2002). Other studies, however, have observed imageability-independent deficits for verbs (Crepaldi et al., 2006). Distributed network accounts suggest that perceptual and functional attributes are differentially weighted for nouns and verbs and that this distinct perceptual weighting gives rise to differential deficits (Bird et al., 2000). Crepaldi et al. (2006) proposed that verbs are directly linked to lexical-semantic information and are therefore less readily retrieved in the absence of an appropriate grammatical context or argument structure. Yet other theories propose that since verbs are directly linked to action, their retrieval is only truly assessed through animations rather than through still pictures.

Though the nature of differential noun/verb deficits is debated, a thorough evaluation of semantic deficits in aphasia will consider naming as a function of grammatical class. Table 12.6 presents a series of assessments and tools that can be effective in examining the presence of such differential deficits.

Considering Factors such as Stimulus Frequency, Familiarity, and Visual Complexity

Throughout the assessments described thus far, it is important to control for factors of frequency, familiarity, typicality and visual complexity of items. Studies have shown that poor control of these factors can lead to misidentified category-specific deficits or grammatical class deficits (Fung et al., 2001; Funnell & Sheridan, 1992; Tippett, Grossman, & Farah, 1996; Tippett, Meier, Blackwood, & Diaz-Asper, 2007). Normed assessments are balanced or systematically vary factors such as these and therefore present the most reliable means of assessment. When standardized assessments are

Table 12.6 Assessments of Noun/Verb Dissociations

Nonstandardized assessments

Naming of action pictures vs. naming of object pictures	Crepaldi et al., 2006; Orpwood & Warrington, 1995
Written spelling of verbs vs. written spelling of nouns	Orpwood & Warrington, 1995

Normed and Standardized Assessments
Probing Noun/Verb Dissociations

Western Aphasia Battery (WAB): Noun naming subtest	Kertesz, 2007
Boston Diagnostic Aphasia Exam (BDAE): Naming of action pictures subtest	Goodglass et al., 2000
Northwestern Assessment of Verbs and Sentences (NAVS): Verb naming and verb comprehension subtests	Thompson, 2011
Northwestern Naming Battery (NNB): Noun naming, verb naming and verb comprehension subtests	Thompson et al., 2012
Object and Action Naming Battery (OANB): Noun and verb comprehension	Druks & Masterson, 2000
Test for the Reception of Grammar (TROG): Noun, verb, and adjective comprehension	Bishop, 1989
Psycholinguistic Assessment of Language Processing in Aphasia (PALPA): Grammatical class reading subtest	Kay et al., 1992

not available, clinicians should be careful to balance factors such as frequency, familiarity, visual complexity, and typicality to limit potential confounds in diagnosis or interpretation of results.

Treatment of Semantic Deficits

There are several treatments that are based on strengthening semantic attributes in order to facilitate lexical retrieval and semantic processing. These treatments can generally be categorized into those that focus on: (1) cueing to improve word retrieval; (2) multimodal therapies; (3) therapies based on various levels of semantic processing, such as contextual priming, utilizing semantic relationships in therapy and semantic feature analysis; and (4) therapies that manipulate stimulus characteristics such as typicality and imageability.

Cueing Therapies

Currently, the most common, and perhaps the least theoretically motivated, are treatments that implement cueing hierarchies. Cues are often presented as correct initial phonemes from category coordinates along with target pictures (Jefferies, Patterson, & Ralph, 2008; Soni, Lambon Ralph, & Woollams, 2012). Semantic cues often take the form of associated words (Freed, Celery, & Marshall, 2004; Lowell, Beeson, & Holland, 1995).

Several recent studies have shown that providing semantic cues is beneficial to patients who present with semantic-based naming deficits (Freed et al., 2004; Linebaugh, Shisler, & Lehner, 2005; Lowell et al., 1995) and, likewise, providing phonological cues is beneficial to patients who present with phonological errors in naming (Herbert, Best, Hickin, Howard, & Osborne, 2001; Hickin, Best, Herbert, Howard, & Osborne, 2001; Linebaugh et al., 2005; Wambaugh, Cameron, Kalinyak-Fliszar, Nessler, & Wright, 2004; Wambaugh et al., 2001). Additionally, studies that have combined phonological and semantic information into cueing hierarchies have resulted in improved word finding (Abel, Schultz, Radermacher, Willmes, & Huber, 2005; Abel, Willmes, & Huber, 2007; Cameron, Wambaugh, Wright, & Nessler, 2006; Conroy, Sage, & Lambon Ralph, 2009; Doesborgh et al., 2004; Fink, Brecher, Schwartz, & Robey, 2002; Herbert, Best, Hickin, Howard, & Osborne, 2003). Interestingly, some studies have shown better recovery of naming in persons with phonologically based anomia after semantically focused training (Raymer, Kohen, & Saffell, 2006; Wambaugh et al., 2001).

While cueing has been shown to produce immediate improvements in naming, cueing treatments are symptomatic in nature and do not specifically target the underlying impairment. Long-lasting effects and generalization of therapy are therefore ambiguous (Howard, Patterson, Franklin, Orchard-Lisle, & Morton, 1985; Marshall, Pound, White-Thomson, & Pring, 1990).

Multimodal Therapies

There are several treatments that have focused on multimodal approaches to facilitate lexical retrieval (Howard, Hickin, Redmond, Clark, & Best, 2006; Howard, et al., 1985; Nickels & Best, 1996). In these treatment approaches, the goal is to identify a modality that is relatively unimpaired, and then to utilize this modality to facilitate access and retrieval in a more impaired modality. Marshall et al. (1990) used this technique in a group of patients with aphasia who had relatively spared single word reading in the context of significantly impaired picture naming. During therapy patients were presented with four written words (the target word, two semantically related words, and one unrelated word) along with a target picture. Researchers observed improvements in the naming of target and semantically related items, suggesting that single word reading paired with picture matching helped reinforce links between semantic and phonological activation (Marshall et al., 1990). Other studies have included written stimuli that range from words to sentences to improve noun production (Visch-Brink, Bajema, & Van De Sandt-Koenderman, 1997).

Rose and Douglas (2008) have shown that understanding objects and shapes within different semantic categories through gesture and verbal output can also influence lexical retrieval. Significant gains were observed in a case study involving gesture, verbal, and combined verbal plus gesture treatment. Similarly, Boo and Rose (2011) examined the combination of semantic and gesture-based treatment for verb retrieval in two individuals with Broca's aphasia. Such therapies demonstrate the importance of assessing various modalities so that they can be utilized in the process of facilitating naming for patients with aphasia.

Therapies Based on Various Levels of Semantic Processing

Repetition Priming and Contextual Priming

Research demonstrating facilitated lexical access after phonological or semantic priming (Baum, 1997; Milberg & Blumstein, 1981; Soni et al., 2012) has led to a line of therapy studies examining repetition priming as a potential therapy for aphasia. While repetition priming has been found to lead to naming improvements in patients with aphasia (Silkes, Dierkes, & Kendall, 2013), several studies have indicated that, similar to cueing strategies, classic repetition priming may have only temporary benefits for patients with aphasia (Howard et al., 1985; Martin & Laine, 2000).

In response to the criticism that repetition priming may have only temporary effects, as well as evidence that therapies that elicit semantic activation are likely to have longer-lasting effects, researchers have examined an alternate form of priming in aphasia: *contextual repetition priming* (Cornelissen et al., 2003; Laine & Martin, 1996; Martin & Laine, 2000; Renvall, Laine, & Martin, 2005). Contextual repetition priming combines effects of mass repetition with principles of spreading activation brought about through semantically and phonologically related words. In this method, target names are repeatedly primed through the presentation of semantically or phonologically similar pictures. In many contextual priming studies, patients are presented with semantically or phonologically related six-picture matrices. During priming trials, patients attempt to repeat each target name immediately after it is produced by an examiner. After multiple priming trials, patients are asked to spontaneously name pictures. Some studies do implement contextual priming without requiring participants to verbalize targets. Word-picture matching tasks and rhyming tasks, for example, can be tailored to include principles of repetition priming (Howard et al., 1985; Marshall et al., 1990).

Research has shown that therapy tailored to an individual's level of impairment is typically more beneficial than treatment that does not match deficit specificity (Martin & Laine, 2000; Nettleton & Lesser, 1991), an additional benefit brought about through contextual priming. Although some patients have shown interference during the semantic context condition (Martin & Laine, 2000), this treatment has shown short-term positive effects for patients with semantic deficits (Cornelissen et al., 2003; Laine & Martin, 1996; Martin, Fink, Laine, & Ayala, 2004; Martin & Laine, 2000; Renvall et al., 2005).

Therapies that Utilize Semantic Relationships in Therapy

Contextual priming studies draw attention to the potential impact of utilizing semantically related versus unrelated words in therapy tasks, a stimulus manipulation that has been explored by other semantically based treatment studies. Davis and Pring (1991), for example, attempted to address the issue of which aspect of semantic treatment, if any, assisted in naming through the comparison of three tasks. In one task patients matched a picture to one of four semantically related written words. The second task utilized unrelated word distractors for the same task, while the third involved repetition of the word in the presence of the target picture alone. Interestingly, a significant improvement was observed for all treatment conditions, suggesting that all variations presented effective treatment methods.

Behrmann and Lieberthal (1989) report a case study that examined semantic treatment based on hierarchical category levels. Items from three semantic categories were selected to be trained on category sorting tasks, using superordinate features of each semantic category, as well as basic-level features. Results indicated significant improvement on all treated items from three semantic categories and significant improvements on untreated items in the trained categories. The patient in this study was able to learn superordinate information relatively easily and demonstrated generalization at this level, but was unable to utilize basic-level object information unless it had been specifically targeted in treatment.

While these studies did not reveal strong advantages of one treatment method over another, they are important to mention, as individual patients with aphasia may present with linguistic strengths and weakness that make them more suitable candidates for one variation of semantic therapy over another.

Semantic Feature Analysis

Another approach that has been extensively examined in the treatment of lexical retrieval deficits is the semantic feature analysis (SFA) method. This approach is based on theoretical models that suggest that lexical concepts are organized within semantic categories and are represented in terms of mutually overlapping semantic features (see *assessing feature and attribute knowledge*). SFA works under the principles of spreading activation (Collins & Loftus, 1975), such that activation of semantic features during treatment leads to activation of the target item as well as its phonological representation.

In the most common version of SFA (Haarbauer-Krupa, Moser, Smith, Sullivan, & Szekeres, 1985) participants are expected to generate semantic features for target items, a process that strengthens the overall lexical-phonological representation of the target item. In the original version of SFA, participants were required to generate six features pertaining to group, action, use, location, properties, and associations. In other variants of this treatment, participants are required to select semantic features from a list of target words. The rationale driving this variant is that a greater diversity of features are presented to the patient, thus spreading activation across a greater network of features (Boyle, 2010).

The evidence supporting the efficacy of semantic feature treatment to improve naming is robust and continues to grow (see Boyle, 2010 for a review). Boyle and Coelho (1995) examined the nature of SFA in one patient with aphasia who was trained on two sets of stimuli. The patient showed improvements on trained items that were maintained even after treatment was terminated. In another study, Law and colleagues examined a combination of semantic feature analysis and semantic priming to improve naming deficits in three patients with aphasia. All three patients showed improvements on trained items as well as untrained items, with long-term gains in improvement observed for one patient (Law, Wong, Sung, & Hon, 2006).

Other case studies have also since reported the beneficial effect of this treatment approach despite mild variations in the treatment regimen in each case (Hashimoto & Frome, 2011; Wambaugh, Mauszycki, Cameron, Wright, & Nessler, 2013). The effect of such feature analysis to improve access to words that are produced in structured discourse tasks has also been examined, and the preliminary results of these case studies have generally been positive (Peach & Reuter, 2010; Rider, Wright, Marshall, & Page, 2008).

The premise of SFA has also been examined in patients with bilingual aphasia, where analysis of semantic features of targets in one language has been found to result in lexical retrieval of those items and improvements to within language targets as well as cross-language translations (Edmonds & Kiran, 2006; Kiran & Iakupova, 2011; Kiran & Roberts, 2010). Overall, the general approach of SFA has proven to be quite efficacious in terms of improving access to trained items as well as generalization to untrained items.

Therapies Targeting Verb Retrieval

While the majority of studies focus on noun retrieval, SFA has also been applied in therapies targeting verb retrieval. Wambaugh and Ferguson (2007) examined the effectiveness of a semantic feature–type treatment for verb retrieval in one individual with aphasia. Again, the principal components of SFA (manipulation of semantic information) were implemented, in this case with verbs as the target. Results showed improved access to naming verbs as well as overall improvements in spoken production. Similarly, Raymer and Ellsworth (2002) examined SFA compared with phonological therapy and repetition as a treatment for verb retrieval. All treatments resulted in verb naming improvement.

Manipulating Stimulus Characteristics Based on Principles of Semantic Organization

Semantic Attributes versus Category Coordinates

In an exploration of additional factors that might impact progress with therapy, Hashimoto, Widman, Kiran, and Richards (2013) recently compared two treatment conditions, one based on shared semantic attributes across items and the other based on category coordinates. While studies in aphasia that have noted a high incidence of coordinate and associate semantic errors often attribute errors to reduced access to attribute-level information, research in nonaphasic individuals has suggested that category coordinates naturally lead to a high degree of semantic interference (Spalek, Damian, & Bolte, 2013). Researchers were therefore interested in determining whether differential effects arose from therapies that included category coordinates (and introduced a high degree of lexical competition) versus therapies that reinforced shared semantic attributes across items.

Overall, both therapy paradigms were observed to produce naming improvements for eight enrolled patients with aphasia. Investigators did observe a higher incidence of semantically related errors following category-based treatment, but this difference was not significant when compared to the feature-based treatment. This study draws attention to the potential to manipulate target items in therapy, focusing on semantic attributes and functional, coordinate, and associative relationships.

Stimulus Typicality

Similar to the SFA approach, other semantic-based treatments focus on strengthening semantic attributes and corresponding phonological representations in a manner based in theoretical principles of semantic organization in order to promote longer-lasting treatment effects (Boyle, 2010; Kiran & Bassetto, 2008). One of these methods is to vary the typicality of stimulus sets (Kiran, 2008; Kiran & Thompson, 2003b; Stanczak, Waters, & Caplan, 2006). This work capitalizes on a large base of normal behavioral studies that detail the organization of semantic categories in terms of semantic attributes such as defining features, shared/overlapping characteristic features, and distinctive features within categories (Cree, McNorgan, & McRae, 2006; Garrard et al., 2001;

Grondin, Lupker, & McRae, 2009). Specifically, the representation of semantic attributes for each category is manifested as *defining* features that all items in the category must necessarily have; *characteristic* features that are strongly associated with the category but that are not absolutely necessary for category membership; and *distinguishing* features, one or more of which in combination identify specific items (e.g., "red breast" for "robin"). In each category, typical items will possess the defining and many overlapping characteristic features, and atypical items will possess the defining features but fewer overlapping characteristic features.

Applied to aphasia therapy, training atypical category exemplars is thought to result in improved access to phonological representations for both atypical and untrained typical examples. Because atypical examples and their features represent a greater variation within the category than typical examples (Plaut, 1996), training of atypical items simultaneously reinforces characteristic and defining features that are relevant to typical examples and thus their phonological representations. Conversely, training typical examples does not result in generalization to untrained atypical examples, since training the overlapping (characteristic) features and defining features only benefits typical examples. Stanczak et al. (2006) applied these principles in a therapy study and found that while typical exemplars were easier to learn than atypical exemplars, training atypical examples was superior in promoting diffuse generalization within the semantic network.

These results are instrumental in extending the Complexity Account of Treatment Efficacy (CATE; Thompson & Shapiro, 2007). Thus far, this work presents a compelling case for training more complex information (atypical items), as within-category generalization to typical items is promoted (Kiran, 2007; Kiran & Bassetto, 2008).

Stimulus Imageability

Similar to the examination of complexity within the context of typicality of category exemplars, Kiran, Sandberg, and Abbott (2009) have examined the nature of training stimulus items varied by their imageability status (see *assessing semantic ability with respect to the imageability of items*). In one study with four patients trained either on abstract or concrete exemplars within contextual categories, Kiran et al. (2009) found that training abstract words in a category resulted in improvement of those words as well as generalization to untrained target concrete words in the same category. However, training concrete words in a category resulted in the retrieval of only the trained concrete words, not generalization to target abstract words. Observed generalization is thought to be based on the more diverse and extensive spreading activation brought about through abstract word training in comparison with a limited spread of activation brought about through training concrete words that share overlapping semantic attributes (Kiran et al., 2009; Newton & Barry, 1997).

Future Directions: Exploring the Neural Mechanisms Underlying Semantic-Based Treatment

In this chapter we have discussed many studies that have used case studies or group studies to examine the efficacy of various therapies. While there is a need for this type of work to continue, researchers are also turning to neuroimaging technologies to further our understanding beyond behavior to the neural mechanisms underlying treatment-induced change (Davis, Harrington, & Baynes, 2006; Heath et al., 2012; Marcotte et al., 2012). Examining neural activation patterns before and after therapy might contribute to information relevant in predicting semantic improvement or identifying appropriate candidates for specific therapies.

Moving towards this type of understanding of the neural mechanisms of therapy, Marcotte et al. (2012) enrolled nine patients with aphasia in a SFA therapy and conducted pre- and post-treatment functional magnetic resonance imaging (fMRI) scans. All participants demonstrated naming improvements for trained and untrained items. Naming outcomes showed no relationship to lesion size, but were negatively correlated with damage to Broca's area. In addition, naming improvements were found to correlate with activation in the left precentral gyrus (PCG; BA 4/6). Interestingly, naming improvements correlated with activation in the left PCG both pre and post treatment, suggesting that activation in this area might be predictive of naming improvement for patients enrolled in SFA. Researchers described the PCG as an area recruited by healthy controls during overt naming tasks (Shuster & Lemieux, 2005), which might also be important for language processing or semantic integration and thus be recruited during SFA.

The first wave of treatment studies based on specific models of semantics have established the feasibility of these different type of treatments; current and future treatments will attempt to understand the neural underpinnings of specific treatments, bringing the field closer to therapy that can be individually tailored with predictable outcomes.

References

Abel, S., Schultz, A., Radermacher, I., Willmes, K., & Huber, W. (2005). Decreasing and increasing cues in naming therapy for aphasia. *Aphasiology, 19*(9), 831–848.

Abel, S., Willmes, K., & Huber, W. (2007). Model-oriented naming therapy: Testing predictions of a connectionist model. *Aphasiology, 21*(5), 411–447.

Barsalou, L.W., Kyle Simmons, W., Barbey, A.K., & Wilson, C.D. (2003). Grounding conceptual knowledge in modality-specific systems. *Trends in Congitive Sciences, 7*(2), 84–91.

Baum, S.R. (1997). Phonological, semantic, and mediated priming in aphasia. *Brain and Language, 60*(3), 347–359. doi:10.1006/brln.1997.1829

Behrmann, M., & Lieberthal, T. (1989). Category-specific treatment of a lexical-semantic deficit: A single case study of global aphasia. *British Journal of Disorders of Communication, 24*(3), 281–299.

Bi, Y., Wei, T., Wu, C., Han, Z., Jiang, T., & Caramazza, A. (2011). The role of the left anterior temporal lobe in language processing revisited: Evidence from an individual with ATL resection. *Cortex, 47*(5), 575–587. doi:10.1016/j.cortex.2009.12.002

Bird, H., Howard, D., & Franklin, S. (2000). Why is a verb like an inanimate object? Grammatical category and semantic category deficits. *Brain and Language, 72*(3), 246–309.

Bishop, D. (1989). *Test for reception of grammar* (2nd ed.). Manchester: University of Manchester Age and Cognitive Performance Research Centre.

Bisiacchi, P., Denes, G., & Semenza, C. (1976). Semantic field in aphasia: An experimental investigation on comprehension of the relations of class and property. *Schweizer Archiv für Neurologie, Neurochirurgie und Psychiatrie, 118*(2), 207–213.

Boo, M., & Rose, M.L. (2011). The efficacy of repetition, semantic, and gesture treatments for verb retrieval and use in Broca's aphasia. *Aphasiology, 25*(2), 154–175. doi:10.1080/02687031003743789Pii 925773566

Boyle, M. (2010). Semantic feature analysis treatment for aphasic word retrieval impairments: What's in a name? *Topics in Stroke Rehabilitation, 17*(6), 411–422. doi:10.1310/Tsr1706–411

Boyle, M., & Coelho, C. (1995). Application of semantic feature analysis as a treatment for aphasic dysnomia. *American Journal of Speech-Language Pathology, 4*, 94–98.

Bozeat, S., Lambon Ralph, M.A., Patterson, K., Garrard, P., & Hodges, J.R. (2000). Non-verbal semantic impairment in semantic dementia. *Neuropsychologia, 38*(9), 1207–1215.

Bozeat, S., Lambon Ralph, M.A., Patterson, K., & Hodges, J.R. (2002). When objects lose their meaning: What happens to their use? *Cognitive, Affective, & Behavioral Neurosciences, 2*(3), 236–251.

Bunn, E.M., Tyler, L.K., & Moss, H.E. (1998). Category-specific semantic deficits: The role of familiarity and property type reexamined. *Neuropsychology, 12*(3), 367–379.

Cameron, R.M., Wambaugh, J.L., Wright, S.M., & Nessler, C.L. (2006). Effects of a combined semantic/phonologic cueing treatment on word retrieval in discourse. *Aphasiology, 20*(2), 269–285.

Capitani, E., Laiacona, M., Mahon, B., & Caramazza, A. (2003). What are the facts of semantic category-specific deficits? A critical review of the clinical evidence. *Cognitive Neuropsychology, 20*(3/4/5/6), 213–261.

Caplan, D., & Bub, D. (1990). *Psycholinguistic assessment of aphasia.* Paper presented at the American Speech and Hearing Association Conference, Seattle, WA.

Caramazza, A., Hillis, A., Rapp, B., & Romani, C. (1990). The multiple semantics hypothesis: Multiple confusions? *Cognitive Neuropsychology, 7*(3), 161–189.

Caramazza, A., & Mahon, B.Z. (2003). The organization of conceptual knowledge: The evidence from category-specific semantic deficits. *Trends in Congitive Sciences, 7*(8), 354–361.

Caramazza, A., & Shelton, J.R. (1998). Domain-specific knowledge systems in the brain the animate-inanimate distinction. *Journal of Cognitive Neuroscience, 10*(1), 1–34.

Cloutman, L., Gottesman, R., Chaudhry, P., Davis, C., Kleinman, J.T., Pawlak, M., . . . Hillis, A. (2009). Where (in the brain) do semantic errors come from? *Cortex, 45,* 641–649.

Cohen, R., Kelter, S., & Woll, G. (1980). Analytical competence and language impairment in aphasia. *Brain and Language, 10*(2), 331–347.

Collins, A.M., & Loftus, E.F. (1975). A spreading activation theory of semantic processing. *Psychological Review, 82,* 407–428.

Conroy, P., Sage, K., & Lambon Ralph, M. (2009). The effects of decreasing and increasing cue therapy on improving naming speed and accuracy for verbs and nouns in aphasia. *Aphasiology, 23*(6), 707–730.

Cornelissen, K., Laine, M., Tarkiainen, A., Jarvensivu, T., Martin, N., & Salmelin, R. (2003). Adult brain plasticity elicited by anomia treatment. *Journal of Cognitive Neuroscience, 15*(3), 444–461.

Cree, G.S., McNorgan, C., & McRae, K. (2006). Distinctive features hold a privileged status in the computation of word meaning: Implications for theories of semantic memory. *Journal of Experimental Psychology. Learning, Memory, and Cognition, 32*(4), 643–658. doi:10.1037/0278–7393.32.4.643

Crepaldi, D., Aggujaro, S., Arduino, L.S., Zonca, G., Ghirardi, G., Inzaghi, M.G., . . . Luzzatti, C. (2006). Noun-verb dissociation in aphasia: The role of imageability and functional locus of the lesion. *Neuropsychologia, 44*(1), 73–89. doi:10.1016/j.neuropsychologia.2005.04.006

Crutch, S.J., Connell, S., & Warrington, E.K. (2009). The different representational frameworks underpinning abstract and concrete knowledge: Evidence from odd-one-out judgements. *Quarterly Journal of Experimental Psychology: QJEP, 62*(7), 1377–1388, 1388–1390. doi:10.1080/17470210802483834

Crutch, S.J., Randlesome, K., & Warrington, E.K. (2007). The variability of country map knowledge in normal and aphasic subjects: Evidence from two new category-specific screening tests. *Journal of Neuropsychology, 1*(Pt 2), 171–187.

Crutch, S.J., & Warrington, E.K. (2007). Semantic priming in deep-phonological dyslexia: Contrasting effects of association and similarity upon abstract and concrete word reading. *Cognitive Neuropsychology, 24*(6), 583–602.

Davis, A., & Pring, T. (1991). Therapy for word-finding deficits: More on the effects of semantic and phonological approaches to treatment with dysphasic patients. *Neuropsychological Rehabilitation, 1*(2), 135–145.

Davis, C., Harrington, G., & Baynes, K. (2006). Intensive semantic intervention in fluent aphasia: A pilot study with fMRI. *Aphasiology, 20*(1), 59–83.

De Renzi, E., Faglioni, P., Scotti, G., & Spinnler, H. (1972). Impairment in associating colour to form, concomitant with aphasia. *Brain, 95*(2), 293–304.

De Renzi, E., & Lucchelli, F. (1994). Are semantic systems separately represented in the brain? The case of living category impairment. *Cortex, 30*(1), 3–25.

Devlin, J.T., Russell, R.P., Davis, M.H., Price, C.J., Wilson, J., Moss, H.E., . . . Tyler, L.K. (2000). Susceptibility-induced loss of signal: Comparing PET and fMRI on a semantic task. *Neuroimage, 11*(6 Pt 1), 589–600. doi:10.1006/nimg.2000.0595

Doesborgh, S., van de Sandt-Koenderman, M.W., Dippel, D.W., van Harskamp, F., Koudstaal, P.J., & Visch-Brink, E.G. (2004). Cues on request: The efficacy of Multicue, a computer program for wordfinding therapy. *Aphasiology, 18*(3), 213–222.

Druks, J., & Masterson, J. (2000). *An object and action naming battery.* Philadelphia, PA: Taylor & Francis.

Edmonds, L.A., & Kiran, S. (2006). Effect of semantic naming treatment on crosslinguistic generalization in bilingual aphasia. *Journal of Speech, Language, and Hearing Research: JSLHR, 49*(4), 729–748. doi:10.1044/1092–4388(2006/053)

Farah, M.J., McMullen, P.A., & Meyer, M.M. (1991). Can recognition of living things be selectively impaired? *Neuropsychologia, 29*(2), 185–193.

Farah, M.J., & Wallace, M.A. (1992). Semantically-bounded anomia: Implications for the neural implementation of naming. *Neuropsychologia, 30*(7), 609–621.

Fink, R., Brecher, A., Schwartz, M.F., & Robey, R.R. (2002). A computer-implemented protocol for treatment of naming disorders: Evaluation of clinician-guided and partially self-guided instruction. *Aphasiology, 16*(10), 1061–1086.

Freed, D., Celery, K., & Marshall, R.C. (2004). Effectiveness of personalised and phonological cueing on long-term naming performance by aphasic subjects: A clinical investigation. *Aphasiology, 18*(8), 743–757. doi:10.1080/02687030444000246

Fung, T.D., Chertkow, H., Murtha, S., Whatmough, C., Peloquin, L., Whitehead, V., & Templeman, F.D. (2001). The spectrum of category effects in object and action knowledge in dementia of the Alzheimer's type. *Neuropsychology, 15*(3), 371–379.

Funnell, E., & Sheridan, J. (1992). Categories of knolwedge—Unfamiliar aspects of living and nonliving things. *Cognitive Neuropsychology, 92*, 135–153.

Gainotti, G., & Lemmo, M.S. (1976). Comprehension of symbolic gestures in aphasia. *Brain and Language, 3*(3), 451–460.

Gainotti, G., Miceli, G., & Caltagirone, C. (1979). The relationship between conceptial and semantic-lexical disorders in aphasia. *International Journal of Neuroscience, 10*, 45–50.

Gainotti, G., Silveri, M.C., Villa, G., & Caltagirone, C. (1983). Drawing objects from memory in aphasia. *Brain, 106*(Pt 3), 613–622.

Garrard, P., & Carroll, E. (2006). Lost in semantic space: a multi-modal, non-verbal assessment of feature knowledge in semantic dementia. *Brain, 129*(Pt 5), 1152–1163. doi:10.1093/brain/awl069

Garrard, P., Ralph, M.A., Hodges, J.R., & Patterson, K. (2001). Prototypicality, distinctiveness, and intercorrelation: Analyses of the semantic attributes of living and nonliving concepts. *Cognitive Neuropsychology, 18*(2), 125–174. doi:10.1080/02643290125857

Goodglass, H., Kaplan, E., & Barresi, B. (2000). *Boston Diagnostic Aphasia Examination—Third Edition (BDAE-3).* Austin, TX: Pro-Ed.

Grondin, R., Lupker, S.J., & McRae, K. (2009). Shared features dominate semantic richness effects for concrete concepts. *Journal of Memory and Language, 60*(1), 1–19. doi:10.1016/j.jml.2008.09.001

Haarbauer-Krupa, J., Moser, L., Smith, G., Sullivan, D.M., & Szekeres, S.F. (1985). Cognitive-rehabilitation therapy: Middle stages of recovery. In M. Ylvisaker (Ed.), *Head injury rehabilitation: Children and adolescents* (pp. 287–310). San Diego, CA: College-Hill Press.

Hampton, J.A. (1995). Testing the prototype theory of concepts. *Journal of Memory and Language, 34*, 686–708.

Hart, J., Jr., Berndt, R.S., & Caramazza, A. (1985). Category-specific naming deficit following cerebral infarction. *Nature, 316*(6027), 439–440.

Hart, J., Jr., & Gordon, B. (1992). Neural subsystems for object knowledge. *Nature, 359*(6390), 60–64. doi:10.1038/359060a0

Hashimoto, N., & Frome, A. (2011). The use of a modified semantic features analysis approach in aphasia. *Journal of Communication Disorders, 44*(4), 459–469. doi:10.1016/j.jcomdis.2011.02.004

Hashimoto, N., Widman, B., Kiran, S., & Richards, M. (2013). A comparison of features and categorical cues to improve naming abilities in aphasia. *Aphasiology, 27*(10), 1252–1279.

Heath, S., McMahon, K.L., Nickels, L., Angwin, A., Macdonald, A. D., van Hees, S., . . . Copland, D.A. (2012). Neural mechanisms underlying the facilitation of naming in aphasia using a semantic task: An fMRI study. *BMC Neuroscience, 13*, 98. doi:10.1186/1471-2202-13-98

Herbert, R., Best, W., Hickin, J., Howard, D., & Osborne, F. (2001). Phonological and orthographic approaches to the treatment of word retrieval in aphasia. *International Journal of Language and Communication Disorders, 36*(Suppl), 7–12.

Herbert, R., Best, W., Hickin, J., Howard, D., & Osborne, F. (2003). Combining lexical and interactional approaches to therapy for word finding deficits in aphasia. *Aphasiology, 17*(12), 1163–1186.

Hickin, J., Best, W., Herbert, R., Howard, D., & Osborne, F. (2001). Treatment of word retrieval in aphasia: Generalisation to conversational speech. *International Journal of Language and Communication Disorders, 36*(Suppl), 13–18.

Hillis, A.E., & Caramazza, A. (1991). Mechanisms for accessing lexical representations for output: Evidence from a category-specific semantic deficit. *Brain and Language, 40*(1), 106–144.

Hillis, A.E., & Caramazza, A. (1995). Cognitive and neural mechanisms underlying visual and semantic processing: implications from "optic aphasia." *Journal of Cognitive Neuroscience, 7*(4), 457–478. doi:10.1162/jocn.1995.7.4.457

Howard, D., Hickin, J., Redmond, T., Clark, P., & Best, W. (2006). Re-visiting "semantic facilitation" of word retrieval for people with aphasia: Facilitation yes but semantic no. *Cortex, 42*(6), 946–962.

Howard, D., & Patterson, K. (1992). *Pyramids and palm trees: A test of semantic access from pictures and words.* Thames Valley: Bury St. Edmunds.

Howard, D., Patterson, K.E., Franklin, S., Orchard-Lisle, V., & Morton, J. (1985). The facilitation of picture naming in aphasia. *Cognitive Neuropsychology, 2*(49–80).

Humphreys, G.W., & Forde, E.M. (2001). Hierarchies, similarity, and interactivity in object recognition: "Category-specific" neuropsychological deficits. *Journal of Behavioral and Brain Science, 24*(3), 453–476; discussion 476–509.

Humphreys, G.W., & Forde, E.M. (2005). Naming a giraffe but not an animal: Base-level but not superordinate naming in a patient with impaired semantics. *Cognitive Neuropsychology, 22*(5), 539–558. doi:10.1080/02643290442000176

Jefferies, E., & Lambon Ralph, M.A. (2006). Semantic impairment in stroke aphasia versus semantic dementia: A case-series comparison. *Brain, 129*(Pt 8), 2132–2147. doi:awl153[pii]10.1093/brain/awl153

Jefferies, E., Patterson, K., & Ralph, M.A. (2008). Deficits of knowledge versus executive control in semantic cognition: insights from cued naming. *Neuropsychologia, 46*(2), 649–658. doi:10.1016/j. neuropsychologia.2007.09.007

Kaplan, E., Goodglass, H., & Weintraub, S. (1983). *Boston Naming Test.* Philadelphia: Lea and Febiger.

Kay, J., Lesser, R., & Coltheart, M. (1992). *Psycholinguistic assessments of language processing in aphasia.* Hove, UK: Lawrence Erlbaum Associates, Ltd.

Kelter, S., Cohen, R., Engel, D., List, G., & Strohner, H. (1976). Aphasic disorders in matching tasks involving conceptual analysis and covert naming. *Cortex, 12*(4), 383–394.

Kelter, J., Cohen, R., Engel, D., List, G., & Strohner, H. (1977). The conceptual structure of aphasic and schizophrenic patients in a nonverbal sorting task. *Journal of Psycholinguist Research, 6*(4), 279–303.

Kertesz, A. (1982). *The Western Aphasia Battery.* Philadelphia: Gruyne & Stratton.

Kertesz, A. (2007). *The Western Aphasia Battery-Revised.* San Antonio, TX: PsychCorp.

Kiran, S. (2007). Semantic complexity in the treatment of naming deficits. *American Journal of Speech-Language Pathology, 16,* 18–29.

Kiran, S. (2008). Typicality of inanimate category exemplars in aphasia treatment: Further evidence for semantic complexity. *Journal of Speech, Language, and Hearing Research: JSLHR, 51*(6), 1550–1568. doi:10.104 4/1092–4388(2008/07–0038)

Kiran, S., & Bassetto, G. (2008). Evaluating the effectiveness of semantic-based treatment for naming deficits in aphasia: What works? *Seminars in Speech and Language, 29*(1), 71–82. doi:10.1055/s-2008-1061626

Kiran, S., & Iakupova, R. (2011). Understanding the relationship between language proficiency, language impairment and rehabilitation: Evidence from a case study. *Clinical Linguistics and Phonetics, 25*(6–7), 565–583. doi:10.3109/02699206.2011.566664

Kiran, S., & Roberts, P.M. (2010). Semantic feature analysis treatment in Spanish-English and French-English bilingual aphasia. *Aphasiology, 24*(2), 231–261. doi:10.1080/02687030902958365 Pii 915031956

Kiran, S., Sandberg, C., & Abbott, K. (2009). Treatment for lexical retrieval using abstract and concrete words in persons with aphasia: Effect of complexity. *Aphasiology, 23*(7), 835–853. doi:10.1080/02687030802588866

Kiran, S., & Thompson, C.K. (2003a). Effect of typicality on online category verification of animate category exemplars in aphasia. *Brain and Language, 85*(3), 441–450.

Kiran, S., & Thompson, C.K. (2003b). The role of semantic complexity in treatment of naming deficits: Training semantic categories in fluent aphasia by controlling exemplar typicality. *Journal of Speech, Language, and Hearing Research: JSLHR, 46*(4), 773–787.

Kittredge, A.K., Dell, G.S., Verkuilen, J., & Schwartz, M.F. (2008). Where is the effect of frequency in word production? Insights from aphasic picture-naming errors. *Cognitive Neuropsychology, 25*(4), 463–492. doi:10.1080/02643290701674851

Kolinsky, R., Fery, P., Messina, D., Peretz, I., Evinck, S., Ventura, P., & Morais, J. (2002). The fur of the crocodile and the mooing sheep: A study of a patient with a category-specific impairment for biological things. *Cognitive Neuropsychology, 19*(4), 301–342. doi:10.1080/02643290143000196

Laiacona, M., Barbarotto, R., & Capitani, E. (1993). Perceptual and associative knowledge in category specific impairment of semantic memory: a study of two cases. *Cortex, 29*(4), 727–740.

Laiacona, M., Capitani, E., & Barbarotto, R. (1997). Semantic category dissociations: A longitudinal study of two cases. *Cortex, 33,* 441–461.

Laine, M., & Martin, N. (1996). Lexical retrieval deficit in picture naming: Implications for word production models. *Brain and Language, 53*(3), 283–314. doi:10.1006/brln.1996.0050

Lambon Ralph, M.A., McClelland, J.L., Patterson, K., Galton, C.J., & Hodges, J.R. (2001). No right to speak? The relationship between object naming and semantic impairment: Neuropsychological evidence and a computational model. *Journal of Cognitive Neuroscience, 13*(3), 341–356.

Law, S.P., Wong, W., Sung, F., & Hon, J. (2006). A study of semantic treatment of three Chinese anomic patients. *Neuropsychological Rehabilitation, 16*(6), 601–629. doi:10.1080/09602010543000046

Levin, N., Ben-Hur, T., Biran, I., & Wertman, E. (2005). Category specific dysnomia after thalamic infarction: a case-control study. *Neuropsychologia, 43*(9), 1385–1390. doi:10.1016/j.neuropsychologia.2004.12.001

Linebaugh, C.W., Shisler, R.J., & Lehner, L. (2005). Cueing hierarchies and word retrieval: A therapy program. *Aphasiology, 19*(1), 77–92.

Lowell, S., Beeson, P.M., & Holland, A.L. (1995). The efficacy of a semantic cueing procedure on naming performance of adults with aphasia. *American Journal of Speech-Language Pathology, 4*(4), 109–114.

Luzzatti, C., & Chierchia, G. (2002). On the nature of selective deficits involving nouns and verbs. *Rivista di Linguistica, 14*(1), 43–71.

Marcotte, K., Adrover-Roig, D., Damien, B., de Preaumont, M., Genereux, S., Hubert, M., & Ansaldo, A.I. (2012). Therapy-induced neuroplasticity in chronic aphasia. *Neuropsychologia, 50*(8), 1776–1786. doi:10.1016/j.neuropsychologia.2012.04.001

Marsh, E.B., & Hillis, A.E. (2005). Cognitive and neural mechanisms underlying reading and naming: Evidence from letter-by-letter reading and optic aphasia. *Neurocase, 11*(5), 325–337.

Marshall, J., Pound, C., White-Thomson, M., & Pring, T. (1990). The use of picture/word matching tasks to assist word retrieval in aphasic patients. *Aphasiology, 4*(2), 167–184.

Martin, N., Fink, R.B., Laine, M., & Ayala, J. (2004). Immediate and short-term effects of contextual priming on word retrieval. *Aphasiology, 18*, 867–898.

Martin, N., & Laine, M. (2000). Effects of contextual priming on impaired word retrieval. *Aphasiology, 14*(1), 53–70.

McCarthy, R.A., & Warrington, E.K. (1988). Evidence for modality-specific meaning systems in the brain. *Nature, 334*(6181), 428–430. doi:10.1038/334428a0

McClelland, J.L., & Rogers, T.T. (2003). The parallel distributed processing approach to semantic cognition. *Nature Reviews. Neuroscience, 4*(4), 310–322. doi:10.1038/nrn1076

Miceli, G., Fouch, E., Capasso, R., Shelton, J.R., Tomaiuolo, F., & Caramazza, A. (2001). The dissociation of color from form and function knowledge. *Nature Neuroscience, 4*(6), 662–667. doi:10.1038/88497

Milberg, W., & Blumstein, S.E. (1981). Lexical decision and aphasia: Evidence for semantic processing. *Brain and Language, 14*(2), 371–385.

Moss, H.E., Tyler, L.K., & Jennings, F. (1997). When leopards lose their spots: Knowledge of visual properties in category-specific deficits for living things. *Cognitive Neuropsychology, 14*(6), 901–950.

Nettleton, J., & Lesser, R. (1991). Therapy for naming difficulties in aphasia: Application of a cognitive neuropsychological model. *Journal of Neurolinguistics, 6*, 139–157.

Newton, P.K., & Barry, C. (1997). Concreteness effects in word production but no word comprehension in deep dyslexia. *Cognitive Neuropsychology, 14*(4), 481–509.

Nickels, L., & Best, W. (1996). Therapy for naming disorders (Part I): Principles, puzzles, and progress. *Aphasiology, 10*(1), 21–47.

Nickels, L., & Howard, D. (1995). Aphasic naming: What matters? *Neuropsychologia, 33*(10), 1281–1303.

Nozari, N., Kittredge, A.K., Dell, G.S., & Schwartz, M.F. (2010). Naming and repetition in aphasia: Steps, routes, and frequency effects. *Journal of Memory and Language, 63*(4), 541–559. doi:10.1016/j.jml.2010.08.001

Orpwood, L., & Warrington, E.K. (1995). Word specific impairments in naming and spelling but not reading. *Cortex, 31*(2), 239–265.

Peach, R.K., & Reuter, K.A. (2010). A discourse-based approach to semantic feature analysis for the treatment of aphasic word retrieval failures. *Aphasiology, 24*(9), 971–990. doi:10.1080/02687030903058629 Pii 915032059

Plaut, D.C. (1996). Relearning after damage in connectionist networks: Toward a theory of rehabilitation. *Brain and Language, 52*(1), 25–82.

Raymer, A.M., & Ellsworth, T.A. (2002). Response to contrasting verb retrieval treatments: A case study. *Aphasiology, 16*, 1031–1045.

Raymer, A.M., Kohen, F.P., & Saffell, D. (2006). Computerised training for impairments of word comprehension and retrieval in aphasia. *Aphasiology, 20*(2–4), 257–268. doi:10.1080/02687030500473312

Renvall, K., Laine, M., & Martin, N. (2005). Contextual priming in semantic anomia: A case study. *Brain and Language, 95*(2), 327–341. doi:10.1016/j.bandl.2005.02.003

Rider, J.D., Wright, H.H., Marshall, R.C., & Page, J.L. (2008). Using semantic feature analysis to improve contextual discourse in adults with aphasia. *American Journal of Speech-Language Pathology, 17*(2), 161–172. doi:10.1044/1058–0360(2008/016)

Rogers, T.T., & McClelland, J.L. (2008). Precis of semantic cognition, a parallel distributed processing approach. *Behavioral and Brain Sciences, 31*, 689–749).

Rosch, E., & Mervis, C. (1975). Family resemblances: Studies in the internal structure of categories. *Cognitive Psychology, 7*, 573–605.

Rose, M., & Douglas, J. (2008). Treating semantic deficits in aphasia with gesture and verbal methods. *Aphasiology, 22*(1), 1–22.

Samson, D., & Pillon, A. (2003). A case of impaired knowledge for fruit and vegetables. *Cognitive Neuropsychology, 20*(3), 373–400. doi:10.1080/02643290244000329

Samson, D., Pillon, A., & De Wilde, V. (1998). Impaired knowledge of visual and non-visual attributes in a patient with a semantic impairment for living entitites: A case of a true category-specific deficit. *Neurocase, 4*(4–5), 273–290.

Sartori, G., & Job, R. (1988). The oyster with four legs: A neuropsychological study on the interaction of visual and semantic information. *Cognitive Neuropsychology, 5*(1), 105–132.

Saygin, A.P., Dick, F., Wilson, S.M., Dronkers, N.F., & Bates, E. (2003). Neural resources for processing language and environmental sounds: Evidence from aphasia. *Brain, 126*(Pt 4), 928–945.

Semenza, C., Denes, G., Lucchese, D., & Bisiacchi, P. (1980). Selective deficit of conceptual structures in aphasia: Class versus thematic relations. *Brain and Language, 10*(2), 243–248.

Shallice, T. (1988). Specialization within the semantic system. *Cognitive Neuropsychology, 5*(1), 133–142.

Shuster, L.I., & Lemieux, S.K. (2005). An fMRI investigation of covertly and overtly produced mono- and multisyllabic words. *Brain and Language, 93*(1), 20–31. doi:10.1016/j.bandl.2004.07.007

Silkes, J., Dierkes, K., & Kendall, D. (2013). Masked repetition priming effects on naming in aphasia: A phase I treatment study. *Aphasiology, 27*(4), 381–397.

Snodgrass, J.G., & Vanderwart, M. (1980). A standardized set of 260 pictures: Norms for name agreement, image agreement, familiarity, and visual complexity. *Journal of Experimental Psychology. Human Learning and Memory, 6*(2), 174–215.

Soni, M., Lambon Ralph, M.A., & Woollams, A.M. (2012). Reptition priming of picture naming in semantic aphasia: The impact of intervening items. *Aphasiology, 26*(1), 44–63.

Spalek, K., Damian, M., & Bolte, J. (2013). Is lexical selection in spoken word production competitive? Introduction to the special issue on lexical competitive in language production. *Language and Cognitive Processes, 28*(5), 597–614.

Spinnler, H., & Vignolo, L.A. (1966). Impaired recognition of meaningful sounds in aphasia. *Cortex, 2*(3), 337–348.

Stanczak, L., Waters, G., & Caplan, D. (2006). Typicality-based learning and generalisation in aphasia: Two case studies of anomia treatment. *Aphasiology, 20*(2–4), 374–383. doi:10.1080/02687030600587631

Strain, E., Patterson, K., & Seidenberg, M.S. (1995). Semantic effects in single-word naming. *Journal of Experimental Psychology. Learning, Memory, Cognition, 21*(5), 1140–1154.

Taylor, K.I., Devereux, B.J., & Tyler, L.K. (2011). Conceptual structure: Towards an integrated neuro-cognitive account. *Language and Cognitive Processes, 26*(9), 1368–1401. doi:10.1080/01690965.2011.568227

Thompson, C.K. (2011). *Northwestern Assessment of Verbs and Sentences.* Evanston, IL: Northwestern.

Thompson, C.K., Lukic, S., King, M.C., Mesulam, M.M., & Weintraub, S. (2012). Verb and noun deficits in stroke-induced and primary progressive aphasia: The Northwestern Naming Battery. *Aphasiology, 26*(5), 632–655. doi:10.1080/02687038.2012.676852

Thompson, C.K., & Shapiro, L.P. (2007). Complexity in treatment of syntactic deficits. *American Journal of Speech-Language Pathololgy, 16*(1), 30–42.

Tippett, L.J., Grossman, M., & Farah, M.J. (1996). The semantic memory impairment of Alzheimer's disease: Category-specific? *Cortex, 32*(1), 143–153.

Tippett, L.J., Meier, S.L., Blackwood, K., & Diaz-Asper, C. (2007). Category specific deficits in Alzheimer's disease: Fact or artefact? *Cortex, 43*(7), 907–920.

Tyler, L.K., & Moss, H.E. (2001). Towards a distributed account of conceptual knowledge. *Trends in Cognitive Science, 5*(6), 244–252.

Varney, N.R. (1980). Sound recognition in relation to aural language comprehension in aphasic patients. *Journal of Neurology, Neurosurgery, and Psychiatry, 43*(1), 71–75.

Visch-Brink, E.G., Bajema, I.M., & Van De Sandt-Koenderman, M.E. (1997). Lexical semantic therapy: BOX. *Aphasiology, 11*(11), 1057–1115.

Wambaugh, J.L., Cameron, R., Kalinyak-Fliszar, M., Nessler, C., & Wright, S. (2004). Retrieval of action names in aphasia: Effects of two cueing treatments. *Aphasiology, 18*(11), 979–1004. doi:10.1080/02687030444000471

Wambaugh, J.L., & Ferguson, M. (2007). Application of semantic feature analysis to retrieval of action names in aphasia. *Journal of Rehabilitation Research and Development, 44*(3), 381–394. doi:10.1682/Jrrd.2006.05.0038

Wambaugh, J.L., Linebaugh, C.W., Doyle, P., Martinez, A.L., Kalinyak-Fliszar, M., & Spencer, K. (2001). Effects of two cueing treatments on lexical retrieval in aphasic patients with different levels of deficit. *Aphasiology, 15*(10/11), 933–950.

Wambaugh, J.L., Mauszycki, S., Cameron, R., Wright, S., & Nessler, C. (2013). Semantic feature analysis: Incorporating typicality treatment and mediating strategy training to promote generalization. *American Journal of Speech-Language Pathology, 22*(2), S334–S369. doi:10.1044/1058–0360(2013/12–0070)

Warrington, E.K., & Crutch, S.J. (2007). Selective category and modality effects in deep dyslexia. *Neurocase, 13*(3), 144–153. doi:10.1080/13554790701440462

Warrington, E.K., & McCarthy, R.A. (1987). Categories of knowledge. Further fractionations and an attempted integration. *Brain, 110*(Pt 5), 1273–1296.

Warrington, E.K., McKenna, P., & Orpwood, L. (1998). Single word comprehension: a concrete and abstract word synonym test. *Neuropsychological Rehabilitation, 8*, 143–154.

Warrington, E.K., & Shallice, T. (1984). Category specific semantic impairments. *Brain, 107*(Pt 3), 829–854.

Whitehouse, P., Caramazza, A., & Zurif, E. (1978). Naming in aphasia: Interacting effects of form and function. *Brain and Language, 6*(1), 63–74.

Zingeser, L.B., & Berndt, R.S. (1990). Retrieval of nouns and verbs in agrammatism and anomia. *Brain and Language, 39*(1), 14–32.

PART 5

Auditory Discrimination and Recognition

13

MODELS OF SPEECH PROCESSING

Michael Grosvald, Martha W. Burton (deceased), and Steven L. Small

Introduction

One of the fundamental questions about language is how listeners map the acoustic signal onto syllables, words, and sentences, resulting in understanding of speech. For normal listeners, this mapping is so effortless that one rarely stops to consider just how it takes place. However, studies of speech have shown that this acoustic signal contains a great deal of underlying complexity. A number of competing models seek to explain how these intricate processes work. Such models have often narrowed the problem to mapping the speech signal onto isolated words, setting aside the complexity of segmenting continuous speech. Continuous speech has presented a significant challenge for many models because of the high variability of the signal and the difficulties involved in resolving the signal into individual words.

The importance of understanding speech becomes particularly apparent when neurological disease affects this seemingly basic ability. Lesion studies have explored impairments of speech sound processing to determine whether deficits occur in perceptual analysis of acoustic-phonetic information or in stored abstract phonological representations (e.g., Basso, Casati, & Vignolo, 1977; Blumstein, Cooper, Zurif, & Caramazza, 1977). Furthermore, researchers have attempted to determine in what ways underlying phonological/phonetic impairments may contribute to auditory comprehension deficits (Blumstein, Baker, & Goodglass, 1977).

In this chapter, we discuss several psycholinguistic models of word recognition (the process of mapping the speech signal onto the lexicon), and outline how components of such models might correspond to the functional anatomy of the brain. We will also relate evidence from brain lesion and activation studies to components of such models. We then present some approaches that deal with speech perception more generally, and touch on a few current topics of debate.

Psycholinguistic Models of Word Recognition

The speech signal contains well-known characteristics that provide constraints on models of word recognition (Frauenfelder & Floccia, 1998; Jusczyk, 1986). First, the fine acoustic details of every word or sentence differ each time it is produced. Thus, one challenge for models of word recognition is to explain how acoustically different tokens of a word, which may vary in myriad ways, are mapped into a single word (from what may be a number of similar words). Among other factors, variation among tokens may occur as a function of who is speaking, that is, the "talker" (e.g., through differences in voice or pronunciation); neighboring words (e.g., through coarticulatory effects); and prosodic context. In addition, the speech signal is continuous, lacking easily discernible discrete boundaries between sounds or words. Thus, any model must account for how diverse phonetic tokens that are part of a continuous signal can be mapped onto discrete units that can be recognized as individual sounds and words.

Different models of word recognition diverge on particular details, especially with regard to the nature of intermediate representations, but there does appear to be general consensus about word recognition that accounts for a wide range of experimental results from the psycholinguistic literature (Frauenfelder & Floccia, 1998).[1] Most models consist of processes by which sublexical units, such as phonetic features or phonemes, are extracted from the acoustic signal and then matched with the appropriate lexical entry.

Sublexical units have been postulated in most models of word recognition, including TRACE (McClelland & Elman, 1986), Cohort (Marslen-Wilson, 1987; Marslen-Wilson & Warren, 1994), and Merge (Norris et al., 2000), to provide a less variable, more abstract form of the acoustic signal. This is done in order to simplify the mapping of sublexical information onto the lexical level.

A primary difference among these models relates to the nature of input representations. Some models, like the Cohort model (Marslen-Wilson, 1987; Lahiri & Marslen-Wilson, 1991; Marslen-Wilson & Warren, 1994) rely on relatively small units like phonetic features that correspond to either acoustic or articulatory characteristics. For example, the feature of "voicing" refers to the presence of vocal cord vibration during the articulation of a speech sound and distinguishes voiceless sounds like /p/ from voiced ones like /b/. Other models, such as TRACE, proposed by McClelland and Elman (1986), rely more heavily on sets or bundles of phonetic features that define more abstract units, called segments or phonemes, that are considered the minimal units of sound distinguishing the meanings of words. For example, the initial phonemes, /p/ and /b/, which share the same place and manner of articulation features, but contrast in terms of voicing, differentiate the words "pear" and "bear."

Different realizations of a given phoneme are not acoustically identical; some (though not all) of this variation tends to be systematic. For example, in English, the same phoneme, /p/, is produced with different phonetic realizations that depend partly on where it occurs in a syllable or word (e.g., with aspiration noise in initial position, as in "pill," and without aspiration after /s/, as in "spill"). Such variations across spoken instances of a given speech sound are said to occur at the phonetic level, while at the more general phonemic level the fine detail of the physical characteristics of the speech signal is not relevant.

The nature of these abstract representations remains controversial. Early evidence indicated that listeners showed poor discrimination between acoustically different members of the same phonetic category (e.g., acoustically different exemplars of /d/, as in the classic categorical perception experiments of Liberman, Harris, Hoffman, & Griffith, 1957), suggesting that listeners perceive speech sounds using abstract phoneme category information and discard much of the fine acoustic detail.

Subsequent studies have indicated that listeners retain more acoustic detail in stored representations of speech than many researchers had initially believed (Kuhl, 1991; Pisoni, 1993). Kuhl and colleagues have argued that listeners maintain within-category distinctions for speech sounds such as vowels. In other words, some sounds within a given speech category (e.g., spoken instances of the vowel /i/) are considered by listeners to be better exemplars of the category than others, and in this sense can be considered more prototypical. Furthermore, these prototypical sounds serve as perceptual magnets, affecting the perception of other similar speech stimuli, whereas nonprototypical sounds do not show such effects. Along these lines, Kuhl (1991) provided evidence that listeners are sensitive to some within-category acoustic detail, and that speech prototypes may serve to organize categories of sounds during perception.

Pisoni (1993) further challenged traditional views of speech perception, arguing that even more acoustic information (including variability from utterances of individual talkers and context effects, such as rate) is preserved from initial perceptual analysis of the speech signal, and in addition provides important information for later recognition of specific talkers (Nygaard, Sommers, & Pisoni, 1995). According to Pisoni (1993), information about specific acoustic characteristics of particular talkers is stored in long-term memory.

Despite these findings, models of speech perception still tend to assume that during perceptual analysis of the signal listeners are able to "normalize" variability in the signal and map acoustic input onto abstract representations such as features (Marslen-Wilson & Warren, 1994) and phonemes (Norris et al., 2000). Some models of speech perception, such as the connectionist TRACE model of McClelland and Elman (1986), incorporate abstract segmental units as well as phonetic features, whereas other models map spectral properties of the acoustic signal directly onto syllables (Klatt, 1979). The motor theory of speech perception posits that these intermediate units correspond to articulatory gestures (Liberman et al., 1967; Liberman & Mattingly, 1985; Galantucci et al., 2006).

The mapping of these input representations onto the word level characteristically involves activation of lexical entries, for which the level of activation is determined by the goodness of fit between the input representation and the lexical representation. Typically, once a threshold of activation has been reached a word is recognized. An example of such a model implemented using the connectionist framework is TRACE (McClelland & Elman, 1986), which has been used to account for a number of effects of lexical influence on phonetic categorization (e.g., Pitt & Samuel, 1993).

Despite the common use of an activation mechanism to represent how words are recognized, models differ in the mechanistic details of the activation process, such as the amount of top-down processing that is permitted from higher levels to lower levels, or the degree to which inhibition between competing representations plays a role. For example, the Merge model maintains that top-down (lexical) information does not influence categorization of lower-level phonetic information (Norris et al., 2000), whereas models such as TRACE allow such feedback (McClelland & Elman, 1986). Other models, such as the neighborhood activation model, emphasize the role of competition among lexical entries in facilitating word recognition (Luce & Pisoni, 1998). In that model, the number of similar words, their degree of phonetic similarity, and frequency of occurrence in a language (similarity-neighborhood) affect the speed and accuracy of word recognition.

Despite such differences among models, the generally accepted view—that the speech signal is analyzed into sublexical units that activate word entries—provides a framework for how the most basic processes of word recognition proceed (Frauenfelder & Floccia, 1998). Although lesion studies have often seemed inconsistent regarding the physical loci of these processes in the brain, more recent results offer some revealing insights. Evidence from a variety of experimental tasks in neuropsychological studies, and from functional neuroimaging of normal adults, reveals a network of regions of the brain that appear to correspond to specific functions postulated in models of speech processing. Below we will consider what specific areas of the brain may be involved in the analysis and mapping of the speech signal onto lexical information. We will argue that although listeners have access to different kinds of sublexical representations, their use depends critically on task demands, and the effects of such task demands are reflected in activation patterns seen in neuroimaging studies.

Evidence from Aphasia

Experiments exploring speech perception in stroke patients with aphasia have focused attention on segmental contrasts within words (e.g., /p/ vs. /b/ in *pear/bear*) or in nonsense syllables (e.g., *pa/ba*) (Basso et al., 1977; Benson, 1988; Blumstein, Cooper, et al., 1977; Carpenter &

Rutherford, 1973; Miceli, Caltagirone, Gainotti, & Payer-Rigo, 1978; Oscar-Berman, Zurif, & Blumstein, 1975; Riedel & Studdert-Kennedy, 1985). Nearly all patients show some impairment in discrimination ("same-different" judgments) and/or labeling or identification (e.g., "Is the first sound a *p* or a *b*?") (Blumstein, 1998). Patterns of errors on these tasks follow those seen in speech production errors. For example, more errors occur in medial or final position in the syllable than in initial position (Blumstein, 1998). Individuals with lesions in the temporal lobe might be expected to show speech discrimination deficits because primary auditory areas are located in the temporal lobe and have direct connections to the auditory association areas. However, individuals with anterior lesions also manifest such impairments. These data have challenged the traditional view that speech perception impairments should be associated solely with posterior lesions in people with aphasia.

Several lines of evidence suggest that speech perception impairments in aphasic individuals do not occur at the stage of extracting sublexical information from the acoustic signal. Patients' performance is generally better on discrimination tasks than on identification tasks, indicating that they are sensitive to acoustic-phonetic differences in the stimuli, but may have difficulty providing accurate responses based on segmental information (Gow & Caplan, 1996). Furthermore, patterns of results in discrimination tasks are similar to those of healthy controls in the location of boundaries between phonetic categories and in the overall shape of the discrimination functions, even in cases where patients cannot label the stimuli (Blumstein, 1998).

Blumstein and colleagues (2000), in an investigation of the effects of phonological priming, offered further evidence that participants with aphasia are able to extract useful acoustic properties from the signal. In a set of priming tasks, aphasic participants presented with pairs of words or nonwords performed a lexical decision on the second member of the pair. The phonological properties of the first member of the pair were systematically varied (e.g., producing either rhyming or unrelated pairs like "pear-bear" vs. "pen-bear"). Both Broca's and Wernicke's aphasic participants showed effects of rhyming primes on lexical decision times, suggesting that both types of aphasic participants are sensitive to phonological similarity (see also Gordon & Baum, 1994). In a second experiment, the researchers tested repetition priming with these same aphasic participants using lexical decision on repeated words occurring at different intervals (i.e., presentation of the same word immediately following the prime, two words following the prime, eight words following the prime, and so on). The results suggested the presence of a second impairment in these participants, namely, maintaining an acoustic form in short-term memory. Unlike normals, the aphasic participants showed neither increased repetition effects at shorter intervals compared to longer intervals nor any repetition effects for nonwords. As long as the lexicon was activated by a real word, aphasic participants showed priming effects. However, the lack of increased repetition effects at shorter intervals suggests that the aphasic participants were "matching" the meaning of the stimulus, not its phonetic form, which may have dissipated in working memory faster for the aphasic participants than for controls. The lack of increased repetition effects at longer intervals and nonword effects were consistent across all aphasic participants.

These findings are also in agreement with other patterns of deficits described in single case studies. For example, Martin, Bredin, and Damian (1999) report a patient able to perform phoneme discrimination at a level similar to that of normals, yet speech discrimination declined with increased interstimulus interval, suggesting a short-term memory deficit. Such short-term memory impairments of maintaining information over time certainly contribute to auditory language comprehension deficits, such as those in which listeners must actively retrieve specific pieces of information over the longer periods of time required by sentence processing (Caplan & Waters, 1995; Martin & Romani, 1994; Miyake, Carpenter, & Just, 1994). In contrast, low-level speech perception impairments may have some limited role in higher-level language comprehension, but do not appear to account for severe auditory language comprehension difficulties (Blumstein, Baker, et al., 1977). Blumstein and colleagues found that the level of performance on identification and discrimination of consonant-vowel syllables that do not require maintenance over long intervals was a poor predictor of auditory comprehension as measured by standard clinical diagnostic tests.

In summary, a number of studies have investigated speech perception in aphasic individuals using different experimental tasks. The results have generally demonstrated that impairments are not due to initial acoustic analysis of the speech signal. Because the patterns of impairment have not clearly corresponded to particular levels of representation in speech perception models and have had unclear localization, they have not played a significant role in models of normal speech perception. Although one might hypothesize that components of sublexical processing could be selectively impaired (e.g., perceptual analysis of the signal vs. segmentation), neuropsychological studies have shown that nearly all aphasic individuals display some impairments in speech perception. These difficulties performing a range of tasks do not generally appear to be due to early stages of sublexical speech processing in which the acoustic information, such as temporal or spectral properties, are extracted from the signal. Thus, even if aphasic participants have left temporal damage, they may be able to perform some speech discrimination tasks because of spared right hemisphere structures.

In an effort to better understand the relationship between location of brain lesions and deficits in language comprehension, Dronkers et al. (2004) conducted a study of 64 participants with aphasia due to left hemisphere stroke, who were asked to choose drawings that best matched the meanings of auditorily presented sentences. The results of a voxel-based lesion-symptom mapping analysis (Bates et al., 2003) identified several relevant left hemisphere regions: posterior middle temporal gyrus, anterior superior temporal gyrus, superior temporal sulcus and angular gyrus, and two frontal regions—Brodmann areas 46 and 47. Of these regions, middle temporal gyrus seemed to be the one most involved in word-level speech comprehension, with the others apparently more involved in comprehension at the sentence level. Interestingly, the analysis found that significant deficits in language comprehension were neither associated with lesions of Broca's area nor Wernicke's area.

Anatomically, the effects of hypometabolism in temporal and temporoparietal regions have been found for patients with various types of aphasia and thus may provide a potential common neural substrate (Metter et al., 1989, 1990). Behaviorally, many people with aphasia have problems with auditory working memory that may play a greater role in speech identification (comparison of stimulus to a stored representation) than speech discrimination (comparison between two exemplars).

People with aphasia may show some impairment in discrimination tasks as well as identification tasks. It remains unclear to what extent hemispheric differences in the posterior temporal lobe play a role in speech perception impairments. However, theories that postulate hemispheric asymmetries predict difficulties with those speech contrasts that rely on rapidly changing frequency information (discussed further in the section on superior temporal regions, below). This could explain why some adults with focal brain lesions in the left hemisphere have difficulties with rapid formant transitions in stop consonants (Ivry & Robertson, 1998).

In broad terms, however, basing our understanding of the underlying neuroanatomy of speech perception on lesion studies alone leaves a number of unanswered questions. The common finding that inferior frontal cortex is activated in phonological tasks and in tasks that are designed to require verbal working memory suggests that the role of working memory requires more attention in explaining impaired performance on certain speech perception tasks.

Functional Neuroanatomy of Speech Perception

In contrast to the lesion data, functional neuroimaging studies of healthy participants have been converging on a set of regions involved in specific functional components of speech perception. From these studies, it is possible to gain insight into why some aphasic participants may have difficulty with particular tasks, such as phoneme identification, and to determine whether processing of different types of sublexical information (e.g., acoustic-phonetic features and phonemes) produces distinct patterns of brain behavior (e.g., patterns of activation, electromagnetic responses). Evidence that listeners are sensitive to sublexical information (acoustic-phonetic features and/or phonemic category information)—as demonstrated through neurobiological responses—will help to clarify what role sublexical information may play in models of speech perception.

Functional neuroimaging studies of speech perception typically rely on one of two task-dependent imaging methods, PET (positron emission tomography) or fMRI (functional magnetic resonance imaging), to reveal areas of the brain that participate in a task, yet when damaged may not necessarily impair performance of language functions. Although PET and fMRI differ in a number of aspects of experimental design and analysis and have different spatial and temporal properties, both methods involve imaging some (presumed) correlate of neural activity during performance of a cognitive task. These methods allow observation of the particular areas of the brain that participate in a cognitive task (for reviews of neuroimaging methods see Burton & Small, 1999; Bandettini, 2009). Magnetoencephalography (MEG) provides highly accurate information about the time-course of processing for relatively small areas of cortex by measuring neuromagnetic responses to stimulation. For that reason, MEG has been used to study speech perception, which takes place within milliseconds in the temporal lobe. Other methods, such as event-related potentials (ERP), that provide highly accurate time-course information but not spatial localization, have also been used to identify stages of speech processing (e.g., Rinne et al., 1999).

Long-standing evidence indicates that three main areas of activity—superior temporal gyrus and sulcus, inferior parietal lobule, and inferior frontal gyrus—perform critical functions during the processing of speech. Figure 13.1 shows the approximate location of these areas on a structural image of the left lateral cortex of a normal subject. More recent data indicate that other brain regions are crucially involved as well, and together with the three regions just mentioned, form networks or processing streams whose configuration can depend at least partly on task demands (Hein & Knight, 2008; Londei et al., 2010; Price, 2012).

Superior Temporal Regions

Some of the most compelling evidence for the role of superior temporal cortex in early speech analysis is the consistent pattern of activation when passive speech is compared to rest or to nonspeech sounds. Although activation in primary auditory cortex and auditory association areas is seen for nonlinguistic as well as for language sounds (for an overview, see Price, 2012), much evidence suggests that during speech perception initial acoustic/phonetic analysis also takes place in these regions. During this process, it appears that phonetic/phonemic information is extracted from the acoustic signal (Binder et al., 1994; Dhankhar et al., 1997; Gage, Poeppel, Roberts, & Hickok, 1998; Kuriki, Okita, & Hirata, 1995; Petersen, Fox, Posner, Mintun, & Raichle, 1988; Poeppel et al., 1996; Price et al., 1992; Wise et al., 1991; Zatorre, Meyer, Gjedde, & Evans, 1996).

Initial research comparing speech and nonspeech perception often contrasted speech to tones, and found greater temporal activity for the speech stimuli, particularly in the left hemisphere. This

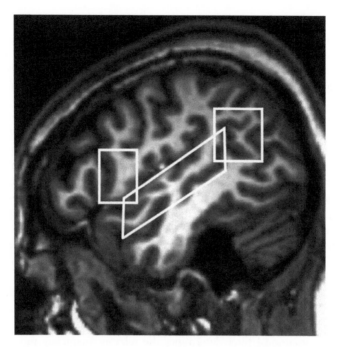

Figure 13.1 Sagittal view of left lateral cortex acquired using structural magnetic resonance imaging. White boxes highlight three areas involved in components of speech processing: the posterior two-thirds of inferior frontal gyrus (Broca's area); superior temporal sulcus and gyrus, including primary auditory cortex; and inferior parietal lobe.

suggested that specialized mechanisms for speech-related processing might be at work (Burton, Blumstein, & Small, 2000; Mummery, Ashburner, Scott, & Wise, 1999), but such studies left open the possibility that preferential activity for speech might be due to the greater acoustic complexity of speech syllables compared to the tone stimuli that had been used. However, a number of subsequent imaging studies comparing speech and nonspeech perception have controlled for acoustic complexity and have found a preferential response to speech in the left posterior superior temporal sulcus (Narain et al., 2003; Giraud et al., 2004; Hugdahl et al., 2003; Benson et al., 2006; Rimol et al., 2006). Such findings are bolstered by the results of Dehaene-Lambertz et al. (2005) and Meyer et al. (2005), who found greater activation in left posterior temporal cortex when distorted (sine-wave) speech was perceived by listeners as language, relative to when it was not. More generally, studies have tended to find that greater sound familiarity and greater acoustic complexity are associated with superior temporal activity that is, respectively, more posterior or more anterior (Price, 2012).

Despite the tendency in some studies for greater left temporal activation than right, and the predilection to discuss more fully the left hemisphere findings, the activation across imaging studies of speech perception has been consistently bilateral (Hickok & Poeppel, 2000). Further evidence for bilateral activation comes from fMRI studies of speech perception in normals and two aphasic patients listening to speech presented at varying rates (Mummery et al., 1999). In normal subjects, increasing rates of speech correlate with greater bilateral superior temporal activation in response to speech stimuli. Participants with left temporal infarction who perform well on single word comprehension tests have right superior temporal activity correlated with the rate of speech presentation, but no significant left temporal activity. Thus, their spared speech comprehension ability could be due to involvement of the right hemisphere, which, in normal controls, is more characteristically involved in prelexical processing of speech.

Based on patterns of bilaterality, some researchers have postulated different roles for the left and right superior temporal cortices in speech signal analysis. One such hypothesis claims that left hemisphere is specialized for processing quickly changing frequency information, such as the rapid transitions that occur in stop consonants, such as /p t k b d g/ (Hesling et al., 2005; Hickok & Poeppel, 2000; Nicholls, 1996; Poeppel, 2003). For example, Belin and colleagues (1998) found significantly greater activation for left auditory cortex than right when subjects were presented with speech-like rapid (e.g., 40 msec) acoustic changes that had identical temporal structure to frequency transitions between consonants and vowels. In contrast, the right hemisphere has been associated with processing of slower-changing information found in some speech sounds, such as fricatives and nasals, compared to the rapid frequency transitions found in stops (Allard & Scott, 1975; Gage et al., 1998) or spectral information (Zatorre, 1997). Slower-changing information may be useful for processing that occurs over longer windows of time, such as prosody or the melody of a sentence. Evidence consistent with this sort of difference in hemispheric processing has been found in a number of subsequent studies (Husain et al., 2006; Rimol et al., 2005; Zaehle et al., 2004).

A related view is that the left hemisphere is more specialized for processing that requires greater temporal precision and the right hemisphere for computations that require greater spectral resolution (Zatorre, Belin, & Penhune, 2002). In still another proposal, double filtering by frequency, it is argued that an attentional filter determines the relevant frequency properties for analysis of the acoustic signal (Ivry & Robertson, 1998). Parts of the signal that occupy comparatively high portions of the frequency spectrum, relative to an anchoring point, are processed in the left hemisphere, whereas relatively low-frequency components of the signal are processed in the right hemisphere.

In summary, a number of proposals seek to explain the apparent differences in the roles of the left and right hemispheres in early acoustic/phonetic analysis. Whether these processes are speech specific remains to be determined. It may be possible for the contralateral hemisphere to compensate for loss when damage occurs; thus, it may be difficult to see evidence of hemispheric differences in aphasia (see also chapter 14, this volume).

Inferior Parietal Regions

Once the initial acoustic analysis is performed, the resulting sound representation must make contact with lexical-semantic information. Inferior parietal regions have consistently been implicated in such processes, often appearing to act in concert with frontal regions, and with the angular and supramarginal gyri appearing to play somewhat different roles.

In Demonet et al. (1992, 1994b), participants made semantic judgments on words and phonological judgments on nonwords, and showed widespread activation in frontal, temporal, and inferior parietal regions. The results indicated that the angular gyri (acting together with left temporal regions) are more involved with semantic processing at the word level, while the supramarginal gyri (together with left inferior frontal cortex) appear to be more involved with tasks requiring phonological decision making.

Other early studies found activation in inferior parietal regions for tasks requiring short-term storage of phonological information (Awh, Smith, & Jonides, 1995; Jonides et al., 1998; Paulesu, Frith, & Frackowiak, 1993; Paulesu et al., 1996). This activation was reported more consistently for tasks that involved stimuli requiring more extensive phonological coding (e.g., nonwords) than with word tasks in which subjects could use a combination of semantic and phonological coding to store verbal material (Jonides et al., 1998). One method of maintaining information in a phonological store is through rehearsal. If this area were part of an auditory-motor (articulatory) integration network that includes inferior frontal regions, the concomitant activity in the inferior frontal lobe due to rehearsal and inferior parietal lobe due to temporary storage could be explained as a single network of regions that participate in speech processing (Hickok & Poeppel, 2000). In a number of studies (Myers et al., 2009; Ravizza et al., 2011; Zevin et al., 2010), for tasks in which working memory demands were minimized, frontoparietal areas associated with verbal short-term memory were also engaged. The results of these and other studies (Davis et al., 2007; Elmer et al., 2011) suggest that this frontoparietal network is involved in auditory and categorization processes that are not language specific (Price, 2012; see also chapters 11 and 14, this volume).

Gow et al.'s (2008) combined MEG, EEG, and MRI study found evidence that interplay between inferior parietal and superior temporal regions underlie a lexical-phonological perceptual phenomenon known as the Ganong effect (Ganong, 1980; Warren, 1970; Samuel & Pitt, 2003). This phenomenon occurs when an acoustically ambiguous language sound (e.g., a fricative sound intermediate between /s/ as in "sin" and /š/ as in "shin") is inserted into a phoneme sequence that may or may not be interpretable as a word, depending on how the ambiguous sound is interpreted (e.g., Chri[s]mas forms a word while Chri[š]mas does not). Listeners in such a situation will tend to interpret the sound in such a way that a real lexical item is perceived, providing evidence that top-down processes influence lower-level phonetic perception. Gow and colleagues' analysis indicated that lexical-level processing taking place in supramarginal gyrus affects phonetic-level processing in posterior superior temporal gyrus. Clarifying the interplay between brain regions is increasingly seen as crucial to an understanding of the human language system, a theme we will return to in the section on processing streams, below.

Inferior Frontal Regions

Activation of the left inferior frontal cortex (particularly the inferior frontal gyrus) has long been attributed to phonological processing in auditory tasks (Demonet et al., 1992; Demonet, Price, Wise, & Frackowiak, 1994a; Zatorre et al., 1992, 1996). Reviews of early PET evidence found that the patterns of activation did not converge as expected (compare Poeppel, 1996, and Demonet, Fiez, Paulesu, Petersen, & Zatorre, 1996), but subsequent researchers have tested phonological processing with increasingly specific cognitive tasks. The results of such studies suggest that there are indeed common underlying speech processes that may specifically activate these regions.

Based on PET data, Zatorre and colleagues (1992, 1996) argue that inferior frontal activation during particular speech tasks reflects segmentation processes in which listeners must separate speech sounds contained within syllables. For example, in pairs of spoken consonant-vowel-consonant sequences where the vowels differ (e.g., "fat"-"tid"), subjects making a "same/different" judgment on the final consonant must separate out the final consonant from a continuous acoustic signal. By using stimuli in which different vowels precede the consonant within the pairs, the need for segmentation is ensured because the consonant transitions vary as a function of preceding vowel context. Furthermore, Zatorre and colleagues (1992, 1996) argued that in performing this segmentation, listeners are required to access articulatory representations. In this account, such recoding of acoustic information to articulatory gestures is said to require Broca's area involvement because of its traditional association with articulatory deficits in neuropsychological studies of aphasic patients. Results of experiments comparing speech discrimination to either pitch discrimination or passive listening have shown activation of the left frontal cortex in the phonetic discrimination task. However, Zatorre and colleagues

(1992, 1996) found no such activation in Broca's area under passive listening conditions to the same stimuli.

The location of activation in the speech discrimination tasks was in the most posterior and superior aspect of Broca's area. This subregion of Broca's area is similar to that reported in several other studies of auditory phonological processing that involved segmentation of speech sounds and comparison of stimuli for a decision (Burton et al., 2000; Demonet et al., 1992; Demonet et al., 1994a). These studies compared activation for tasks involving phoneme monitoring for sequences of sounds or consonant segmentation to passive or sensory tasks. This area differs from the regions cited in studies of semantic tasks that have argued for Broca's area activation (Poldrack et al., 1999). Functional specialization of different subregions of Broca's area seems likely to explain—at least in part—why multiple functions have historically been attributed to Broca's area as a whole (Dronkers, 1998).

A related question is whether listeners are always required to access segmental information in speech discrimination tasks. In segmentation tasks like those used by Zatorre and colleagues (1992, 1996), in which there are multiple differences among the segments in the stimuli, it appears likely that subjects must compare entire segments in order to make a same/different judgment. In contrast, if segments differ by only one phonetic feature, such as voicing, there may be no need for segmentation, since the subject only has to perceive a single phonetic difference between the stimulus pairs to make a decision. Burton et al. (2000) investigated this issue using an overt speech discrimination task in which subjects were required to make a same/different judgment about phonetic segments in initial position. It was expected that Broca's area would be involved only when the subject had to perform a task requiring articulatory recoding. Significantly more frontal activation was seen for tasks requiring overt segmentation (e.g., "dip-doom" pairs) compared to those that did not (e.g., "dip-tip" pairs). Thus, phonetic judgments may invoke different neural mechanisms depending on task demands.

Importantly, Burton and colleagues (2000) found significant superior temporal gyrus activation (with a trend toward left-lateralization) regardless of whether the speech task required segmentation. Thus, frontal areas might not typically be recruited in the processing of speech for purposes of at least some speech discrimination tasks (i.e., those that do not require segmentation) and may not necessarily be invoked on a more global level for auditory language comprehension, a situation in which listeners may not need to identify individual sounds to accomplish word recognition. These results also suggest that posterior brain structures participate in initial perceptual analysis of the signal that is necessary for the subsequent mapping of acoustic/phonetic patterns onto higher levels of language, such as meaning.

Although functional neuroimaging studies of speech focusing on frontal activity have typically concentrated on segmental phonological tasks, imaging studies have suggested that suprasegmental information such as pitch contour may also activate inferior frontal cortex in discrimination tasks (Gandour et al., 2000; Gandour, Wong, & Hutchins, 1998; Gandour, 2007). Pitch cues can be used to distinguish lexical meaning in tone languages, such as Mandarin Chinese or Thai. Cross-linguistic studies provide the opportunity to compare perception of the same pitch contrasts under circumstances in which the pairs of speech stimuli are linguistically distinctive (e.g., two Thai words varying in lexical tones that have different meanings) to cases where they are not (e.g., English). When a pitch discrimination condition was compared to a filtered speech control task in which semantic and phonological information was eliminated, but other suprasegmental information was preserved, Gandour and colleagues found that only Thai speakers showed inferior frontal activation. Similar to English speakers, Chinese listeners with experience in tonal language, but not the particular tone distinctions in Thai, did not show activation in Broca's area. These findings indicate that Broca's area subserves not only segmental, but also suprasegmental processing.

In response to a number of findings in both spoken and written language, Bornkessel-Schlesewsky and Schlesewsky have developed a model called the extended argument dependency model (Bornkessel & Schlesewsky, 2006; Bornkessel-Schlesewsky & Schlesewsky, 2009). This model is informed by—and attempts to account for—the fact that qualitatively similar phenomena can elicit different processing consequences in different languages, or the reverse. The basic intuition behind the model is that the flow of language processing is broadly similar cross-linguistically, but differences arise due to the kinds of information that are available, relevant, or prominent in different languages. For example, word order is relatively fixed in English but flexible in Czech; case is rudimentary or nonexistent in languages like English and Mandarin Chinese but much more important in German and Russian. This leads to differences in how languages encode information such as agency (i.e., "who did what to whom"). The result is that the same sentence—modulo translation—can elicit one kind of processing consequence in one language (e.g., a particular ERP waveform) but not in another.

Processing Streams

In addition to providing a better understanding of how specific brain regions contribute to linguistic processing, recent work has also led to a growing appreciation of how brain regions operate together. Much of the current work on processing "streams" in language comprehension has its origins in the visual processing literature. Frequently these are tied to some degree to known anatomical pathways. For example, two visual processing pathways in macaque, one "ventral" and the other "dorsal," appear to have different functions (Ungerleider & Mishkin, 1982). The ventral stream projects from visual cortex (striate and prestriate) to inferior temporal areas and is important for object recognition ("what"), while the dorsal stream connects visual cortex to inferior parietal areas and is important for spatial localization ("where") and visual-motor transformations ("how"). These two pathways may therefore reflect a fundamental distinction between perception- or sensory-oriented processing on the one hand and action-oriented processing on the other (Goodale & Milner, 1992).

Rauschecker and colleagues (Rauschecker, 1998; Rauschecker & Tian, 2000) proposed that, like visual processing, auditory processing is also segregated into dorsal and ventral streams. Support for these "ventral/what" and "dorsal/where" streams has been found in connectivity studies of structure/function relations (Saur et al., 2008) and in statistical relations among regions (i.e., "functional connectivity") (Obleser et al., 2007; Londei et al., 2010; Leff et al., 2008; Schofield et al., 2009; Osnes et al., 2011; Eickhoff et al., 2009; Nath & Beauchamp, 2011). There is also evidence that the anatomical pathways subserving these "what" and "how" functions converge in frontal regions (Romanski et al., 1999; Scott & Johnsrude, 2003). Much subsequent work has attempted to elucidate the structure of these processing streams and to clarify their roles in language processing (e.g., Bornkessel-Schlesewsky & Schlesewsky, 2013; Bornkessel-Schlesewsky, Schlesewsky, Small, & Rauschecker, 2014; Friederici, 2012; Hickok & Poeppel, 2004, 2007; Rauschecker & Scott, 2009).

Although anatomical and functional details of these pathways are not yet fully understood, the general dorsal versus ventral distinction is now widely recognized, and much ongoing work seeks to clarify their respective roles. For example, DeWitt and Rauschecker's (2012) meta-analysis of functional imaging studies related to auditory processing found specific evidence of hierarchically organized linguistic processing along the ventral pathway. Processing related to progressively more temporally complex linguistic sounds (i.e., phonemes and words) appears to be localized to areas progressively further along the ventral stream, with left mid-superior temporal gyrus implicated in short-timescale sound form (phoneme-level) processing, and processing related to the integration of such items into longer forms (words) occurring in left anterior superior temporal gyrus (STG). Accordingly, there is a tendency toward greater invariance further along this processing stream. Poeppel et al. (2008) also argue that auditory analysis in at least two different timescales, corresponding to approximately the feature/segment and syllable/word levels, occurs during speech processing.

In addition to supporting auditory-motor mapping, the dorsal pathway also appears to be involved in syntactic processing (Bornkessel-Schlesewsky & Schlesewsky, 2013; Bornkessel-Schlesewsky, Schlesewsky, Small, & Rauschecker, 2014; Friederici et al., 2006; Wilson et al., 2010), a qualitatively different function. In light of these and other findings, Friederici (2012) presents a model with two separate dorsal streams, one joining temporal and premotor cortex via inferior parietal cortex and the superior longitudinal fasciculus, the other linking temporal cortex with Brodmann area 44 via the arcuate fasciculus. The ventral pathway may support simple syntactic processing, in addition to its more generally recognized role in auditory-semantic mapping. Friederici's (2012) model incorporates two ventral streams to accommodate this. At the same time, Friederici (2012) acknowledges some limitations of her model—for example, in not specifying a clear role for the right hemisphere in language processing. The work discussed earlier that attempts to account for apparent hemispheric differences in early acoustic/phonetic analysis (Hesling et al., 2005; Hickok & Poeppel, 2000; Ivry & Robertson, 1998; Nicholls, 1996; Poeppel, 2003; Zatorre, Belin, & Penhune, 2002) may suggest at least a partial solution to that problem. More generally, as we learn more about the functional and structural complexity of the human language system, no doubt further refinements leading to still better models will be possible.

Motor Region Involvement in Speech Perception

As noted earlier, the motor theory of speech perception (Liberman et al., 1967; Liberman & Mattingly, 1985; Galantucci et al., 2006) posits that the percepts of speech are the articulatory gestures used in producing that speech or, more specifically, the neural commands that produced those gestures. Another way of expressing this idea is that understanding speech requires simulation of that speech on the part of the listener. It has been debated whether motor simulation is strictly necessary for speech perception or might simply be helpful in some situations. Though the former view appears untenable (Hickok et al., 2011; Pulvermüller & Fadiga, 2010; Rogalsky et al., 2011; Scott, McGettigan, & Eisner, 2009, 2013; Skipper et al., 2006; Tremblay & Small, 2011a, 2011b), evidence does suggest that motor regions may play a role in speech perception in particular contexts, such as under challenging perceptual conditions, or when useful visual input is present (Callan et al., 2010; Gow & Segawa, 2009; Hasson et al., 2007; Osnes et al., 2011; Skipper et al., 2005; Tremblay & Small, 2011b).

This topic has received renewed attention with the discovery of so-called "mirror neurons." These neurons, first discovered in macaque, were so named because they fire selectively when the animal carries out certain kinds of manual or oral actions, as well as when the animal observes others executing those same actions (Gallese et al., 1996; Rizzolatti et al., 1996). Therefore, this "mirror" property could, in principle, enable a perceiver to relate others' actions with the perceiver's own motor plans. Mirror neurons were first found in a ventral premotor region of macaque, area F5, and were later discovered in a parietal region, area 7b (Gallese et al., 2002). Broca's area has sometimes been considered the human homologue of area F5, and these findings have led to speculation about the role a human frontparietal mirror neuron system might play in action understanding in general, language processing in particular, and in the evolution of language itself (Arbib, 2005; Rizzolatti & Arbib, 1998).

Two pertinent topics in this line of research are the role of visual information in speech processing, and the likelihood that substantially overlapping networks are involved in speech production and perception (e.g., Poeppel & Monahan, 2008; Pulvermüller & Fadiga, 2010; Rossi et al., 2011; Scott, McGettigan, & Eisner, 2013; Skipper et al., 2006; Skipper et al., 2007). It has long been known that speech perception can be aided (Sumby & Pollack, 1954), or even altered, by accompanying visible facial movements. The latter situation occurs, for instance, in the well-known McGurk effect, in which auditory "pa" and visual "ka" syllables fuse to induce the perception of a "ta" syllable (McGurk & MacDonald, 1976).

Skipper, Nusbaum, and Small (2006) propose a model in which available visual information (the latter of which can include both facial movements and co-speech gestures) aids in the perception of speech by helping the listener compute a hypothesized motor plan for the heard utterance. This computed motor plan can influence what the listener perceives. Such computations are performed by a dorsal-stream mirror neuron system whose basic "building blocks" are paired inverse and forward models. While inverse models map perceived actions to motor plans hypothesized to cause such actions, forward models map (simulated) motor commands to predicted sensory consequences. One function of such a system is to delimit the set of possible interpretations of the incoming language signal. This is consistent with the view that activity in inferior frontal or premotor regions during speech processing may be due at least in part to the operation of top-down mechanisms that constrain the output of bottom-up processing in temporal cortex (Dehaene-Lambertz et al., 2005; Price, 2012; Zekveld et al., 2006).

Conclusion

Although differing in some details, particularly with regard to the nature of sublexical representations, models of word recognition have broadly converged in overall structure: sublexical information is extracted from the speech signal and mapped onto a lexical level via some kind of activation method. Because of the similarities of these models, they are often difficult to evaluate against each other solely on the basis of psycholinguistic evidence. Nevertheless, functional neuroimaging evidence suggests that different brain areas are recruited for the processing of distinct types of sublexical information, and provides support for the basic framework of these models. More generally, functional neuroimaging studies of normal subjects are converging upon a number of brain regions associated with different aspects of speech processing, and are offering greater insight into how these regions operate in concert.

Knowledge about the function of brain regions in components of normal speech processing has contributed to understanding the nature of some aphasic deficits. Specifically, aphasic individuals with damage to anterior structures may have difficulty with tasks that require explicit segmentation of the speech signal. For example, they may have trouble with phoneme identification tasks, which require such segmentation. However, because other auditory speech comprehension tasks may not require explicit segmentation of speech information, these patients may have relatively good speech comprehension. In contrast, aphasic individuals with damage in the posterior temporo-parietal junction may have difficulty performing an identification task because of difficulty integrating the auditory and articulatory information in the inferior parietal component of the network. Thus, both types of patients may do poorly on tasks involving explicit identification of speech sounds, but for different reasons, which is congruent with evidence from neuroimaging studies of control subjects and is consistent with the framework of models of word recognition that we have presented here.

A number of challenges remain in understanding the nature of breakdown of speech processing in aphasia. It is unlikely that an aphasic person would have damage only affecting as specific an area as described by the functional neuroimaging studies. For example, in the frontal lobe, few people with chronic aphasia have damage only affecting Broca's area (Dronkers, 2000), and it is even less likely that such a lesion would only damage a subregion of Broca's area. Thus, understanding other functions, such as the role of verbal working memory (cf. Jacquemot & Scott, 2006), will be crucial to understanding how damage in a particular area affects language comprehension.

Acknowledgment

This research was supported in part by the National Institutes of Health under grant NIH DC R01–3378 to the senior author (SLS). Their support is gratefully acknowledged.

Note

1 In addition to psycholinguistic models, a number of computational models have been developed to perform automatic speech recognition in many cases using hidden Markov models (Deng & Erler, 1992; Krogh & Riis, 1999; Watrous, 1990). Many of these neural network models employ the same types of subphonetic (e.g., features) and phonemic representations to achieve high levels of success in recognizing isolated words. However, because these models typically have not attempted to account for a wide range of psycholinguistic data, we will not discuss them further.

References

Allard, F., & Scott, B.L. (1975). Burst cues, transition cues, and hemispheric specialization with real speech sounds. *Quarterly Journal of Experimental Psychology, 27*, 487.

Arbib, M.A. (2005). From monkey-like action recognition to human language: An evolutionary framework for neurolinguistics. *Behavioral and Brain Sciences, 28*, 105–124.

Awh, E., Smith, E.E., & Jonides, J. (1995). Human rehearsal processes and the frontal lobes: PET evidence. *Annals of the New York Academy of Sciences, 769*, 97–117.

Bandettini, P.A. (2009). What's new in neuroimaging methods? *Annals of the New York Academy of Sciences, 1156(1)*, 260–293.

Basso, A., Casati, G., & Vignolo, L. (1977). Phonemic identification defect in aphasia. *Cortex, 13*, 85–95.

Bates, E., Wilson, S., Saygin, A.P., Dick, F., Sereno, M., Knight, R.T., & Dronkers, N.F. (2003). Voxel-based lesion-symptom mapping. *Nature Neuroscience, 6(5)*, 448–450.

Belin, P., Zilbovicius, M., Crozier, S., Thivard, L., Fontaine, A., Masure, M.C., & Samson, Y. (1998). Lateralization of speech and auditory temporal processing. *Journal of Cognitive Neuroscience, 10*, 536–540.

Benson, D. (1988). Classical syndromes of aphasia. In F. Boller & J. Grafman (Eds.), *Handbook of neuropsychology*. New York: Elsevier.

Benson, R.R., Richardson, M., Whalen, D.H., & Lai, S. (2006). Phonetic processing areas revealed by sine-wave speech and acoustically similar non-speech. *Neuroimage, 31*, 342–353.

Binder, J.R., Rao, S.M., Hammeke, T. A., Yetkin, F.Z., Jesmanowicz, A., Bandettini, P. A., Wong, E.C., Estkowski, L.D., Goldstein, M.D., Haughton, V.M., & Hyde, J.S. (1994). Functional magnetic resonance imaging of human auditory cortex. *Annals of Neurology, 35*, 662–672.

Blumstein, S.E. (1998). Phonological aspects of aphasia. In M. Sarno (Ed.), *Acquired aphasia*. New York: Academic Press.

Blumstein, S.E., Baker, E., & Goodglass, H. (1977). Phonological factors in auditory comprehension in aphasia. *Neuropsychologia, 15*, 19–30.

Blumstein, S.E., Cooper, W., Zurif, E., & Caramazza, A. (1977). The perception and production of voice-onset time in aphasia. *Neuropsychologia, 15*, 371–383.

Blumstein, S.E., Milberg, W., Brown, T., Hutchinson, A., Kurowski, A., & Burton, M.W. (2000). The mapping from sound structure to the lexicon in aphasia: Evidence from rhyme and repetition priming. *Brain and Language, 72*, 75–99.

Bornkessel, I., & Schlesewsky, M. (2006). The extended argument dependency model: A neurocognitive approach to sentence comprehension across languages. *Psychological Review, 113(4)*, 787.

Bornkessel-Schlesewsky, I., & Schlesewsky, M. (2009). The role of prominence information in the real-time comprehension of transitive constructions: A cross-linguistic approach. *Language and Linguistics Compass, 3*(1), 19–58.

Bornkessel-Schlesewsky, I., & Schlesewsky, M. (2013). Reconciling time, space and function: A new dorsal-ventral stream model of sentence comprehension. *Brain and Language, 125*(1), 60–76.

Bornkessel-Schlesewsky, I., Schlesewsky, M., Small, S.L., & Rauschecker, J.P. (2014). Neurobiological roots of language in primate audition: Common computational properties. *Trends in Cognitive Sciences*, in revision.

Burton, M., Blumstein, S., & Small, S.L. (2000). The role of segmentation in phonological processing: An fMRI investigation. *Journal of Cognitive Neuroscience, 12*, 679–690.

Burton, M., & Small, S.L. (1999). An introduction to fMRI. *The Neurologist, 5*, 145–158.

Callan, D., Callan, A., Gamez, M., Sato, M.A., Kawato, M. (2010). Premotor cortex mediates perceptual performance. *Neuroimage, 51*, 844–858.

Caplan, D., & Waters, G.S. (1995). Aphasic disorders of syntactic comprehension and working memory capacity. *Cognitive Neuropsychology, 12*, 637–649.

Carpenter, R., & Rutherford, D. (1973). Acoustic cue discrimination in adult aphasia. *Journal of Speech and Hearing Research, 16*, 534–544.

Davis, M.H., Coleman, M.R., Absalom, A.R., Rodd, J.M., Johnsrude, I.S., Matta, B.F., Owen, A.M., & Menon, D.K. (2007). Dissociating speech perception and comprehension at reduced levels of awareness. *Proceedings of the National Academy of Sciences of the United States of America, 104*, 16032–16037.

Dehaene-Lambertz, G., Pallier, C., Serniclaes, W., Sprenger-Charolles, L., Jobert, A., & Dehaene, S. (2005). Neural correlates of switching from auditory to speech perception. *Neuroimage, 24*, 21–33.

Demonet, J.-F., Chollet, F., Ramsay, S., Cardebat, D., Nespoulous, J.-L., Wise, R., Rascol, A., & Frackowiak, R.S. (1992). The anatomy of phonological and semantic processing in normal subjects. *Brain, 115*, 1753–1768.

Demonet, J.-F., Fiez, J.A., Paulesu, E., Petersen, S.E., & Zatorre, R.J. (1996). PET studies of phonological processing: A critical reply to Poeppel. *Brain and Language, 55*, 352–379.

Demonet, J.-F., Price, C., Wise, R., & Frackowiak, R.S. (1994a). Differential activation of right and left posterior sylvian regions by semantic and phonological tasks: A positron emission tomography study in normal human subjects. *Neuroscience Letters, 182*, 25–28.

Demonet, J.-F., Price, C, Wise, R., & Frackowiak, R.S. (1994b). A PET study of cognitive strategies in normal subjects during language tasks: Influence of phonetic ambiguity and sequence processing on phoneme monitoring. *Brain, 117*, 671–682.

Deng, L., & Erler, K. (1992). Structural design of hidden Markov model speech recognizer using multivalued phonetic features: Comparison with segmental speech units. *Journal of the Acoustical Society of America, 92*, 3058–3067.

DeWitt, I., & Rauschecker, J.P. (2012). Phoneme and word recognition in the auditory ventral stream. *Proceedings of the National Academy of Sciences of the United States of America, 109*(8), E505–E514.

Dhankhar, A., Wexler, B.E., Fulbright, R.K., Halwes, T., Blamire, A.M., & Shulman, R.G. (1997). Functional magnetic resonance imaging assessment of the human brain auditory cortex response to increasing word presentation rates. *Journal of Neurophysiology, 77*, 476–483.

Dronkers, N.F. (1998). Symposium: The role of Broca's area in language. *Brain and Language, 65*, 71–72.

Dronkers, N.F. (2000). The pursuit of brain-language relationships. *Brain and Language, 71*, 59–61.

Dronkers, N.F., Wilkins, D.P., Van Valin, R.D., Redfern, B.B., & Jaeger, J.J. (2004). Lesion analysis of the brain areas involved in language comprehension. *Cognition, 92*(1), 145–177.

Eickhoff, S.B., Heim, S., Zilles, K., & Amunts, K. (2009). A systems perspective on the effective connectivity of overt speech production. *Philosophical Transactions of the Royal Society A: Mathematical, Physical and Engineering Sciences, 367*(1896), 2399–2421.

Elmer, S., Meyer, M., Marrama, L., & Jancke, L. (2011). Intensive language training and attention modulate the involvement of fronto-parietal regions during a nonverbal auditory discrimination task. *European Journal of Neuroscience, 34*, 165–175.

Frauenfelder, U., & Floccia, C. (1998). The recognition of spoken word. In A. Friederici (Ed.), *Language comprehension*. New York: Springer.

Friederici, A.D. (2012). The cortical language circuit: From auditory perception to sentence comprehension. *Trends in Cognitive Sciences, 16*(5), 262–268.

Friederici, A.D., Bahlmann, J., Heim, S., Schubotz, R.I., & Anwander, A. (2006). The brain differentiates human and non-human grammars: Functional localization and structural connectivity. *Proceedings of the National Academy of Sciences of the United States of America, 103*(7), 2458–2463.

Gage, N., Poeppel, D., Roberts, T.P.L., & Hickok, G. (1998). Auditory evoked M100 reflects onset acoustics of speech sounds. *Brain Research, 814*, 236–239.

Galantucci, B., Fowler, C.A., Turvey, M.T. (2006). The motor theory of speech perception reviewed. *Psychonomic Bulletin & Review, 13*, 361–377.

Gallese, V., Fadiga, L., Fogassi, L., & Rizzolatti, G. (1996). Action recognition in the premotor cortex. *Brain, 119*(2), 593–609.

Gallese, V., Fogassi, L., Fadiga, L. & Rizzolatti, G. (2002). Action representation and the inferior parietal lobule. In W. Prinz & B. Hommel (Eds.), *Attention and performance*. New York: Oxford University Press.

Gandour, J. (2007). Neural substrates underlying the perception of linguistic prosody. *Tones and Tunes, 2*, 3–25.

Gandour, J., Wong, D., Hsieh, L., Weinzapfel, B., Van Lancker, D., & Hutchms, G.D. (2000). A crosslinguistic PET study of tone perception. *Journal of Cognitive Neuroscience, 12*, 207–222.

Gandour, J., Wong, D., & Hutchins, G. (1998). Pitch processing in the human brain is influenced by language experience. *Neuroreport, 9*, 2115–2119.

Ganong, W.F. (1980). Phonetic categorization in auditory word perception. *Journal of Experimental Psychology: Human Perception and Performance, 6*(1), 110–125.

Giraud, A.L., Kell, C., Thierfelder, C., Sterzer, P., Russ, M.O., Preibisch, C., & Kleinschmidt, A. (2004). Contributions of sensory input, auditory search and verbal comprehension to cortical activity during speech processing. *Cerebral Cortex, 14*, 247–255.

Goodale, M.A., & Milner, A.D. (1992). Separate visual pathways for perception and action. *Trends in Neurosciences, 15(1)*, 20–25.

Gordon, J., & Baum, S. (1994). Rhyme priming in aphasia: The role of phonology in lexical access. *Brain and Language, 47*, 661–683.

Gow, D.W., Jr., & Caplan, D. (1996). An examination of impaired acoustic-phonetic processing in aphasia. *Brain and Language, 52*, 386–407.

Gow, D.W., Jr., & Segawa, J.A. (2009). Articulatory mediation of speech perception: A causal analysis of multi-modal imaging data. *Cognition, 110*(2), 222–236.

Gow, D.W., Jr., Segawa, J.A., Ahlfors, S.P., & Lin, F.H. (2008). Lexical influences on speech perception: A Granger causality analysis of MEG and EEG source estimates. *Neuroimage, 43*(3), 614–623.

Hasson, U., Skipper, J.I., Nusbaum, H.C., & Small, S.L. (2007). Abstract coding of audiovisual speech: Beyond sensory representation. *Neuron, 56*, 1116–1126.

Hein, G., & Knight, R.T. (2008). Superior temporal sulcus—it's my area: Or is it? *Journal of Cognitive Neuroscience, 20*(12), 2125–2136.

Hesling, I., Dilharreguy, B., Clément, S., Bordessoules, M., & Allard, M. (2005). Cerebral mechanisms of prosodic sensory integration using low-frequency bands of connected speech. *Human Brain Mapping, 26*(3), 157–169.

Hickok, G., Costanzo, M., Capasso, R., & Miceli, G. (2011). The role of Broca's area in speech perception: Evidence from aphasia revisited. *Brain and Language, 119*, 214–220.

Hickok, G., & Poeppel, D. (2000). Towards a functional neuroanatomy of speech perception. *Trends in Cognitive Sciences, 4*, 131–138.

Hickok, G., & Poeppel, D. (2004). Dorsal and ventral streams: A framework for understanding aspects of the functional anatomy of language. *Cognition, 92*, 67–99.

Hickok, G., & Poeppel, D. (2007). The cortical organization of speech processing. *Nature Reviews Neuroscience, 8*(5), 393–402.

Hugdahl, K., Thomsen, T., Ersland, L., Rimol, L. M., & Niemi, J. (2003). The effects of attention on speech perception: An fMRI study. *Brain and Language, 85*, 37–48.

Husain, F.T., Fromm, S.J., Pursley, R.H., Hosey, L.A., Braun, A.R., & Horwitz, B. (2006). Neural bases of categorization of simple speech and nonspeech sounds. *Human Brain Mapping, 27*, 636–651.

Ivry, R., & Robertson, L. (1998). *The two sides of perception*. Cambridge, MA: MIT Press.

Jacquemot, C., & Scott, S.K. (2006). What is the relationship between phonological short-term memory and speech processing? *Trends in Cognitive Sciences, 10(11)*, 480–486.

Jonides, J., Schumacher, E.H., Smith, E.E., Koeppe, R. A., Awh, E., Reuter-Lorenz, P. A., Marshuetz, C., & Willis, C.R. (1998). The role of parietal cortex in verbal working memory. *Journal of Neuroscience, 18*, 5026–5034.

Jusczyk, P. (1986). Speech perception. In K. Boff, K. Kaufman, & J. Thomas (Eds.), *Handbook of perception and human performance: Cognitive processes and performance* (Vol. 2). New York: Wiley.

Klatt, D. (1979). Speech perception: A model of acoustic-phonetic analysis and lexical access. In R. Cole (Ed.), *Perception and production of fluent speech*. Hillsdale, NJ: Lawrence Erlbaum.

Krogh, A., & Riis, S. (1999). Hidden neural networks. *Neural Computation, 11*, 541–563.

Kuhl, P.K. (1991). Human adults and human infants show a "perceptual magnet effect" for the prototypes of speech categories, monkeys do not. *Perception and Psychophysics, 50*, 93–107.

Kuriki, S., Okita, Y., & Hirata, Y (1995). Source analysis of magnetic field responses from the human auditory cortex elicited by short speech sounds. *Experimental Brain Research, 104*, 144–152.

Lahiri, A., & Marslen-Wilson, W. (1991). The mental representation of lexical form: A phonological approach to the recognition lexicon. *Cognition, 38*, 245–294.

Leff, A.P., Schofield, T.M., Stephan, K.E., Crinion, J.T., Friston, K.J., & Price, C.J. (2008). The cortical dynamics of intelligible speech. *Journal of Neuroscience, 28(49)*, 13209–13215.

Liberman, A.M., Cooper, F.S., Shankweiler, D.P., & Studdert-Kennedy, M. (1967). Perception of the speech code. *Psychological Review, 74*, 431.

Liberman, A.M., Harris, K.S., Hoffman, H.S., & Griffith, B.C. (1957). The discrimination of speech sounds within and across phoneme boundaries. *Journal of Experimental Psychology, 54*, 358–368.

Liberman, A.M., & Mattingly, I.G. (1985). The motor theory of speech revised. *Cognition, 21*, 1–36.

Londei, A., D'Ausilio, A., Basso, D., Sestieri, C., Gratta, C.D., Romani, G.L., & Belardinelli, M.O. (2010). Sensory-motor brain network connectivity for speech comprehension. *Human Brain Mapping, 31(4)*, 567–580.

Luce, P.A., & Pisoni, D.B. (1998). Recognizing spoken words: The neighborhood activation model. *Ear and Hearing, 19*, 1–36.

Marslen-Wilson, W.D. (1987). Functional parallelism in spoken word-recognition. *Cognition, 25(1)*, 71–102.

Marslen-Wilson, W., & Warren, P. (1994). Levels of perceptual representation and process in lexical access: Words, phonemes, and features. *Psychological Review, 101*, 653–675.

Martin, R.C., Breedin, S.D., & Damian, M.F. (1999). The relation of phoneme discrimination, lexical access, and short-term memory: A case study and interactive activation account. *Brain and Language, 70*, 437–482.

Martin, R.C., & Romani, C. (1994). Verbal working memory and sentence comprehension: A multiple-components view. *Neuropsychology, 8*, 506–523.

McClelland, J.L., & Elman, J.L. (1986). The TRACE model of speech perception. *Cognitive Psychology, 18*, 1–86.

McGurk, H., & MacDonald, J. (1976). Hearing lips and seeing voices. *Nature, 264*, 746–748.

Metter, E.J., Hanson, W.R., Jackson, C.A., Kempler, D., Van Lancker, D., Mazziotta, J.C., & Phelps, M.E. (1990). Temporoparietal cortex in aphasia: Evidence from positron emission tomography. *Archives of Neurology, 47(11)*, 1235.

Metter, E.J., Kempler, D., Jackson, C., Hanson, W.R., Mazziotta, J.C., & Phelps, M.E. (1989). Cerebral glucose metabolism in Wernicke's, Broca's, and conduction aphasia. *Archives of Neurology, 46*, 27–34.

Meyer, M., Zysset, S., von Cramon, D.Y., & Alter, K. (2005). Distinct fMRI responses to laughter, speech, and sounds along the human peri-sylvian cortex. *Cognitive Brain Research, 24*, 291–306.

Miceli, G., Caltagirone, C., Gainotti, G., & Payer-Rigo, P. (1978). Discrimination of voice versus place contrasts in aphasia. *Brain and Language, 6*, 47–51.

Miyake, A., Carpenter, P., & Just, M. (1994). A capacity approach to syntactic comprehension disorders: Making normal adults perform like aphasic patients. *Cognitive Neuropsychology, 11*, 671–717.

Mummery, C.J., Ashburner, J., Scott, S.K., & Wise, R.J. (1999). Functional neuroimaging of speech perception in six normal and two aphasic subjects. *Journal of the Acoustical Society of America, 106*, 449–457.

Myers, E.B., Blumstein, S.E., Walsh, E., & Eliassen, J. (2009). Inferior frontal regions underlie the perception of phonetic category invariance. *Psychological Science, 20*, 895–903.

Narain, C., Scott, S.K., Wise, R.J., Rosen, S., Leff, A., Iversen, S.D., & Matthews, P.M. (2003). Defining a left-lateralized response specific to intelligible speech using fMRI. *Cerebral Cortex, 13*, 1362–1368.

Nath, A.R., & Beauchamp, M.S. (2011). Dynamic changes in superior temporal sulcus connectivity during perception of noisy audiovisual speech. *Journal of Neuroscience, 31(5)*, 1704–1714.

Nicholls, M. (1996). Temporal processing asymmetries between the cerebral hemispheres: Evidence and implications. *Laterality, 1*, 97–137.

Norris, D., McQueen, J.M., & Cutler, A. (2000). Merging phonetic and lexical information in phonetic decision-making. *Behavioral and Brain Sciences, 23*, 299–325.

Nygaard, L.C., Sommers, M.S., & Pisoni, D.B. (1995). Effects of stimulus variability on perception and representation of spoken words in memory. *Perception and Psychophysics, 57*, 989–1001.

Obleser, J., Wise, R.J., Dresner, M.A., & Scott, S.K. (2007). Functional integration across brain regions improves speech perception under adverse listening conditions. *Journal of Neuroscience, 27*(9), 2283–2289.

Osnes, B., Hugdahl, K., & Specht, K. (2011). Effective connectivity analysis demonstrates involvement of premotor cortex during speech perception. *Neuroimage, 54*(3), 2437–2445.

Oscar-Berman, M., Zurif, E., & Blumstein, S. (1975). Effects of unilateral brain damage on the processing of speech sounds. *Brain and Language, 2,* 345–355.

Paulesu, E., Frith, C.D., & Frackowiak, R.J. (1993). The neural correlates of the verbal component of working memory. *Nature, 362,* 342–345.

Paulesu, E., Frith, U., Snowling, M., Gallagher, A., Morton, J., Frackowiak, R.S.J., & Frith, C.D. (1996). Is developmental dyslexia a disconnection syndrome? Evidence from PET scanning. *Brain, 199,* 143–157.

Petersen, S.E., Fox, P.T., Posner, M.I., Mintun, M.A., & Raichle, M.E. (1988). Positron emission tomographic studies of the cortical anatomy of single-word processing. *Nature, 331,* 585–589.

Pisoni, D.B. (1993). Long-term memory in speech perception: Some new findings on talker-variability, speaking rate, and perceptual learning. *Speech Communication, 13,* 109–125.

Pitt, M.A., & Samuel, A.G. (1993). An empirical and meta-analytic evaluation of the phoneme identification task. *Journal of Experimental Psychology: Human Perception and Performance, 19,* 699–725.

Poeppel, D. (1996). A critical review of PET studies of phonological processing. *Brain and Language, 55,* 317–351.

Poeppel, D. (2003). The analysis of speech in different temporal integration windows: Cerebral lateralization as 'asymmetric sampling in time.' *Speech Communication, 41*(1), 245–255.

Poeppel, D., Idsardi, W.J., & van Wassenhove, V. (2008). Speech perception at the interface of neurobiology and linguistics. *Philosophical Transactions of the Royal Society B: Biological Sciences, 363*(1493), 1071–1086.

Poeppel, D., & Monahan, P.J. (2008). Speech perception cognitive foundations and cortical implementation. *Current Directions in Psychological Science, 17*(2), 80–85.

Poeppel, D., Yellin, E., Phillips, C., Roberts, T.P., Rowley, H.A., Wexler, K., & Marantz, A. (1996). Task-induced asymmetry of the auditory evoked M100 neuromagnetic field elicited by speech sounds. *Brain Research: Cognitive Brain Research, 4,* 231–242.

Poldrack, R.A., Wagner, A.D., Prull, M.W., Desmond, J.E., Glover, G.H., & Gabrieli, J.D. (1999). Functional specialization for semantic and phonological processing in the left inferior prefrontal cortex. *Neuroimage, 10,* 15–35.

Price, C., Wise, R., Ramsey, S., Friston, K., Howard, D., & Patterson, K. (1992). Regional response differences within the human auditory cortex when listening to words. *Neuroscience Letters, 146,* 179–182.

Price, C.J. (2012). A review and synthesis of the first 20 years of PET and fMRI studies of heard speech, spoken language and reading. *Neuroimage, 62*(2), 816–847.

Pulvermüller, F., & Fadiga, L. (2010). Active perception: Sensorimotor circuits as a cortical basis for language. *Nature Reviews Neuroscience, 11*(5), 351–360.

Rauschecker, J.P. (1998). Cortical processing of complex sounds. *Current Opinion in Neurobiology, 8*(4), 516–521.

Rauschecker, J.P., & Scott, S.K. (2009). Maps and streams in the auditory cortex: Nonhuman primates illuminate human speech processing. *Nature Neuroscience, 12*(6), 718–724.

Rauschecker, J.P., & Tian, B. (2000). Mechanisms and streams for processing of "what" and "where" in auditory cortex. *Proceedings of the National Academy of Sciences, 97*(22), 11800–11806.

Ravizza, S.M., Hazeltine, E., Ruiz, S., Zhu, D.C., (2011). Left TPJ activity in verbal working memory: Implications for storage- and sensory-specific models of short term memory. *Neuroimage, 55,* 1836–1846.

Riedel, K., & Studdert-Kennedy, M. (1985). Extending formant transitions may not improve aphasies' perception of stop consonant place of articulation. *Brain and Language, 24,* 223–232.

Rimol, L.M., Specht, K., Weis, S., Savoy, R., & Hugdahl, K. (2005). Processing of sub-syllabic speech units in the posterior temporal lobe: An fMRI study. *Neuroimage, 26,* 1059–1067.

Rimol, L.M., Specht, K., & Hugdahl, K. (2006). Controlling for individual differences in fMRI brain activation to tones, syllables, and words. *Neuroimage, 30,* 554–562.

Rinne, T., Alho, K., Alku, P., Holi, M., Sinkkonen, J., Virtanen, J., Bertrand, O., & Näätänen, R. (1999). Analysis of speech sounds is left-hemisphere predominant at 100–150 ms after sound onset. *Neuroreport, 10,* 1113–1117.

Rizzolatti, G., & Arbib, M.A. (1998). Language within our grasp. *Trends in Neurosciences, 21,* 188–194.

Rizzolatti, G., Fadiga, L., Gallese, V., & Fogassi, L. (1996). Premotor cortex and the recognition of motor actions. *Cognitive Brain Research, 3,* 131–141.

Rogalsky, C., Love, T., Driscoll, D., Anderson, S.W., & Hickok, G. (2011). Are mirror neurons the basis of speech perception? Evidence from five cases with damage to the purported human mirror system. *Neurocase, 17*(2), 178–187.

Romanski, L.M., Tian, B., Fritz, J., Mishkin, M., Goldman-Rakic, P.S., & Rauschecker, J.P. (1999). Dual streams of auditory afferents target multiple domains in the primate prefrontal cortex. *Nature Neuroscience, 2*(12), 1131–1136.

Rossi, E., Schippers, M., & Keysers, C. (2011). Broca's area: Linking perception and production in language and actions. In S. Han & E. Pöppel, (Eds.), *Culture and neural frames of cognition and communication.* Berlin, Heidelberg: Springer Berlin Heidelberg.

Samuel, A.G., & Pitt, M.A. (2003). Lexical activation (and other factors) can mediate compensation for coarticulation. *Journal of Memory and Language, 48*(2), 416–434.

Saur, D., Kreher, B.W., Schnell, S., Kümmerer, D., Kellmeyer, P., Vry, M.S., Umarova, R., Musso, M., Glauche, V., Abel, S., Huber, W., Rijntjes, M., Hennig, J., & Weiller, C. (2008). Ventral and dorsal pathways for language. *Proceedings of the National Academy of Sciences, 105*(46), 18035–18040.

Schofield, T.M., Iverson, P., Kiebel, S.J., Stephan, K.E., Kilner, J.M., Friston, K.J., Crinion, J.T., Price, C.J., & Leff, A.P. (2009). Changing meaning causes coupling changes within higher levels of the cortical hierarchy. *Proceedings of the National Academy of Sciences, 106*(28), 11765–11770.

Scott, S.K., & Johnsrude, I.S. (2003). The neuroanatomical and functional organization of speech perception. *Trends in Neurosciences, 26*(2), 100–107.

Scott, S.K., McGettigan, C., & Eisner, F. (2009). A little more conversation, a little less action—candidate roles for the motor cortex in speech perception. *Nature Reviews Neuroscience, 10*(4), 295–302.

Scott, S.K., McGettigan, C., & Eisner, F. (2013). The neural basis of links and dissociations between speech perception and production. In J.J. Bolhuis & M. Everaert (Eds.), *Birdsong, speech, and language: Exploring the evolution of mind and brain.* Cambridge, MA: MIT Press.

Skipper, J.I., Nusbaum, H.C., & Small, S.L. (2005). Listening to talking faces: motor cortical activation during speech perception. *Neuroimage, 25*, 76–89.

Skipper, J.I., Nusbaum, H.C., & Small, S.L. (2006). Lending a helping hand to hearing: Another motor theory of speech perception. In M.A. Arbib (Ed.), *Action to language via the mirror neuron system.* Cambridge, MA: Cambridge University Press.

Skipper, J.I., van Wassenhove, V., Nusbaum, H.C., & Small, S.L. (2007). Hearing lips and seeing voices: How cortical areas supporting speech production mediate audiovisual speech perception. *Cerebral Cortex, 17*, 2387–2399.

Sumby, W.H., & Pollack, I. (1954). Visual contribution of speech intelligibility in noise. *Journal of the Acoustical Society of America, 26*, 212–215.

Tremblay, P., & Small, S.L. (2011a). From language comprehension to action understanding and back again. *Cerebral Cortex, 21(5)*, 1166–1177.

Tremblay, P., & Small, S.L. (2011b). On the context-dependent nature of the contribution of the ventral premotor cortex to speech perception. *Neuroimage, 57*, 1561–1571.

Ungerleider, L., & Mishkin, M. (1982). Two cortical visual systems. In M.A. Goodale, D.J. Ingle, & R.J. Mansfield (Eds.), *Analysis of visual behavior* (pp. 549–586). Cambridge, MA: MIT Press.

Warren, R.M. (1970). Perceptual restoration of missing speech sounds. *Science, 167(3917)*, 392–393.

Watrous, R.L. (1990). Phoneme discrimination using connectionist networks. *Journal of the Acoustical Society of America, 87*, 1753–1772.

Wilson, S.M., Dronkers, N.F., Ogar, J.M., Jang, J., Growdon, M.E., Agosta, F., Henry, M.L., Miller, B.L., & Gorno-Tempini, M.L. (2010). Neural correlates of syntactic processing in the nonfluent variant of primary progressive aphasia. *Journal of Neuroscience, 30*(50), 16845–16854.

Wise, R., Chollet, F., Hadar, U., Friston, K., Hoffner, E., & Frackowiak, E. (1991). Distribution of cortical neural networks involved in word comprehension and word retrieval. *Brain, 114*, 1803–1817.

Zaehle, T., Wustenberg, T., Meyer, M., & Jancke, L. (2004). Evidence for rapid auditory perception as the foundation of speech processing: a sparse temporal sampling fMRI study. *European Journal of Neuroscience, 20*, 2447–2456.

Zatorre, R. (1997). Cerebral correlates of human auditory processing: Perception of speech and musical sounds. In J. Syka (Ed.), *Acoustical signal processing in the central auditory system.* New York: Plenum Press.

Zatorre, R.J., Belin, P., & Penhune, V.B. (2002). Structure and function of auditory cortex: Music and speech. *Trends in Cognitive Sciences, 6*, 37–46.

Zatorre, R.J., Evans, A.C., Meyer, E., & Gjedde, A. (1992). Lateralization of phonetic and pitch discrimination in speech processing. *Science, 256*, 846–849.

Zatorre, R., Meyer, E., Gjedde, A., & Evans, A. (1996). PET studies of phonetic processing of speech: Review, replication, and reanalysis. *Cerebral Cortex, 6*, 21–30.

Zekveld, A.A., Heslenfeld, D.J., Festen, J.M., & Schoonhoven, R. (2006). Top-down and bottom-up processes in speech comprehension. *Neuroimage, 32*, 1826–1836.

Zevin, J.D., Yang, J., Skipper, J.I., McCandliss, B.D., (2010). Domain general change detection accounts for "dishabituation" effects in temporal–parietal regions in functional magnetic resonance imaging studies of speech perception. *Journal of Neuroscience, 30*, 1110–1117.

14

NEUROBIOLOGICAL BASES OF AUDITORY PROCESSING

Deepti Ramadoss and Dana Boatman

The human auditory system transforms continuous acoustic signals into neural representations that enable listeners to perceive and attach meanings to sounds. Although the neural mechanisms underlying human auditory perception are not fully understood, recent advances in research and technology have enhanced our knowledge. In this chapter, we provide a brief overview of sound processing in the human auditory system, from the ear to the brain.

The auditory system is divided conceptually into two contiguous components: the peripheral and central auditory systems. The peripheral auditory system encompasses the outer ear, middle ear, and inner ear. The central auditory system is a complex array of ascending, descending, and crossing pathways that extend from the brainstem to the cortex. We will focus on central auditory mechanisms involved in processing complex sounds, such as speech. We begin with a brief review of the peripheral auditory system.

Peripheral Auditory System

Outer Ear

The outer ear, also called the pinna or auricle, captures sound waves from the environment and funnels them down the ear canal to the middle ear (Figure 14.1). Coupled with the head, the pinna and ear canal play an important role in localizing sounds in the environment. The resonant properties of the ear canal serve to amplify frequencies in the range of 2500–3000 Hz that are common to speech sounds. Abnormalities of the outer ear resulting from trauma, obstruction of the ear canal, or congenital malformations can impede sound transmission to the middle ear.

Middle Ear

The middle ear is separated from the outer ear by the ear drum, or tympanic membrane (TM), a small, fibrous, oval-shaped structure. Sound waves travel down the ear canal and impinge on the TM, setting it into motion. The movement of the TM vibrates three small bones in the middle ear—the malleus, incus, and stapes—collectively known as the ossicles. The ossicles form a chain that extends across the air-filled middle ear cavity from the ear drum to the inner ear. Sound vibrations are transmitted to the inner ear through the motion of the stapes footplate in the oval window of the inner ear.

Peripheral Auditory System

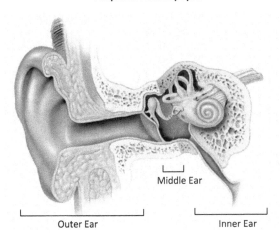

Middle Ear

Outer Ear

Inner Ear

Adapted from online

Figure 14.1 Schematic showing cross-section of human peripheral auditory system, with divisions into outer, middle, and inner ear. Adapted from online. From Handbook of Sensory Physiology, Volume 5, Auditory System, by W.D. Keidel and W.D. Neff (1976). Reproduced with permission of Springer.

Middle ear disorders, including infections (otitis media) or otosclerosis, can impede normal function of the TM and ossicles, reducing sound transmission to the inner ear. The resulting hearing loss is classified as conductive in nature and is often reversible. Conductive hearing loss can affect perception of speech sounds, especially consonants, which are typically softer (e.g., lower amplitude) than vowels.

Inner Ear and Auditory Nerve

The inner ear is located in the petrous portion of the temporal bone and contains structures for both hearing and balance. The inner ear structure associated with hearing is the cochlea: a snail-shaped, bony structure with three spiral fluid-filled chambers. Sound transduction is performed in the organ of Corti housed in the membranous, endolymph-filled, middle chamber of the cochlea, the scala media. At the base of the organ of Corti is the basilar membrane, which contains rows of hair cells that are involved in transducing sound energy into neural impulses. The mechanical movement of the stapes in the oval window generates waves in the cochlear fluids that, in turn, displace the basilar membrane. There are two main types of hair cells on the basilar membrane: inner hair cells (one row) that are involved directly in sound transduction and outer hair cells (two to three rows) that contract and expand in response to sound, serving mainly as mechanical amplifiers (Brownell et al., 1985).

One of the primary functions performed by the cochlea is frequency analysis: the decomposition of sounds into their individual frequency components. Hair cells on the basilar membrane are organized by frequency (tonotopic), with high frequencies represented at the basal end and low frequencies represented at the apical end (von Békésy, 1960). Overlying the basilar membrane is a flexible, gel-like structure called the tectorial membrane whose mechanical properties include gradient stiffness along the length of the cochlea (Gueta et al., 2006). Displacement of the basilar membrane by cochlear fluid waves causes the tectorial membrane to shear across the tips (stereocilia) of the hair cells. The shearing motion triggers a change in the hair cell membrane potential (depolarization) and the release of neurotransmitters that, in turn, cause auditory nerve fibers that synapse at the base of the hair cells to fire. Sound frequency and intensity are encoded by the particular populations of auditory nerve fibers that fire and their firing rates (Viemeister, 1988). The cell bodies of auditory nerve fibers form the spiral ganglion. Their axons relay neural impulses from the peripheral to the central auditory system. As auditory nerve fibers leave the cochlea, they combine with fibers from the vestibular organ to form the eighth cranial nerve, also known as the vestibulocochlear nerve. Excitatory neurotransmitters such as glutamate and aspartate appear to play an important role in transmission of neural impulses along the auditory nerve (Caspary et al., 1981; Glowatzki et al., 2006).

Hearing loss associated with damage to hair cells or other disorders of the cochlea and/or auditory nerve is classified as sensorineural and is often not reversible. Common causes of sensorineural hearing loss include aging, noise exposure, and ototoxic drugs. Hearing high-frequency sounds may be disproportionately impaired because the corresponding hair cells are located at the opening of the cochlea (basal end), and therefore are more vulnerable to damage.

Central Auditory System

The central auditory system comprises the brainstem, thalamus, and cortex (Figure 14.2). Output from the cochlea is transmitted in the form of neural impulses to the central auditory system by the auditory nerve, which enters the brainstem at the junction between the pons and medulla at the level of the cochlear nucleus.

Brainstem

There are four main auditory centers, or relay stations, located on each side of the brainstem: the cochlear nucleus, the superior olivary complex, the lateral lemniscus, and the inferior colliculus.

Cochlear Nucleus

The cochlear nucleus (CN) is the first major structure in the central auditory system and an obligatory synapse in the ascending auditory system. The CN is the only structure in the central auditory system that receives input from only one ear: the ipsilateral cochlea. The CN has three main divisions that differ in cell type and distribution but are all tonotopically organized: the anteroventral CN (spherical and globular bushy cells), posteroventral CN (stellate and octopus cells), and dorsal CN (fusiform cells). CN neurons have frequency-intensity tuning curves similar to those of auditory nerve fibers, thereby preserving the frequency-specific information extracted by the cochlea. CN neurons also encode precise stimulus timing and intensity information needed for sound localization performed by higher-level auditory centers, including the superior olivary complex and inferior colliculus (Young et al., 1988; Oertel, 1991; Oertel et al., 2000). Like the auditory nerve, the CN also encodes acoustic features used by listeners to discriminate and identify vowel sounds, including formant frequencies, duration, and intensity (Sachs & Young, 1979; Delgutte, 1980; May et al., 1998). The majority of CN fibers project contralaterally to the superior olivary complex, lateral lemniscus, and inferior colliculus.

Superior Olivary Complex

The superior olivary complex (SOC) is located medial to the CN, in the caudal portion of the pons. The SOC has three major divisions (nuclei): medial nucleus of the trapezoid body, medial

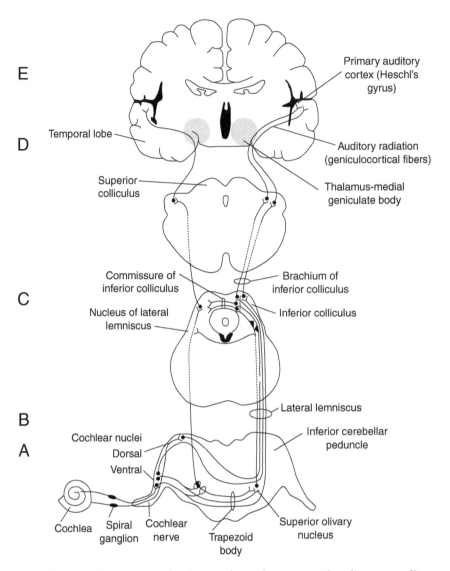

Figure 14.2 Schematic of human central auditory pathways, beginning with auditory nerve fiber synapse on cochlear nuclei. A. Medulla. B. Pons. C. Midbrain. D. Thalamus. E. Cerebral Cortex. Adapted from Neuroscience: Communicative Disorders, by Subhash C. Bhatnagar and Orlando J. Andy (1995). Lippincott Williams & Wilkins.

superior olivary nucleus, and lateral superior olivary nucleus. The SOC receives binaural input and is thought to play an important role in sound localization. Specifically, inter-aural timing differences used to localize low-frequency sounds are processed in the medial superior olive (Yin & Chan, 1990), while inter-aural intensity differences used to localize high-frequency sounds are processed by the lateral superior olive (Joris & Yin, 1995). One of the main efferent (descending) auditory pathways, the olivocochlear bundle, originates in the SOC and projects back to the cochlea, serving to protect the ear from loud sounds (Maison & Liberman, 2000; Rajan, 2000) and to improve sound detection in noise (Giraud et al., 1997; de Boer & Thornton, 2008). The SOC projects contralaterally and ipsilaterally via the lateral lemniscus to higher levels of the central auditory system.

Lateral Lemniscus

The lateral lemniscus (LL) is a large fiber tract projecting from the rostral portion of the pons to the inferior colliculus. The LL contains both ascending and descending auditory fibers and three nuclei. The main source of input to the LL is the contralateral dorsal CN and both the ipsilateral and contralateral SOC. Communication between both LL occurs via the commissure of Probst. The LL serves as a relay station from the CN and SOC to the inferior colliculi, and LL nuclei have been implicated in other aspects of auditory processing, including temporal and spatial discrimination (Metzner & Radtke-Schuller, 1987; Covey & Casseday, 1991; Ito et al., 1996).

Inferior Colliculus

The inferior colliculus (IC) is located on the dorsal side of the midbrain and is the largest auditory structure in the brainstem. Most ascending auditory pathways synapse in the IC, although a small number project directly to the thalamus. The central nucleus of the IC is auditory specific and tonotopically organized. Recordings from single neurons in the central nucleus show sharp tuning curves, suggesting that the IC plays a role in enhancing frequency resolution (Ehret & Merzenich, 1988; Egorova & Ehret, 2008). Some IC neurons respond selectively to the rate or direction of frequency-modulated (FM) sweeps (Geis & Borst, 2013)—an important cue for perceiving consonant-vowel transitions in speech. IC neurons also respond to binaural temporal and spatial cues (Ehret, 1997) and may contribute to phase encoding of speech cues (Warrier et al., 2011). The central nucleus of the IC is considered the primary generator of wave V of the auditory brain response (ABR) (Starr & Hamilton, 1976) and has been implicated in processing complex sounds, such as speech and music (Russo et al., 2004; Mussachia et al., 2008; Skoe & Kraus, 2010). Other areas of the IC process both auditory and somatosensory input. Output from the central (auditory) nucleus of the IC projects ipsilaterally and contralaterally to the medial geniculate body of the thalamus.

In summary, auditory processing in the brainstem serves to preserve and transmit tonotopic information, process binaural cues for sound localization, and process acoustic cues, such as frequency modulations, that listeners use to perceive pitch, music, and speech.

Thalamus

The auditory division of the thalamus, the medial geniculate body (MGB), is an obligatory relay station between the IC and auditory cortex (de Ribaupierre, 1997). The MGB is located on the dorsolateral surface of the thalamus approximately 1 cm from the IC and is subdivided into ventral, dorsal, and medial divisions. The ventral division, which is characterized by sharply tuned neuronal responses and strong tonotopic organization, projects directly to ipsilateral primary auditory cortex. Neurons in the ventral MGB are also responsive to binaural stimulation and inter-aural intensity differences (Aitkin & Webster, 1972; Ivarsson et al., 1988). The medial and dorsal divisions of the MGB show weaker tonotopic organization and have neurons that respond preferentially to complex acoustic stimuli (de Ribaupierre, 1997). The medial MGB projects to both primary and non-primary auditory cortices, and has been implicated in auditory attention (He, 2003). The MGB is one of the generators of the middle latency response (MLR), reflecting detection of changes in acoustic aspects of speech sounds; that is, acoustic-phonetic change (Giard et al., 1990; Kraus et al., 1994a; Kraus et al., 1994b). More recently, it has been shown that attention-dependent modulation of the MGB is behaviorally relevant for speech recognition (von Kriegstein et al., 2008; Diaz et al., 2012).

The MGB projects ipsilaterally to auditory cortex via the auditory radiations: white matter fibers that traverse the posterior limb of the internal capsule. Auditory radiations from the ventral

MGB project to primary auditory cortex, while those from the dorsal and medial divisions of the MGB project to primary and non-primary auditory cortices.

To summarize, the subcortical auditory system plays an important role in processing and transmitting complex sound information between the auditory periphery and the cortex. The auditory brainstem and the MGB of the thalamus are involved in analyzing acoustic features of speech, as well as preserving and transmitting tonotopic information and binaural spatial cues.

Auditory Cortex

Auditory cortex is housed in the temporal lobe, in particular the superior temporal gyrus (STG), of both cerebral hemispheres. Auditory cortex encompasses multiple subdivisions or fields, including a core, belt, and parabelt region (Figure 14.3), and shares reciprocal connections with other cortical regions within and outside the temporal lobe (Hackett, 2011). The first cortical area to receive auditory input from the thalamus is primary auditory cortex.

Primary Auditory Cortex

In the human brain, primary auditory cortex is located inside the Sylvian fissure, overlaying Heschl's gyrus on the transverse temporal, or supratemporal, plane of the STG (Figure 14.3). The primary auditory cortex maps to the auditory core, an oval-shaped area approximately 2.5 cm in length (Artacho-Pérula et al., 2004; Da Costa et al., 2011) that corresponds to Brodmann area 41. Neurophysiology and architectonic studies in animals have shown that the auditory core has a number of primary sensory characteristics, including a well-developed layer IV (koniocortex), dense thalamic inputs, and maximal responsiveness to simple tone stimuli. The auditory core receives input from the ventral division of the medial geniculate body of the thalamus and from the auditory core in the contralateral hemisphere through the corpus callosum (Hackett et al., 1998; Kaas et al., 1999). Callosal commissural inputs originate predominantly in homologous tonotopic areas (Luethke et al., 1989; Morel et al., 1993) and regulate (excitatory inputs) neuronal responses in the auditory core (Carrasco et al., 2013).

The auditory core has been subdivided into two to three fields, the largest of which is AI, which has traditionally been considered primary auditory cortex and is tonotopically organized with low frequencies represented anterolaterally and high frequencies represented posteromedially (Merzenich & Brugge, 1973; Morel et al., 1993). The adjacent rostral area (R) shows a gradient tonotopic organization sharing a low-frequency border with AI (Merzenich & Brugge, 1973; Morel et al., 1993). A third rostral-temporal subdivision (RT) has been identified, although its functional properties remain poorly characterized (Kaas & Hackett, 2000; Petkov et al., 2006; Humphries et al., 2010). In addition to encoding frequency-specific information, neurons in the auditory core are also responsive to temporal information (Steinschneider et al., 1995; Lu et al., 2001) and spectral complexity (Sadagopan & Wang, 2009) and show learning-induced plasticity (Fritz et al., 2003).

Over the past decade, brain imaging studies have confirmed tonotopic organization of primary auditory cortex in humans (Formisano et al., 2003; Talvage et al., 2004; Woods & Alain, 2009) and have identified two to three distinct tonotopic gradients in the auditory core, compatible with animal studies (Humphries et al., 2010; Langers & van Dijk, 2012). All subdivisions of the auditory core share reciprocal connections, and each division projects to immediately adjacent areas of the auditory belt (Kaas & Hackett, 2000).

Auditory Belt

The auditory belt is a narrow, 2–4 mm band that encircles the auditory core on the transverse temporal plane and corresponds to Brodmann area 42 (Figure 14.3). The medial border of the

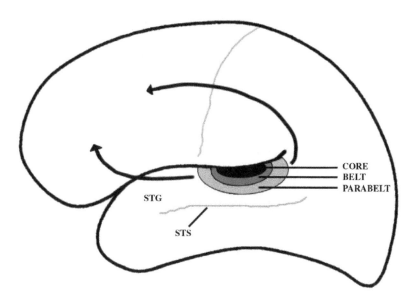

Figure 14.3 Schematic of lateral left hemisphere showing auditory cortex in the temporal lobe. Concentric rings represent auditory core, belt, and parabelt areas in the superior temporal gyrus (STG). Arrows denote two main functional pathways: ventral 'what' (or 'how') pathway and dorsal 'where' pathway. Light gray lines represent the central sulcus and the superior temporal sulcus (STS).

auditory belt abuts the insula; the lateral border is adjacent to the auditory parabelt. The auditory belt has six to eight reciprocally connected fields that receive input directly from adjacent regions in the auditory core and from dorsal and medial divisions of the MGB (Kaas et al., 1999). Although the auditory belt shows evidence of tonotopic organization, neurons in this region also respond to spectrally complex sounds, such as bandpass noise (Rauschecker et al., 1995; Wessinger et al., 2001; Rauschecker & Tian, 2004). While relatively little is known about the function of the auditory belt, it appears to serve as an intermediate processing stage between the core and parabelt (Morel & Kaas, 1992).

Auditory Parabelt

The auditory parabelt, also known as auditory association cortex or Brodmann area 22, is located on the lateral aspect of the posterior STG adjacent to the auditory belt (Figure 14.3). The two main divisions of the parabelt are the rostral field (RPB) and caudal field (CPB). Neurons in the auditory parabelt respond preferentially to complex sounds, in contrast to simple tones, consistent with the view that the parabelt is not tonotopically organized (Woods et al., 2009). However, recent evidence based on functional imaging suggests that non-primary auditory areas, including the parabelt, may be tonotopically organized in humans (Striem-Amit et al., 2011). The auditory parabelt receives direct inputs from the adjacent belt region and from the dorsal and medial divisions of the medial geniculate body of the thalamus (Kaas et al., 1999). The auditory core does not project directly to the parabelt, but instead, indirectly through the belt, consistent with the traditional hierarchical model of cortical auditory processing (Boatman et al., 1995; Rauschecker et al., 1995; Kaas et al., 1999; Wessinger et al., 2001; Okada et al., 2010). The auditory core is the first cortical region to receive input and responds preferentially to simple acoustic stimuli (e.g., pure tones), while the belt and parabelt regions respond preferentially to increasingly complex stimuli. Hierarchical organization of human auditory cortex appears to be evident as early as three months of age, suggesting that a dedicated neural network for auditory speech processing is present in the human brain at birth (Dehaene-Lambertz & Baillet, 1998).

Auditory association cortex is part of what has traditionally been referred to as Wernicke's area based on early stroke studies that associated lesions in this area with impaired auditory comprehension (Wernicke, 1874; Luria, 1976). Structural and functional lesion studies and brain imaging studies have also implicated the auditory parabelt in phonological and lexical-semantic processing (Blumstein et al., 1977; Miceli et al., 1978; Binder et al., 1994; Boatman & Miglioretti, 2005; Woods et al., 2011; chapters 8 and 11, this volume). A network of pathways connects auditory association cortex to other cortical areas, suggesting that this region is a gateway to higher-level language processing. Multiple connections between auditory cortex and the frontal lobe have also been identified (Hackett et al., 1998; Romanski et al., 1999). These connections appear to support two parallel processing streams (Figure 14.3): (1) a dorsal 'where' pathway that projects from the posterior temporal lobe through parietal cortex to dorsal prefrontal cortex and is implicated in processing auditory spatial information (Clarke et al., 2000; Rauschecker & Tian, 2000) and (2) a ventral 'what' (or 'how') pathway that projects through the anterior temporal lobe to the inferior frontal lobe and ventral prefrontal areas and supports auditory object and pattern recognition, including speech (Rauschecker & Tian, 2000; Nelken, 2003; Rauschecker & Scott, 2009).

Planum Temporale

The planum temporale (PT) is a triangular-shaped structure located posterior to Heschl's gyrus on the transverse temporal plane. The PT has been associated with a variety of auditory functions, including speech and language processing (Steinmetz et al., 1991; Foundas et al., 1994), pitch processing (Griffiths et al., 1998), spatial hearing (Smith et al., 2009), and sensory-motor integration for speech (Hickok & Saberi, 2012). The PT is reportedly larger in the language-dominant (left) hemisphere than the non-dominant hemisphere (Geschwind & Levitsky, 1968; Steinmetz et al., 1991; Foundas et al., 1994, Binder et al., 1996) and is less asymmetric in individuals with dyslexia (Galaburda et al., 1985) and autism (Rojas et al., 2002).

Planum Polare

The planum polare is located anterior to Heschl's gyrus on the transverse temporal plane and extends anteriorly to the temporal pole (Destrieux et al., 2010). The role of the planum polare in auditory processing remains poorly understood although it has been implicated in higher-level music processing, especially analysis of pitch and temporal structure (Brown et al., 2004; Baumann et al., 2007).

Corticofugal (Efferent) Auditory Pathways

Auditory cortex projects back to the subcortical auditory system through a series of descending (efferent) corticofugal auditory pathways that share many of the same relay stations as the ascending auditory pathways. Efferent connections project both ipsilaterally and contralaterally (Imig & Morel, 1983). The thalamus receives approximately as many efferent as afferent inputs forming a cortico-thalamic feedback loop (de Ribaupierre, 1997). The primary function of efferent auditory pathways is inhibitory, or protective. Examples include decreasing neuronal responses to loud sounds and to background noise, thereby increasing the signal-noise ratio and optimizing the neuronal response to biologically significant signals, including speech (Musiek & Lamb, 1992; Giraud et al., 1997; de Boer & Thornton, 2008), as well as facilitating sound localization in noise (Andéol et al., 2011).

Functional Lateralization of Auditory Cortex

The left hemisphere has traditionally been associated with language processing, including speech perception (Wernicke, 1874; Wada et al., 1975; Steinmetz et al., 1991). Because the majority of ascending auditory projections from each ear cross at the level of the superior olivary complex in the brainstem, auditory cortex in the left hemisphere receives strongest input from the contralateral right ear. This manifests as a right-ear advantage for speech on tests of dichotic listening (simultaneous presentation of two different stimuli to each ear), demonstrating greater efficiency of the contralateral (right ear) pathway to the language-dominant (left) hemisphere (Kimura, 1961; Mononen & Seitz, 1977). The left hemisphere is also thought to process auditory information on fast (short) timescales (20–40 ms) making it well suited for capturing the rapid, brief acoustic cues characteristic of consonant sounds (Poeppel, 2003; Boemio et al., 2005).

Conversely, the right hemisphere is thought to preferentially process auditory information on longer (150–250 ms) timescales (Poeppel, 2003) and is, therefore, well-suited for supporting perception of pitch (Zatorre et al., 2002), music (Peretz & Zatorre, 2005), environmental sounds (Schnider et al., 1994; Thierry et al., 2003), and prosody (chapter 24, this volume). Prominent right hemisphere responses to auditory spatial cues have also been reported (Tiitinen et al., 2006).

Despite the traditional view that speech perception is lateralized to the left hemisphere, there is growing evidence that the non-dominant (right) hemisphere can also support auditory language processing. Neuroimaging studies with normal subjects typically report bilateral activation during speech perception (Wise et al., 1991; Zatorre et al., 1992; Binder et al., 1994; Tobey et al., 2003; Okada & Hickok, 2006; Obleser et al., 2008). Moreover, lesions involving the right hemisphere have been associated with impaired auditory language function (Coslett et al., 1984; Eustache et al., 1990). Functional deactivation of the right hemisphere by intracarotid sodium amobarbital injection (Wada test) for pre-surgical language lateralization testing has also resulted in impaired auditory language processing (McGlone, 1984; Boatman et al., 1998). Right hemisphere recruitment has also been documented in recovery of auditory language functions, including comprehension, in patients with aphasia (Cummings et al., 1979; Coslett & Monsul, 1994; Hillis, 2006; Schlaug et al., 2010) and after left hemispherectomy in children up to 14 years of age (Boatman et al., 1999).

In summary, the human auditory system comprises a complex array of ascending, descending, and crossing pathways that process and transmit auditory information from the ear to the brain. Although our understanding of the neurobiological bases of human auditory processing has improved over the past decade, determining the precise neural mechanisms underlying a listener's ability to perceive and comprehend spoken speech and other complex sounds in the environment remains a challenge for future research.

Acknowledgments

This work was supported by NIH grants DC05645 and DC010028 (DB) and the Johns Hopkins Science of Learning Initiative. Special thanks to Dr. Steven Eliades for assistance with the manuscript.

References

Aitkin, L.M., & Webster, W.R. (1972). Medial geniculate body of the cat: Organization and responses to tonal stimuli of neurons in ventral division. *Journal of Neurophysiology, 35*(3), 365–380.

Andéol, G., Guillaume, A., Micheyl, C., Savel, S., Pellieux, L., & Moulin, A. (2011). Auditory efferents facilitate sound localization in noise in humans. *Journal of Neuroscience, 31*(18), 6759–6763.

Artacho-Pérula, E., Arbizo, J., Arroyo-Jimenez, M.de M., Marcos, P., Martinez-Marcos, A., Blaizot, X., & Insauti, R. (2004). Quantitative estimation of the primary auditory cortex in human brains. *Brain Research, 1008*(1), 20–28.

Baumann, S., Koeneke, S., Schmidt, C.F., Meyer, M., Lutz, K., & Jancke, L. (2007). A network for audio-motor coordination in skilled pianists and non-musicians. *Brain Research, 1161*, 65–78.

Binder, J.R., Frost, J.A., Hammeke, T.A., Rao, S.M., & Cox, R.W. (1996). Function of the left planum temporale in auditory and linguistic processing. *Brain, 119*(4), 1239–1247.

Binder, J.R., Rao, S.M., Hammeke, T.A., Yetkin, F.Z., Jesmanowicz, A., Bandettini, P.A., Wong, E.C., Estkowski, L.D., Goldstein, M.D., Haughton, V.M., & Hyde, J.S. (1994). Functional magnetic resonance imaging of human auditory cortex. *Annals of Neurology, 35*(6), 637–638.

Blumstein, S., Cooper, W., Zurif, E., & Caramazza, A. (1977). The perception and production of voice-onset time in aphasia. *Neuropsychologia, 15*(3), 371–383.

Boatman, D., Freeman, J., Vining, E., Pulsifer, M., Miglioretti, D., Minahan, R., Carson, B., Brandt, J., & McKhann, G. (1999). Language recovery after left hemispherectomy in children with late onset seizures. *Annals of Neurology, 46*(4), 579–586.

Boatman, D., Hart, J., Lesser, R., Honeycutt, N., Anderson, N., Miglioretti, D., & Gordon, B. (1998). Right hemisphere speech perception revealed by amobarbital injection and electrical interference. *Neurology, 51*(2), 458–464.

Boatman, D., Lesser, R., & Gordon, B. (1995). Auditory speech processing in the left temporal cortex: An electrical interference study. *Brain and Language, 51*(2), 269–290.

Boatman, D.F., & Miglioretti, D.L. (2005). Cortical sites critical for speech discrimination in normal and impaired listeners. *Journal of Neuroscience, 25*(23), 5475–5480.

Boemio, A., Fromm, S., Braun, A., & Poeppel, D. (2005). Hierarchical and asymmetric temporal sensitivity in human auditory cortices. *Nature Neuroscience, 8*(3), 389–395.

Brown, S., Martinez, M.J., Hodges, D.A., Fox, P.T., & Parsons, J.M. (2004). The song system of the human brain. *Cognitive Brain Research, 20*(3), 363–375.

Brownell, W.E., Bader C.R., Bertrand, D., & De, R.Y. (1985). Evoked mechanical responses of isolated cochlear outer hair cells. *Science, 227*(4683), 194–196.

Carrasco, A., Brown, T.A., Kok, M.A., Chabot, N., Kral, A., & Lomber, S.G. (2013). Influence of core auditory cortical areas on acoustically evoked activity in contralateral primary auditory cortex. *Journal of Neuroscience, 33*(2), 776–789.

Caspary, D.M., Havey, D.C., & Faingold, C.L. (1981). Glutamate and aspartate: Alteration of thresholds and response patterns of auditory neurons. *Hearing Research, 4*(3–4), 325–333.

Clarke, S., Bellman, A., Meuli, R.A., Assal, G., & Steck, A.J. (2000). Auditory agnosia and auditory spatial deficits following left hemispheric lesions: Evidence for distinct processing pathways. *Neuropsychologia, 38*(6), 797–807.

Coslett, B., Brashear, H., & Heilman, K. (1984). Pure word deafness after bilateral primary auditory cortex infarcts. *Neurology, 34*(3), 347–352.

Coslett, B., & Monsul, N. (1994). Reading with the right hemisphere: Evidence from transcranial magnetic stimulation. *Brain and Language, 46*(2), 198–211.

Covey, E., & Casseday, J.H. (1991). The monaural nuclei of the lateral lemniscus in an echolocating bat: Parallel pathways for analyzing temporal features of sound. *Journal of Neuroscience, 11*(11), 3456–3470.

Cummings, J., Benson, D., Walsh, M., & Levine, H. (1979). Left-to-right transfer of language dominance: A case study. *Neurology, 29*(11), 1547–1550.

Da Costa, S., van der Zwaag, W., Merques, J.P., Frackowiak, R.S.J., & Clarke, S. (2011). Human primary auditory cortex follows the shape of Heschl's gyrus. *Journal of Neuroscience, 31*(40), 14067–14075.

de Boer, J., & Thornton, A.R.D. (2008). Neural correlates of perceptual learning in the auditory brainstem: Efferent activity predicts and reflects improvement at a speech-in-noise discrimination task. *Journal of Neuroscience, 28*(19), 4929–4937.

de Ribaupierre, F. (1997) Acoustical information processing in the auditory thalamus and cerebral cortex. In G. Ehret & R. Romand (Eds.), *The central auditory system* (pp. 259–316). Oxford: Oxford University Press.

Dehaene-Lambertz, G., & Baillet, S. (1998). A phonological representation in the infant brain. *NeuroReport, 9*(8), 1885–1888.

Delgutte, B. (1980). Representation of speech-like sounds in the discharge patterns of auditory-nerve fibers. *Journal of the Acoustical Society of America, 68*(3), 843–857.

Destrieux, C., Fischl, B., Dale, A., & Halgren, E. (2010). Automatic parcellation of human cortical gyri and sulci using standard anatomical nomenclature. *NeuroImage, 53*(1), 1–15.

Diaz, B., Hintz, F., Kiebel, S.J., & von Kriegstein, K. (2012). Dysfunction of the auditory thalamus in developmental dyslexia. *Proceedings of the National Academy of Sciences USA, 109*(34), 13841–13846.

Egorova, M., & Ehret, G. (2008). Tonotopy and inhibition in the midbrain inferior colliculus shape spectral resolution of sounds in neural critical bands. *European Journal of Neuroscience, 28*(4), 675–692.

Ehret, G. (1997). The auditory midbrain, a "shunting yard" of acoustical information processing. In G. Ehret & R. Romand (Eds), *The central auditory system* (pp. 259–316). Oxford: Oxford University Press.

Ehret, G., & Merzenich, M.M. (1988). Complex sound analysis (frequency resolution, filtering and spectral integration) by single units of the inferior colliculus of the cat. *Brain Research Reviews, 13*(2), 139–163.

Eustache, F., Lechevalier, B., Viader, F., & Lambert, J. (1990). Identification and discrimination disorders in auditory perception: a report on two cases. *Neuropsychologia, 28*(3), 257–270.

Formisano, E., Kim, D., Salle, F.D., van de Moortele, P., Ugurbil, K., & Goebel, R. (2003). Mirror-symmetric tonotopic maps in human primary auditory cortex. *Neuron, 40*(4), 859–869.

Foundas, A., Leonard, C., Gilmore, R., Fennel, E., & Heilman, K.M. (1994). Planum temporale asymmetry and language dominance. *Neuropsychologia, 32*(10), 1225–1231.

Fritz, J., Shamma, S., Elhilali, M., & Klein, D. (2003). Rapid task-related plasticity of spectrotemporal receptive fields in primary auditory cortex. *Nature Neuroscience, 6*(11), 1216–1223.

Galaburda, A., Sherman, G., Rosen, G., Aboitiz, F., & Geschwind, N. (1985). Developmental dyslexia: Four consecutive patients with cortical anomalies. *Annals of Neurology, 18*(2), 222–233.

Geis, H.R.A.P., & Borst, J.G.G. (2013). Intracellular responses to frequency modulated tones in the dorsal cortex of the mouse inferior colliculus. *Frontiers in Neural Circuits, 7*(7), 1–19. doi:10.3389/fncir.2013.00007

Geschwind, N., & Levitsky, W. (1968). Human brain: left-right asymmetries in temporal speech region. *Science, 161*(3837), 186–187.

Giard, M.H., Perrin, F., Pernier, J., & Bouchet, P. (1990). Brain generators implicated in the processing of auditory stimulus deviance: A topographic event-related potential study. *Psychophysiology, 27*(6), 627–640.

Giraud, A.L., Garnier, S., Micheyl, C., Lina, G., Chays, A., & Chéry-Croze, S. (1997). Auditory efferents involved in speech-in-noise intelligibility. *NeuroReport, 8*(7), 1779–1783.

Glowatzki, E., Cheng, N., Hiel, H., Yi, E., Tanaka, K., Ellis-Davies, G.C.R., Rothstein, J.D., & Bergles, D.E. (2006). The glutamate-aspartate transporter GLAST mediates glutamate uptake at inner hair cell afferent synapses in the mammalian cochlea. *Journal of Neuroscience, 26*(29), 7659–7664.

Griffiths, T.D., Büchel, C., Frackowiak, R.S.J., & Patterson, R.D. (1998). Analysis of temporal structure in sound by the human brain. *Nature Neuroscience, 1*(5), 422–427.

Gueta, R., Barlam, D., Shneck, R. Z., & Rousso, I. (2006). Measurement of the mechanical properties of isolated tectorial membrane using atomic force microscopy. *Proceedings of National Academy of Sciences of USA, 103*(40), 14790–14795.

Hackett, T.A. (2011). Information flow in the auditory cortical network. *Hearing Research, 271*(1–2), 133–146.

Hackett, T.A., Stepniewaska, I., & Kaas, J.H. (1998). Subdivisions of auditory cortex and ipsilateral cortical connections of the parabelt auditory cortex in macaque monkeys. *Journal of Comparative Neurology, 394*, 475–495.

He, J. (2003). Corticofugal modulation of the auditory thalamus. *Experimental Brain Research, 153*, 579–590.

Hickok, G., & Saberi, K. (2012). Redefining the functional organization of the planum temporale region: Space, objects, and sensory-motor integration. In D. Poeppel, T. Overath, A.N. Popper, & R.R. Fay (Eds.), *The human auditory cortex. Springer handbook of auditory research*, vol. 43 (pp. 333–350). New York: Springer.

Hillis, A. (2006). The right place at the right time? *Brain, 129*, 1351–1356.

Humphries, C., Liebenthal, E., & Binder, J.R. (2010). Tonotopic organization of human auditory cortex. *NeuroImage, 50*(3), 1202–1211.

Imig, T., & Morel, A. (1983). Organization of the thalamocortical auditory system in the cat. *Annual Review of Neuroscience, 6*, 95–120.

Ito, M., van Adel, B., & Kelly, J.B. (1996). Sound localization after transection of the commissure of Probst in the albino rat. *Journal of Neurophysiology, 76*(5), 3493–3502.

Ivarsson, C., de Ribaupierre, Y., & de Ribaupierre, F. (1988). Influence of auditory localization cues on neuronal activity in the auditory thalamus of the cat. *Journal of Neurophysiology, 59*(2), 586–606.

Joris, P.X., & Yin, T.C. (1995). Envelope coding in the lateral superior olive. I. Sensitivity to interaural time differences. *Journal of Neurophysiology, 73*(3), 1043–1062.

Kaas, J.H., & Hackett, T.A. (2000). Subdivisions of auditory cortex and processing streams in primates. *Proceedings of National Academy of Sciences of USA, 97*(22), 11793–11799.

Kaas, J.H., Hackett, T.A., & Tramo, M.J. (1999). Auditory processing in primate cerebral cortex. *Current Opinion in Neurobiology, 9*(2), 164–170.

Kimura, D. (1961). Cerebral dominance and the perception of verbal stimuli. *Canadian Journal of Psychology, 15*(3), 166–171.

Kraus, N., Carrell, T., King, C., Littman, T., & Nicol, T. (1994a). Discrimination of speech-like contrasts in the auditory thalamus and cortex. *Journal of Acoustic Society of America, 96*(5), 2758–2768.

Kraus, N., McGee, T., Littman, T., Nicol, T., & King, C. (1994b). Nonprimary auditory thalamic representation of acoustic change. *Journal of Neurophysiology, 72*(3), 1270–1277.

Langers, D.R.M., & van Dijk, P. (2012). Mapping the tonotopic organization in human auditory cortex with minimally salient acoustic stimulation. *Cerebral Cortex, 22*, 2024–2038.

Lu, T., Ling, L., & Wang, X. (2001). Temporal and rate representations of time-varying signals in the auditory cortex of awake primates. *Nature Neuroscience, 4*(11), 1131–1138.

Luethke, L.E., Krubitzer, L.A., & Kaas, J.H. (1989). Connections of primary auditory cortex in the New World monkey, Saguinus. *Journal of Comparative Neurology, 285*(4), 487–513.

Luria, A. (1976). *Basic problems of neurolinguistics*. Paris: Mouton.

Maison, S.F., & Liberman, C.M. (2000). Predicting vulnerability to acoustic injury with a noninvasive assay of olivocochlear reflex strength. *Journal of Neuroscience, 20*(12), 4701–4707.

May, B.J., le Prell, G.S., & Sachs, M.B. (1998). Vowel representations in the ventral cochlear nucleus of the cat: Effects of level, background noise and behavioral state. *Journal of Neurophysiology, 79*(4), 1755–1767.

McGlone, J. (1984). Speech comprehension after unilateral injection of sodium amytal. *Brain and Language, 22*(1), 150–157.

Merzenich, M., & Brugge, J. (1973) Representation of the cochlear partition on the superior temporal plane of the macaque monkey. *Brain Research, 50*(2), 275–296.

Metzner, W., & Radtke-Schuller, S. (1987). The nuclei of the lateral lemniscus in the rufous horseshoe bat, *Rhinolophus rouxi. Journal of Comparative Physiology, 160*(3), 395–411.

Miceli, G., Caltagirone, C., Gainotti, G., & Payer-Rigo, P. (1978). Discrimination of voice versus place contrasts in aphasia. *Brain and Language, 6*(1), 47–51.

Mononen, L.J., & Seitz, M.R. (1977). An AER analysis of contralateral advantage in the transmission of auditory information. *Neuropsychologia, 15*(1), 165–173.

Morel, A., Garraghty, P.E., & Kaas, J.H. (1993). Tonotopic organization, architectonic fields, and connections of auditory cortex in macaque monkeys. *Journal of Comparative Neurology, 335*(3), 437–459.

Morel, A., & Kaas, J. (1992). Subdivisions and connections of auditory cortex in owl monkeys. *Journal of Comparative Neurology, 318*(1), 437–459.

Musiek, F., & Lamb, L. (1992). Neuroanatomy and neurophysiology of central auditory processing. In J. Katz, N. Stecker, & D. Henderson (Eds.), *Central auditory processing: A transdisciplinary view* (pp. 11–38). Mosby Year Book. St. Louis: Mosby.

Mussachia, G., Strait, D., & Kraus, N. (2008). Relationships between behavior, brainstem and cortical encoding of seen and heard speech in musicians and non-musicians. *Hearing Research, 241*(1–2), 34–42.

Nelken, I., Fishback, A., Las, L., Ulanovsky, N., & Farkas, D. (2003). Primary auditory cortex of cats: Feature detection or something else? *Biological Cybernetics, 89*(5), 397–406.

Obleser, J., Eisner, F., & Kotz, S.A. (2008). Bilateral speech comprehension reflects differential sensitivity to spectral and temporal features. *Journal of Neuroscience, 28*(32), 8116–8124.

Oertel, D. (1991). The role of intrinsic neuronal properties in the encoding of auditory information in the cochlear nuclei. *Current Opinion in Neurobiology, 1*(2), 221–228.

Oertel, D., Ramazan, B., Gardner, S.M., Smith, P.H., & Joris, P.X. (2000). Detection of synchrony in the activity of auditory nerve fibers by octopus cells of the mammalian cochlear nucleus. *Proceedings of National Academy of Sciences of USA, 97*(22), 11773–11779.

Okada, K., & Hickok, G. (2006). Identification of lexical-phonological networks in the superior temporal sulcus using functional magnetic resonance imaging. *NeuroReport, 17*(12), 1293–1296.

Okada, K., Rong, F., Venezia, J., Matchin, W., Hsieh, I-H., Saberi, K., Serences, J.T., & Hickok, G. (2010). Hierarchical organization of human auditory cortex: Evidence from acoustic invariance in the response to intelligible speech. *Cerebral Cortex, 20*(10), 2486–2495.

Peretz, I., & Zatorre, R.J. (2005). Brain organization for music processing. *Annual Review of Psychology. 56*, 89–114.

Petkov, C.I., Kayser, C., Augath, M., & Logothetis, N.K. (2006). Functional imaging reveals numerous fields in the monkey auditory cortex. *PLoS Biology, 4*, e215. doi:10.1371/journal.pbio.0040215

Poeppel, D. (2003). The analysis of speech in different temporal integration windows: Cerebral lateralization as 'asymmetric sampling in time.' *Speech Communication, 41*(1), 245–255.

Rajan, R. (2000). Centrifugal pathways protect hearing sensitivity at the cochlea in noisy environments that exacerbate the damage induced by loud sound. *Journal of Neuroscience, 20*(17), 6684–6693.

Rauschecker, J.P., & Scott, S.K. (2009). Maps and streams in the auditory cortex: Nonhuman primates illuminate human speech processing. *Nature Neuroscience, 12*(6), 718–724.

Rauschecker, J.P., & Tian, B. (2000). Mechanisms and streams for processing of "what" and "where" in auditory cortex. *Proceedings of National Academy of Sciences USA, 97*(22), 11800–11806.

Rauschecker, J.P., & Tian, B. (2004). Processing of band-passed noise in the lateral auditory belt cortex of the rhesus monkey. *Journal of Neurophysiology, 91*(6), 2578–2589.

Rauschecker, J.P., Tian, B., & Hauser, M. (1995). Processing of complex sounds in macaque nonprimary auditory cortex. *Science, 268*(5207), 111–114.

Rojas, D.C., Bawn, S.D., Benkers, T.L., Reite, M.L., & Rogers, S.L. (2002). Smaller left hemisphere planum temporale in adults with autistic disorder. *Neuroscience Letters, 328*(3), 237–240.

Romanski, L.M., Bates, J.F., & Goldman-Rakic, P.S. (1999). Auditory belt and parabelt projections to the prefrontal cortex in the rhesus monkey. *Journal of Comparative Neurology, 403*(2), 141–157.

Russo, N., Nicol, T., Musacchia, G., & Kraus, N. (2004). Brainstem responses to speech syllables. *Clinical Neurophysiology, 115*(9), 2021–2030.

Sachs, M.B., & Young, E.D. (1979). Encoding of steady-state vowels in the auditory nerve: Representation in terms of discharge rate. *Journal of Acoustic Society of America, 66*(2), 470–479.

Sadagopan, S., & Wang, X. (2009). Nonlinear spectrotemporal interactions underlying selectivity for complex sounds in auditory cortex. *Journal of Neuroscience, 29*(36), 11192–11202.

Schlaug, G., Norton, A., Marchina, S., Zipse, L., & Wan, C.Y. (2010). From singing to speaking: Facilitating recovery from nonfluent aphasia. *Future Neurology, 5*(5), 657–665.

Schnider, A., Benson, D.F., Alexander, D.N., & Schnider-Klaus, A. (1994). Non-verbal environmental sound recognition after unilateral hemispheric stroke. *Brain, 117*(2), 281–287.

Skoe, E., & Kraus, N. (2010). Auditory brainstem response to complex sounds: A tutorial. *Ear and Hearing, 31*(3), 302–324.

Smith, K.R., Hsieh, I.H., Saberi, K., & Hickok, G. (2009). Auditory spatial and object processing in the human planum temporale: No evidence for selectivity. *Journal of Cognitive Neuroscience, 22*(4), 632–639.

Starr, A., & Hamilton, A.E. (1976). Correlation between confirmed sites of neurological lesions and abnormalities of far-field auditory brainstem responses. *Electroencephelography and Clinical Neurophysiology, 41*(6), 595–608.

Steinschneider, M., Schroeder, C., Arezzo, J., & Vaughan, H. (1995). Physiological correlates of voice onset time in primary auditory cortex (A1) of the awake monkey: Temporal response patterns. *Brain and Language, 48*(3), 326–340.

Steinmetz, H., Volkmann, J., Jäncke, L., & Freund, H-J. (1991). Anatomical left-right asymmetry of language related temporal cortex is different in left- and right-handers. *Annals of Neurology, 29*(3), 315–319.

Striem-Amit, E., Hertz, U., & Amedi, A. (2011). Extensive cochleotopic mapping of human auditory cortical fields obtained with phase-encoding fMRI. *PLoS One, 6*(3), e17832. doi:10.1371/journal.pone.0017832

Talvage, T.M., Sereno, M.I., Melcher, J.R., Ledden, P.J., Rosen, B.R., & Dale, A.M. (2004). Tonotopic organization in human auditory cortex revealed by progressions in frequency sensitivity. *Journal of Neurophysiology, 91*(3), 1282–1296.

Thierry, G., Giraud, A., & Price, C. (2003). Hemispheric dissociation in access to the human semantic system. *Neuron, 38*(3), 499–506.

Tiitinen, H., Salminen, N.H., Palomäki, K.J., Mäkinen, V.T., Alku, P., & May, P.J.C. (2006). Neuromagnetic recordings reveal the temporal dynamics of auditory spatial processing in the human cortex. *Neuroscience Letters, 396*(1), 17–22.

Tobey, E.A., Devous, Sr. M.D., & Rolan, P.S. (2003). Functional brain imaging of speech perception via electrical stimulation. *25th Conference Proceedings IEEE Engineering in Medicine and Biology Society, 3*, 1991–1994.

Viemeister, N. (1988). Psychophysical aspects of auditory intensity coding. In G. Edelman, W. Gall, & W. Cowan (Eds.), *Auditory function: Neurobiological bases of hearing* (pp. 213–241). New York: John Wiley & Sons.

von Békésy, G. (1960). *Experiments in hearing.* New York: McGraw-Hill.

von Kriegstein, K., Patterson, R.D., & Griffiths, T.D. (2008). Task-dependent modulation of medial geniculate body is behaviorally relevant for speech recognition. *Current Biology, 18*(23), 1855–1859.

Wada, J.A., Clarke, R., & Hamm, A. (1975). Cerebral hemispheric asymmetry in humans. *Archives of Neurology, 32*(4), 239–246.

Warrier, C.M., Abrams, D.A., Nicol, T.G., & Kraus, N. (2011). Inferior colliculus contributions to phase encoding of stop consonants in an animal model. *Hearing Research, 282*(1–2), 108–118.

Wernicke, C. (1874). The symptom complex of aphasia. Reprinted in English in *Proceedings of Boston Studies in Philosophy of Science,* 1968; *4,* 34–97.

Wessinger, C.M., Van Meter, J., Tian, B., Van Lare, J., Pekar, J., & Rauschecker, J.P. (2001). Hierarchical organization of the human auditory cortex revealed by functional magnetic resonance imaging. *Journal of Cognitive Neuroscience, 13*(1), 1–7.

Wise, R., Chollet, F., Hadar, U., Friston, K., Hoffner, E., & Frackowiak, R. (1991). Distribution of cortical neural networks involved in word comprehension and word retrieval. *Brain, 114*(4), 1803–1817.

Woods, D.L., & Alain, C. (2009). Functional imaging of human auditory cortex. *Current Opinion in Otolaryngology & Head and Neck Surgery, 17*(5), 407–411.

Woods, D.L., Herron, T.J., Cate, A.D., Kang, X., & Yund, E.W. (2011). Phonological processing in human auditory cortical fields. *Frontiers in Human Neuroscience, 5,* 42. doi:10.3389/fnhum.2011.00042

Woods, D.L., Stecker, G.C., Rinne, T., Herron, T.J., Cate, A.D., Yund, E.W., Liao, I., & Kang, X. (2009). Functional maps of human auditory cortex: effects of acoustic features and attention. *PLoS One, 4*(4), e5183. doi:10.1371/journal.pone.0005183

Yin, T.C., & Chan, J.C. (1990). Interaural time sensitivity in medial superior olive of cat. *Journal of Neurophysiology, 64*(2), 465–488.

Young, E., Shofner, W., White, J., Robert, J., & Voigt, H. (1988). Response properties of cochlear nucleus neurons in relationship to physiological mechanisms. In G. Edelman, W. Gall, & W. Cowan (Eds.), *Auditory function: Neurobiological bases of hearing* (pp. 213–241). New York: John Wiley & Sons.

Zatorre, R.J., Belin, P., & Penhune, V.B. (2002). Structure and function of auditory cortex: Music and speech. *Trends in Cognitive Sciences, 6*(1), 37–46.

Zatorre, R.J., Evans, A.C., Meyer, E., & Gjedde, A. (1992). Lateralization of phonetic and pitch discrimination in speech processing. *Science, 256*(5058), 846–849.

15

DIAGNOSIS AND TREATMENT OF AUDITORY DISORDERS

Stephanie Nagle, Deepti Ramadoss, and Dana Boatman

Auditory disorders can arise from the peripheral auditory system or the central auditory system. Peripheral auditory disorders impact hearing, while disorders of the central auditory system affect higher-level auditory functions, including sound recognition and comprehension. Auditory disorders can be developmental or acquired. Developmental and acquired disorders of the peripheral auditory system are typically associated with structural abnormalities of the outer, middle, and/ or inner ear. Developmental disorders of the central auditory system occur in the absence of structural abnormalities, while acquired central auditory disorders are commonly associated with structural lesions. We will focus on acquired disorders of the central auditory system at the level of the cerebral cortex. Because the peripheral and central auditory systems are physically contiguous, disorders of the peripheral system can affect central auditory processing. This is especially relevant for people who have had strokes who, in addition to speech comprehension difficulties, may have preexisting hearing loss. Therefore, comprehensive auditory evaluations should assess both peripheral and central auditory functions. We begin by reviewing the diagnosis and treatment of peripheral hearing loss.

Disorders of the Peripheral Auditory System

Hearing loss is characterized by elevated (abnormal) sound detection thresholds based on a hearing test, or audiological evaluation, that uses acoustically calibrated equipment in a sound-treated booth (for discussion, see Martin & Clark, 2011). Pure tones are used to determine frequency-specific air conduction thresholds (250–8000 Hz) and bone conduction thresholds (500–4000 Hz) for each ear separately. Sound is transmitted (conducted) through the air-filled outer ear and middle ear to the fluid-filled inner ear. Sound can also be transmitted directly to the inner ear by bone conduction. In bone conduction testing, the outer ear and middle ear are bypassed, and the inner ear is stimulated directly using a bone conduction vibrator. In addition to pure tone testing, routine audiological evaluations include word recognition testing at suprathreshold levels and evaluation of middle ear function by tympanometry. Hearing thresholds worse (i.e., greater) than 20–25 dB at two or more frequencies suggest hearing loss. Comparison of air and bone conduction thresholds is used to determine the type of hearing loss: conductive, sensorineural, or mixed.

Conductive Hearing Loss

Conductive hearing loss refers to elevated (abnormal) air-conduction thresholds that are at least 10 dB worse than the normal bone conduction thresholds at two or more tone frequencies. The main effect of conductive hearing loss is sound attenuation. If the presentation level is sufficiently high (loud), individuals with conductive hearing loss often perform within normal limits on speech recognition tests. Conductive hearing losses usually do not exceed 65 dB (moderate-severe) and are often reversible. The gap between elevated air-conduction thresholds and normal bone conduction thresholds is consistent with outer or middle ear pathology. The most common middle ear pathology is otitis media, which results in the buildup of fluid or negative pressure in the middle ear that interferes with normal transmission of sound to the inner ear. Otitis media can also be identified based on measures of middle ear compliance represented graphically by a tympanogram. Tympanograms show the relative compliance (and impedance) of the tympanic membrane and ossicles of the middle ear and can help identify the presence of middle ear fluid (flat tympanogram). Otitis media affects very young to school-age children more than adults and can result in a fluctuating conductive hearing loss.

Another middle ear pathology in adults is otosclerosis, which is often hereditary (Moumoulidis et al., 2007) and has a higher incidence in women (Morrison & Bundey, 1970; Niedermeyer et al., 2001). Otosclerosis is a progressive, unilateral or bilateral disease resulting in new growth of spongy bone on the middle ear ossicles, especially the stapes footplate. Fixation of the stapes footplate in the oval window damps the amplitude of sound transmitted to the inner ear. Early signs of otosclerosis include a low-frequency conductive hearing loss and a notch in the audiogram around 2000 Hz (referred to as Carhart's notch) with elevated bone conduction thresholds. In contrast to otitis media, Individuals with otosclerosis typically have normal tympanograms, although peak compliance may be reduced.

Other conductive pathologies include disarticulation of the ossicles, as can occur with head trauma; congenital malformations of the middle and outer ear; tympanic membrane perforations; and middle ear tumors, including glomus tumors, which arise from glomus bodies in tympanic branches of ninth and tenth cranial nerve, and cholesteatomas that arise from epithelial tissue of the tympanic membrane.

Treatment of conductive hearing loss usually targets the underlying pathology. Otitis media may be treated with a course of antibiotics. For who suffer from chronic otitis media, pressure-equalizing (PE) tubes can be surgically inserted into the tympanic membrane to permit drainage of middle ear fluid. If otitis media is left untreated, the tympanic membrane can rupture. Because children with conductive hearing losses are at risk for speech and language disorders, preferential classroom seating is often recommended. If the conductive hearing loss is relatively stable, hearing aids may be helpful in compensating for sound attenuation. Most other middle ear pathologies are treated surgically to help restore hearing. Stapedectomy/stapedotomy remains the surgical procedure of choice for treatment of otosclerosis. Stapedectomy involves prosthetic replacement of a fixated stapes; stapedotomy involves inserting a small piston-like prosthesis that mimics footplate movement. Surgery is also indicated to correct ossicular fractures or dislocations and for removal of middle ear tumors.

Sensorineural Hearing Loss

Sensorineural hearing loss is characterized by abnormal (elevated) air *and* bone conduction thresholds and may be sensory (e.g., cochlear) or neural (retrocochlear) in origin. Sensorineural hearing loss is often associated with damage to the hair cells in the cochlea from noise exposure, ototoxic drugs (e.g., aminoglycosides), or normal aging (presbycusis). Hair cells associated with high-frequency hearing (e.g., > 1000 Hz) are more vulnerable because of their location at the basal end of the cochlea. Individuals with a high-frequency sensorineural hearing loss often have difficulty discriminating consonant sounds, which are softer than vowel sounds, especially in the presence of background noise. Low-frequency sensorineural hearing loss can also occur and is characteristic of Meniere's disease. Meniere's disease is a cochlear pathology characterized by endolymphatic hydrops, abnormal generation of endolymph fluid in the scala media, and may be accompanied by sudden attacks of vertigo and/or tinnitus.

Routine hearing tests do not distinguish between sensory *versus* neural hearing loss. To further localize the origin of sensorineural hearing loss, clinicians use otoacoustic emissions (OAEs), which assess the integrity of outer hair cell motility. The absence of OAEs is consistent with cochlear (i.e., sensory) hearing loss.

Treatment for sensorineural hearing loss depends largely on the underlying etiology. There are multiple treatment options for people with Meniere's disease, including medication, low-sodium diet, surgery, and gentamycin injection. Individuals with presbycusis who have no other medical complications may benefit from hearing aids. Over the past decade, advances in hearing aid technology have made hearing aids smaller, more comfortable, and programmable. Automatic noise reduction algorithms and feedback-cancelling features are now routinely included in even the most basic hearing aids. Binaural amplification is usually recommended for people with bilateral hearing loss, even if hearing in one ear is better than the other ear (Silverman & Silman, 1990). Monoaural amplification can lead to decreased speech understanding in the better ear and can adversely affect sound localization, which relies in part on interaural intensity differences. Despite amplification, some people with sensorineural hearing loss continue to demonstrate poor speech recognition abilities. In such cases, a central auditory processing disorder may also be present. Individuals with severe-profound sensorineural hearing loss and intact eighth nerve function, who have shown no measurable benefit from hearing aids, may be candidates for a cochlear implant. Cochlear implants are surgically implanted electrodes in the cochlea that electrically stimulate the auditory nerve to transmit auditory information to the brain.

Individuals presenting with sensorineural hearing loss accompanied by other clinical symptoms such as unilateral tinnitus, dizziness, extreme difficulty understanding speech in noise, and/or aural fullness require further evaluation to rule out retrocochlear pathologies or other medical conditions. Retrocochlear pathologies include tumors of the eighth cranial nerve, referred to as acoustic neuromas, as well as auditory neuropathy/dys-synchrony disorder (ANSD). Most acoustic neuromas are unilateral and arise from schwann cells in the sheath covering the vestibular branch of the eighth nerve and, therefore, are more accurately termed vestibular schwannomas. As these tumors grow, they expand into the cerebellopontine angle exerting pressure on the eighth nerve and other cranial nerves, including the trigeminal nerve (cranial nerve V). Brainstem auditory evoked response (BAER/ABR) testing, which assesses neural integrity of the eighth cranial nerve and auditory nuclei in the brainstem, can identify vestibular schwannomas. Although most clinical centers now rely on MRI studies, combining BAER/ABR and MRI studies may be effective for early identification of eighth nerve tumors (Josey et al., 1988). Surgical treatment is indicated for most individuals with eighth nerve tumors. A potential complication of surgery is damage to the auditory and/or facial nerve; the risk of this occurring depends on the size and location of the tumor.

Combining OAE with BAER/ABR testing can be useful in the differential diagnosis of retrocochlear pathology. For example, in ANSD otoacoustic emissions are usually present/normal, while ABR results are markedly abnormal. ANSD is generally diagnosed in childhood, and is characterized by asynchronous or disordered depolarization of the auditory nerve and/or synaptic abnormalities at the hair cell-auditory nerve synapse. ANSD causes varying degrees of hearing loss, extreme difficulty processing speech in background noise, and other related speech and language impairments. Treatment for ANSD is not standardized at this time, and may include a trial with hearing aids, educational accommodations, or cochlear implants.

Mixed Hearing Loss

Individuals with mixed hearing loss have a combined conductive and sensorineural hearing loss. In this case, both air and bone conduction thresholds are elevated (abnormal), with air conduction thresholds at least 10 dB worse than bone conduction thresholds. Mixed hearing loss is common in elderly people with established sensorineural hearing loss who then develop middle ear infections or obstruction of the ear canal (e.g., impacted cerumen). In general, the conductive portion of a mixed hearing loss is treated first (as described above). Once the air-bone gap has closed and thresholds are stable, the sensorineural hearing loss can be re-evaluated and remediation options determined.

Additional Hearing Tests

Hearing thresholds can be screened at bedside or in a clinical exam room using a portable audiometer or tuning fork tests. Vibrating tuning forks generate single-frequency tones (e.g., 256 Hz, 512 Hz) and can be used to screen both air conduction (held up to the outer ear) and bone conduction (held against the mastoid) thresholds. Three tuning fork tests are: the Rinne, the Weber, and the Schwabach. The Rinne test compares individuals' hearing sensitivity by air *versus* bone conduction; examinees are asked whether the tuning fork's tone is louder when presented via air conduction or bone conduction. Louder air conduction (positive Rinne) is associated with both sensorineural hearing loss and normal hearing, while louder bone conduction (negative Rinne) is consistent with conductive hearing loss. The Schwabach tuning fork test compares the patient's *versus* the clinician's hearing by bone conduction. Once the patient can no longer detect the tone, the clinician places the tuning fork on his/her own mastoid to determine whether the patient has a normal Schwabach (no tone heard by clinician) or a diminished Schwabach (tone still audible to clinician). An obvious limitation of this test is the assumption that the examiner has normal hearing. For the Weber test, the patient determines whether the tone produced by a tuning fork placed at midline on the forehead lateralizes to one ear (unilateral hearing loss) or is perceived as equally loud in both ears (normal hearing or bilateral hearing loss). In the former case, the tone may lateralize to the ear with unilateral conductive hearing loss, or to the ear opposite the sensorineural hearing loss. Tuning fork tests are used only as screening tests and do not provide detailed diagnostic information (e.g., degree of hearing loss).

Disorders of the Central Auditory System

Auditory disorders can arise from abnormalities at any level of the central auditory system, but are perhaps best documented in people with cortical lesions. Three main classes of cortical auditory disorders have been identified: receptive aphasia, auditory agnosia, and cortical deafness.

Receptive (Auditory) Aphasias

The hallmark of receptive aphasia is impaired language comprehension, in particular, spoken language comprehension. Receptive aphasia is associated with lesions of the language-dominant (left) hemisphere, including the posterior temporal lobe and parietal lobe. There are three types of receptive aphasia: Wernicke's aphasia, transcortical sensory aphasia, and the receptive component of global aphasia.

Wernicke's Aphasia

Wernicke's aphasia is characterized by severe impairment of spoken language comprehension, with fluent speech output. In addition to poor comprehension, individuals with Wernicke's aphasia also have impaired repetition and naming abilities (Hillis, 2007). The spontaneous speech of people with Wernicke's aphasia is typically fluent but meaningless, with numerous phonological and semantic paraphasias. Because people with Wernicke's aphasia are unable to monitor their speech output for meaning or phonological accuracy, they may also use neologisms (invented words). Traditionally, Wernicke's aphasia has been associated with lesions of the posterior perisylvian region, including the temporal and parietal lobes. In most cases, Wernicke's area (Brodmann area 22) in the posterior temporal lobe is involved (Naeser & Hayward, 1978; see also chapters 8 and 11, this volume). However, Wernicke's aphasia has also been associated with subcortical lesions (Naeser et al., 1982). The auditory impairments characteristic of Wernicke's aphasics may reflect abnormal phonological or acoustic analysis/decoding, deficits in semantic processing, or a combination thereof (Robson et al., 2012).

Transcortical Sensory Aphasia

Transcortical sensory aphasia is a rare form of receptive aphasia that is characterized by impaired auditory comprehension, with intact repetition and fluent speech. Comprehension of written and spoken speech is usually severely impaired and affected individuals may also have echolalia. Sparing of repetition distinguishes transcortical sensory aphasia from other receptive aphasias and is thought to reflect disruption of access from phonology to lexical-semantic processing. This view is supported by their relatively intact performance on phonological tasks, despite poor auditory comprehension. Although their speech output is typically fluent, it is often paraphasic. Likewise, in transcortical sensory aphasia, the ability to read aloud may be relatively spared despite poor reading comprehension. This rare receptive aphasia has traditionally been associated with lesions that spare and isolate Wernicke's area from more posterior language areas (Geschwind et al., 1968; Kertesz et al., 1982). However, studies have also identified transcortical sensory aphasia in individuals with frontal lobe lesions and/or lesions of Wernicke's area (Otsuki et al., 1998; Boatman et al., 2000). Transcortical sensory aphasia is differentiated from other receptive aphasias by the sparing of repetition, and from other transcortical aphasias by impaired auditory comprehension with fluent speech output.

Global Aphasia

Individuals with global aphasia have both receptive and expressive language disorders. The receptive component of global aphasia is similar to Wernicke's aphasia. Language comprehension deficits in people with global aphasia may be less severe than their expressive deficits. In most cases phonological processing is also compromised. Traditionally, global aphasia has been associated with damage to the anterior and posterior language areas (Hayward et al., 1977; Kertesz et al., 1979). However, there are also reports of global aphasia with sparing of Wernicke's area (Mazzochi & Vignolo, 1979; Basso et al., 1985; Vignolo et al., 1986). In a number of cases, subcortical involvement has been documented, suggesting that receptive aphasia is not associated exclusively with posterior cortical lesions.

Differentiating between the three main types of receptive aphasia is based on performance on receptive language tests and standardized aphasia test batteries, such as the Boston Diagnostic Aphasia Examination (Goodglass & Kaplan, 1972; Goodglass et al., 2000), the Western Aphasia Battery (Kertesz, 1982; Kertesz, 1996), or the European Aachen Aphasia Test (Huber et al., 1983).

In addition to testing individuals' language comprehension abilities, it is important to evaluate phonological processing, since this basic auditory language function may also be compromised. Most phonological processing tests require listeners to discriminate pairs of words that are phonologically contrasted (e.g., pat-bat) or to identify auditory stimuli by repetition, orthographic matching, or picture matching. It is also important to assess auditory processing in other aphasic individuals, not just those with receptive aphasia, since more subtle auditory disorders, including phonological deficits, may be present (Blumstein et al., 1977).

Accurate diagnosis is important for effective rehabilitation. Functional neuroimaging is used increasingly to investigate the mechanisms and substrates involved in aphasia and language recovery (Hillis, 2006). Functional imaging is also used to predict long-term outcomes in aphasia (for review, see Meinzer et al., 2011). Aural rehabilitation therapies designed for individuals with receptive aphasia focus largely on recovery of lexical-semantic information, and are usually implemented by a speech-language pathologist or audiologist. Rehabilitation therapy for individuals with Wernicke's aphasia may begin with common semantic categories, such as those involved in everyday activities. The initial goal is often improvement of single-word comprehension, followed by increasingly more complex spoken language structures (phrases). For transient aphasias, such as transcortical sensory aphasia, aural rehabilitation may not be useful. For those with phonological processing disorders, there are many aural therapy programs, including software programs, designed to improve phonological processing skills. Typically, these programs focus on improving the listener's ability to decode speech sounds (phonemes) from the incoming acoustic signal, to discriminate them from other similar phonemes, and to identify them by their corresponding orthographic representations, or by use of pictures. Training in speech reading (lip reading) may also be helpful for those with phonological processing disorders. Modifying speech rates has been shown to be useful for improving speech understanding in individuals with auditory agnosia, but not for with receptive aphasias (Blumstein et al., 1985). Although the potentially confounding effects of spontaneous recovery and heterogeneity among individuals make it difficult to assess rehabilitation programs during the early stages of language recovery, individualized therapies are considered important for continued functional recovery (Kertesz, 1997).

Auditory Agnosia

Auditory agnosia is characterized by impaired sound recognition, in the context of normal peripheral hearing. Individuals with auditory agnosia can detect sounds but may be unable to differentiate speech, environmental sounds, or music. Auditory agnosia is associated with bilateral lesions of the temporal lobe and/or insula (Habib et al., 1995) and can be further subdivided into auditory verbal agnosia (pure word deafness) and auditory non-verbal agnosia.

Auditory Verbal Agnosia

Auditory verbal agnosia, or pure word deafness, refers to a selective impairment in the ability to recognize or understand spoken speech. In contrast to transcortical sensory aphasia, repetition and phonological processing are always impaired in pure word deafness. Written comprehension and oral reading are usually spared. Although most individuals with auditory verbal agnosia can differentiate speech from environmental sounds or music, they often report that speech sounds like a foreign language (Albert & Bear, 1974). Sparing of written language comprehension (reading) distinguishes pure word deafness from Wernicke's aphasia and points to an underlying auditory disorder rather than a higher-level language disorder (aphasia). However, because pure word deafness and Wernicke's aphasia share a number of similarities, it remains unclear whether these are distinct disorders or variants of the same disorder (i.e., Wernicke's aphasia).

Pure word deafness is associated with bilateral lesions of auditory cortex (e.g., Auerbach et al., 1982; Coslett et al., 1984; Tanaka et al., 1987; Poeppel, 2001) or deep unilateral left hemisphere lesions that disrupt auditory radiations from the thalamus and contralateral auditory cortex (Kussmaul, 1877; Lichtheim, 1885; Takahashi et al., 1992; Stefanatos et al., 2005). Studies of pure word deafness have identified two subtypes: a phonetic-phonological decoding deficit (Praamstra et al., 1991) and a more basic (pre-phonologic) auditory deficit (Albert & Bear, 1974; Chocholle et al., 1975; Auerbach et al., 1982; Best & Howard, 1994; Godefroy et al., 1995). Individuals with unilateral left hemisphere lesions appear more likely to have phonological decoding deficits as evidenced by impaired discrimination of consonant contrasts but not vowel contrasts (Denes & Semenza, 1975; Saffran et al., 1976), while individuals with bilateral lesions often exhibit more basic auditory processing deficits (Albert & Bear, 1974; Auerbach et al., 1982; Best & Howard, 1994; Godefroy et al., 1995).

Auditory Non-Verbal Agnosia

Auditory non-verbal agnosia is characterized by the inability to recognize previously familiar environmental sounds despite normal peripheral hearing and absence of aphasia. This disorder is rarer than pure word deafness, but may also be underreported since speech comprehension remains intact and recognition of environmental sounds is not routinely evaluated. In addition to impaired recognition of environmental sounds, people with auditory non-verbal agnosia may also have impaired pitch discrimination (Spreen et al., 1965). A selective impairment in the processing of musical information (e.g., pitch, prosody) is referred to as auditory amusia. Although most cases of auditory non-verbal agnosia are associated with bilateral involvement (L'Hermitte et al., 1971; Albert et al., 1972; Kazui et al., 1990), it may also occur with unilateral right hemisphere lesions (Spreen et al., 1965; Clarke et al., 1996).

Auditory agnosia, including pure word deafness, is often transient and may resolve spontaneously or progress to a more mild receptive aphasia. Because these individuals often experience spontaneous recovery (Kertesz, 1997), long-term aural rehabilitation may not be indicated. When rehabilitation is indicated, language-based therapies may not be as useful as therapies that focus on lower-level auditory processing skills. For example, individuals who have difficulty processing frequency information may benefit from pitch discrimination training using steady-state and frequency-modulated tones. Similarly, individuals who have difficulty processing auditory events that occur in rapid succession (a feature of spoken speech) may benefit from recent software programs that train people to detect auditory stimuli that are systematically sequenced at shorter and shorter intervals. Individuals with auditory agnosia may show improved auditory comprehension at slower speech rates (Neisser, 1976). Emphasis on speech reading (lip reading) skills may further supplement information lost during auditory processing by exploiting visual articulatory cues (Auerbach et al., 1982). Because written language comprehension is usually spared, this modality can be used for communication as well as for re-establishing access to lexical-semantic information from audition. Finally, auditory comprehension can often be improved in cases of auditory agnosia by increasing reliance on contextual information.

Cortical Deafness

Cortical deafness is characterized by the inability to detect or recognize sounds despite normal hearing and language abilities (Vignolo, 1969). Individuals with cortical deafness are often indifferent to sound and may report that they are deaf (Michel et al., 1980; Garde & Cowey, 2000). However, objective measures of peripheral hearing, including OAEs and BAER/ABR, typically yield relatively normal findings. Individuals with cortical deafness can understand written language and have intact speech output. Cortical deafness is associated with bilateral lesions of the temporal lobes, including Heschl's gyrus, and/or bilateral damage to the underlying white matter and auditory radiations. Cortical auditory evoked potentials are usually abnormal or absent bilaterally (Michel et al., 1980).

Other Cortical Auditory Disorders

In addition to focal cortical lesions, auditory disorders are associated with more diffuse cortical neuropathologies, such as Alzheimer's disease. The main pathological changes associated with Alzheimer's disease include accumulation of microscopic neurofibrillary tangles and amyloid plaques, which tend to primarily involve the temporal lobe and hippocampus. It is not surprising, therefore, that people with Alzheimer's disease have impaired auditory comprehension. It has been suggested that the language comprehension deficits of people with Alzheimer's disease resemble those of individuals with transcortical sensory aphasia or, in the later stages, Wernicke's aphasia (Cummings et al., 1985; Murdoch et al., 1987). Impaired auditory comprehension coupled with evidence of phonological paraphasias in the speech productions of people with Alzheimer's disease raise the question of an underlying receptive phonological processing deficit (Croot et al., 2000; but see also Biassou et al., 1995).

Cortical auditory disorders have also been associated with epilepsy. For example, Landau-Kleffner syndrome, a childhood epilepsy syndrome, is characterized initially by the disproportionate impairment of auditory comprehension relative to other language abilities (Landau & Kleffner, 1957; Rapin et al., 1977; Seri et al., 1998). Likewise, individuals with temporal lobe epilepsies often demonstrate auditory processing difficulties, especially under adverse listening conditions such as background noise (Boatman et al., 2006; Wied et al. 2007; Boatman et al. 2008). One potential explanation is that abnormal cortical electrical activity associated with seizures may add "noise" to the system, rendering it less capable of compensating for degradation of the speech signal in poor listening environments.

Neural Plasticity in the Adult Auditory System

Traditionally, neural plasticity has been associated with the developing nervous system and is thought to decrease inversely with age (Lenneberg, 1967; Krashen & Harshman, 1972). However, there is growing evidence of neural plasticity in the mature auditory system as well. Neural plasticity has been documented in studies of adult auditory cortex after (1) hearing loss, (2) re-introduction of sound to deafened systems, (3) increased sound input to impaired systems, and (4) with behavioral training, as described below.

Changes in the functional organization of auditory cortex resulting from hearing loss have been documented in adult animals and humans (e.g., Rajan et al., 1993; Dietrich et al., 2001). In such cases, auditory cortex reorganizes to become maximally responsive to the remaining intact cochlear frequencies; moreover, the cortical representations of frequencies adjacent to those associated with the hearing loss may expand (e.g., McDermott et al., 1998; Thai-Van et al., 2002; Thai-Van et al., 2003). These changes are referred to as deprivation induced plasticity (see Syka, 2002 for discussion).

Re-introduction of sound into the deafened adult auditory system can also induce reorganization and plasticity (Fallon et al., 2008). When the onset of deafness occurs after language development (post-lingual), cochlear implants can induce reorganization of auditory cortex (Giraud et al., 2001, Pantev et al., 2006). Cochlear implant users who became deaf before developing language (pre-lingual), show less reorganization of auditory cortex (Naito et al., 1997). The extent of reorganization in the adult system also appears to be related to age and duration of deafness (Fallon et al., 2008).

Increasing sensory (sound) input to the impaired hearing system can induce functional reorganization. Auditory electrophysiological responses recorded from individuals with hearing aids indicate improved neural function as compared to individuals without hearing aids (Korczak et al., 2005; Munro et al., 2007).

Behavioral training can also modify the functional organization of adult auditory cortex, as shown in animal studies (e.g., Fritz et al., 2003; Bao et al., 2004; Polley et al., 2006). In human adults, behavioral training leads to improved perceptual performance (e.g., Sweetow & Palmer, 2005), and electrophysiological studies following auditory training have demonstrated neural plasticity as well (e.g., Kraus et al., 1995; Atienza et al., 2002; Tremblay & Kraus, 2002; Reinke, et al., 2003; Gottselig et al., 2004; Russo et al., 2004; Alain et al., 2007). These studies indicate that training and aural rehabilitation can induce neuroplastic changes in the adult auditory system.

Acknowledgment

This work was supported by NIH-NIDCD grant DC010028 and by a grant from the Johns Hopkins University Science of Learning Institute.

References

Alain, C., Snyder, J.S., He, Y., & Reinke, K.S. (2007). Changes in auditory cortex parallel rapid perceptual learning. *Cerebral Cortex, 17*(5), 1074–1084.

Albert, M.L., & Bear, D. (1974). Time to understand: a case study of word deafness with reference to the role of time in auditory comprehension. *Brain, 97*(2), 373–384.

Albert, M.L., Sparks, R., von Stockert, T., & Sax, D. (1972). A case study of auditory agnosia: linguistic and non-linguistic processing. *Cortex, 8*(4), 427–433.

Atienza, M., Cantero, J.L., & Dominguez-Marin, E. (2002). The time course of neural changes underlying auditory perceptual learning. *Learning and Memory, 9*(3), 138–150.

Auerbach, S.H., Allard, T., Naeser, M., Alexander, M.P., & Albert, M.L. (1982). Pure word deafness: analysis of a case with bilateral lesions and a defect at the prephonemic level. *Brain, 105*(2), 271–300.

Bao, S., Chang, E.F., Woods, J., & Merzenich, M.M. (2004). Temporal plasticity in the primary auditory cortex induced by operant perceptual learning. *Nature Neuroscience, 7*(9), 974–981.

Basso, A., Lecours, A.R., Morashini, S., & Vanier, M. (1985). Anatomoclinical correlations of the aphasias as defined through computerized tomography: exceptions. *Brain and Language, 26*(2), 201–229.

Best, W., & Howard, D. (1994). Word sound deafness resolved? *Aphasiology, 8*(3), 223–256.

Biassou, N., Grossman, M., Onishi, K., Mickanin, J., Hughes, E., Robinson, K.M., & D'Esposito, M. (1995). Phonologic processing deficits in Alzheimer's disease. *Neurology, 45*(12), 2165–2169.

Blumstein, S.E., Baker, E., & Goodglass, H. (1977). Phonological factors in auditory comprehension in aphasia. *Neuropsychologia, 15*(1), 19–30.

Blumstein, S.E., Katz, B., Goodglass, H., Shrier, R., & Dworetsky, B. (1985). The effects of slowed speech on auditory comprehension in aphasia. *Brain and Language, 24*(2), 246–265.

Boatman, D., Gordon, B., Hart, J., Selnes, O., Miglioretti, D., & Lenz, F. (2000). Transcortical sensory aphasia: revised and revisited. *Brain, 123*(8), 1634–1642.

Boatman, D., Lesser, R., Crone, N., Krauss, G., Lenz, F., & Miglioretti, D. (2006). Speech recognition impairments in with intractable right temporal lobe epilepsy. *Epilepsia, 47*(8), 1397–1401.

Boatman, D.F., Trescher, W.H., Smith, C., Ewen, J., Los, J., Wied, H.M., Gordon, B., Kossoff, E.H., Gao, Q., & Vining, E.P. (2008). Cortical auditory dysfunction in benign rolandic epilepsy. *Epilepsia, 49*(6), 1018–1026.

Chocholle, R., Chedru, F., Bolte, M.C., Chain, F., & L'Hermitte, F. (1975). Etude psychoacoustique d'un cas de 'surdite corticale.' *Neuropsychologia, 13*(2), 163–172.

Clarke, S., Bellman, A., Ribaupierre, F.D., & Assal, G. (1996). Non-verbal auditory recognition in normal subjects and brain-damaged patients. *Neuropsychologia, 34*(6), 587–603.

Coslett, H.B., Brashear, H.R., & Heilman, K.M. (1984). Pure word deafness after bilateral primary auditory cortex infarcts. *Neurology, 34*(3), 347–352.

Croot, K., Hodges, J.R., Xuereb, J., & Patterson, K. (2000). Phonological and articulatory impairment in Alzheimer's disease: a case series. *Brain and Language, 75*(2), 277–309.

Cummings, J.L., Benson, D.F., Hill, M.A., & Read, S. (1985). Aphasia in dementia of the Alzheimer type. *Neurology, 35*(3), 394–397.

Denes, G., & Semenza, C. (1975). Auditory modality-specific anomia: evidence from a case of pure word deafness. *Cortex, 11*(4), 401–411.

Dietrich, V., Nieschalk, M., Stoll, W., Rajan, R., & Pantev, C. (2001). Cortical reorganization in patients with high frequency cochlear hearing loss. *Hearing Research, 158*(1–2), 95–101.

Fallon, J.B., Irvine, D.R.F., & Shephard, R.K. (2008). Cochlear implants and brain plasticity. *Hearing Research, 238*(1–2), 110–117.

Fritz, J., Shamma, S., Elhilali, M., & Klein, D. (2003). Rapid task-related plasticity of spectrotemporal receptive fields in primary auditory cortex. *Nature Neuroscience, 6*(11), 1216–1223.

Garde, M.M., & Cowey, A. (2000). "Deaf hearing": unacknowledged detection of auditory stimuli in a patient with cerebral deafness. *Cortex, 36*(1), 71–80.

Geschwind, N., Quadfasel, F.A., & Segarra, J.M. (1968). Isolation of the speech area. *Neuropsychologia, 6*(4), 327–340.

Giraud, A.L., Truy, E., & Frackowiak, R. (2001). Imaging plasticity in cochlear implant patients. *Audiology and Neurotology, 6*(6), 381–393.

Godefroy, O., Leys, D., Furby, A., De Reuck, J., Daems, C., Rondepierre, P., Debachu, B., Deleume, J.F., & Desaulty, A. (1995). Psychoacoustical deficits related to bilateral subcortical hemorrhages. A case with apperceptive auditory agnosia. *Cortex, 31*(1), 149–159.

Goodglass, H., & Kaplan, E. (1972). *Assessment of aphasia and related disorders.* Philadelphia: Lea and Febiger.

Goodglass, H., Kaplan, E., & Barresi, B. (2000). *Boston diagnostic aphasia examination* (3rd ed.). San Antonio, TX: The Psychological Corporation.

Gottselig, J.M., Brandeis, D., Hofer-Tinguely, G., Borbely, A.A., & Achermann, P. (2004). Human central auditory plasticity associated with tone sequence learning. *Learning & Memory, 11*(2), 162–171.

Habib, M., Daquin, G., Milandre, L., Royere, M.L., Rey, M., Lanteri, A., & Khalil, R. (1995). Mutism and auditory agnosia due to bilateral insular damage—role of the insula in human communication. *Neuropsychologia, 33*(3), 327–339.

Hayward, R.W., Naeser, M.A., & Zatz, L.M. (1977). Cranial computed tomography in aphasia. *Radiology, 123*(3), 653–660.

Hillis, A.E. (2006). The right place at the right time? *Brain, 129*(6), 1351–1356.

Hillis, A.E. (2007). Aphasia: progress in the last quarter of a century. *Aphasia: Views and Reviews, 69*(2), 200–213.

Huber, W., Poeck, K., Weniger, D., & Willmes, K. (1983). *Aachener-aphasie test.* Gottingen: Hogrefe.

Josey, A.F., Glasscock, M.E., & Musiek, F.E. (1988). Correlation of ABR and medical imaging in patients with cerebellopontine angle tumors. *American Journal of Otology, 9*, 12–16.

Kazui, S., Naritomi, H., Sawada, T., Inoue, N., & Okuda, J. (1990). Subcortical auditory agnosia. *Brain and Language, 38*(4), 476–487.

Kertesz, A. (1982). *Western aphasia battery.* New York: Grune and Stratton.

Kertesz, A. (1996). *Western aphasia battery—revised.* San Antonio, TX: Pearson.

Kertesz, A. (1997). Recovery of aphasia. In T.E. Feinburg & M.J. Farah (Eds.), *Behavioral neurology and neuropsychology.* New York: McGraw-Hill.

Kertesz, A., Harlock, W., & Coates, R. (1979). Computer tomographic localization of lesion size and prognosis in aphasia and nonverbal impairment. *Brain and Language, 8*(1), 34–50.

Kertesz, A., Sheppard, M. A., & MacKenzie, R. (1982). Localization in transcortical sensory aphasia. *Archives of Neurology, 39*(8), 475–478.

Korczak, P.A., Kurtzberg, D., & Stapells, D.R. (2005). Effects of sensorineural hearing loss and personal hearing aids on cortical event-related potential and behavioral measures of speech sound processing. *Ear and Hearing, 26*(2), 165–185.

Krashen, S., & Harshman, R. (1972). Lateralization and the critical period. *Journal of Acoustical Society of America, 52*(1A), 174–174.

Kraus, N., McGee, T., Carrell, T. D., King, C., Tremblay, K., & Nicol, T. (1995). Central auditory system plasticity associated with speech discrimination training. *Journal of Cognitive Neuroscience, 7*(1), 25–32.

Kussmaul, A. (1877). Disturbances of speech. In H. von Ziemssen (Ed.), *Cyclopedia of the practice of medicine* (pp. 581–875). New York: William Wood.

L'Hermitte, F., Chain, F., Escourolle, R., Ducarne, B., Pillon, B., & Chedru, F. (1971). Etude des troubles perceptifs auditifs dans les lésions temporales bilatérales. *Revue Neurologique, 124*, 329–351.

Landau, W.M., & Kleffner, F.R. (1957). Syndrome of acquired aphasia with convulsive disorder in children. *Neurology, 7*(8), 523–530.

Lenneberg, E.H. (1967). *Biological foundations of language.* New York: John Wiley.

Lichtheim, L. (1885). On aphasia. *Brain, 7*, 433–484.

Martin, F., & Clark, J.G. (2011). *Introduction to audiology* (11th ed.). San Antonio: Pearson.

Mazzochi, F., & Vignolo, L.A. (1979). Localizations of lesions in aphasia: clinical-CT correlations in stroke patients. *Cortex, 15*(4), 627–654.

McDermott, H.J., Lech, M., Kornblum, M.S., & Irvine, D.R. (1998). Loudness perception and frequency discrimination in subjects with steeply sloping hearing loss: possible correlates of neural plasticity. *Journal of the Acoustical Society of America, 104*(4), 2314–2325.

Meinzer, M., Harnish, S., Conway, T., & Crosson, B. (2011). Recent developments in functional and structural imaging of aphasia recovery after stroke. *Aphasiology, 25*(3), 271–290.

Michel, F., Peronnet, F., & Schott, B. (1980). A case of cortical deafness: clinical and electrophysiological data. *Brain and Language, 10*(2), 367–377.

Morrison, A.W., & Bundey, S.E. (1970). The inheritance of otosclerosis. *Journal of Laryngology and Otology, 84*(9), 921–932.

Moumoulidis, I., Axon, P., Baguley, D., & Reid, E. (2007). A review on the genetics of otosclerosis. *Clinical Otolaryngology, 32*(4), 239–247.

Munro, K.J., Pisareva, N.P., Parker, D.J., & Purdy, S.C. (2007). Asymmetry in the auditory brainstem response following experience of monaural amplification. *NeuroReport, 18*(17), 1871–1874.

Murdoch, B.E., Chenery, H.J., Wilks, V., & Boyle, R. (1987). Language disorders in dementia of the Alzheimer type. *Brain and Language, 31*(1), 122–137.

Naeser, M.A., & Hayward, R.W. (1978). Lesion localization in aphasia with cranial computed tomography and the B.D.A.E. *Neurology, 28*(6), 545–551.

Naeser, M.A., Alexander, M.P., Helm-Estabrooks, N., Levine, H.L., Laughlin, M.A., & Geschwind, N. (1982). Aphasia with predominantly subcortical lesion sites: description of three capsular/putaminal aphasia syndromes. *Archives of Neurology, 39*(1), 2–14.

Naito, Y., Hirano, S., Honjo, I., Okazawa, H., Ishizu, K., Takahashi, H., Fujiki, N., Shiomi, Y., Yonekura, Y., & Konishi, J. (1997). Sound- induced activation of auditory cortices in cochlear implant users with post- and prelingual deafness demonstrated by positron emission tomography. *Acta Otolaryngologica, 117*(4), 490–496.

Neisser, U. (1976). *Cognition and reality*. San Francisco: Freeman.

Niedermeyer, H.P., Arnold, W., Schwub, D., Busch, R., Wiest, I., & Sedlmeier, R. (2001). Shift of the distribution of age in patients with otosclerosis. *Acta Otolaryngologica, 121*(2), 197–199.

Otsuki, M., Soma, Y., Koyama, A., Yoshimura, N., Furkawa, H., & Tsuji, S. (1998). Transcortical sensory aphasia following left frontal infraction. *Journal of Neurology, 245*(2), 69–76.

Pantev, C., Dinnesen, A., Ross, B., Wollbrink, A., & Knief, A. (2006). Dynamics of auditory plasticity after cochlear implantation: a longitudinal study. *Cerebral Cortex, 16*(1), 31–36.

Poeppel, D. (2001). Pure word deafness and the bilateral processing of the speech code. *Cognitive Science, 25*(5), 679–693.

Polley, D.B., Steinberg, E.E., & Merzenich, M.M. (2006). Perceptual learning directs auditory cortical map reorganization though top-down influences. *The Journal of Neuroscience, 26*(18), 4970–4982.

Praamstra, P., Hagoort, P., Maassen, B., & Crul, T. (1991). Word deafness and auditory cortical function: a case history and hypothesis. *Brain, 114*(3), 1197–1225.

Rajan, R., Irvine, D.R.F., Wise, L.Z., & Heil, P. (1993). Effect of unilateral partial cochlear lesions in adult cats on the representation of lesioned and unlesioned cochleas in primary auditory cortex. *Journal of Comparative Neurology, 338*(1), 17–49.

Rapin, I., Mattis, S., Rowan, A.J., & Golden, G.G. (1977). Verbal auditory agnosia in children. *Developmental Medicine and Child Neurology, 19*(2), 192–207.

Reinke, K.S., He, Y., Wang, C., & Alain, C. (2003). Perceptual learning modulates sensory evoked response during vowel segregation. *Brain Research: Cognitive Brain Research, 17*(3), 781–791.

Robson, H., Sage, K., & Lambon Ralph, M.A. (2012). Wernicke's aphasia reflects a combination of acoustic-phonological and semantic control deficits: A case-series comparison of Wernicke's aphasia, semantic dementia and semantic aphasia. *Neuropsychologia, 50*(2), 266–275.

Russo, N.M., Nicol, T.G., Zecker, S.G., Hayes, E.A., & Kraus, N. (2004). Auditory training improves neural timing in the human brainstem. *Behavioral Brain Research, 156*(1), 95–103.

Saffran, R., Marin, O., & Yeni-Komshan, G. (1976). An analysis of speech perception in word deafness. *Brain and Language, 3*(2), 209–228.

Seri, S., Cerquiglini, A., & Pisani, F. (1998). Spike-induced interference in auditory sensory processing in Landau-Kleffner syndrome. *Electroencephalography and Clinical Neurophysiology, 108*(5), 506–510.

Silverman, C.A., & Silman, S. (1990). Apparent auditory deprivation from monaural amplification and recovery with binaural amplification: two case studies. *Journal of the American Academy of Audiology, 1*(4), 175–180.

Spreen, O., Benton, A.L., & Fincham, R. (1965). Auditory agnosia without aphasia. *Archives of Neurology, 13*, 84–92.

Stefanatos, G.A., Gershkoff, A., & Madigan, S. (2005). On pure word deafness, temporal processing and the left hemisphere. *Journal of the International Neuropsychological Society, 11*(4), 456–470.

Sweetow, R., & Palmer, C. (2005) Efficacy of individual auditory training in adults: a systematic review of the evidence. *Journal of the American Academy of Audiology, 16*(7), 494–504.

Syka, J. (2002). Plastic changes in the central auditory system after hearing loss, restoration of function, and during learning. *Physiological Reviews, 82*(3), 601–636.

Takahashi, N., Kawamura, M., Shinotou, H., Hirayama, K., Kaga, K., & Shindo M. (1992). Pure word deafness due to left hemisphere damage. *Cortex, 28*(2), 295–303.

Tanaka, Y., Yamadori, A., & Mori, E. (1987). Pure word deafness following bilateral lesions: a psychophysical analysis. *Brain, 110*(2), 381–403.

Thai-Van, H., Micheyl, C., Moore, B. C., Collet, L. (2003). Enhanced frequency discrimination near the hearing loss cut-off: a consequence of central auditory plasticity induced by cochlear damage? *Brain, 126*(10), 2235–45.

Thai-Van, H., Micheyl, C., Norena, A., & Collet, L. (2002). Local improvement in auditory frequency discrimination is associated with hearing-loss slope in subjects with cochlear damage. *Brain, 125*(3), 524–37.

Tremblay, K.L., & Kraus, N. (2002). Auditory training induces asymmetrical changes in cortical neural activity. *Journal of Speech, Language, and Hearing Research, 45*(3), 564–572.

Vignolo, L.A. (1969). Auditory agnosia: a review and report of recent evidence. In A.L. Benton (Ed.), *Contributions to clinical neuropsychology*. Chicago: Aldine.

Vignolo, L.A., Boccardi, E., & Caverni, L. (1986). Unexpected CT-scan finding in global aphasia. *Cortex, 22*(1), 55–69.

Wied, H., Morrison, P., Gordon, B., Zimmerman, A., Vining, E., & Boatman, D. (2007). Cortical auditory dysfunction in childhood epilepsy: Electrophysiologic evidence. *Current Pediatric Reviews, 3*(4), 317–327.

PART 6

Sentence Processing

16

SENTENCE COMPREHENSION DEFICITS

Independence and Interaction of Syntax, Semantics, and Working Memory

Randi C. Martin and Yingying Tan

Findings during the 1970s demonstrated impaired sentence comprehension in aphasic patients who had good single word comprehension (e.g., Caramazza & Zurif, 1976; von Stockert & Bader, 1976). For example, a patient might understand the meanings of *girl, boy, kiss, red*, and *hair*, but be unable to determine for an object-extracted relative clause sentence such as "*The boy that the girl kissed had red hair*" who is doing the kissing and who has red hair.[1] Difficulties in establishing the roles played by nouns based on syntactic structure were found even for simple active and passive sentences such as "*The cat was chasing the dog*" or "*The dog was chased by the cat*" (Schwartz, Saffran, & Marin, 1980). These sentences are termed reversible, since either noun can play the role of agent (i.e., person carrying out the action) or theme (i.e., person or object being acted upon). The same patients did not have difficulty understanding sentences with similar structures that were nonreversible, such as "*The car that the woman drove was an import*" or "*The apple was eaten by the boy.*" Thus, the patients were able to integrate word meanings into a sentence meaning when such could be done on the basis of semantic plausibility but were impaired when they had to use syntactic structure to understand the relations in the sentence. These findings generated a good deal of excitement among researchers in and outside the field of aphasia because they seemed to provide strong evidence for the disruption of a syntactic processing module that was independent of semantics (e.g., see Caramazza & Berndt, 1978; Jackendoff, 1993, chap. 11). However, since these early studies, additional results have complicated the interpretation of these findings and their implications for sentence processing.

The early findings on sentence comprehension deficits seemed in tune with psycholinguistic theories of sentence processing from the 1960s that assumed a deterministic set of rules for parsing; that is, a set of rules such as phrase structure rules and transformations for assigning the syntactic structure to a sentence (Fodor & Garrett, 1967). These rules were assumed to be purely syntactic in nature and were applied to a sequence of words on the basis of the syntactic category of the words (e.g., noun, verb, adjective) and not on the basis of the meaning of the words. If the entire set of rules were disrupted due to brain damage, one would expect patients with such a deficit to perform poorly on any task involving syntactic processing. One influential paper hypothesized that individuals with Broca's aphasia had a global deficit in syntactic knowledge, which accounted for both their agrammatic speech (i.e., speech with simplified grammatical structure, marked by the omission of function word and inflections) and their asyntactic comprehension (e.g., difficulties understanding reversible sentences) (Berndt & Caramazza, 1980). However, this proposal has encountered numerous difficulties. For one, dissociations have been found between agrammatic speech and asyntactic comprehension (Berndt, Mitchum, & Haendiges, 1996; Martin & Blossom-Stach, 1986; Miceli, Mazzucchi, Menn, & Goodglass, 1983). Several studies showed that some aphasic patients with near chance performance on reversible passive sentences using a sentence-picture matching paradigm or enactment (i.e., acting out the action with toy objects) did well when they were asked to judge the grammatical acceptability of sentences, even for sentences with complex structures (Linebarger, 1995; Linebarger, Schwartz, & Saffran, 1983). The patients were able to detect errors such as the omission or substitution of function words and inflections, the elements most affected in their speech. Based on these findings, Linebarger and colleagues (Linebarger, 1995; Linebarger, Schwartz, Romania, Kohn, & Stephens, 2000; Linebarger et al., 1983) hypothesized that the patients' difficulties were not with syntactic parsing, but rather with the mapping between the grammatical roles that entities played in a sentence and their thematic roles with respect to the verb (i.e., roles such as agent, theme, and recipient). For example, for a sentence such as "*The car that the truck splashed was green*," the patient would be able to determine that this sentence is grammatical, and that "*truck*" is the grammatical subject and "*car*" is the grammatical object of "*splashed*." However, they would be unable to determine that "*car*" should be mapped as the agent of "*splashed*" and "*truck*" should be mapped as the theme.

However, if patients were completely unable to carry out the mapping process, they should have performed poorly on all sentence types, whether or not the sentence had a canonical subject-verb-object (SVO) structure. In fact, although aphasic patients often do show some impairment in the comprehension of reversible sentences with canonical word orders, they typically show a greater impairment for noncanonical word orders—as in passive sentences, cleft object (e.g., "*It was the boy that the girl kissed*"), and object-extracted relative clause sentences (Berndt et al., 1996; Schwartz et al., 1980). Perhaps some notion of "strength" of a syntactic analysis can be introduced here to help explain this pattern of results. Some recent models of sentence comprehension assume that multiple syntactic interpretations of an ambiguous string may be generated in parallel with different strengths assigned to each that depend on the frequency with which each is encountered (Boland, 1997), and that these frequencies play a role in comprehension (Mitchell, Cuetos, Corley, & Brysbaert, 1995). Under this view, in even unambiguous sequences such as "*The boy that the girl kissed*" the assignment of "*boy*" to object position with respect to the embedded verb would have a relatively weak strength (in normal subjects as well as in patients) because of the overall infrequency of this type of object-extracted relative clause construction. One could further surmise that although syntactic analysis is being carried out by the patients, the strengths throughout the system that supports syntactic processing have been weakened due to brain damage, a problem that combines with a mapping deficit to create particular difficulties in mapping for infrequently encountered structures. This explanation thus assumes that these patients have two deficits rather than one.

Verb-Specific Deficits

Whereas Linebarger et al. (1983, 2000) hypothesized a deficit in a general mapping process, other findings suggest that such mapping difficulties may be tied to the representations of particular verbs. A case (LK) demonstrating the dissociation between syntactic structural analysis and a verb-specific mapping deficit was reported by Breedin and Martin (1996). LK performed at chance in choosing between two pictures to match a verb when the distracter picture depicted a "reverse-role" verb. Reverse-role pairs included verbs like *buy-sell, chase-flee*, and *borrow-lend*, where the thematic roles of the participants were the same but their mapping to grammatical roles with respect to the verb differed for the words within the pair. LK's poor performance on the reverse-role pairs could not be attributed to difficulty with semantically complex verbs, as he performed significantly better (92% correct) when asked to discriminate one of the reverse-role verbs from a semantically related verb that was equally complex (e.g., *buy* vs. *trade*). LK's difficulty seemed to be specifically in discriminating between verbs that had very similar semantic representations but different mappings between grammatical and thematic roles, which Breedin and Martin attributed to disruptions affecting the representations of particular verbs. In the case of the verbs *lend* and *borrow*, for example, LK appeared to know that these verbs imply that someone owns some object and that this owner allows someone else to temporarily take possession, but lacked the knowledge that in the case of *lend* the agent role is assigned to the permanent owner, whereas in *borrow* the agent is the person temporarily taking possession.

Berndt, Haendiges, Mitchum, and Sandson (1997) provided evidence that difficulties with verb representation may underlie some patients' difficulty in comprehending reversible sentences. In their study, aphasic patients who showed worse verb than noun retrieval in single word and sentence production also showed comprehension deficits for reversible relative to nonreversible sentences. Patients who showed better verb than noun retrieval or equivalent noun and verb retrieval performed well on comprehension of both reversible and nonreversible sentences. More recently, Wu, Waller, and Chatterjee (2007) demonstrated that some aphasic patients could, like LK in Breedin and Martin (1996), understand the action implied by individual verbs but have difficulty mapping verb thematic roles even in simple active reversible sentences (e.g., "*The circle kicked the square*"). Interestingly, this deficit dissociated from an understanding of thematic relations with respect to a locative preposition (e.g., "*The square is above the circle*") both behaviorally and in terms of the underlying neural damage (i.e., left lateral temporal for verb and left inferior frontal-parietal for prepositions). Unlike the Berndt et al. study, however, verb production was not tested, and thus one cannot tell if these patients would also have had difficulty producing single verbs in isolation.

Recently, Miozzo, Rawlins, and Rapp (2014) uncovered a dissociation in the mapping of syntax to thematic role assignment for verbs versus nonverbal lexical categories (i.e., prepositions and adjectival comparatives such as "*darker than*"). Two patients were found to have great difficulty in assigning thematic roles to the nonverbal elements than to verbs, even when the overall meaning of the sentences was quite similar. For example, they did well in sentence-picture matching for sentences such as "*The plate covers the napkin*" but did poorly for sentences such as "*The plate is on the napkin.*" Their difficulty with thematic role assignment for nonverbal lexical elements relative to verbs was consistent across production and comprehension and across several different tasks tapping comprehension. Miozzo, Rawlins, and Rapp interpreted these findings as consistent with linguistic theories that hypothesize that thematic role assignment depends on specialized structures and processes for nonverbal elements, different from those involved with verbs.

Disruptions of Specific Aspects of Syntactic Parsing

In studies from the 1980s, Caplan and colleagues (Caplan & Hildebrandt, 1988; Hildebrandt, Caplan, & Evans, 1987) examined sentence processing deficits from the point of view of Chomsky's (1982) government and binding theory, comparing patients' comprehension of sentences with and without referential dependencies. Referential dependencies refer to noun phrases that depend on the linkage with another noun phrase for their interpretation—such as the linkage between a reflexive and its referent or between a "trace" and the noun phrase that was moved from that position. A "trace" (**t**) is a construct from linguistic theory that indicates the position from which a noun phrase has been moved during a transformation. For instance, in a relative clause sentence such as "*The boy$_i$ that the girl kissed* **t**$_i$ *, . . .,*" correct understanding of such sentence relies on the correct processing of traces. The "*boy*" plays the role of object with respect to the verb "*kissed*" in the relative clause, but has been moved out of this deep structure position to its surface structure position in the main clause. This movement is hypothesized to leave behind a trace that links it from its position in the main clause to this empty position in the relative clause. This trace provides the syntactic cue for assigning the object role to the noun phrase *"boy."* Some researchers have attributed aphasic patients' deficits in sentence comprehension to their failure in tracking moved constituents—that is, their failure to either represent or process traces in their representations of syntactic structure (trace deletion hypothesis; Grodzinsky, 1990; Grodzinsky, Piñango, Zurif, & Drai, 1999).

In the Hildebrandt, Caplan, and Evans (1987) study, patient KG was tested on a wide range of sentence types involving moved elements (and traces) and other types of referential dependencies. KG showed a striking deficit on an enactment task for many of the structures involving moved elements. However, his performance was affected by the complexity of the sentence involving these elements—with good performance for relatively simpler sentences like cleft object sentences with transitive verbs and two nouns (e.g., *"It was the monkey that the elephant kicked")* and poorer performance for more complex sentences like cleft object sentences with dative verbs and three nouns (e.g., *"It was the monkey that the elephant gave to the goat")* and object-extracted relative clauses. Also, he performed well on simple sentences involving either missing subjects (termed PRO; e.g., *"Jim promised Dan [PRO]to shave")* or reflexive pronouns (e.g., *"Dan shaved himself"),* but he performed poorly on sentences combining both (e.g., *"Dan promised Jim to shave himself").*[2] This effect of complexity rules out the possibility that KG has a complete disruption of knowledge of, for instance, the processing of empty noun phrases like traces. Caplan and colleagues thus interpreted this pattern of results as indicating a capacity limitation specific to syntactic parsing, hypothesizing that several factors contribute to capacity demands during parsing, including (1) having to postulate empty noun phrases (relative to the processing of overt noun phrases), (2) having to hold a noun phrase without a thematic role assignment while assigning thematic roles to other noun phrases, and (3) searching over a long distance in the syntactic structure to determine the mapping of referential dependencies. Although KG could handle one of these capacity demands, when two or more were combined his performance broke down. It should be noted that KG's capacity constraint for syntactic parsing could not be attributed to a general verbal memory span deficit, as his performance on a variety of span tasks was within normal range.

Caplan and Hildebrandt (1988) reported several other case studies of patients with mild or more severe deficits on their syntactic comprehension battery. Among the mildly impaired patients, the pattern of deficits across sentence types differed. For instance, patient GS had difficulty with a variety of relative clause constructions involving object movement, but not with sentences termed NP-raising constructions (e.g., *"Joe seems to Patrick to be praying")* where the subject of the main verb *"Joe"* must be interpreted as the subject of the embedded verb phrase *"to be praying."* Patient JV showed the opposite dissociation. The highly specific deficits demonstrated in these patients suggest that there are different parsing operations associated with comprehending these various linguistic constructions that may be selectively affected by brain damage. Caplan and Hildebrandt (1988) made various suggestions regarding what these operations might be (see pp. 198–199 for a summary), but they implied that parsing theories are not well specified enough to accommodate all of their findings.

However, before drawing conclusions about the disruption of specific parsing mechanisms, it is necessary to demonstrate consistent deficits for particular structures across various tasks, as some researchers have found considerable variation in performance on the same sentence structures across different tasks such as sentence-picture matching and sentence anomaly judgments (Cupples & Inglis, 1993; Linebarger, Schwartz, & Saffran, 1983). In fact, in more recent studies, Caplan and colleagues (Caplan, Michaud, & Hufford, 2013; Caplan, DeDe, & Michaud, 2006) reported little consistency in patients' performance across different comprehension tasks (i.e., sentence-picture matching, enactment) on similar structures to those tested in Caplan and Hildrebandt (1988), using two different sentence types to assess each syntactic feature (i.e., cleft object and object-extracted relative clauses to test processing of traces). They concluded that task demands need to be taken into account in any theory of parsing deficits, though they did not explicate how such task effects could be accounted for. There are problematic aspects, however, to their approach to assessing consistency. In order to claim a deficit for a particular structure, patients were required to perform above chance for a baseline sentence (e.g., cleft subject sentence) but at chance or below for a corresponding experimental sentence with a more difficult structure (e.g., cleft object).[3] One issue concerns the reliability of the dependent measures, as the determination of "above chance" or "chance" performance might depend on a difference in only one item correct (e.g., 8/10 above chance vs. 7/10 chance). Patients might show a similar pattern of worse performance on experimental than baseline sentences across both sentence types tapping a particular syntactic feature and across both tasks but not be counted as showing consistent performance because performance on the experimental task fell above chance for one task but not the other, although the difference in performance was slight. Consider the data from two patients (50001, 50002) shown in Table 16.1 from Caplan et al. (2006), who were claimed to show either only a sentence type–specific, task-specific deficit (50001) or sentence type–specific (CO), task-independent deficit (50002) despite showing consistently worse performance on the experimental than baseline sentences across both sentence types used to tap a particular syntactic feature and across both tasks (a difference of identical magnitude between experimental and baseline for all comparisons for 50001). If these authors had correlated the difference in experimental and baseline sentences across all subjects, no doubt significant correlations would have been obtained—which would suggest consistency. Thus, while some case studies have demonstrated dramatic task effects on the processing of syntactic structure (e.g., Cupples & Inglis, 1993), there may be, in general, more consistency across tasks for more patients than has been claimed.

Online Syntactic Processing in Aphasic Patients

The above discussion focused on syntactic processing deficits in aphasic patients as revealed through performance accuracy on different sentence structures. Some researchers have argued that aphasic individuals' deficits in sentence comprehension may be due to slowed processing, rather than to impaired syntactic representations (Haarmann & Kolk, 1991; Kolk, 1995; Swinney & Zurif, 1995). For instance, patients' comprehension may fail if syntactic computation processes are slowed because earlier sentence constituents may have faded from working memory by the time a later structure has been analyzed. This problem should be particularly evident for complex syntactic structures where slowed processing would have the greatest effect. If the slowed-processing hypothesis is correct, then one would anticipate that "online" effects would be delayed relative to

Table 16.1 Performance (Proportion Correct) on Object-Extracted and Baseline Structures Based on Mean Normal Performance. CO: cleft object. CS: cleft subject. SO: subject-modifying object relative clause. SS: subject-modifying subject relative clause.

	Cleft Sentences				Relative Clauses			
	Sentence-Picture Matching		Enactment		Sentence-Picture Matching		Enactment	
Subject	CO at/below	CS above	CO above	CS above	SO at/below	SS above	SO at/below	SS at/below
50001	70	90	80	100	60	80	30	50
50002	at/below 60	above 80	above 80	above 100	at/below 50	above 90	at/below 40	above 100

those for controls.[4] Recently, Thompson and colleagues have addressed online processing using an eye-tracking-while-listening paradigm (Dickey, Choy, & Thompson, 2007; Dickey & Thompson, 2009; Meyer, Mack, & Thompson, 2012; Thompson & Choy, 2009). For example, Dickey, Choy, and Thompson (2007) traced subjects' eye movements as they listened to brief stories while looking at a display with four objects. They responded aloud to comprehension probes following each story. Based on prior results from healthy young subjects (Sussman & Sedivy, 2003), participants were expected to look to the object of the verb in a wh- question immediately following the verb, implying that subjects were filling the empty NP position (often termed the "gap") with the appropriate direct object. For example, in a story context in which a boy kissed a girl, subjects were expected to look to a picture of the girl when hearing the verb in the question "*Who did the boy kiss (gap) that day at school?*" The other pictures included the subject ("*boy*"), the location ("*school*"), and a nonmentioned object ("*door*"). Similar results were predicted when subjects heard a cleft object sentence instead of a wh- questions (e.g., "*It was the girl who the boy kissed (gap) that day at school*")—that is, with subjects looking to the girl following "*kissed.*" As predicted by both the slowed processing and syntactic impairment hypotheses, the aphasic participants as a group were impaired relative to controls in accuracy of response to comprehension probes. However, for the wh- questions, the proportion of looks to the picture of the direct object and the timing of these looks were equivalent to that for the controls, suggesting that they had successful automatic comprehension of these wh- questions—which argues against both hypotheses. Interestingly, the patients showed different fixation patterns for trials eliciting correct and incorrect responses. On correct trials, they, like controls, only looked at the moved-element picture (e.g., "*girl*"), following the verb, whereas on incorrect trials, they looked at the moved-element picture first then at the subject competitor (e.g., "*boy*"). In subsequent studies, Thompson and colleagues extended the finding for questions with wh- movement to object-extracted relative clause structures, passives, and pronominal reference resolution (Dickey & Thompson, 2009; Thompson & Choy, 2009). The results were not as clear cut as for the Dickey et al. study, in that the aphasic individuals looks to the appropriate referent were sometimes somewhat delayed relative to controls (in object relative constructions; Dickey & Thompson, 2009) and, for other constructions, there was no clear reactivation of an earlier noun phrase in either the patient or control findings (in passives, Dickey & Thompson, 2009; see also results for cleft objects, Dickey et al., 2007). Nonetheless, Thompson and colleagues argue that aphasic individuals show evidence of at least relatively rapid correct syntactic interpretation even though they may show comprehension errors for end-of-sentence probes. They suggest that comprehension deficits occur because the representations patients construct for these syntactic structures are not strong enough to inhibit competition from other sources on all trials.

While the results from Thompson and colleagues are intriguing, there are some problematic aspects of these studies. For one, the aphasic patients whom they tested showed a huge variation in their offline sentence comprehension (e.g., scoring from 0–100% correct on answers to the wh-questions in the Dickey et al., 2007, study), consistent with numerous previous studies of variation in comprehension of syntactic information in individuals with Broca's aphasia producing agrammatic speech (Berndt, Mitchum, & Haendiges, 1996; Kolk & Van Grunsven, 1985). Therefore, when separating the data into correct and incorrect trials, performance on correct trials would be dominated by those participants who performed well. Thus, it is perhaps not surprising that the results for correct sentences implied (relatively) rapid online processing. That is, those patients contributing most to the correct trial data may have no syntactic processing deficit of any kind, in which case normal online processing would follow. In contrast, performance on incorrect trials would be dominated by those who did poorly on the comprehension probes. For those sentence types in which the patients showed early looks to the appropriate NP for the incorrect trials, such may have resulted because of strategic factors (e.g., they had been looking at the subject "*girl*" when hearing "*who the girl kissed*" and the only other relevant picture to look at following the verb was the theme—that is, "*boy*"). However, they may have soon realized that they were unsure as to who was kissing whom, thus resulting in subsequent looks to the subject.

Another study of online sentence processing by Caplan and Waters (2003) also reported evidence suggestive of preserved rapid online processing in aphasic patients in conjunction with poor offline processing. This study also reported wide variation in comprehension accuracy; however, the results were broken down into those for good versus poor comprehenders, based on performance on pretests of sentence comprehension. The good comprehenders showed normal online effects in self-paced listening for both object clefts and object-extracted relative clause sentences (e.g., "*The man that the fire injured called the doctor*"). More interestingly, the poor comprehenders also showed normal online effects for cleft object sentences, even those sentences on which they made a comprehension error. Specifically, they showed longer listening times for the embedded clause verb in the cleft object than in the cleft subject sentences. In contrast, on the object-extracted relatives, they failed to show normal online effects for sentences on which they made either correct or incorrect judgments. This normal slowing for the cleft object verb may indeed reflect preserved syntactic processing for this structure. On the other hand, it may reflect confusion over how to assign subject and object roles when there are two nouns preceding the verb, as is the case in the cleft object sentences, contrasting with the cleft subject sentences (e.g., "*It was the boy who kissed the girl*") in which there is only one noun preceding the verb, which the aphasic participants might take as the subject based on a linear subject-verb-object strategy (Caplan & Futter, 1986). Caplan and Waters argue against this kind of interpretation on the grounds that the effect at the verb was of similar magnitude for patients and controls, but it is hard to know what size of effect should be expected from confusion about grammatical role assignment.

Independence and Interactions of Syntax and Semantics

In contrast to the early emphasis on purely syntactic factors in sentence parsing, more recent linguistic and psycholinguistic research has uncovered the importance of lexical and semantic factors. For example, Spivey-Knowlton and Sedivy (1995) showed that preferences for attachment of a prepositional phrase to a verb or to a noun (as in the ambiguous "*He saw the girl with the binoculars*") depended on whether the verb was a perception verb (*saw*) or an action verb (e.g., *hit*). Later findings indicated that lexical-semantic and even discourse-level semantics influence initial parsing decisions (Boland, 1997; Kim & Osterhout, 2005; Kuperberg, 2007; Kuperberg, Caplan, Sitnikova, Eddy, & Holcomb, 2006; MacDonald, Pearlmutter, & Seidenberg, 1994; Trueswell & Tanenhaus, 1994; Trueswell, Tanenhaus, & Garnsey, 1994; Van Berkum, Brown, & Hagoort, 1999). For example, consider sentences beginning with "*The evidence examined . . .*" versus "*The woman examined . . .*" In both cases, *examined* could be either the main verb or part of a reduced relative clause construction (e.g., "*The evidence examined by the lawyer . . .*" or "*The woman examined by the lawyer . . .*"). Trueswell and colleagues (1994) found that both the likelihood of the initial noun as an agent and its likelihood as a theme of the verb influenced whether initial parsing decisions favored the main verb versus reduced relative interpretation of the verb. Thus, in these examples, *examined* would be more likely to be given the reduced relative interpretation when "*evidence*" is the head noun compared to when "*woman*" is the head noun, since "*evidence*" is unlikely as an agent of *examine*.

The emerging consensus is that syntactic and semantic systems generate constraints independently but that many constraints (syntactic, lexical, semantic, and discourse) act simultaneously to determine initial sentence interpretation. These findings on the influence of nonsyntactic factors on syntactic parsing do not rule out the possibility that *knowledge* of general syntactic constraints is represented autonomously from lexically specific syntactic information and semantic information. However, they do indicate that during sentence processing, syntactically based rules do not play some overriding role that is unaffected by other sources of information.

Independence of Syntax and Semantics

Preserved Syntax and Disrupted Semantics

Whereas syntactic and semantic processing work together to determine sentence comprehension, evidence from neuropsychological studies shows that semantic and syntactic information may be represented independently. Evidence for selective preservation of syntax in the presence of semantic disruptions comes from a number of studies of patients with Alzheimer's dementia or progressive aphasia (Breedin & Saffran, 1999; Hodges, Patterson, & Tyler, 1994; Kempler, Curtiss, & Jackson, 1987; Schwartz & Chawluk, 1990; Schwartz, Marin, & Saffran, 1979). One example of this dissociation comes from a study by Hodges and colleagues (1994) of patient PP, a semantic dementia case who showed impaired performance on a variety of semantic tasks, including picture naming, picture-word matching, and attribute judgments. PP's syntactic abilities were assessed in a word monitoring task developed by Marslen-Wilson and Tyler (1980), which has been used extensively in studies of healthy subjects and brain-damaged patients (Grossman, Rhee, & Moore, 2005; Karmiloff-Smith et al., 1998; Marslen-Wilson & Tyler, 1980; Peelle, Cooke, Moore, Vesely, & Grossman, 2007; Tyler, 1992; Tyler, Moss, Patterson, & Hodges, 1997; Tyler et al., 2010). In this paradigm, subjects hear a target word followed by a sentence and are asked to respond as soon as they hear the target word in the sentence. A number of studies have demonstrated that subjects' times to detect the target words depend on the semantic and syntactic well-formedness of the sentence materials. Healthy control subjects are faster to detect target words in a grammatically well-formed sentence than in a sentence with a grammatical or semantic error(s) preceding the target word (Grossman et al., 2005; Marslen-Wilson & Tyler, 1980). In Hodges and colleagues' study, patient PP's times to detect a target word were faster for grammatically well-formed sentences compared to sentences with scrambled word order, indicating a sensitivity to grammatical structure. However, unlike normal subjects, PP showed no such reaction time advantage for semantically and grammatically well-formed prose relative to grammatically well-formed but semantically anomalous prose; that is, she failed to benefit from semantic meaningfulness. This pattern of findings, in which there is an effect of grammatical structure but not of meaningfulness, suggests that PP's deficit selectively affected her ability to process semantic information during sentence comprehension while sparing her ability to process syntax.

The evidence from Hodges and colleagues indicates that patients with severe semantic deficits (as for PP with semantic dementia) may be able to access the syntactic properties of individual words (e.g., word class) and may be able to process phrase structure. Work by Breedin and Saffran (1999) further suggests that such patients can also carry out thematic role assignments based on sentence structures and verb argument structure. They used modified versions of standard sentence-picture matching tasks in which patients saw a picture of two animals involved in some semantically reversible action (e.g., "*The lion was chased by the tiger*"), then heard a sentence describing the action and were asked to point to one of the animals in the sentence (e.g., "*Show me lion*"). Patients in these studies showed a preserved ability to indicate the correct animal when the sentence correctly described the action, but consistently chose the wrong animal on all trials when the sentence reversed the roles of the animals. For example, when hearing the stimulus "*The tiger was chased by the lion. Show me lion*" paired with a picture of a tiger chasing a lion, the patient chose the tiger. Thus, these patients were not making their choices based on lexical-semantics, but instead based on the thematic role that the named entity played in the sentence. In this sentence, "*lion*" is the grammatical object of the *by* phrase, but plays the thematic role of agent. The patient chose the entity in the picture that appeared to be the agent of the verb. This ability to determine grammatical and thematic roles for noun entities was demonstrated for complex sentence structures, including passive, subject cleft, and object cleft sentences. These results provide a dramatic demonstration that some patients with severe semantic deficits can process grammatical structure, including mapping of grammatical structure onto thematic roles, even when the semantics of single words *are* severely disrupted.

Preserved Semantics and Disrupted Syntax

Other studies reported dissociations in the opposite direction—that is, with patients showing preserved semantic processing but impaired syntactic processing (Ostrin & Tyler, 1995). Ostrin and Tyler (1995) reported a case (JG) who showed a marked disruption of all syntactic abilities together with relatively preserved lexical-semantic abilities. In a standard sentence-picture matching paradigm, JG showed an asyntactic comprehension pattern with poor performance when the distracter picture depicted a reversal of agent and object, but good performance when the distracter picture included a lexical substitution. Unlike the patients reported in Linebarger et al. (1983), he performed poorly on a grammaticality judgment task. In online word and sentence processing tasks, he also showed a dissociation between disrupted syntactic and preserved semantic processing. In a series of word-monitoring tasks involving the processing of words in sentence contexts, JG was insensitive to a variety of grammatical violations—violations of subcategorization frame, violations of inflectional and derivational morphology, and, in a previous study (Tyler, 1992), violations of word order. In a later study using a lexical decision task, JG failed to show normal morphological priming effects for regular past tense words (e.g., jumped—jump), though he showed semantic priming (Marslen-Wilson & Tyler, 1997). These cases thus showed the reverse pattern as the case reported by Hodges and colleagues (1994).

Interactions between Syntax and Semantics

Although the neuropsychological findings indicate that at least some aspects of semantic and syntactic information are represented independently, findings from healthy subjects indicate that during sentence comprehension semantics and syntax interact, as discussed earlier (Boland, 1997; Hagoort, 2003; MacDonald et al., 1994; Spivey & Tanenhaus, 1998; Trueswell & Tanenhaus, 1994). Some models of syntactic parsing, however, continue to assume a predominant role for syntactic information, and assume that such interaction only occurs when the syntax is ambiguous (Boland, 1997; Spivey & Tanenhaus, 1998). A number of recent findings indicate, however, that semantic factors can override syntactic information even when there is no ambiguity. For instance, Ferreira, Bailey, and Ferraro (2002) showed that healthy young subjects judged simple unambiguous passive sentences like "*The dog was bitten by the man*" as semantically plausible 25% of the time, though they rarely made such a mistake for an active version ("*The man bit the dog*"). Also, Van Dyke (2007) showed that, for syntactically unambiguous sentences, an embedded clause noun phrase (which could not be the subject of the main clause verb) caused interference in determining the subject of the main clause verb when the noun phrase was semantically plausible as the subject. For instance for the sentence, "*The resident who was living near the dangerous neighbor/warehouse complained about the rent*," comprehenders showed greater interference in terms of longer reaction times and more errors in determining the main clause subject (i.e., "*resident*") when the embedded clause subject was "*neighbor*" compared to "*warehouse*," even though there is no syntactic ambiguity regarding which noun phrase is the main clause subject. Thus, these findings suggest that syntax does not always play a predominant role in determining sentence interpretation (see also findings from event-related potentials leading to the same conclusions; Kim & Osterout, 2005; Kuperberg, 2007).

Consistent with the assumptions of interactive models, Saffran, Schwartz, and Linebarger (1998) reported that aphasic individuals with asyntactic comprehension patterns on sentence-picture matching tasks showed an exaggerated effect of semantic constraints on thematic role mapping in a sentence anomaly task. Two types of sentences were used: (1) verb constrained and

(2) proposition based. In the verb-constrained sentences, one of the nouns was plausible as a filler of only one thematic role of the verb, but the other noun was plausible in either role. For example, in the implausible sentence "*The cat barked at the puppy,*" a puppy can bark or be barked at, but a cat can only be barked at. In the proposition-based sentences, both nouns could fill either role; however, for the implausible versions, the overall proposition was implausible. For example, in the implausible sentence "*The insect ate the robin,*" both robins and insects can eat and be eaten, but it is implausible for something as small as an insect to eat a robin. Normal controls were less accurate at detecting implausible sentences in the verb-constrained relative to the proposition-based condition (4.7% errors vs. 1.3% errors, respectively), reflecting some tendency to interpret the implausible verb-constrained sentences by assigning nouns to their most semantically plausible slot, even though the syntax indicated otherwise. The patients showed an exaggeration of this disparity between the verb-constrained and proposition-based conditions (45.7% errors vs. 22.9% errors, respectively), reflecting a large effect of thematic role plausibility on assignment of nouns to roles. Thus, for even a simple active sentence such as "*The deer shot the hunter*" the patients often said that the sentence was plausible, presumably because role assignments had been made on the basis of semantic constraints rather than on the basis of syntactic structure of the sentence. However, their relatively preserved performance on the proposition-based sentences indicates that these patients were not completely insensitive to syntactic structure. The results imply a weakened, though not totally disrupted, influence of syntactic structure and a stronger role of semantic influences on sentence comprehension, supporting a mapping deficit explanation for these patients.

Other evidence of an interaction between semantic and syntactic influences comes from Tyler's (1989) word monitoring studies of an agrammatic aphasic patient, DE, who had shown evidence in a previous study of difficulty in structuring prose materials syntactically (Tyler, 1985). Tyler's (1989) study showed that DE was sensitive to local syntactic violations (e.g., "*slow very kitchen*") in sentences that were otherwise well formed syntactically, but semantically anomalous. However, for meaningful prose sentences, the patient's sensitivity to the local syntactic violations disappeared. Tyler concluded that for meaningful materials the patient's analysis focused on the use of word meaning and pragmatic inference to construct an interpretation of the sentence and made little use of at least some aspects of syntactic structure.

Working Memory and Sentence Comprehension

Aphasic patients often have very restricted verbal short-term memory (STM) spans, with spans of only one to three words, which contrast with spans of five or six words for neurally healthy individuals (De Renzi & Nichelli, 1975). Patients' restricted memory spans and the fact that syntactic deficits are graded rather than all-or-none (Kolk & Van Grunsven, 1985) have led some researchers to hypothesize that aphasic patients' comprehension deficits are not due to specific disruptions of parsing or other sentence processing mechanisms, but rather due to restrictions in working memory (WM) capacity (Grossman et al., 2005; Kolk & Van Grunsven, 1985; Miyake, Carpenter, & Just, 1994). A role for WM in sentence processing seems highly plausible as it is often the case that later parts of a sentence have to be integrated with earlier parts across some intervening material. The ubiquitous presence of long-distance syntactic dependencies (i.e., one-to-one correspondences between two syntactically bound elements at some distance from each other, e.g., subject—verb) indicates that some type of memory representation is needed for successful sentence comprehension. Accordingly, Gibson (1998) has argued that one central processing demand in sentence comprehension involves retrieving prior discourse entities in a sentence to integrate with new entities and the consequent need for the temporary maintenance of these prior entities (Gibson, 1998, 2000).

Some researchers have argued that the memory capacities tapped by standard STM or WM tasks support this kind of integration by holding partial results of earlier processing (Daneman &

Carpenter, 1980; Daneman & Hannon, 2007; Fedorenko, Gibson, & Rohde, 2006, 2007; Gordon, Hendrick, & Levine, 2002; Just & Carpenter, 1992). The role of WM in sentence comprehension, however, is a controversial topic, with researchers disagreeing as to whether WM is one general capacity or consists of separate capacities for different components, and whether any of these components plays an important role in sentence processing (Caplan, Michaud, & Hufford, 2013; Caplan & Waters, 1999; Just & Carpenter, 1992; Martin, 2005, 2006; Martin & He, 2004; Martin & Romani, 1994; Martin, Shelton, & Yaffee, 1994). Below we outline research on the role of different components of WM in sentence processing.

Phonological Short-Term Memory

Findings from early neuropsychological studies suggested that sentence comprehension relies heavily on the retention of phonological codes, since patients with poor phonological storage capacity (as measured by a simple span task, such as digit span) showed deficits in sentence comprehension (Baddeley & Wilson, 1988; Caramazza, Basili, Koller, & Berndt, 1981; Saffran & Marin, 1975; Vallar & Baddeley, 1984). A deficit specific to phonological codes has been seen as consistent with Baddeley's well-known working memory model, which assumes that verbal retention depends on a phonological loop dedicated to the maintenance and rehearsal of phonological representations. In a recent study of 47 acute stroke cases (i.e., testing within approximately 48 hours of the patient's ischemic event), Pettigrew and Hillis (2014) found significant correlations between STM span (combining digit and word span) and reversible sentence comprehension for a number of different sentence types, even when using a strict control for multiple comparisons. However, as Pettigrew and Hillis indicated, they did not manipulate phonological factors on their span tasks, and thus it is unclear whether the acute patients' deficits on span tasks were specifically due to phonological retention deficits or deficits in the retention of other types of information, such as semantic codes (see multiple code approaches, below).[5]

In contrast to these findings, other studies have demonstrated that patients with very restricted phonological STM span can nonetheless show excellent sentence comprehension even for complex syntactic structures (Caplan & Waters, 1999; Hanten & Martin, 2000; Martin, 1987; Martin & Romani, 1994; Waters, Caplan, & Hildebrandt, 1991). For instance, Friedmann and Gvion (2003) showed that three participants with conduction aphasia with very reduced STM span showed preserved comprehension of subject- and object-extracted relative clause structures, with performance unaffected by the distance between the gap and the filler (see Figure 16.1 for results). Interestingly, these same patients were very impaired in reinterpreting the meaning of an ambiguous word, with the impairment increasing with distance between the ambiguous word and the disambiguating information. Thus, they concluded that retrieval of semantic and syntactic information, required in understanding the relative clause structures, did not rely on phonological storage whereas retrieval of a lexical representation did. Recently, Caplan et al. (2013) provided further evidence against a role for phonological storage, reporting an absence of a correlation between typical phonological effects on memory span (i.e., phonological similarity and word length effects) and sentence comprehension performance for 61 aphasic patients. Thus, there appears to be a broad consensus that phonological storage is not crucial for sentence interpretation (see Caplan et al., 2013, for a review).

General Working Memory Capacity

In contrast to claims about the role of a specialized phonological store, some researchers have claimed that there is a general WM capacity common to all kinds of verbal tasks, including sentence comprehension (Daneman & Carpenter, 1980; Daneman & Hannon, 2007; Fedorenko

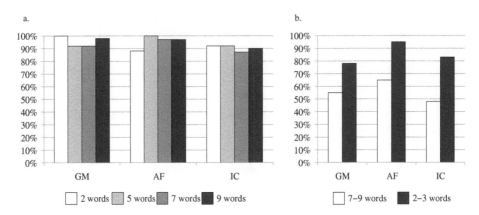

Figure 16.1 In experiment 1 (a), Friedmann and Gvion (2003) manipulated the distance between the antecedent and the gap by adding adjunct prepositional phrases and adjectives following the noun (2, 5, 7, or 9 words). Three participants with conduction aphasia showed a high level of performance on both subject and object-extracted relative clauses and showed no influence of the number of intervening words. In experiment 2 (b), Friedmann and Gvion used sentences with a temporary lexical ambiguity that later was disambiguated to the less dominant meaning, and thus required the reactivation of the original word in order to reaccess all meanings for reanalysis. For these sentences, the patients showed a large effect of the distance between the ambiguous word and the disambiguating information (2–3 words or 7–9 words), with very poor performance for the long-distance disambiguation.

et al., 2006, 2007; Gordon et al., 2002; Just & Carpenter, 1992; King & Just, 1991). In the Just and Carpenter (1992) view, this capacity is used both for carrying out language processes and storing the results of these processes (e.g., access to and storage of word meanings and thematic role assignments). Studies relating general WM capacity and comprehension have typically used a complex span task, such as reading span (Daneman & Carpenter, 1980) and operation span (Turner & Engle, 1989) to measure individuals' WM capacity. Different from simple span tasks, in which subjects passively repeat back a list of random digits/letters/words, complex span tasks impose simultaneous processing (e.g., reading a sentence aloud in the reading span task and solving a math equation in the operation task) and storage demands (e.g., actively maintaining the to-be-remembered information). Some have claimed the WM capacity tapped by complex span measures predicts an individual's performance in sentence comprehension, especially when the sentence is complex or there is an external memory load (Daneman & Carpenter, 1980; Daneman & Hannon, 2007; Fedorenko et al., 2006, 2007; Just & Carpenter, 1992). However, in a review and critique of the literature, Caplan and Waters (1999; see also Evans, Caplan, & Waters, 2011) argued that there was little evidence of a relation between "online" syntactic comprehension and WM capacity as measured by either simple or complex span tasks for either healthy individuals or brain-damaged patients. In contrast, however, they noted a relation between "offline" sentence processing (e.g., answering probe questions following the sentences) and standard WM tests. In the recent study of 61 aphasic patients, which, as mentioned earlier, failed to show a relation between phonological storage and comprehension, Caplan, Michaud, and Hufford (2013) did find a relation between span measures and sentence comprehension for end-of-sentence measures of comprehension (e.g., sentence-picture matching accuracy), but did not find such a relation for online measures (i.e., self-paced reading times). Effects of WM specifically on syntactic processing were assessed by correlating performance on span measures with the difference in performance on syntactically complex (e.g., object clefts) versus baseline sentences (e.g., subject clefts). Such correlations were only obtained for a few sentence types on certain tasks. Moreover, as they acknowledged, some of the effects may have been artifactual—for example, resulting from ceiling or floor effects. Thus, as they suggest, it seems more plausible that the correlations between span and overall sentence comprehension (combining across baseline and complex structures) resulted from task factors, like checking a sentence against two closely related pictures or refreshing a sentence in mind, while acting out the action, rather than to playing a critical role in online syntactic processing. Thus, Caplan et al. (2013) suggested that these results strengthened Caplan and Waters' (1999) claim that the online syntactic processing is supported by a specialized verbal WM system that cannot be tapped by standard simple or complex span tasks, while the use of the products of online comprehension processes to perform a task is supported by a general verbal WM system shared with other verbal tasks. In a recent review, Caplan and Waters (2013) further postulated that the specialized verbal WM system supporting online parsing and interpretation is a form of procedural memory, which is an aspect of long-term working memory (Caplan et al., 2013; Caplan & Waters, 2013).

Multiple Codes in Verbal Short-Term Memory

A different specialized capacity approach is the multiple-components model put forward by Martin and colleagues (Hamilton, Martin, & Burton, 2009; Martin, 2005; Martin & He, 2004; Martin & Romani, 1994; Martin, Tan, & Van Dyke, 2011). These authors have provided evidence that some types of STM deficits tapped by span tasks do cause sentence comprehension difficulties for patients—specifically, deficits in retaining lexical-semantic information rather than in retaining phonological information. In this multiple-components approach, Martin and colleagues argued that verbal working memory should be broken down into three separate capacities for the retention of phonological, semantic, and syntactic information. Supporting evidence has been obtained from both neuropsychological (Martin & He, 2004; Martin & Romani, 1994) and neuroimaging studies (Hamilton, Martin, & Burton, 2009; Martin, Wu, Freedman, Jackson, & Lesch, 2003). In distinguishing between patients with phonological and semantic STM deficits, performance was evaluated on a variety of STM tasks (e.g., Martin, Shelton, & Yaffee, 1994). Patients with a phonological STM deficit failed to show standard phonological effects on memory span (e.g., phonological similarity and word length) and did better with word than nonword lists, whereas patients with a semantic STM deficit showed phonological effects and failed to show the normal advantage for words over nonwords. Also, patients with a phonological STM deficit performed better on a probe recognition task tapping semantic retention (category probe) than a task tapping phonological retention (rhyme probe task), whereas patients with a semantic STM deficit showed the reverse pattern. On the rhyme probe task, patients judged whether a probe word rhymed with any word in a preceding list (e.g., *pain-book*, probe: *game*). On the category probe task, patients judged whether a probe word was in the same category as any of the list items (e.g., *snow-dress*, probe: *jacket*). Importantly, the patients showing these STM deficits did not show deficits in phonological or semantic processing of individual words.

Patients with difficulty retaining lexical-semantic information have difficulty comprehending sentences in which the integration of individual word meanings into propositional representations is delayed (Martin & He, 2004; Martin & Romani, 1994). For instance, in a sentence with several prenominal adjectives, such as "*the rusty old red pail*," the integration of the first adjective with the noun ("*rusty*" with "*pail*") is delayed in comparison to a sentence in which the adjectives appear postnominally (e.g., "*The pail was old, red, and rusty . . .*"). Thus, the meaning of the adjectives in the prenominal case must be maintained in a lexical-semantic form for some time prior to integration. Similar arguments can be made for sentences in which several nouns precede (e.g., "*The vase, the mirror, and the platter cracked*") or follow a verb (e.g., "*The movers cracked the platter, the mirror, and the vase*"). When the nouns precede the verb, their assignment to thematic roles with respect to the verb is delayed in comparison to when the nouns appear after the verb. Martin and Romani (1994) and Martin and He (2004) reported that two patients whose span deficits appeared to be due to lexical-semantic retention deficits (ML and AB) scored near chance on a sentence anomaly task when two or three adjectives preceded a noun or two or three nouns preceded the verb, but performed at a much higher level when the adjectives followed the noun or the nouns followed the verb. (See Table 16.2 for example stimuli and Figure 16.2 for results.) A patient with a phonological retention deficit (EA) did not show this pattern, instead showing a pattern within the range of controls for the before/after manipulation.

Table 16.2 Examples of Distance 1 and Distance 3 Sentences from Anomaly Judgment Task of Martin & Romani (1994)

	Sensible	*Anomalous*
Distance 1 *Adj-N* Before After	The rusty pail was lying on the beach. The pail was rusty but she took it to the beach anyway.	The rusty swimsuit was lying on the beach. The swimsuit was rusty by she took it to the beach anyway.
N-V Before After	The platter cracked during the move. The movers cracked the platter.	The cloth cracked during the move. The movers cracked the cloth.
Distance 3 *Adj-N* Before	The rusty, old, red pail was lying on the beach.	The rusty, old, red swimsuit was lying on the beach.
After	The pail was old, red, and rusty but she took it to the beach anyway.	The swimsuit was old, red, and rusty by she took it to the beach anyway.
N-V Before	The platter, the vase, and the mirror cracked during the move.	The cloth, the vase, and the mirror cracked during the move.
After	The movers cracked the vase, the mirror, and the platter.	The movers cracked the vase, the mirror, and the cloth.

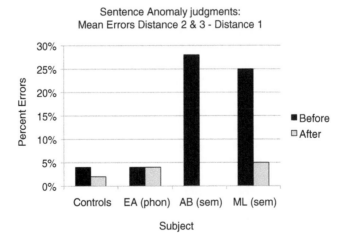

Figure 16.2 Difference in percent errors for [(mean of distance 2 and 3) – distance 1] on sentence anomaly judgments. "After" condition allows for immediate integration, whereas "before" condition involves delayed integration. Patients AB and ML show a semantic STM deficit, whereas patient EA shows a phonological STM deficit.

Regarding the dissociation between syntactic STM capacity and other systems, an interesting contrast between retention of lexical-semantic information and syntactic information during sentence processing was uncovered (Martin & Romani, 1994). The patients with the semantic retention deficits were unaffected by the distance between two words that signaled that a sentence was ungrammatical (e.g., near condition: "*Susan didn't leave and neither was Mary*" vs. far condition: "*Susan didn't leave, despite many hints from her tired hosts, and neither was Mary*"). In contrast, one patient (MW), who showed preserved semantic and phonological retention on STM tasks and who had not shown the interaction between before/after and distance in the sentence anomaly task, did perform significantly worse in the far than near condition in the grammaticality judgments (see Table 16.3.for results). Thus, these findings suggest a further dissociation between the capacities involved in retaining syntactic information and those involved in retaining lexical-semantic and phonological information.

Martin et al. (2003) found neuroimaging evidence supporting the distinction between phonological and semantic STM using the rhyme probe task and a synonym probe task (similar to the category probe task but requiring subjects to judge whether a probe word was a synonym of any list word). They found that an area in the inferior parietal lobe showed greater activation in a rhyme probe task than in a synonym probe task, while the semantic STM manipulation caused greater activation in a left frontal region. More recently, Hamilton, Martin, and Burton (2009) modified the semantic anomaly judgment paradigm described above (using adjectives before or after a noun; Martin & He, 2004) and found greater activation in the left inferior frontal gyrus (LIFG) and middle frontal gyri for the phrases with the adjectives before compared to after the noun. Importantly, brain areas previously found to support phonological STM were not sensitive to this contrast.

The role of semantic versus phonological STM capacity in comprehension has recently been investigated for a wider range of sentence structures, where the emphasis has been on potential interference in memory rather than the load imposed by sentences due to delayed integration. Specifically, interference in integrating a verb with is subject was investigated for sentences in which potentially interfering material intervened between the subject and verb (Tan, Martin, & Van Dyke, 2013). For example, in the sentence "*The customer who said the clerk was rude stomped out of the store*," when encountering "*stomped*," the comprehender would attempt to locate a subject for this verb that is semantically plausible and that is a syntactic subject. The intervening noun phrase "*clerk*" provides both semantic and syntactic interference, since "*clerk*" is semantically plausible as the agent of the verb and is also a syntactic subject. Prior studies with healthy young

Table 16.3 Comparison of Semantic Anomaly and Grammaticality Judgments for Patients AB, ML, and MW (Percent Correct)

	Anomaly Judgments (Distances 2 and 3)		
	Before	*After*	*Difference*
AB (semantic)	61	83	22 ($p < .01$)
ML (semantic)	62	79	17 ($p < .01$)
MW (normal span)	75	74	−1 (ns)
	Memory-stressed grammaticality judgments		
	Intervening	*ATB*	*Difference*
AB (semantic)	87	91	4 (ns)
ML (semantic)	88	91	3 (ns)
MW (normal span)	77	85	8 ($p < .01$)

subject have shown that both semantic and syntactic interference occur as revealed by longer online processing times and greater comprehension errors for sentence with high relative to low interference (Lewis, Vasishth, & Van Dyke, 2006; Van Dyke, 2007; Van Dyke & Lewis, 2003; Van Dyke & McElree, 2011).

Tan, Martin, and Van Dyke (2013) used sentences like those below (based on Van Dyke, 2007) to investigate patients' sensitivity to semantic and syntactic interference and the relation of STM abilities to their ability to resolve this interference. Semantic interference was manipulated by varying whether the intervening noun was semantically plausible as the agent of the verb (e.g., *neighbor* vs. *warehouse*). Syntactic interference was manipulated by varying whether the embedded noun phrase was a syntactic subject or the object of a preposition.

1. Low semantic/low syntactic: "*The resident who was living near the dangerous warehouse complained about the rent.*"
2. High semantic/low syntactic: "*The resident who was living near the dangerous neighbor complained about the rent.*"
3. Low semantic/high syntactic: "*The resident who thought the warehouse was dangerous complained about the rent.*"
4. High semantic/high syntactic: "*The resident who thought the neighbor was dangerous complained about the rent.*"

Tan et al. (2013) demonstrated exaggerated semantic and syntactic interference for 10 aphasic patients on comprehension accuracy relative to controls (see Figure 16.3 for results). Moreover, the degree of semantic interference was related to patients' semantic STM capacity (as measured by category probe), with lower capacity related to greater interference, but was unrelated to their phonological STM capacity (as measured by rhyme probe). The degree of syntactic interference was unrelated to both semantic and phonological STM capacity. Thus, these findings are consistent with the idea that there are separable phonological, semantic, and syntactic capacities, with only the latter two playing an important role in sentence comprehension.

Alternative Accounts of the Role of General Cognitive Capacities in Sentence Comprehension and Their Application to Comprehension Deficits

Recently, some researchers have shifted the emphasis away from the role of WM storage capacity towards the role of other general cognitive capacities in sentence comprehension. One motivation for this shift is the rise of WM models that eschew the notion of buffers and instead argue that WM consists of the activated portion of long-term memory—termed embedded processes models (Cowan, 1999). According to the embedded processes view, among activated long-term representations, only an extremely limited number of items are maintained in a highly accessible state (i.e., in the focus of attention). The capacity of the focus of attention has been argued by some to encompass only one or two chunks of information (McElree, 2006; Lewis, 1996; though see Cowan, who argues for a capacity of three to four chunks), which should be within the capacity of most individuals, including many aphasic patients. According to researchers taking the embedded processes approach, information outside the focus must be retrieved through the use of retrieval cues that are matched in parallel to memory representations (Cowan, 1999; Cowan et al., 2005; McElree, 2006). Interference occurs when these cues provide a partial match to inappropriate information. For example, in a short-term recognition paradigm in which subjects judge whether a probe word occurred in the immediately preceding list, the probe might share phonological features with an item in a preceding list, causing difficulty in rejecting that item as appearing on the current list (Barde, Schwartz, Chrysikou, & Thompson-Schill, 2010; Hamilton & Martin, 2007).

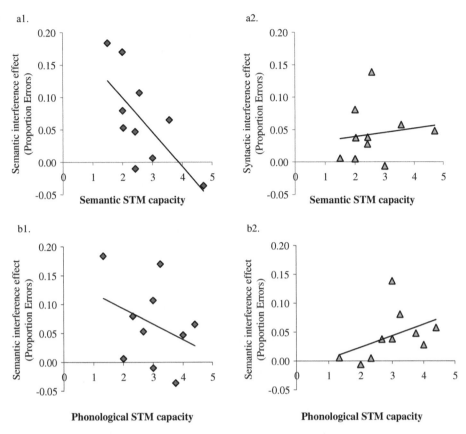

Figure 16.3 Semantic and syntactic interference effects for statement verification (Tan, Martin, & Van Dyke, 2013). a1 & a2: Semantic and syntactic interference in percent errors relative to semantic STM capacity, respectively. b1 & b2: Semantic and syntactic interference effects in percent errors relative to phonological STM capacity, respectively. After partialling out vocabulary (as measured by the Peabody Picture Vocabulary Test), only the correlation between the magnitude of semantic interference effect and semantic STM capacity was significant (as shown in a1).

Researchers taking the embedded processes approach to sentence comprehension (Lewis & Vasishth, 2005; Lewis et al., 2006; Van Dyke, 2007; Van Dyke & Lewis, 2003; Van Dyke & McElree, 2006, 2011) call into question the memory capacity–based explanations of variation in sentence comprehension ability and have suggested instead that the observed correlations between WM capacity and sentence comprehension performance actually derive from other factors, such as executive control ability (especially, the ability to resolve interference), word knowledge, and reading skills, which affect both the capacity measures and the sentence measures (Acheson, Wells, & MacDonald, 2008; MacDonald & Christiansen, 2002; Novick, Trueswell, & Thompson-Schill, 2005; Perfetti, 2007; Reali & Christiansen, 2007; Van Dyke & Johns, 2012; Wells, Christiansen, Race, Acheson, & MacDonald, 2009).

Executive Control and Comprehension

A growing number of studies with both neurally healthy and brain-damaged patients support a role of executive control abilities in sentence comprehension (Hamilton & Martin, 2007; Martin,

Vuong, & Hull, 2007; Novick, Kan, Trueswell, & Thompson-Schill, 2009; Novick et al., 2005; Vuong & Martin, 2011, 2014). For instance, Vuong and Martin (2014) found that healthy young subjects' ability to recover from a syntactic garden path (e.g., "*While the man coached the woman attended the party . . .*") related to their general executive control abilities as measured by the Stroop task. In a review of aphasic sentence processing deficits, Novick, Trueswell, and Thompson-Schill (2005) proposed a link between executive control abilities and conflict resolution during sentence comprehension and hypothesized that the LIFG is crucial for conflict resolution for both nonparsing tasks (like the Stroop task) as well as for parsing. They make the strong claim that deficits in sentence processing following damage to Broca's area (which is part of the LIFG), actually derive from deficits in conflict resolution. Novick and colleagues (2009) provided evidence for their hypothesis in a case study of patient with restricted damage to LIFG. This patient (IG) showed an inflated error rate in tasks that measured resistance to proactive interference and had difficulty in language production and comprehension tasks when there was semantic, conceptual, or syntactic competition, such as in naming pictures with low name agreement (e.g., couch/sofa/loveseat) or in carrying out spoken instructions that required subjects to revise their early interpretation because of temporary ambiguity (e.g. "*Put the apple on the napkin into the box*," where the prepositional phrase "*on the napkin*" is initially ambiguous between being a modifier or a goal indicating where to put the apple). Vuong and Martin (2011) have also reported that patients with LIFG damage who demonstrated attentional control deficits on nonsentence tasks had difficulty in resolving lexical ambiguities during sentence processing (e.g., "*He drank the port*"). Several studies on Parkinson's disease (PD) patients have also demonstrated a correlation between patients' deficits in sentence processing and their deficits in executive control (Colman, Koerts, Stowe, Leenders, & Bastiaanse, 2011; Hochstadt, 2009; Hochstadt, Nakano, Lieberman, & Friedman, 2006).

Language Knowledge Accounts

Another account of individual differences in sentence comprehension, namely the experience-based account, claims that the distinction commonly drawn between language processing ability and verbal WM capacity is artificial because all these tasks are just different measures of language processing skills (MacDonald & Christiansen, 2002). MacDonald et al. (2002) argued that skilled sentence comprehension is affected by variation in subjects' exposure to language and some biological differences that affect processing accuracy. Supporting evidence includes findings showing that comprehension success is related to experience-based factors, such as individuals' receptive vocabulary size or phonological decoding ability (Perfetti, 2007; Van Dyke & Johns, 2012), which may reflect variation in individuals' exposure to spoken and written words, and expertise in complex syntactic structures and knowledge of probabilistic constraints that govern online language comprehension (MacDonald & Christiansen, 2002; Reali & Christiansen, 2007; Wells et al., 2009). Moreover, Van Dyke and Johns (2012) showed that working memory did not contribute to the prediction of comprehension ability when controlling for IQ, whereas vocabulary size did. According to this view, then, variation in patients' comprehension deficits would be attributed to the degree of disruption of lexical, semantic, and syntactic knowledge, rather than to variation in working memory or executive control abilities. While the contributions of knowledge deficits are no doubt important, without a specific model it is hard to see how such an approach can explain the relation between, for example, semantic STM capacity and sentence comprehension for patients who do not have semantic knowledge deficits, nor the relation between executive control abilities as measured by Stroop and other nonlanguage tasks and the ability to revise sentence interpretations. Moreover, IQ and WM measures are correlated and many have claimed that a major component of IQ is WM capacity (Engle et al., 1999). Thus, controlling for IQ would have reduced the contribution of WM to prediction, since the overlap between IQ and WM would not be reflected in the WM weight.

Summary and Directions for Future Research

Findings in the 1970s and 1980s showing sentence comprehension deficits in aphasic patients with good single word comprehension were first interpreted as due to a complete disruption of syntactic parsing, which seemed consonant with theories at the time postulating a deterministic set of parsing rules. Since that time, our notions of sentence comprehension mechanisms have been elaborated substantially in terms of the factors affecting comprehension success. Findings from aphasia support these elaborated views, as a wide range of studies have demonstrated that sentence comprehension deficits may derive from many sources, including disruptions in the representation of verbs (e.g., Berndt, Mitchum, Haendiges, & Sandson, 1997; Breedin & Martin, 1996; Miozzo, Rawlins, & Rapp, 2014; Wu, Waller, & Chatterjee, 2007), difficulties in mapping grammatical roles to thematic roles (e.g., Linebarger et al., 1983; Linebarger, Schwartz, Romania, Kohn, & Stephens, 2000), and disruptions of the cognitive mechanisms involved in working memory (e.g., Caplan & Waters, 1999; Grossman et al., 2005; Martin & He, 2004; Martin & Romani, 1994; Pettigrew & Hillis, 2014) and interference resolution (e.g., Hamilton & Martin, 2007; Novick, Pan, Trueswell, & Thompson-Schill, 2009; Vuong & Martin, 2011).

Even though many factors affect comprehension, most current sentence processing theories maintain the assumption of separable syntactic parsing and semantic processing components, but assume that both processes proceed in parallel and interact in determining sentence meaning. A number of patient studies support the contention that there are separable semantic and syntactic components as some patients show a pattern of disrupted syntactic processing but preserved semantic processing or the reverse. However, disruptions in syntactic processing are rarely total. Patients typically display a graded breakdown in performance, with poorer performance on more complex constructions. Even for the most complex constructions, patients may show above-chance performance on comprehension tasks. Moreover, their success at carrying out syntactic computations may vary depending on the extent to which parsing decisions are supported or contradicted by semantic constraints. These results suggest that the output of syntactic parsing mechanisms may be weakened rather than totally disrupted. This weakening has the greatest effect on structures that are less common.

To the extent that there are different mental components involved in different parsing operations localized in different neural tissue, one might expect to see patients with deficits in specific syntactic parsing procedures and not others. Caplan and Hildebrandt (1988) presented some evidence that highly specific disruptions might be observed, though it is unclear whether such disruptions are consistent across tasks. Recently, Miozzo, Rawlins, and Rapp (2014) obtained some evidence for a consistent deficit in specific syntactic processing mechanisms underlying sentence comprehension where thematic roles were assigned by verbs versus nonverbal constructions.

Considerable research has been directed toward the role of general cognitive mechanism in sentence comprehension deficits—specifically focusing on the role of working memory and executive control (e.g., Caplan & Waters, 1999; Caplan et al., 2013; Martin & He, 2004; Novick, et al., 2009). With regard to working memory, the neuropsychological evidence supports the conclusion that the capacity involved in lexical-semantic retention plays a critical role in sentence comprehension when integration of word meanings is delayed, and syntactic STM is crucial when maintaining unintegrated syntactic information is required. There is greater controversy on whether phonological retention capacity plays a role in online sentence comprehension, or whether its role is restricted to postcomprehension processes involved in relating a meaning to an action.

Recent embedded processes and experience-based approaches to comprehension, which provide a challenge to any type of working memory account, have yet to be investigated in any depth with patient populations. With respect to executive control, a number of studies have demonstrated an important role for conflict resolution abilities in the comprehension of sentences with lexical or syntactic ambiguities, both in studies with healthy participants and aphasic patients.

Has neuropsychological research lived up to its early promise in contributing to our under-standing of sentence comprehension processes? The topics of interest for normal and impaired populations differed for many years—with studies with healthy individuals focusing on the relative independence and timing of syntactic and semantic factors in resolving syntactic ambiguities (e.g., Spivey & Tanenhaus, 1998), and studies of brain-damaged patients concentrating on the difficulty of various syntactic structures (e.g., Caplan & Hildebrandt, 1988). Recently, a greater convergence on topics of interest has occurred, with those studying both populations investigating the role of working memory and executive control, and neuropsychological findings have been influential in focusing the debate.

Despite a prominent role for general cognitive mechanisms in sentence comprehension and sentence comprehension deficits, deficits specific to syntactic and semantic knowledge and pro-cessing should be observed that cannot be attributed to these general cognitive deficits, assuming that different brain regions support the general cognitive mechanism and the representations of syntactic and semantic knowledge (e.g., see Hagoort, 2005, for one proposal along these lines). While case studies showing specific deficits in syntactic processing have been reported, much remains to be learned about the organization of these systems and their neural basis—which might be uncovered through closer examination of specific syntactic processes. Thus, while much has been learned about sentence processing from the study of brain-damaged patients, much remains to be addressed. The findings from the patient research should provide an important set of con-straints in making progress toward a comprehensive model of sentence comprehension.

Notes

1 Regarding the linguistic terminology, relative clause (RC) is a kind of subordinate clause that typically defines or modifies a noun or noun phrase. Relative clauses usually start with the relative pronouns who, that, which, whose, etc. In subject-extracted relative clause (SRCs), e.g., "*The boy that [gap] kissed the girl had red hair*," the noun that is modified by the RC (*boy*) is also the subject of the relative clause verb (*kiss*), and is linked to a phonological empty element (often termed the "gap") in the verb's subject position. In object-extracted relative clauses (ORCs), such as "*The boy that the girl kissed [gap] had red hair*," the noun that is modified by the RC (*boy*) is the object of the relative clause verb (*kiss*), and is linked to an empty element in object position. Cleft sentence is a kind of construction in which some element in a sentence is moved from its normal position into a separate clause to put it into focus. In a subject cleft sentence, e.g., "*It is the boy that kissed the girl*," the noun that is moved (*boy*) is the subject of the subordinate clause verb (*kiss*). In an object cleft sentence, e.g., "*It is the boy that the girl kissed*," the noun that is moved (*boy*) is the object of the subordinate clause verb.

2 PRO, like a trace, is a hypothetical empty element. It differs from a trace in that no movement from a deep structure position is presumed to be involved with PRO.

3 Caplan, DeDe, & Michaud (2006) also determined the range of normal performance based on the mean proportion correct and standard deviation of the control subjects. However, inconsistent results across tasks were also obtained when the criterion for good performance was scoring within normal range and the criterion for poor performance was scoring below normal range.

4 Online effects refer to word-by-word effects that occur as a sentence is being processed. Offline effects refer to end-of-sentence effects, such as in choosing a picture to match a sentence.

5 Pettigrew and Hillis (2014) also suggested that the stronger findings of a relation between STM and com-prehension for acute than chronic cases might result because the acute stroke individuals have not had a chance to develop strategies for sentence comprehension that might be employed by chronic cases (as a result, perhaps, of treatment).

References

Acheson, D., Wells, J., & MacDonald, M. (2008). New and updated tests of print exposure and reading abilities in college students. *Behavior Research Methods, 40*, 278–289.

Baddeley, A.D., & Wilson, B. (1988). Comprehension and working memory: A single case neuropsychological study. *Journal of Memory and Language, 27*, 479–498.

Barde, L.H.F., Schwartz, M.F., Chrysikou, E.G., & Thompson-Schill, S.L. (2010). Reduced short-term memory span in aphasia and susceptibility to interference: Contribution of material-specific maintenance deficits. *Neuropsychologia, 48*, 909–920.

Berndt, R.S., & Caramazza, A. (1980). A redefinition of the syndrome of Broca's aphasia: Implications for a neuropsychological model of language. *Applied Linguistics, 1*, 225–278.

Berndt, R.S., Haendiges, A.N., Mitchum, C.C., & Sandson, J. (1997). Verb retrieval in aphasia. 2. Relationship to sentence processing. *Brain and Language, 56*, 107–137.

Berndt, R.S., Mitchum, C.C., & Haendiges, A.N. (1996). Comprehension of reversible sentences in "agrammatism": A meta-analysis. *Cognition, 58*, 289–308.

Berndt, R.S., Mitchum, C.C., Haendiges, A.N., & Sandson, J. (1997). Verb retrieval in aphasia. 1. Characterizing single word impairments. *Brain and Language, 56*, 68–106.

Boland, J.E. (1997). The relationship between syntactic and semantic processes in sentence comprehension. *Language and Cognitive Processes, 12*, 423–484.

Breedin, S.D., & Martin, R.C. (1996). Patterns of verb impairment in aphasia: An analysis of four cases. *Cognitive Neuropsychology, 13*, 51–92.

Breedin, S.D., & Saffran, E.M. (1999). Sentence processing in the face of semantic loss: A case study. *Journal of Experimental Psychology: General, 128*, 547.

Caplan, D., DeDe, G., & Michaud, J. (2006). Task-independent and task-specific syntactic deficits in aphasic comprehension. *Aphasiology, 20*, 893–920.

Caplan, D., & Futter, C. (1986). Assignment of thematic roles to nouns in sentence comprehension in an agrammatic patient. *Brain and Language, 27*, 117–134.

Caplan, D., & Hildebrandt, N. (1988). *Disorders of syntactic comprehension.* Cambridge, MA: MIT Press.

Caplan, D., Michaud, J., & Hufford, R. (2013). Short-term memory, working memory, and syntactic comprehension in aphasia. *Cognitive Neuropsychology, 30*, 77–109.

Caplan, D., & Waters, G. (2003). On-line syntactic processing in aphasia: Studies with auditory moving window presentation. *Brain and Language, 84*, 222–249.

Caplan, D., & Waters, G. (2013). Memory mechanisms supporting syntactic comprehension. *Psychonomic Bulletin & Review, 20*, 243–268.

Caplan, D., & Waters, G.S. (1999). Verbal working memory and sentence comprehension. *Behavioral and Brain Sciences, 22*, 77–94.

Caramazza, A., Basili, A.G., Koller, J.J., & Berndt, R.S. (1981). An investigation of repetition and language processing in a case of conduction aphasia. *Brain and Language, 2*, 235–271.

Caramazza, A., & Berndt, R.S. (1978). Semantic and syntactic processes in aphasia: A review of the literature. *Psychological Bulletin, 85*, 898.

Caramazza, A., & Zurif, E.B. (1976). Dissociation of algorithmic and heuristic processes in language comprehension: Evidence from aphasia. *Brain and Language, 3*, 572–582.

Chomsky, N. (1982). *Some concepts and consequences of the theory of government and binding.* Cambridge, MA: MIT Press.

Colman, K.S., Koerts, J., Stowe, L.A., Leenders, K.L., & Bastiaanse, R. (2011). Sentence comprehension and its association with executive functions in patients with Parkinson's disease. *Parkinson's Disease, 2011*, 1–15.

Cowan, N. (1999). An embedded-process model of working memory. In A. Miyake & P. Shah (Eds.), *Models of working memory* (pp. 62–101). Cambridge: Cambridge University Press.

Cowan, N., Elliott, E.M., Scott Saults, J., Morey, C.C., Mattox, S., Hismjatullina, A., & Conway, A.R. (2005). On the capacity of attention: Its estimation and its role in working memory and cognitive aptitudes. *Cognitive Psychology, 51*, 42–100.

Cupples, L., & Inglis, A.L. (1993). When task demands induce "asyntactic" comprehension: A study of sentence interpretation in aphasia. *Cognitive Neuropsychology, 10*, 201–234.

Daneman, M., & Carpenter, P.A. (1980). Individual differences in working memory and reading. *Journal of Verbal Learning and Verbal Behavior, 19*, 450–466.

Daneman, M., & Hannon, B. (2007). What do working memory span tasks like reading span really measure? In N. Osaka, R.H. Logie, & M. D'Esposito (Eds.), *The cognitive neuroscience of working memory* (pp. 21–42). Oxford, England: Oxford University Press.

De Renzi, E., & Nichelli, P. (1975). Verbal and non-verbal short-term memory impairment following hemispheric damage. *Cortex, 11*, 341–354.

Dickey, M.W., Choy, J.J., & Thompson, C.K. (2007). Real-time comprehension of wh-movement in aphasia: Evidence from eyetracking while listening. *Brain and Language, 100*, 1–22.

Dickey, M.W., & Thompson, C.K. (2009). Automatic processing of wh- and NP-movement in agrammatic aphasia: Evidence from eyetracking. *Journal of Neurolinguistics, 22*, 563–583.

Engle, R.W., Tuholski, S.W., Laughlin, J. E., & Conway, A.R.A. (1999). Working memory, short-term memory, and general fluid intelligence: A latent-variable approach. *Journal of Experimental Psychology: General, 128*, 309–331.

Evans, W.S., Caplan, D., & Waters, G. (2011). Effects of concurrent arithmetical and syntactic complexity on self-paced reaction times and eye fixations. *Psychonomic Bulletin & Review, 18*, 1203–1211.

Fedorenko, E., Gibson, E., & Rohde, D. (2006). The nature of working memory capacity in sentence comprehension: Evidence against domain-specific working memory resources. *Journal of Memory and Language, 54*, 541–553.

Fedorenko, E., Gibson, E., & Rohde, D. (2007). The nature of working memory in linguistic, arithmetic and spatial integration processes. *Journal of Memory and Language, 56*, 246–269.

Ferreira, F., Bailey, K.G.D., & Ferraro, V. (2002). Good-enough representations in language comprehension. *Current Directions in Psychological Science, 11*, 11–15.

Fodor, J.A., & Garrett, M. (1967). Some syntactic determinants of sentential complexity. *Perception & Psychophysics, 2*, 289–296.

Friedmann, N., & Gvion, A. (2003). Sentence comprehension and working memory limitation in aphasia: A dissociation between semantic-syntactic and phonological reactivation. *Brain and Language, 86*, 23–39.

Gibson, E. (1998). Linguistic complexity: Locality of syntactic dependencies. *Cognition, 68*, 1–76.

Gibson, E. (2000). The dependency locality theory: A distance-based theory of linguistic complexity. In Y. Miyashita, A. Mirantz, & W. O'Neil (Eds.), *Image, language, brain* (pp. 95–126). Cambridge, MA: MIT Press.

Gordon, P.C., Hendrick, R., & Levine, W.H. (2002). Memory-load interference in syntactic processing. *Psychological Science, 13*, 425–430.

Grodzinsky, Y. (1990). *Theoretical perspectives on language deficits.* Cambridge, MA: MIT Press.

Grodzinsky, Y., Piñango, M.M., Zurif, E., & Drai, D. (1999). The critical role of group studies in neuropsychology: Comprehension regularities in Broca's aphasia. *Brain and Language, 67*, 134–147.

Grossman, M., Rhee, J., & Moore, P. (2005). Sentence processing in frontotemporal dementia. *Cortex, 41*, 764–777.

Haarmann, H.J., & Kolk, H.H.J. (1991). Syntactic priming in Broca's aphasics: Evidence for slow activation. *Aphasiology, 5*, 247–263.

Hagoort, P. (2003). Interplay between syntax and semantics during sentence comprehension: ERP effects of combining syntactic and semantic violations. *Journal of Cognitive Neuroscience, 15*, 883–899.

Hagoort, P. (2005). On Broca, brain, and binding: A new framework. *Trends in Cognitive Sciences, 9*, 416–423.

Hamilton, A.C., & Martin, R.C. (2007). Proactive interference in a semantic short-term memory deficit: Role of semantic and phonological relatedness. *Cortex, 43*, 112–123.

Hamilton, A.C., Martin, R.C., & Burton, P.C. (2009). Converging functional magnetic resonance imaging evidence for a role of the left inferior frontal lobe in semantic retention during language comprehension. *Cognitive Neuropsychology, 26*, 685–704.

Hanten, G., & Martin, R.C. (2000). Contributions of phonological and semantic short-term memory to sentence processing: Evidence from two cases of closed head injury in children. *Journal of Memory and Language, 43*, 335–361.

Hildebrandt, N., Caplan, D., & Evans, K. (1987). The man left without a trace: A case study of aphasic processing of empty categories. *Cognitive Neuropsychology, 4*, 257–302.

Hochstadt, J. (2009). Set-shifting and the on-line processing of relative clauses in Parkinson's disease: Results from a novel eye-tracking method. *Cortex, 45*, 991–1011.

Hochstadt, J., Nakano, H., Lieberman, P., & Friedman, J. (2006). The roles of sequencing and verbal working memory in sentence comprehension deficits in Parkinson's disease. *Brain and Language, 97*, 243–257.

Hodges, J.R., Patterson, K., & Tyler, L.K. (1994). Loss of semantic memory: Implications for the modularity of mind. *Cognitive Neuropsychology, 11*, 505–542.

Jackendoff, R. (1993). *Patterns in the mind: Language and human nature.* New York: Harvester Wheatsheaf.

Just, M.A., & Carpenter, P.A. (1992). A capacity theory of comprehension: Individual differences in working memory. *Psychological Review, 99*, 122–149.

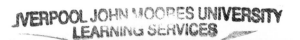
LIVERPOOL JOHN MOORES UNIVERSITY
LEARNING SERVICES

Karmiloff-Smith, A., Tyler, L.K., Voice, K., Sims, K., Udwin, O., Howlin, P., & Davies, M. (1998). Linguistic dissociations in Williams syndrome: Evaluating receptive syntax in on-line and off-line tasks. *Neuropsychologia, 36,* 343–351.

Kempler, D., Curtiss, S., & Jackson, C. (1987). Syntactic preservation in Alzheimer's disease. *Journal of Speech, Language and Hearing Research, 30,* 343.

Kim, A., & Osterhout, L. (2005). The independence of combinatory semantic processing: Evidence from event-related potentials. *Journal of Memory and Language, 52,* 205–225.

King, J., & Just, M.A. (1991). Individual differences in syntactic processing: The role of working memory. *Journal of Memory and Language, 30,* 580–602.

Kolk, H.H.J. (1995). A time-based approach to agrammatic production. *Brain and Language, 50,* 282–303.

Kolk, H.H.J., & Van Grunsven, F. (1985). Agrammatism as a variable phenomenon. *Cognitive Neuropsychology, 2,* 347–384.

Kuperberg, G.R. (2007). Neural mechanisms of language comprehension: Challenges to syntax. *Brain Research, 1146,* 23–49.

Kuperberg, G.R., Caplan, D., Sitnikova, T., Eddy, M., & Holcomb, P.J. (2006). Neural correlates of processing syntactic, semantic, and thematic relationships in sentences. *Language and Cognitive Processes, 21,* 489–530.

Lewis, R.L. (1996). Interference in short-term memory: The magical number two (or three) in sentence processing. *Journal of Psycholinguistic Research, 25,* 93–115.

Lewis, R.L., & Vasishth, S. (2005). An activation-based model of sentence processing as skilled memory retrieval. *Cognitive Science, 29,* 375–419.

Lewis, R.L., Vasishth, S., & Van Dyke, J.A. (2006). Computational principles of working memory in sentence comprehension. *Trends in Cognitive Sciences, 10,* 447–454.

Linebarger, M.C. (1995). Agrammatism as evidence about grammar. *Brain and Language, 50,* 52–91.

Linebarger, M.C., Schwartz, M.F., Romania, J.R., Kohn, S.E., & Stephens, D.L. (2000). Grammatical encoding in aphasia: Evidence from a "processing prosthesis." *Brain and Language, 75,* 416–427.

Linebarger, M.C., Schwartz, M.F., & Saffran, E.M. (1983). Sensitivity to grammatical structure in so-called agrammatic aphasics. *Cognition, 13,* 361–392.

MacDonald, M.C., & Christiansen, M.H. (2002). Reassessing working memory: Comment on Just and Carpenter (1992) and Waters and Caplan (1996). *Psychological Review, 109,* 35–54.

MacDonald, M.C., Pearlmutter, N.J., & Seidenberg, M.S. (1994). The lexical nature of syntactic ambiguity resolution. *Psychological Review, 101,* 676.

Marslen-Wilson, W., & Tyler, L.K. (1980). The temporal structure of spoken language understanding. *Cognition, 8,* 1–71.

Marslen-Wilson, W.D., & Tyler, L.K. (1997). Dissociating types of mental computation. *Nature, 387,* 592–593.

Martin, R.C. (1987). Articulatory and phonological deficits in short-term memory and their relation to syntactic processing. *Brain and Language, 32,* 159–192.

Martin, R.C. (2005). Components of short-term memory and their relation to language processing: Evidence from neuropsychology and neuroimaging. *Current Directions in Psychological Science, 14,* 204–208.

Martin, R.C. (2006). The neuropsychology of sentence processing: Where do we stand? *Cognitive Neuropsychology, 23,* 74–95.

Martin, R.C., & Blossom-Stach, C. (1986). Evidence of syntactic deficits in a fluent aphasic. *Brain and Language, 28,* 196–234.

Martin, R.C., & He, T. (2004). Semantic short-term memory and its role in sentence processing: A replication. *Brain and Language, 89,* 76–82.

Martin, R.C., & Romani, C. (1994). Verbal working memory and sentence comprehension: A multiple-components view. *Neuropsychology, 8,* 506.

Martin, R.C., Shelton, J.R., & Yaffee, L.S. (1994). Language processing and working memory: Neuropsychological evidence for separate phonological and semantic capacities. *Journal of Memory and Language, 33,* 83–111.

Martin, R.C., Tan, Y., & Van Dyke, J. (2011). Working memory, retrieval interference, and sentence comprehension deficits in aphasia. *Procedia—Social and Behavioral Sciences, 23,* 98–99.

Martin, R.C., Vuong, L., & Hull, R. (2007). Impaired vs. preserved inhibitory processes in a patient with a semantic short-term memory deficit. *Brain and Language, 103,* 169–170.

Martin, R.C., Wu, D.H., Freedman, M.L., Jackson, E.F., & Lesch, M. (2003). An event-related fMRI investigation of phonological versus semantic short-term memory. *Journal of Neurolinguistics, 16,* 341–360.

McElree, B. (2006). Accessing recent events. *Psychology of Learning and Motivation, 46,* 155–200.

Meyer, A.M., Mack, J.E., & Thompson, C.K. (2012). Tracking passive sentence comprehension in agrammatic aphasia. *Journal of Neurolinguistics, 25,* 31–43.

Miceli, G., Mazzucchi, A., Menn, L., & Goodglass, H. (1983). Contrasting cases of Italian agrammatic aphasia without comprehension disorder. *Brain and Language, 19,* 65–97.

Miozzo, M., Rawlins, K., & Rapp, B. (2014). How verbs and non-verbal categories navigate the syntax/semantics interface: Insights from cognitive neuropsychology. *Cognition, 133,* 621–640.

Mitchell, D.C., Cuetos, F., Corley, M.M., & Brysbaert, M. (1995). Exposure-based models of human parsing: Evidence for the use of coarse-grained (nonlexical) statistical records. *Journal of Psycholinguistic Research, 24,* 469–488.

Miyake, A., Carpenter, P.A., & Just, M.A. (1994). A capacity approach to syntactic comprehension disorders: Making normal adults perform like aphasic patients. *Cognitive Neuropsychology, 11,* 671–717.

Novick, J.M., Kan, I.P., Trueswell, J.C., & Thompson-Schill, S.L. (2009). A case for conflict across multiple domains: Memory and language impairments following damage to ventrolateral prefrontal cortex. *Cognitive Neuropsychology, 26,* 527–567.

Novick, J.M., Trueswell, J.C., & Thompson-Schill, S.L. (2005). Cognitive control and parsing: Reexamining the role of Broca's area in sentence comprehension. *Cognitive, Affective, & Behavioral Neuroscience, 5,* 263–281.

Ostrin, R.K., & Tyler, L.K. (1995). Dissociations of lexical function: Semantics, syntax, and morphology. *Cognitive Neuropsychology, 12,* 345–389.

Peelle, J.E., Cooke, A., Moore, P., Vesely, L., & Grossman, M. (2007). Syntactic and thematic components of sentence processing in progressive nonfluent aphasia and nonaphasic frontotemporal dementia. *Journal of Neurolinguistics, 20,* 482–494.

Perfetti, C. (2007). Reading ability: Lexical quality to comprehension. *Scientific Studies of Reading, 11,* 357–383.

Pettigrew, C., & Hillis, A.E. (2014). Role for memory capacity in sentence comprehension: Evidence from acute stroke. *Aphasiology.* Advance online publication. doi:10.1080/02687038.2014.919436

Reali, F., & Christiansen, M.H. (2007). Processing of relative clauses is made easier by frequency of occurrence. *Journal of Memory and Language, 57,* 1–23.

Saffran, E.M., & Marin, O.S.M. (1975). Immediate memory for word lists and sentences in a patient with deficient auditory short-term memory. *Brain and Language, 2,* 420–433.

Saffran, E.M., Schwartz, M.F., & Linebarger, M.C. (1998). Semantic influences on thematic role assignment: Evidence from normals and aphasics. *Brain and Language, 62,* 255–297.

Schwartz, M.F., & Chawluk, J.B. (1990). Deterioration of language in progressive aphasia: A case study. In M.F. Schwartz (Eds.), *Modular deficits in Alzheimer-type dementia* (pp. 245–296). Cambridge, MA: MIT Press.

Schwartz, M.F., Marin, O.S.M., & Saffran, E.M. (1979). Dissociations of language function in dementia: A case study. *Brain and Language, 7,* 277–306.

Schwartz, M.F., Saffran, E.M., & Marin, O.S.M. (1980). The word order problem in agrammatism: I. Comprehension. *Brain and Language, 10,* 249–262.

Spivey-Knowlton, M., & Sedivy, J. (1995). Resolving attachment ambiguities with multiple constraints. *Cognition, 55,* 226–267.

Spivey, M.J., & Tanenhaus, M.K. (1998). Syntactic ambiguity resolution in discourse: Modeling the effects of referential context and lexical frequency. *Journal of Experimental Psychology: Learning, Memory, and Cognition, 24,* 1521.

Sussman, R.S., & Sedivy, J. (2003). The time-course of processing syntactic dependencies: Evidence from eye movements. *Language and Cognitive Processes, 18,* 143–163.

Swinney, D., & Zurif, E. (1995). Syntactic processing in aphasia. *Brain and Language, 50,* 225–239.

Tan, Y., Martin, R.C., & Van Dyke, J. (2013). Verbal WM capacities in sentence comprehension: Evidence from aphasia. *Procedia—Social and Behavioral Sciences, 94,* 108–109.

Thompson, C.K., & Choy, J.J. (2009). Pronominal resolution and gap filling in agrammatic aphasia: Evidence from eye movements. *Journal of Psycholinguistic Research, 38,* 255–283.

Trueswell, J.C., & Tanenhaus, M.K. (1994). Toward a lexicalist framework for constraint-based syntactic ambiguity resolution. In L. Frazier & K. Rayner (Eds.), *Perspectives on sentence processing* (pp. 155–179). Mahwah, NJ: Lawrence Erlbaum.

Trueswell, J.C., Tanenhaus, M.K., & Garnsey, S.M. (1994). Semantic influences on parsing: Use of thematic role information in syntactic ambiguity resolution. *Journal of Memory and Language, 33,* 285–318.

Turner, M.L., & Engle, R.W. (1989). Is working memory capacity task dependent? *Journal of Memory and Language, 28,* 127–154.

Tyler, L.K. (1985). Real-time comprehension processes in agrammatism: A case study. *Brain and Language, 26,* 259–275.

Tyler, L.K. (1989). Syntactic deficits and the construction of local phrases in spoken language comprehension. *Cognitive Neuropsychology, 6,* 333–355.

Tyler, L.K. (1992). *Spoken language comprehension: An experimental approach to disordered and normal processing.* Cambridge, MA: MIT Press.

Tyler, L.K., Moss, H.E., Patterson, K., & Hodges, J. (1997). The gradual deterioration of syntax and semantics in a patient with progressive aphasia. *Brain and Language, 56,* 426–476.

Tyler, L.K., Shafto, M.A., Randall, B., Wright, P., Marslen-Wilson, W.D., & Stamatakis, E.A. (2010). Preserving syntactic processing across the adult life span: The modulation of the frontotemporal language system in the context of age-related atrophy. *Cerebral Cortex, 20,* 352–364.

Vallar, G., & Baddeley, A.D. (1984). Phonological short-term store, phonological processing and sentence comprehension: A neuropsychological case study. *Cognitive Neuropsychology, 1,* 121–141.

Van Berkum, J.J., Brown, C.M., & Hagoort, P. (1999). Early referential context effects in sentence processing: Evidence from event-related brain potentials. *Journal of Memory and Language, 41,* 147–182.

Van Dyke, J. (2007). Interference effects from grammatically unavailable constituents during sentence processing. *Journal of Experimental Psychology: Learning, Memory and Cognition, 33,* 407–430.

Van Dyke, J., & Johns, C.L. (2012). Memory interference as a determinant of language comprehension. *Language and Linguistics Compass, 6,* 193–211.

Van Dyke, J., & Lewis, R.L. (2003). Distinguishing effects of structure and decay on attachment and repair: A cue-based parsing account of recovery from misanalyzed ambiguities. *Journal of Memory and Language, 49,* 285–316.

Van Dyke, J., & McElree, B. (2006). Retrieval interference in sentence comprehension. *Journal of Memory and Language, 55,* 157–166.

Van Dyke, J., & McElree, B. (2011). Cue-dependent interference in comprehension. *Journal of Memory and Language, 65,* 247–263.

von Stockert, T.R., & Bader, L. (1976). Some relations of grammar and lexicon in aphasia. *Cortex, 12,* 49–60.

Vuong, L.C., & Martin, R.C. (2011). LIFG-based attentional control and the resolution of lexical ambiguities in sentence context. *Brain and Language, 116,* 22–32.

Vuong, L.C., & Martin, R.C. (2014). Domain-specific executive control and the revision of misinterpretations in sentence comprehension. *Language, Cognition and Neuroscience, 29,* 312–325.

Waters, G., Caplan, D., & Hildebrandt, N. (1991). On the structure of verbal short-term memory and its functional role in sentence comprehension: Evidence from neuropsychology. *Cognitive Neuropsychology, 8,* 81–126.

Wells, J.B., Christiansen, M.H., Race, D.S., Acheson, D.J., & MacDonald, M.C. (2009). Experience and sentence processing: Statistical learning and relative clause comprehension. *Cognitive Psychology, 58,* 250–271.

Wu, D., Waller, S., & Chatterjee, A. (2007). The functional neuroanatomy of thematic role and locative relational knowledge. *Journal of Cognitive Neuroscience, 19,* 1542–1555.

17

MODELS OF SENTENCE PRODUCTION

Cynthia K. Thompson, Yasmeen Faroqi-Shah, and Jiyeon Lee

Producing a sentence involves stringing words together to convey a message one wants to communicate while also adhering to the grammatical rules of a particular language (Levelt, 1989). An important property of sentence generation is *productivity* in that speakers create novel utterances that can be as unique as their thoughts by selecting from a variety of words and sentence structures. Incredibly, adult speakers produce 16–20 grammatical sentences per minute, seemingly automatically without conscious thought! Not surprisingly, the mechanisms underlying sentence production include a number of complex processes. It is important to point out at the outset that these processes are not completely understood and many are underspecified in terms of how they function and interact with one another. In this chapter we summarize psycholinguistic models of sentence production and discuss component processes engaged for sentence production. We also discuss data supporting these models and their components derived from both cognitively healthy and aphasic speakers.

1   Overview of Sentence Production Models

There is broad agreement across models of sentence production that several major component processes or levels of processing are involved, including message conceptualization, accessing relevant lexical material, sentence building (i.e., concatenation [sequencing] of lexical material into grammatical sentences), morphophonological processes, and articulatory encoding. Models of sentence production differ, however, with regard to whether or not these component processes are engaged serially or in parallel and whether or not there is interaction between them.

1.1   Serial Models

Early models conceptualized the component processes engaged for sentence production in a largely serial, top-down architecture, proceeding from the speaker's communicative intention to overt speech (Bock & Levelt, 1994; Garrett, 1975, 1980, 1982, 1988; Levelt, 1989, 1993, 1999). At each level in the model, distinct data sets are surveyed and processes are engaged to form grammatical utterances that convey the speaker's intent. The result is essentially a modular system, with language processes separate from general cognitive processes (Fodor, 1983) as well as distinct from each other within levels of sentence production.

The components (levels) of processing originally posed by Garrett (1975), nearly four decades ago, included: (1) a *message level* required for generating what is to be said, (2) a *functional level* concerned with selecting major lexical concepts for conveying the intended message and assigning grammatical roles or syntactic functions, (3) a *positional level* involved in assembling phonologically realized words and morphemes into a sentence frame, and (4) a *sound level* associated with programming articulatory processes. The major source of data used to develop Garrett's model came from speech errors produced by cognitively healthy speakers (Cutler, 1982; Dell & Reich, 1981; Fay & Cutler, 1977; Fromkin, 1971; Garrett, 1975).

Spontaneously produced speech errors, also called *slips of the tongue*, provide clues into how speech is produced. For instance, an error such as "bed rus" (for "red bus"), called a *spoonerism* by Reverend Dr. Spooner, involves the exchange of initial consonants between words. Also known as a *phoneme exchange* error, such errors suggest that the target lexical items (i.e., in the example above, the adjective *red* and noun *bus*), as well as associated phonological material, are selected prior to ordering words into the sentence frame. Similarly *word exchange* errors (e.g., "His *mind* came to *name*?" for "His *name* came to *mind*?"), *morpheme exchange* errors (e.g., "The randomiz*ed* samp*ly* data" for "the randomly sampled data") and *phoneme anticipatory* errors (e.g., "The *mest* of the mangos" for "the best of the mangos") suggest that lexicalization (i.e., going from meaning to sound) occurs prior to word string assembly. But other speech error phenomenon suggest otherwise. For example, the *tip-of-the-tongue* (TOT) state (Vigliocco, Antonini, & Garrett, 1997), in which speakers know the meaning of the word to be expressed (concept), can access syntactic information about it (e.g., that the target word is a noun or a verb), and information about the word form is available (e.g., the speaker knows the first letter and perhaps the number of syllables), suggests that word string assembly may proceed without completely accessing all lexical material. For example, consider the sentence: "Before the train gets into Chicago, there's a stop at . . . oh what's the name of that town, it starts with a 'g,' has two syllables . . . oh yea, Glenview." Such an utterance indicates that lexicalization and syntactic planning may not be serial processes. (We address this issue in more depth below.)

Hesitations during sentence production, including filled and unfilled pauses, false starts, repetitions, and parenthetical remarks (e.g., "well I mean") are another source of data used to understand sentence production processes. The type of interruption or dysfluency and where during the flow of speech it occurs provides clues about lexical-semantic and syntactic processes. Garrett (1982) suggested that dysfluencies reflect delays created by momentary inaccessibility of essential information, transient increases in processing load, and/or advanced planning of upcoming structural units. Pauses (i.e., moments of silence longer than 200 to 250 ms), for example, may be associated with planning large chunks of language or retrieving the phonological form of words (particularly words of low frequency or that are otherwise less predictable in the context) (Goldman-Eisler, 1968; Levelt, 1989; Petrie, 1987).

Subsequent sentence production models have expanded and refined the levels of sentence production and component processes posed by Garrett (1982), while retaining the idea that sentence production engages hierarchical top-down processes, with content-related operations such as thematic role assignment preceding structural operations such as word order. For example, Bock and Levelt's (1994) model considers both functional and positional processes within the process of grammatical encoding, as shown in Figure 17.1. Their model also further specifies processes involved at the positional level, including constituent assembly and inflectional processes. In Levelt's (1999) model two core systems are included (Figure 17.2). The first, a *rhetorical/semantic/syntactic system*, involves conceptual preparation and grammatical encoding. By interacting with knowledge of the external and internal world and the mental lexicon, this system generates the surface structure of sentences. The second core, the *phonological/phonetic system*, includes morphophonological encoding, phonetic encoding, and articulatory processes. In a more recent model, Griffin and Crew (2012) retained the message, grammatical, and phonological levels of Bock and Levelt (1994) and further introduced a prearticulatory stage of phonological buffering (as shown in Figure 17.3).

Griffin and Crew also added the process of incrementality, which addresses the relative timing of conceptual, grammatical, and phonological processes for individual elements of a sentence (see also Bock & Levelt, 1994; Kempen & Hoenkemp, 1987). Eye-tracking-while-speaking methods have provided increased granularity in sentence production research by providing a real-time measure of sentence formulation (Griffin & Bock, 2000; Meyer & Lethaus, 2004; Lee & Thompson, 2011a, 2011b). The rationale behind this approach is that eye movements are time-locked with speech preparation. In a typical experiment, speakers are asked to describe scenes presented on a computer monitor while their eye fixations to particular parts of the scene are recorded. It turns out that speakers' eye gazes precede production. That is, they look at the to-be-mentioned part of the scene (i.e., people or objects) about one second before speech (Griffin, 2004). This pattern suggests that it is not necessary to completely encode all elements of an utterance prior to production. So, for a simple subject-verb-object (SVO) sentence in English, the sentential subject is first accessed and undergoes phonological encoding, at which time the verb undergoes grammatical encoding and the object is accessed from the mental lexicon.

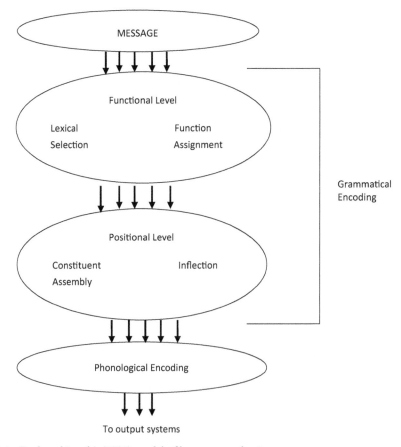

Figure 17.1 Bock and Levelt's (1994) model of language production.

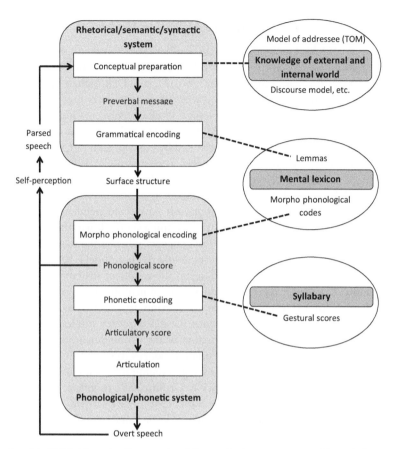

Figure 17.2 Levelt's (1999) blueprint for a speaker. The speaker's representational knowledge is represented by ellipses.

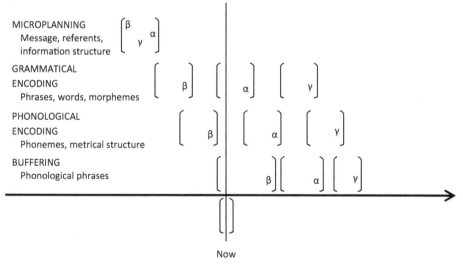

Figure 17.3 Griffin and Crew's (2012) overview of language production processes for producing a simple utterance. Elements of sentence production are denoted by Greek letters and the time course of grammatical and phonological encoding associated with each element is indicated by subscripted brackets. This model illustrates the relative timing of encoding individual message elements (α, β, γ).

1.2 Interactive Activation Models

In contrast to serial models of sentence production, other models contend that content and structural processes proceed roughly in parallel with bidirectional interaction between them (Chang et al., 2006; Ferriera, 2010). For example, Dell (1986), Martin, Dell, Saffran, and Schwartz (1994), Stemberger (1995), and others argue that lexical access during sentence production involves interaction between conceptual, lexical, and phonological levels of representation in a feedforward and feedback fashion. In interactive activation (IA) models, also referred to as connectionist models, targeted and related sets of semantic features, activated by conceptual input, feed forward to lexical and phonological levels to activate the target as well as related nodes. When nodes are primed at each level, feedback is sent back to the source node as well as related nodes.

Chang et al. (2006) proposed an interactive *dual-path model* of sentence production. This model fractionates the sentence production system into two relatively independent components, a *meaning system* and a *sequencing system* (Figure 17.4). The meaning system learns the association between the message and thematic roles of different lexical concepts, whereas the sequencing system learns to sequence these roles and insert morphosyntactic markers. This model is based on what is known about acquisition of syntax in children as well as on the results of structural (syntactic) priming studies (Bock, 1986). In its most typical version, structural priming involves a *prime* sentence of a specific syntactic type. After hearing the prime, participants are required to repeat it, and then to describe a picture, unrelated to the prime sentence. Results of several studies show that cognitively healthy people tend to reuse the syntactic structure of the prime during the picture description trial, reflecting implicit learning. Structural priming produces robust effects, even with variations of the classic paradigm and lasts for as many as 10 intervening filler sentences between prime and target (Bock, Dell, Chang, & Onishi, 2007; Bock & Griffin, 2000; Branigan, Pickering, & Cleland, 2000; Cleland & Pickering, 2003; Potter & Lombardi, 1998). The dual-path model emphasizes the interdependence between the acquisition of syntactic knowledge by implicit learning and use of this knowledge during sentence production.

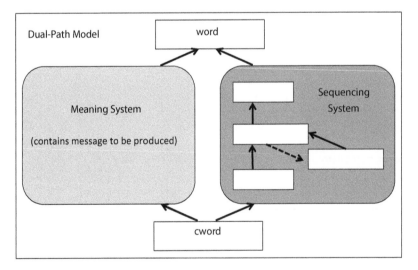

Figure 17.4 Chang, Dell, and Bock's (2006) dual-path model of language production. The two paths refer to the meaning and sequencing systems, with the latter system being a simple recurrent network. This model emphasizes the interconnection between language learning and language use. The prefix c- denotes a comprehended word.

2 Component Processes of Sentence Production

Regardless of whether or not sentence production involves serial processing, parallel processing, or a combination of both, virtually all models of sentence production describe crucial component processes. In the next section, we discuss these processes.

2.1 Generating the Message

Prior to producing a sentence, generation of a nonlinguistic message is required. This stage of sentence production is considered to be the interface between thought and language (Bock, 1990; Garrett, 1988) and is represented in all models of sentence production (see Figures 17.1–17.4). Levelt (1999) refers to this processing level as "conceptual preparation," whereas Chang et al. (2006) refer to it as the "meaning system." Message generation involves both *macroplanning* and *microplanning*. Macroplanning, the focus of studies on discourse and pragmatics (see Garnham, 2010, for review), is influenced by the communicative context, for example, the conversational participants, social situation, what has already been expressed in the discourse, and the speakers' general goals (to be funny, sarcastic, untruthful, etc.). Microplanning is associated with casting the propositional form of the message—for example, specification of referents and predication (i.e., who did what to whom), modification (i.e., attributes of referents; such as beautiful, happy), quantification (e.g., some or all), and mood (i.e., declarative, imperative, or interrogative). Although message generation is concerned with both macro- and microplanning, the latter serves as the starting point of sentence generation (Levelt, 1993). During microplanning at the message level speakers may simplify the content of the message (for children or elderly listeners) or encode additional details to minimize listener ambiguity. For example, Ferreira, Slevc, and Rogers (2005) asked participants to describe object pairs that were either of the same type (two mammalian bats), were homophones (mammalian bat and baseball bat), or were unrelated. Participants avoided potential ambiguities for the listener by inserting additional detail such as, *the big bat* or *the bat and baseball bat*. Microplanning yields a set of semantic and pragmatic specifications of the speaker's communicative intention and provides the raw material for subsequent processes.

2.2 Grammatical Encoding

All models of sentence production include mechanisms for selection of words that match the speakers' intended message as well as processes for concatenation of words based on the phrase structure rules of the language being spoken. Ferreira (2010) refers to two primary processes engaged for grammatical encoding: *content processes* (i.e., those associated with translation of thoughts to words [i.e., lexicalization]) and *structure processes* (i.e., processes engaged for multiword encoding), respectively (Figure 17.5). We discuss these in some detail below.

2.2.1 Content Processes

Lexicalization involves access to both meaning and form—that is, translation of the semantic representation of a word into its phonological form. The precise stages involved, the independence of these stages, and the time course of lexicalization, however, is unclear and has been under debate for some years (Caramazza, 1997; Dell, 1986; Rapp & Goldrick, 2000). It could be argued, however, that sentence production *must* include access to the mental lexicon and processes for word selection and production. Indeed, all models of production include units corresponding to words.

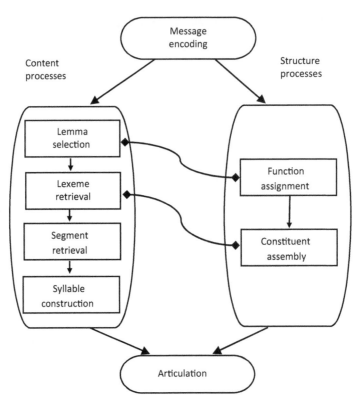

Figure 17.5 Ferreira's (2010) framework of language production shows concurrent encoding of lexical and syntactic content. Arrows indicate the general flow of information, and diamonds indicate melding of content and structural representations.

Levelt (1989) proposed the concept of the *lemma*, suggesting that all words in the mental lexicon are represented by lemmas, which are specified both semantically and syntactically (see also Kempen & Huijbers, 1983). That is, each lemma is marked for form class (e.g., noun, verb), gender, case marking, and other grammatical information. Others suggest, however, that syntactic information is not encoded within lemmas (Caramazza, 1997). Rather, the flow of information is from a lexical-semantic network to a separate lexical-syntactic network, where grammatical information is accessed. An often-cited source of evidence supporting a lemma level of representation comes from tip-of-the-tongue (TOT) data showing that Italian speakers in the TOT state are able to report grammatical gender, but not phonological information, about target words, indicating that syntactic and phonological information are independent (Badecker, Miozzo, and Zanuttini, 1995; Viggliocco et al., 1997). However, Caramazza and colleagues report cases of Italian speakers in the TOT state who show the opposite pattern: they can sometimes report phonological, but *not* gender information (Caramazza & Miozzo, 1997; Miozzo & Caramazza, 1997). These data suggest that access to phonological information is not necessarily mediated by access to syntactic information.

In addition to contacting lemma information, lexicalization also requires access to the phonological form of words, referred to as *lexemes*. For example, evidence from picture-word interference paradigms suggests that speakers encode both semantic and phonological information during preparation of object names (Glaser, 1992; Glaser & Dungelhoff, 1984; Hashimoto & Thompson, 2009; Mack et al., 2013; Roelofs, 1992; Schriefers, Meyer, & Levelt, 1990; Thompson et al., 2012). Participants name pictures of objects presented with either visual or auditory distractor words. Naming reaction times (RTs) are recorded under all conditions. Results of such experiments have shown that when the distractor word is semantically related to the target picture (e.g., *bed—chair*) interference in activation of the target word ensues, resulting in longer RTs as compared to when semantically unrelated distractor words (e.g., *fish—chair*) are presented (Glaser & Dungelhoff, 1984; Schriefers et al., 1990; Thompson et al., 2012). This pattern of performance can be explained as follows: when two lemmas (i.e., a distractor word and a target picture) are simultaneously activated, the probability of selecting the target is diminished. This is called "conceptual intrusion" (Levelt, 1989). When the distractor and target are semantically related, activation of the two semantically related lemmas creates even greater interference, resulting in slowed activation of the target (associative intrusion). Several studies show this pattern when semantically related distractors are presented prior to (e.g., −150 ms) or simultaneously with (0 ms) the target picture.

The effects of presenting phonologically related distractor words also have been tested using this paradigm (Mack et al., 2013; Hashimoto & Thompson, 2009; Schrifers et al., 1990). Results show a phonological facilitation effect (i.e., faster naming) when phonologically related distractors are presented. For example, naming a picture of a *rake* is faster when a distractor word like *rain* versus *book* is presented. The phonological facilitation effect occurs when a phonologically related distractor is presented at the same time (i.e., 0 ms) or immediately after the picture to be named (e.g., stimulus onset asynchrony [SOA] of +150 ms). The phonological facilitation effect, however, is less likely to be seen when the phonological distractor is presented prior to the target picture (i.e., at −150 ms). These findings suggest that semantic processing precedes phonological processing. Thompson et al. (2012) and Mack et al. (2013) replicated these findings in cognitively healthy older participants as well as in people with primary progressive aphasia.

Importantly, however, not all studies have found these patterns (Jescheniak & Schriefers, 1998). Rather, some studies show that semantically related distractors interfere with picture naming when presented both prior to the target (−150 ms before) and after the target picture (+150 ms) while phonologically related distracters facilitate picture naming at 0 ms and +150 ms. Hashimoto and Thompson (2009) also found this pattern in people with aphasia. These findings provide support for interaction among levels of lexical representation during lexicalization, rather than a strict serial—semantic to phonological—processing order.

Some speech error data also support interactive activation. Mixed errors, such as *rat* for *cat*, have been found to occur more frequently than would be expected based on chance (Dell & Reich, 1981). The observation that phonologically erred productions are often real words, known as the lexical bias effect, also coincides with the idea that feedback from the phonological level to the lexical level occurs, since retrieval of the phonological form, without feedback to the lexical level, would not result in real-word errors.

Paraphasias—or word substitution—made by people with aphasia (as well as cognitively healthy people) also provide insight into the temporal schema existing between semantic and phonological representations. Paraphasias often are related semantically to target words (e.g., *cat* for *dog*), phonologically related (i.e., errors involving phonological substitutions, additions, or deletions; e.g., *pentil* for *pencil*), or unrelated (e.g., neologistic paraphasic errors in which the form produced bears no resemblance to the target word form, such as *flanginlangin* for *hammer*[1]) (Gainnotti, Miceli, Caltagirone, Silveri, & Masullo, 1981; Kay & Ellis, 1987; Schwartz, 1987). A simple explanation for these error patterns, based on serial models of lexical processing, is that semantic and phonological errors arise from difficulty at the semantic and phonological processing levels, respectively, and that neologistic paraphasic errors reflect semantic errors, confounded by superimposed phonological errors. Caramazza and Hillis (1990) argue, however, that the source of semantic errors may be associated with faulty phonological processes, the assumption being that a semantic representation activates all related lexemes in proportion to their similarity, or number of semantic features in common with the activated semantic representation.

Dell, Saffran, and colleagues developed a computational model for naming and repetition based on interactive two-step (i.e., semantic and phonological) activation (Dell, Martin, & Schwartz, 2007; Dell, Schwartz, Martin, Saffran, & Gagnon, 1997; Foygel & Dell, 2000). This model is designed to accommodate lexical access errors of both typical speakers and those with aphasia by assuming that lexical errors in aphasia are not qualitatively different from errors made by typical speakers. In the interactive two-step model, lexical knowledge is distributed in a network of semantic, word, and phonological units with excitatory and bidirectional connections between them. The weights of these units and their connection strengths can be altered to account for paraphasic errors of various types (Foygel & Dell, 2000; Nozari, Kittredge, Dell, & Schwartz, 2010) and have shown a good fit with actual patient data (Schwartz, Dell, Martin, Gahl, & Sobel, 2006). (See also chapter 7, this volume, for discussion of models of lexical access.)

2.2.2   Structure Processes

Production of a syntactically well-formed sentence involves ordering of lexical items to express relationships between entities to convey a message. The complexity of syntactic processes is evident from the fact that speakers can choose from a variety of syntactic structures to express a message. A fundamental question of syntactic planning is when and how these different sentence structures become available to the speaker and what determines which sentence structure is eventually produced. Based on **lexicalist** syntactic approaches to sentence production, structure processes are lexically driven at least to some extent in that lexical entries contain not only semantic information, but also grammatical information used for sentence planning. For example, verb lemmas carry grammatical information, including subcategorization frames, which denote the grammatical environments in which words may occur as well as gender, tense, and other information. For example, accessing passive-bias verbs (e.g., *get*) often leads to production of passivized sentence structures (Ferreira, 1994).

A radical alternative to the lexicalist approach is the **constructivist** approach (Goldberg, 1995, 2003). On this account lexical entries include no grammatically relevant information. This means, for example, for verbs, that thematic specifications do not exist in the lexicon, and therefore that syntactic structure building is not guided by the thematic information associated with them. Rather, structure building is free, restricted only by word knowledge (Borer, 2005). Following Pinker (1989), the constructional approach assumes that a sentence structure is predictable from the verb's semantic representation, and therefore different sentence structures reflect differences in the verb meaning or in the discourse function (see 1, from Goldberg, 2003).

1.   a. He sliced the bread. (transitive)
    b. Pat sliced the carrots into the salad. (causative motion)
    c. Pat sliced Chris a piece of pie. (ditransitive)
    d. Pat sliced the box open. (resultative)
    e. Emeril sliced and diced his way to stardom. (way construction)

However, as noted by Ramchand (2008), this view is problematic for explaining subcategorization frames and argument structure requirements for verbs, as illustrated in 2–4. Depending on the verb selected, different syntactic environments are required for grammatically well-formed sentences. Considering the verbs *sneeze, visit*, and *know*, only the verb *sneeze* can be produced without a direct object or internal (theme) argument, as in 2a, and only the complement verb *know* can be produced with a sentential complement, as in 4c. On lexicalist views, this information about verbs (and other syntactic information) is encoded within the representation of the verb, and hence guides the grammatical structure of sentences.

2. a. The man sneezed.
    b. *The man sneezed [the doctor].

3. a. *The man visited.
    b. The man visited [the doctor].
    c. *The man visited [the doctor was wrong].

4. a. *The man knew.
    b. The man knew [the doctor].
    c. The man knew [the doctor was wrong].

2.2.2.1   Function Assignment

A crucial process for sentence construction is linking lexical items to their relational or grammatical functions (e.g., subject/nominative, object/accusative). In early models, this process is referred to as function assignment (Bock & Levelt, 1994). Consider, for example, the sentence "The man visited the doctor." To formulate this sentence, concepts for *man, doctor*, and *visit* and corresponding lemmas are selected from the lexicon. *Man* is then linked to the subject/nominative function, and *doctor* is linked to the object/accusative function. In configurational languages such as English, function assignment corresponds with the ordering of words in sentences because agents are more likely to be placed in sentence initial position (i.e., in the subject position). In contrast, in nonconfigurational languages, functions are denoted by case marking. Function assignment is hence an interface between lexical and syntactic processes.

Function assignment is influenced by inherent properties of selected items such as the animacy and concreteness of lexical elements, discourse-related factors such as topic prominence and focus, and the argument structure of verbs. The importance of animacy in function assignment has been elucidated in experiments using a sentence-recall paradigm. For example, Bock and Warren (1985) showed that animate and concrete elements are more likely to be assigned to sentence initial position than inanimate or abstract elements. Similarly, McDonald, Bock, and Kelly (1993) noted a tendency for production of animate nouns as subjects in transitive sentences. The prominence of particular elements in the discourse also may affect function assignment in that those that are more prominent are more likely to be assigned the subject function. This postulate has been tested in experiments using queries about pictures. For example, presented with a scene such as a girl chasing a *boy* and a query about the *boy* (e.g., "What is going on with the boy?"), participants are likely to assign the subject role to the *boy* in their answers, resulting in production of a passive sentence (e.g., "The boy is being chased by the girl"). When questioned about the *girl*, the *girl* receives subject status, resulting in an active sentence (e.g., "The girl is chasing the boy") (Bates & Devescovi, 1989; Bock, 1977).

Function assignment errors, called role reversals, are frequently seen in normal speech (e.g., "*He* wants *us* to do something else" rather than "*We* want *him* to do something else," from Bock, 1995). Such errors also are common in aphasic speakers. A classic example is Martin and Blossom-Stach's (1986) Wernicke's aphasic patient who produced sentences with acceptable surface form, but with function assignment errors, such as "*The pupil* gave *her* an A+" for the target "*She* gave *the pupil* an A+." Function assignment deficits in aphasia are more common in semantically reversible sentences (where both nouns are animate) as compared to nonreversible sentences (one noun is animate and the other inanimate) (Martin & Blossom-Stach, 1986; Saffran, Schwartz, & Marin, 1980). This pattern suggests that when two animate nouns are selected from the lexicon the animacy rule does not assist in assignment of the subject function, resulting in role-reversal errors (see Bock & Warren, 1985). Function assignment errors also are found in aphasic individuals for sentences with complex syntax such as passives (Caramazza & Miceli, 1991; Faroqi-Shah & Thompson, 2003; Cho & Thompson, 2010; Martin & Blossom-Stach, 1986). In an elicited sentence production task where a constraint was placed on the first noun with which to begin sentences, Faroqi-Shah and Thompson (2003) found that agrammatic aphasic speakers produced function assignment errors, frequently producing active for passive sentence targets, with reversed function assignments (e.g., "*The boy* lifted *the fireman*" was produced instead of "*The boy* was lifted by *the fireman*"). Similarly, in a structural priming experiment, Cho and Thompson (2010) found that when passive sentences are primed, role reversals were the most common error, even though using this paradigm agrammatic aphasic speakers showed better ability to produce passive sentences as compared to in their spontaneous speech attempts. That is, when they repeated the prime sentence "the tiger was licked by the lion" prior to production of the target sentence, aphasic participants produced sentence with correct passive morphology but still with role-reversal errors (e.g., "The *man* is poked by the *woman*" for the target "The *woman* is poked by the *man*"), whereas in picture description and other tasks these patients showed inability to produce passive sentences.

Verbs, in particular, are integrally involved in function assignment and syntactic planning. As noted above, lemma and lexicalist syntactic theories posit that verbs are stored in the lexicon together with syntactic information. In addition, when a particular verb is selected for production, the argument structure properties (i.e., participant roles or event structure) of that verb also are accessed. Thus, transitive verbs such as *visit*, as in 3 above, are produced with two arguments, as in "The man visited the doctor," whereas complement verbs such as *know* can occur with an internal argument that is a noun (e.g., "The man knew *the doctor*") or a sentential complement (e.g., "The man knew *that the doctor was wrong about the diagnosis*"). Verbs are also semantically associated with their most typical arguments, which likely aids in both lexical selection and sentence formulation. For instance, using a lexical priming study in which participants made animacy decisions, Ferretti, McRae, and Hatherell (2001) showed that verb primes facilitate processing of typical agents, patients/themes, and instruments associated with them (e.g., arresting/policeman, arresting/criminal, cutting/scissors). There is also evidence for a reverse priming effect of verb facilitation using typical agents/patients and themes as primes (Edmonds & Mizrahi, 2011; McRae, Hare, Elman, & Ferretti, 2005).

The properties of verbs also influence sentence type. That is, the thematic roles assigned to selected arguments impact which argument will occupy the subject position of the sentence (Fillmore, 1968; Grimshaw, 1990). This *thematic hierarchy* ranks agent, experiencer, instrument, and patient/theme arguments, respectively, in decreasing order of semantic prominence (Grimshaw, 1990). Thus, when agents or experiencers compete with the theme for the subject position, the theme is likely to lose. For example, unaccusative verbs with alternating transitivity, such as *open*, select for both an agent and a theme as shown in 4. However, because speakers (and listeners) prefer agents to be in the subject position, structures like 4a are more common than 4b.

4.   a. The boy $_{AGENT}$ opened the door $_{THEME}$.
     b. The door $_{THEME}$ opened.

This phenomenon is also relevant for psych verbs (i.e., verbs with an experiencer argument). Consider the verbs *admire* and *amuse*, as in 5 below.

5. a. The children EXPERIENCER admired the clown THEME.
    b. The clown THEME amused the children EXPERIENCER.
    c. The children EXPERIENCER were amused by the clown THEME.

Although both verbs select for experiencer and theme arguments, *admire* is a subject experiencer verb, requiring that the experiencer occupy the subject position, as in 5a, whereas *amuse* is an object-experiencer verb, requiring that the experiencer occupy the object position. Notably, however, because themes make unpopular sentential subjects, object-experiencer verbs are more likely to be produced in passivized sentences, as in 5c. Thus, verbs like *amuse* are passive-bias verbs. Notably, this bias has been documented in both cognitively healthy and aphasic speakers (Gahl et al., 2003; Ferreria, 1994; Thompson & Lee, 2009).

Research also has shown that verb production is often impaired in people with aphasia and that the argument structure characteristics of verbs play an important role. That is, verbs with complex argument structure entries are more difficult to produce than those with simpler entries (Thompson, 2003). This pattern is particularly characteristic of agrammatic aphasic speakers, who experience difficulty with syntactic aspects of language, including sentence production. Interestingly, this pattern has been reported in patients across languages (Bastiannse & Jonkers, 1998 [Dutch]; Dragoy & Bastiannse, 2010 [Russian]; Kiss, 2000 [Hungarian]; Kim & Thompson, 2000, 2004, and Kemmerer & Tranel, 2000 [English]; and Luzzatti et al., 2002 [Italian]) and is prevalent in both monolingual and bilingual aphasic speakers (Faroqi-Shah & Waked, 2010; Poncelet, Majerus, Raman, Warginaire, & Weekes, 2007; also see Faroqi-Shah, 2012 and Mätzig, Druks, Masterson, & Vigliocco, 2009 for review). For example, in a case study, Faroqi-Shah and Waked (2010) reported a trilingual (Arabic, French, English) person with aphasia, who showed a consistent verb deficit in all three languages, with a sparing of noun retrieval.

Agrammatic aphasic individuals, unlike cognitively healthy adults or persons with anomic aphasia, also have difficulty producing verbs with more complex argument structure properties, such as unaccusatives and psych verbs (Bastiaanse & van Zonneveld, 2005; Kegl, 1995; Lee & Thompson, 2003; Luzzatti et al., 2002; Thompson & Lee, 2009). Studies also show a close association between verb retrieval abilities and sentence production in people with aphasia (Berndt, Haendiges, Mitchum, & Sandson, 1997; Druks & Carroll, 2005; Faroqi-Shah & Thompson, 2003; Thompson, Riley, den Ouden, Meltzer-Asscher, & Lukic, 2013). When participants are provided with the verb to be used in a sentence, their sentence production ability improves significantly, especially for active sentences, confirming the crucial role of verb retrieval in sentence production (Faroqi-Shah & Thompson, 2003).

2.2.2.2 *Constituent Assembly*

The process of assembling lexical items into a sentence structure is sometimes called *constituent assembly*. It is generally accepted that language production proceeds incrementally (Bock & Levelt, 1994; Kempen & Hoenkemp, 1987; Levelt, 1989). That is, speakers do not formulate an entire utterance before speaking. Rather, they initiate speech once a minimal chunk of an utterance is grammatically encoded, and the subsequent part of the utterance is prepared as speaking unfolds in time. At the level of constituent assembly, incremental production implies that not all lexical items need to be selected before the entire syntactic structure of the utterance is generated. The size of sentence planning units, however, is not completely clear. Research to date has focused on how far ahead an utterance is prepared before speech, yielding two threads of evidence. Some studies suggest that planning ensues on the basis of availability of individual lexical items (lemmas; i.e., word-by-word or linear incrementality; de Smedt, 1990, 1996; Kempen & Heonkemp, 1987; Griffin, 2001; Levelt, 1989, 1999; Schriefers et al., 1998), while others indicate that larger linguistic units or structures are formulated prior to phonological encoding (i.e., *structural or hierarchical incrementality*; Allum & Wheeldon, 2009; Ford, 1982; Garrett, 1982; Konopka, 2012; Meyer, 1996; van de Velde, Meyer, & Konopka, 2014; Ferreira, 2000; Lee, Brown-Schmidt, & Watson, 2013; Lindsley, 1975).

2.2.2.2.1   *Word-by-Word (Linear) Incrementality*

Word-by-word incrementality ascertains that speakers formulate sentences one word (or lemma) at a time. Also referred to as *rapid incrementality* (Ferreira, 2000; Ferreira & Swets, 2002) and *elemental planning* (Bock et al., 2004), this view proposes that sentence structure reflects the order of lexical items activated and that the speaker begins speaking without advanced grammatical planning. This means that the grammatical encoder needs to retrieve only the first lemma before phonological encoding begins, and the retrieved lemma takes the highest position in the sentence structure (i.e., the subject position) as a default. The remainder of the sentence structure is then formulated during speech. The approach allows rapid initiation of speech and little reliance on the syntactic (memory) buffer. However, speakers may encounter difficulties during speech due to a limited look-ahead mechanism (e.g., when the grammatical encoder fails to prepare the next piece of an utterance even after the phonological encoder finishes its job). In this case, there may be lags between the two processes, resulting in pauses or other disfluencies during speech (Griffin, 2001; Kempen & deSmedt, 1987).

The influence of lexical accessibility on sentence structure supports the word-by-word incrementality. As discussed in section 2.2.2.1 ('Function Assignment'), speakers tend to build sentence structures so that a more accessible (activated) word is mentioned earlier in the sentence (i.e., in the subject position). For example, Bock (1986) showed that speakers produce a passive sentence to mention a semantically primed theme noun earlier (e.g., "the plant was carried by the girl") instead of producing an active sentence (e.g., "the girl carried the plant"), which is more frequent and simpler structure in the English language. This pattern suggests that the grammatical encoder begins building the sentence structure as the first lemma (theme) becomes available, placing it in the subject position, and the rest of the sentence structure is formulated accordingly following grammatical constraints of the language.

Other evidence for word-by-word incremental planning comes from eye-tracking production studies, requiring participants to produce sentences as they view visual scenes. Results show that speakers' eyes fixate sequentially on different parts of the picture, with speech following these fixations (Griffin, 2001; Griffin & Spieler, 2006; Griffin & Mouzon, 2004; Spieler & Griffin, 2006). For example, Griffin (2001) and Spieler and Griffin (2006) examined younger and older participants' eye movements as they performed a sentence production task, describing the location of three pictured objects in a predefined sentence structure (e.g., "the clock and the needle are above the cup"). The second and third objects in the array were manipulated for codability, or the number of labels the item can be given (e.g., items like *needle* have high codability, whereas items like *cup* have lower codability; i.e., *cup* can be labeled as *cup, mug,* or *stein*). Low codability items are known to be more difficult in terms of lemma selection as compared to those with high codability. Results showed a codability effect for both participant groups, with longer gaze durations to objects with lower codability compared to objects with higher codability. However, codability effects occurred only during speech rather than before speech onset, suggesting that prior to production speakers prepare the lemma for only the first object to be mentioned in sentences. These findings were replicated by Lee, Yoshida, and Thompson (submitted) in their study with young and older cognitively healthy speakers. In addition, a group of agrammatic aphasic speakers showed the same codability effects on their gaze durations, indicating word-by-word incremental planning when retrieving words and assembling them into a prespecified sentence structure.

Experiments using the word-interference paradigm also suggest that constituent assembly occurs on a word-by-word basis (Schriefers, Teruel, & Meinshausen, 1998; Smith & Wheeldon, 1999). Schriefers et al. (1998) examined the scope of advanced planning in German-speaking participants, asking them to describe simple transitive scenes using either verb-subject-object (VSO) or subject-object-verb (SOV) sentences. On each production trial, a related or unrelated distractor verb was superimposed on target pictures, both at a stimulus onset asynchrony of 0 ms. Based on the idea that semantically related verb distractors would compete with production of target verbs, speech onset times for the two sentence types were measured. Results showed a word-interference effect in the VSO condition, but not in the SOV condition, indicating that the advanced grammatical encoding does not require prespeech verb lemma encoding.

2.2.2.2.2 *Structural (Hierarchical) Incrementality*

In structural incrementality, sentence formulation is guided by a larger linguistic unit, resulting in advanced retrieval of multiple lemmas constrained by the hierarchical relational structure of a sentence. This kind of advanced planning allows the speaker to "look ahead" to the upcoming structure, which may help avoid difficulties associated with word-by-word incremental production. Conversely, speakers have to hold more linguistic information in a syntactic buffer prior to phonological encoding, which could result in delayed production and nonfluent speech. Previous studies have shown that the scope of planning can be as large as a complex noun phrase (Allum & Wheeldon, 2007, 2009; Smith & Wheeldon, 1999; Wheeldon et al., 2013), up to the verb (Ferreira, 2000; Lindsley, 1975, 1976), or a sentential clause (Garrett, 1982; Ford, 1982; Meyer, 1996). Here we focused on two lines of evidence suggesting "verb-centered" and "clause-based" incrementality.

One line of evidence suggests that speakers must retrieve at least up to the verb lemma prior to speech onset (Ferreira, 2000; Lindsley, 1975, 1976; Kempen & Huijbers, 1983; Lee, Yoshida, & Thompson, submitted). For example, according to Ferreira (2000)'s TAG (tree-adjoining grammars) approach, the retrieval of a lexical head projects an elementary syntactic tree, including its head and argument slots (see also Levelt, 1989, 1999). When the lexical head is the verb, it projects a syntactic tree for the entire clause with its argument slots. As illustrated in Figure 17.6, the noun lemma (e.g., the first lemma, *John*) is selected and projects its maximal projection, an NP. However, because its grammatical function (i.e., subject or object) is unknown, building a sentence (S) node cannot occur. Only when the verb lemma is retrieved, with its NP argument slots, the sentence frame becomes apparent to the speaker and the retrieved NP can be attached to the tree (Ferreira, 2000). Accordingly, phonological encoding of the subject NP begins only after the verb lemma is retrieved. Importantly, the object does not need to be retrieved before phonological encoding begins. Rather, the object NP can be grammatically encoded during speech.

The results of several experimental studies (and paradigms) support the notion that verb information is accessed prior to articulation of the subject noun. For example, in an early study, Lindsley (1975) compared speech onset latencies associated with production of several different structures (i.e., S, SV, SVO), using the same set of action pictures with transitive verbs. When participants produced the subject noun only in an (S) form (e.g., "the man"), participants showed shorter speech onset latencies as compared to when they produced subject-verb (SV) utterances ("the man greets"), reflecting the time required for grammatical encoding of the subject and verb versus only the subject NP only. Further, results showed that when speech onset latencies for subject-verb (SV) and subject-verb-object (SVO) utterances were compared, no significant differences were found, indicating that object preplanning does not occur.

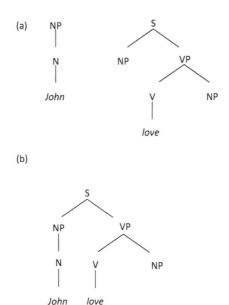

Figure 17.6 Illustration of structural verb-centered incrementality. Phonological encoding of the subject NP (*John*) begins only after the verb lemma is retrieved.

In another study, Kempen and Huijbers (1983) examined Dutch-speaking participants' production of subject-verb or verb-subject utterances in a two-part study. In each part participants used different verbs to describe the same depicted actions. The verb change resulted in increased speech onset latencies in both types of utterances, with a larger effect for verb-subject utterances compared to subject-verb utterances. These findings indicate that lexical processing of the verb occurs before speech onset, but that in the case of subject-verb utterances verb preplanning is incomplete, suggesting that the verb lemma, but not its form (lexeme), is selected before speech onset.

Another set of studies suggests that sentence planning occurs in clause-sized units; that is, that speakers plan not only the schematic structure of the clause but also retrieve all the lemmas prior to speaking (Garrett, 1976, 1980, 1982; Ford, 1978; Ford & Holmes, 1982, Meyer, 1996). Word exchange errors occurring within the same clause (e.g., "Did *the pupil* gave an A+ to *her*?" instead of "Did she give an A+ to the pupil?") suggest that, because the exchanged elements (words) are simultaneously available for insertion into the sentence, sentence planning proceeds in clause-sized units. Ford (1978), measuring pauses during narrative production as an indicator for the planning unit, found that speakers produce pauses at clausal boundaries. The tendency for speakers to repeat syntactic structures in natural conversation and in structural priming also support frame-based sentence production models (Bock, 1986). Lastly, Meyer (1996), using an auditory picture-word interference paradigm, asked participants to describe two objects using the frame "The A is next to B." Participants heard an auditory distracter that was semantically related to A or B. Semantic interference effects, as measured by increased speech onset times when the distractor word was related compared to unrelated, were found for both A and B, indicating that speakers retrieved the lemmas for the entire sentence prior to speech onset.

Recently, Lee and Thompson conducted a series of studies examining the time course of sentence planning in agramamtic speakers. Using the verb's syntactic information as part of advanced planning appears to be a critical process for sentence production in agrammatic aphasia, at least when sentences involve function assignment (Lee & Thompson, 2011a, 2011b; Lee, Yoshida, &

Thompson, submitted). In one study, Lee and Thompson (2011a) examined production of simple sentences with unergative and unaccusative verbs (e.g., "the black dog is *barking*" and "the black tube is *floating*," respectively). Using written words presented on a computer screen, as shown in Figure 17.7, eye movements to the words were recorded as speakers produced sentences. Results showed differential gaze patterns in the vicinity of the subject NP between conditions (i.e., parallel looks to the noun and adjective for unergative vs. sequential looks to the unaccusative). Given that unaccusative verbs have a more complex argument structure representation compared to unergative verbs, with a theme argument in the subject position, these eye gaze differences were taken to suggest increased difficulty in lexco-phrasal integration associated with unaccusative verbs. Interestingly, the different gaze patterns were significant before speech onset for agrammatic speakers, whereas the difference was significant after speech onset for healthy speakers. A parallel pattern was also found in Lee and Thompson (2011b), examining production of sentences with verb arguments (e.g., "the mother is applying lotion to the baby") and adjuncts (e.g., "the mother is choosing the lotion for the baby"). Their agrammatic speakers' eye movement patterns showed "normal" patterns of different processing between verb arguments and adjuncts, but they again showed the difference before speech onset, suggesting early use of verb information, while controls showed the difference during speech.

In a follow-up study using a lexical verb priming paradigm, Lee, Yoshida, and Thompson (submitted) examined whether verb argument structure (VAS) is encoded prior to speech onset or not. The study targeted production of simple active sentences using verbs with alternating transitivity (e.g., *roll*), which select for two argument structure options: either an agent, theme for a transitive sentence (e.g., "the man is rolling the tire") or a theme only for an unaccusatives frame (e.g., "the tire is rolling"). Production of these sentences was primed using nonalternating transitives (e.g., *fix*) and nonalternating unaccusative verbs (e.g., *bloom*). Both verb types have a single, obligatory argument structure, with nonalternating transitives selecting an agent, theme grid and nonalternating unaccusatives selecting only a theme. As illustrated in Figure 17.8, participants orally read the prime verb and then produced a target sentence describing what is happening in the picture. Each target sentence was elicited twice, following a consistent and an inconsistent VAS prime. Because prime verbs automatically activate the verb's argument structure (Shapiro et al., 1987, 1990; 1993; Friedmann et al., 2008, and others), it was predicted that if speakers encode VAS before speech onset, the preactivated argument structure of the prime verb would facilitate advanced planning processes, resulting in faster speech onset latencies as compared to the inconsistent prime verb condition.

Results showed that in both transitive and unaccusative target sentences, when the target picture was preceded by a consistent VAS prime, as opposed to an inconsistent VAS prime, agrammatic speakers showed significantly faster speech onset times, suggesting that they consistently encoded VAS before production. However, interestingly, both young and older cognitively healthy speakers showed significant VAS priming effects only for transitive sentences, but not for unaccusative

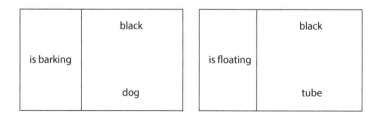

Figure 17.7   Stimuli used to study eye movements during unaccusative and unergative sentence production (from Lee & Thompson, 2011a).

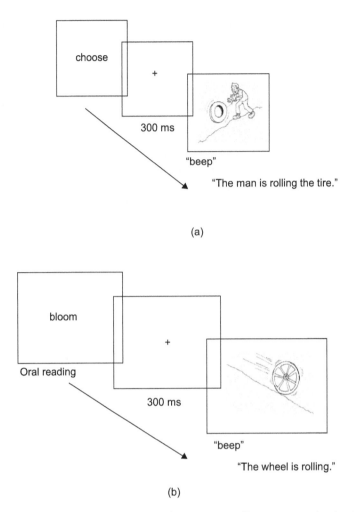

Figure 17.8 Sample trials, priming transitive (a) and unaccusatives (b) sentence production. From Lee, Yoshida, & Thompson (submitted).

sentences. In addition, as mentioned in the 'word-by-word incrementality' section above, the same agrammatic speakers followed word-by-word planning when they produced multiword utterances in a predefined sentence structure (Lee, Yoshida, & Thompson, submitted). These findings, together with the findings from Lee and Thompson (2011a, 2011b) suggest that agrammatic sentence production follows verb-centered grammatical encoding across various sentence types involving function assignment (Ferreira, 2000; Lindsley 1975, 1976; Kempen & Huijbers, 1983). However, for healthy speakers, encoding verb information is not an obligatory part of advanced grammatical encoding effects (Bock, 1987; Griffin & Bock, 2000; Griffin, 2001; Spieler & Griffin, 2006; Schriefers et al., 1998).

2.3 Morphophonological Encoding

Sentence production also requires morphological and phonological processes, which refer to a wide range of operations that finalize the grammatical elements of a sentence and their word structure (phonological form).

2.3.1 Morphological Encoding

Morphological encoding includes selection and retrieval of functional morphemes that not only convey elements of the message (such as negation, tense-aspect, and numerosity), but also fulfill intrasentential agreement (such as subject-verb and pronoun-antecedent) and language-specific well-formedness constraints (such as determiners for noun phrases in English). Additionally, there is some evidence that derivational morphemes are represented in decomposed form and thus could undergo composition during language production (e.g., Clahsen, Sonnenstuhl, & Blevins, 2003). Hence, morphological planning is at the interface of semantic, syntactic, and lexical processes: it includes a complex yet precise set of operations that output a complete, well-formed sentence conveying the speaker's intention.

Models of sentence production differ on the precise details of morphological encoding, and when it occurs during sentence production. However, there is consensus across models that these processes are considered to be at least somewhat distinct from lexical retrieval processes (Bock & Levelt, 1994; Chang et al., 2006; Garrett, 1980). For example, individuals with agrammatic aphasia show selective impairment of open-class versus closed-class (function) words in both spontaneous production and in reading (Biassou, Obler, Nespoulous, Dordain, & Harris, 1997; Friederici & Schonle, 1980; Gardner & Zurif, 1975; Nespoulous et al., 1988), supporting the distinction between words that serve lexical versus morphological functions. Morpheme stranding errors, such as "He has already *trunked* two *packs*" for "He has already packed two trunks," also suggest that lexical items and their morphological counterparts are inserted into the sentence structure at different time points (see also Lane & Ferreira, 2010).

The relationship between morphological and syntactic processes has been debated. While Garrett (1980, 1982, 1988) proposed that syntactic fragments are preloaded with morphological elements (e.g., "He has ____ ____ed ____ ____s"), Lapointe and Dell (1989) proposed that phrasal fragments only contain attachment sites for function words, but not function words themselves. They pointed out that word exchange errors such as "I'm sending *a brother* to my email" for "I'm sending *an* email to my brother" (from Dell & Sullivan, 2004) show adjustment for the phonological form of the determiner in the first noun phrase (*a brother* instead of *an brother* from the originally intended *an email*). Such phonological adjustments suggest initial retrieval of function word slots rather than the function words themselves. Further evidence for the relative independence of syntactic structure and morpheme retrieval comes from structural syntactic priming studies: while speakers are influenced by the syntactic structure of a preceding sentence (e.g., passive or double object dative), they do not reproduce functional morphemes of the prime sentence (Bock, 1982; Pickering & Branigan, 1998). For example, Bock (1989) tested whether closed class words are essential elements of syntactic structure by comparing the priming effects of double object datives, which can be produced by *to* or *for* ("The cheerleader offered/saved her friend a seat") and prepositional datives ("The cheerleader offered a seat to/saved a seat for her friend"). Speakers reproduced the syntactic structure (DO or PO), irrespective of the closed class element in the prime (*to* or *for*), suggesting the dissociation of sentence structure from morphological elements.

Findings from languages in which determiners are marked for gender and/or number suggest also that the process of selecting and inserting function words into syntactic frames is competitive (Janssen & Caramazza, 2003; Schriefers, 1993; Spalek & Schriefers, 2005). For example, Spalek and Schriefers (2005) elicited noun phrases (determiner plus noun) in Dutch. The key manipulation was the number of different determiners with which a noun could occur (e.g., *het* in singular, *de* in plural or *de* for both singular and plural). They found longer naming latencies for nouns that may occur with multiple determiners, suggesting the availability of, and competition between, different determiners.

The processes engaged in selection and retrieval of free and bound (inflectional) morphology also are likely distinct. Although most reports of agrammatic aphasia have found deficits in production of both (Saffran, Berndt, & Schwartz, 1989), there are reports of dissociations in aphasic individuals' ability to produce them (Miceli, Silyeri, Romani, & Caramazza, 1989; Rochon, Saffran, Berndt, & Schwartz, 2000; Saffran, Berndt, & Schwartz, 1989; Thompson, Fix, & Gitelman, 2002). For example, Thompson et al.'s (2002) participant was selectively impaired in production of inflectional morphemes, including plurals, past tense, and subject-verb agreement, but was unimpaired in production of function words such as auxiliaries and determiners. In addition, among inflected forms, numerous studies have reported greater vulnerability of morphological processes for tense marking compared to subject-verb agreement or auxiliary verb agreement (Clahsen & Ali, 2009; Faroqi-Shah & Thompson, 2007; Friedman & Grodzinsky, 1997; Kok, van Doorn, & Kolk, 2007; Nanousi, Masterson, Druks, & Atkinson, 2006).

2.3.1.1   Agreement Morphology

In English, grammatical agreement is most commonly implemented between pronouns and their antecedents (for gender, number, etc.) and between a verb and its subject. Agreement, especially subject-verb agreement, has been extensively examined, especially by eliciting attraction errors (Eberhard et al., 2005; Bock & Miller, 1991; Bock, Nicol, & Cutting, 1991; Vigliocco & Nicol, 1998; for bilinguals, see Hatzidaki, Branigan, & Pickering, 2011). Attraction errors refer to incorrect number marking on a pronoun or verb when the head noun and local noun differ in number features (e.g., "The key to the cabinets fell, didn't they?"). Bock (2004) describes three core facets of computation of agreement: meaning, marking, and morphing (see also Eberhard et al., 2005). Meaning denotes the elements of the message that need to be represented in the sentence, such as conceptual number (in the above example, the number of keys that actually fell). Such message elements were referred to as diacritical features in older models (Levelt, 1989). Marking is the process that transmits the abstract conceptual element onto the verb (or pronoun as the case may be), something like a short-term buffer. Bock and colleagues propose a marking process because conceptual number is not transparently indicated by verbs: *does* is not one instance of doing and *do* is not many doings or many persons doing something. Or an action that involves multiple movements (e.g., drumming) is not denoted by a plural affix (similarly the plural *you* may refer to one person or many people). Morphing is the process of ensuring that the final morphological expression of the verb (or pronoun) expresses the concept and is well-formed. The morphing process resolves any constraints imposed by the mental lexicon with the marking of the subject noun phrase and determines if the verb will be singular or plural.

2.3.1.2   Tense Morphology and Verb Regularity

Research on how speakers convey temporal information (tense and aspect) has been somewhat intertwined with issues concerning the representation of regular and irregular inflections because some past tense and past participle verbs are irregularly inflected in languages such as English and German. While accounts such as meaning, marking, and morphing can accommodate computation of tense inflection, the main contention is in how morphing differs for regular and irregular inflections. Single-mechanism models of inflectional morphology propose that the same kinds of probabilistic mappings between form (e.g., *sang, danced*) and meaning (past tense) are learned with exposure to language and are used for regular and irregular inflections (Joanisse & Seidenberg, 1992; Rumelhart & McClelland, 1986; Woollams, Joanisse, & Patterson, 2009). Dual-mechanism models propose differences in the lexical representations: regular verbs represent only the verb stem (e.g., *dance__*) and affixes (-*d, -s, -ing, -n*, etc.) are retrieved separately. In contrast, lexical entries of irregular verbs include a representation of the irregular verb form and verb stem (e.g., *sing__*, *sang*) (Clahsen, 1999; Pinker & Prince, 1991; Stemberger, 2004). Thus, regular inflections are produced by affixation and irregulars involve whole word access. Individual neuropsychological case studies have shown a dissociation between regular and irregular inflections (Marslen-Wilson & Tyler, 1997; Ullman et al., 1997), especially worse performance on irregulars for persons with lexical impairments such as semantic dementia (Almor et al., 2002), supporting dual-mechanism accounts. Cholin, Rapp, and Miozzo (2010) proposed a stem-based assembly (SAM) based on detailed analysis of a German-speaking aphasic person's productions, suggesting that affixes are activated during the production of both regular *and* irregularly inflected verbs. A competitive process and possibly a blocking mechanism ensures that irregular verbs are not over-regularized (e.g., *singed*).

2.3.2 Phonological Encoding

Phonological encoding refers to processes that intervene between identifying word(s) in the mental lexicon that can express one's message and the full phonetic description of the word(s) (Butterworth, 1992). Most authors agree that phonological encoding includes two distinct subprocesses: the first involves retrieval of a stored representation from the mental lexicon, referred as *phonological lexical representations* (PLR) by Butterworth (1992) and *lexemes* by others (Kempen and Huijbers, 1983; Levelt, 1989), as noted above (see section 2.2.1). This lexeme is thought to be abstract and minimally contain information about the syllabic structure and stress pattern of the word (Butterworth, 1992; Goldrick & Rapp, 2007; Levelt, 1989; Roelofs, 1997; Shattuck-Hufnagel, 1987). For example, the lexeme of *sheep* specifies that it is monomorphemic and consists of three phonological segments, /sh/, /i/, and /p/. Lexemes are also assumed to be underspecified in that they lack predictable (and therefore redundant) phonological patterns. For example, all nasal consonants are voiced in English, hence voicing for a nasal segment would not be specified in the lexeme. The second phonological subprocess is postlexical and involves elaborating the content of lexeme representations with predictable, rule-bound phonological processes such as voicing for nasal consonants and the allomorphic variation of plurals (s/z as in dogs/cats) in English. Postlexical planning yields a detailed phonetic description, which is later turned into a motor plan for articulation.

3   Conclusion

Cognitive models of sentence production have been significantly revised and refined since Garrett proposed the original framework in 1975. Despite numerous modifications, the basic tenets of ensuing speech production models remain largely unchanged, and include levels of processing, including abstract conceptualization of ideas to be expressed; grammatical encoding; and morphophonological processes. We have reviewed both psycholinguistic and neurolinguistic data supporting these processes. In particular, speech error data indicate that an impressively regular set of linguistic restrictions apply during sentence production. Further, experimental data in several domains support distinctions among processing levels and serve to elucidate the nature of component processes. Finally, patterns of breakdown and recovery of sentence production seen in individuals with aphasia, to the extent that they represent focal/discrete disruption of the normal language production system, further support the framework developed from studies of neurologically healthy persons. However, as should be evident from our discussion, there are several facets of each sentence production process that require further specification and elaboration. One crucial issue that needs further resolution is the temporal relationship between processing levels and the nature of interaction between them. Further, there is emerging evidence for the influence of cognitive processes on sentence production, including domain-general cognitive processes, such as executive functions, and attention- and domain-specific mechanisms, such as verbal working memory (Murray, Holland, & Beeson, 1998; Shao, Roelofs, & Meyer, 2012; Slevc, 2011).We anticipate that future sentence production models will incorporate this interplay between cognitive and linguistic processing. Further research of the type discussed here, as well as computational modeling and other innovative methods of experimentation, will lead to a greater understanding of the sentence production process.

Note

1 A paraphasic error produced by LS, a fluent aphasic speaker, studied by Thompson.

References

Allum, P. H., & Wheeldon, L. (2007). Planning scope in spoken sentence production: The role of grammatical units. *Journal of Experimental Psychology: Learning, Memory, and Cognition, 33*(4), 791–810.

Allum, P.H., & Wheeldon, L.R. (2009). Scope of lexical access in spoken sentence production: Implications for the conceptual–syntactic interface. *Journal of Experimental Psychology: Learning, Memory, and Cognition, 35*, 1240–1255.

Almor, A., Kempler, D., Anderson, E., MacDonald, M.C., Hayes, U.L., & Hintiryan, H. (2002). The production of regularly and irregularly inflected nouns and verbs in Alzheimer's and Parkinson's patients. *Brain and Language, 83*, 149–151.

Badecker, W., Miozzo, M., & Zanuttinni, R. (1995). The two-stage model of lexical retrieval: Evidence from a case of anomia with selective preservation of grammatical gender. *Cognition, 57*, 193–216.

Bastiaanse, R., & Jonkers, R. (1998). Verb retrieval in action naming and spontaneous speech in agrammatic and anomic aphasia. *Aphasiology, 12*(11), 951–969.

Bastiaanse, R., & van Zonneveld, R. (2005). Sentence production with verbs of alternating transitivity in agrammatic Broca's aphasia. *Journal of Neurolinguistics, 18*(1), 57–66.

Bates, E., & Devescovi, A. (1989). Crosslinguistic studies of sentence production. In B. MacWhinney & E. Bates (Eds.), *The crosslinguistic study of sentence processing.* Cambridge: Cambridge University Press.

Berndt, R.S., Haendiges, A.N., Mitchum, C.C., & Sandson, J. (1997). Verb retrieval in aphasia. 2. Relationship to sentence processing. *Brain and Language, 56*(1), 107–137.

Biassou, N., Obler, L.K., Nespoulous, J.L., Dordain, M., & Harris, K.S. (1997). Dual processing of open- and closed-class words. *Brain and Language*, 57(3), 360–373.

Bock, J. K. (1982). Toward a cognitive psychology of syntax: Information processing contributions to sentence formulation. *Psychological Review, 89*(1), 1.

Bock, J.K. (2004). Psycholinguistically speaking: Some matters of meaning, marking, and morphing. In B.H. Ross (Ed.), *The psychology of learning and motivation* (vol. 44, pp. 109–144). San Diego, CA: Elsevier.

Bock, K. (1977). The effect of a pragmatic presupposition on syntactic structure in question answering. *Journal of Verbal Learning and Verbal Behavior, 16*, 723–734.

Bock, K. (1986). Syntactic persistence in language production. *Cognitive Psychology, 18*, 355–387.

Bock, K. (1987). An effect of accessibility of word forms on sentence structures. *Journal and Memory and Language, 26*, 119–137.

Bock, K. (1989). Closed-class immanence in sentence production. *Cognition, 31*, 163–186.

Bock, K. (1990). Structure in language. *American Psychologist, 45*(11), 1221–1236.

Bock, K. (1995). Sentence production: From mind to mouth. In J.L. Miller & P.D. Eimas (Eds.), *Speech, language, and communication.* San Diego, CA: Academic Press.

Bock, K., Dell, G.S., Chang, F., & Onishi, K.H. (2007). Persistent structural priming from language comprehension to language production. *Cognition, 104*(3), 437–458.

Bock, K., Eberhard, K.M., & Cutting, J.C. (2004). Producing number agreement: How pronouns equal verbs. *Journal of Memory and Language, 51*(2), 251.

Bock, K., & Griffin, Z.M. (2000). The persistence of structural priming: Transient activation or implicit learning? *Journal of Experimental Psychology-General, 129*(2), 177–192.

Bock, K., & Levelt, W. (1994). Language production: Grammatical encoding. In M.A. Gernsbacher (Ed.), *Handbook of psycholinguistics.* San Diego, CA: Academic Press.

Bock, K., & Miller, C.A. (1991). Broken agreement. *Cognitive Psychology, 23*, 45–93.

Bock, K., Nicol, J. & Cutting, J.C. (1999). The ties that bind: Creating number agreement in speech. *Journal of Memory and Language, 40*, 330–346.

Bock, K., & Warren, R.K. (1985). Conceptual accessibility and syntactic structure in sentence formulation. *Cognition, 21*, 47–67.

Borer, H. (2005). *The normal course of events. Structuring sense*, vol. II. Oxford: Oxford University Press.

Branigan, H.P., Pickering, M.J., & Cleland, A.A. (2000). Syntactic co-ordination in dialogue. *Cognition, 75*, B13–B25.

Butterworth, B. (1992). Disorders of phonological encoding. *Cognition, 42*, 261–286.

Caramazza, A. (1997). How many levels of processing are there in lexical access? *Cognitive Neuropsychology, 14*, 177–208.

Caramazza, A., & Hillis, A.E. (1990). Where do semantic errors come from? *Cortex, 26*, 95–122.

Caramazza, A., & Miceli, G. (1991). Selective impairment of thematic role assignment in sentence processing. *Brain and Language, 41*, 402–436.

Caramazza, A., & Miozzo, M. (1997). The relation between syntactic and phonological knowledge in lexical access: Evidence from the tip-of-the-tongue phenomenon. *Cognition, 64*, 309–343.

Chang, F., Dell, G.S., & Bock, K. (2006). Becoming syntactic. *Psychological Review, 113*, 234–272.

Cho, S., & Thompson, C.K. (2010). What goes wrong during passive sentence production in agrammatic aphasia: An eyetracking study. *Aphasiology, 24*(12), 1576–1592.

Cholin, J., Rapp, B., & Miozzo, M. (2010). When do combinatorial mechanisms apply in the production of inflected words? *Cognitive Neuropsychology, 27*, 1–26.

Clahsen, H. (1999). Lexical entries and rules of language: A multidisciplinary study of German inflection. *Behavioral and Brain Sciences, 22*, 991–1060.

Clahsen, H., & Ali, M. (2009). Formal features in aphasia: Tense, agreement, and mood in English agrammatism. *Journal of Neurolinguistics, 22*, 436–450.

Clahsen, H., Sonnenstuhl, I., & Blevins, J.P. (2003). Derivational morphology in the German mental lexicon: A dual mechanism account In H.R. Baayen & R. Schreuder (Eds.), *Morphological structure in language processing* (Vol. 151, pp. 125–140). Berlin: Walter de Gruyter.

Cleland, A.A., & Pickering, M.J. (2003). The use of lexical and syntactic information in language production: Evidence from the priming of noun-phrase structure. *Journal of Memory and Language, 49*, 214–230.

Cutler, A. (1982). The reliability of speech error data. In A. Cutler (Ed.), *Slips of the tongue and language production*. Amsterdam: Mouton.

Dell, G. (1986). A spreading activation theory of retrieval in sentence production. *Psychological Review, 93*, 283–321.

Dell, G.S., & Reich, P.A. (1981). Stages in sentence production: An analysis of speech error data. *Journal of Verbal Learning and Behavior, 20*, 611–629.

Dell, G.S., Martin, N., & Schwartz, M.F. (2007). A case-series test of the interactive two-step model of lexical access: Predicting word repetition from picture naming. *Journal of Memory and Language, 56*(4), 490–520.

Dell, G.S., Schwartz, M.F., Martin, N., Saffran, E.M., & Gagnon, D.A. (1997). Lexical access in aphasic and nonaphasic speakers. *Psychological Review, 104*(4), 801–838.

Dell, G., & Sullivan, J.M. (2004). Speech errors and language production: Neuropsychological and connectionist perspectives. *The Psychology of Learning and Motivation, 44*, 63–108.

De Smedt, K. (1990). IPF: An incremental parallel formulator. In R. Dale, C. Mellish, & M. Zocks (Eds.), *Current research in natural language generation* (pp. 167–192). London: Academic Press.

De Smedt, K. (1996). Computational models of incremental grammatical encoding In A. Dijkstra & K. de Smedt (Eds.), *Computational psycholinguistics: AI and connectionist models of human language processing* (pp. 279–307). London: Taylor & Francis.

Dragoy, O., & Bastiaanse, R. (2010). Verb production and word order in Russian agrammatic speakers. *Aphasiology, 24*(1), 28–55.

Druks, J., & Carroll, E. (2005). The crucial role of tense for verb production. *Brain and Language, 94*, 1–18.

Eberhard, K.M., Cutting, J.C., and Bock, K. (2005). Making sense of syntax: Number agreement in sentence production. *Psychological Review, 112*, 531–559.

Edmonds, L.A., & Mizrahi, S. (2011). Online priming of agent and patient thematic roles and related verbs in younger and older adults. *Aphasiology, 25*(12), 1488–1506.

Faroqi-Shah, Y. (2012). Grammatical category deficits in bilingual aphasia. In M.R. Gitterman, M. Goral, & L.K. Obler (Eds.), *Aspects of multilingual aphasia*. Clevedon, UK: Multilingual Matters.

Faroqi-Shah, Y., & Thompson, C.K. (2003). Effect of lexical cues on the production of active and passive sentences in Broca's and Wernicke's aphasia. *Brain and Language, 85*(3), 409.

Faroqi-Shah, Y., & Thompson, C.K. (2007). Verb inflections in agrammatic aphasia: Encoding of tense features. *Journal and Memory and Language, 56*(1), 129–151.

Faroqi-Shah, Y., & Waked, A. (2010). Grammatical category dissociation in multilingual aphasia. *Cognitive Neuropsychology, 27,* 181–203. doi:10.1080/02643294.2010.509340

Fay, D., & Cutler, A. (1977). Malapropisms and the structure of the mental lexicon. *Linguistic Inquiry, 8,* 505–520.

Ferreira, F. (1994). Choice of passive verb is affected by verb type and animacy. *Journal of Memory and Language, 33,* 715–736.

Ferreira, F. (2000). Syntax in language production: An approach using tree-adjoining grammars. In L. Wheeldon (Ed.), *Aspects of language production* (pp. 291–330). Philadelphia: Psychology Press.

Ferreira, F., & Swets, B. (2002). How incremental is language production? Evidence from the production of utterances requiring the computation of arithmetic sums. *Journal of Memory and Language, 46*(1), 57–84.

Ferreira, V.S. (2010). Language production. *Wiley Interdisciplinary Reviews: Cognitive Science, 1*(6), 834–844.

Ferreira, V.S., Slevc, L.R., & Rogers, E.S. (2005). How do speakers avoid ambiguous linguistic expressions? *Cognition, 96*(3), 263–284.

Ferretti, T.R., McRae, K., & Hatherell, A. (2001). Integrating verbs, situation schemas and thematic role concepts. *Journal of Memory and Language, 44,* 516–547.

Fillmore, C.J. (1968). The case for case. In E. Bach & R.T. Harms (Eds.), *Universals in linguistic theory* (pp. 1–88). New York: Holt, Rinehart and Winston.

Fodor, J.A. (1983). *Modularity of mind.* Cambridge, MA: MIT Press.

Ford, M. (1978). *Planning units and syntax in sentence production* (Doctoral dissertation), University of Melbourne, Australia.

Ford, M. (1982). Sentence planning units: Implications for the speaker's representation of meaningful relations underlying sentences. In J. Bresnan (Ed.), *The mental representation of grammatical relations* (pp. 797–827). Cambridge, MA: MIT Press.

Foygel, D., & Dell, G.S. (2000). Models of impaired lexical access in speech production. *Journal of Memory and Language, 43*(2), 182–216.

Friederici, A.D., & Schnole, P.W. (1980). Computational dissociation of two vocabulary types. *Neuropsychologia, 13,* 181–190.

Friedmann, N., & Grodzinksy, Y. (1997). Tense and agreement in agrammatic production: Pruning the syntactic tree. *Brain and Language, 56*(3), 397.

Friedmann, N., Taranto, G., Shapiro, L.P., & Swinney, D. (2008). The leaf fell (the leaf): The online processing of unaccusatives. *Linguistic Inquiry, 39*(3), 355–377.

Fromkin, V.A. (1971). The non-anomalous nature of anomalous utterances. *Language, 47,* 27–52.

Gahl, S., Menn, L., Ramsberger, G., Jurafsky, D.S., Elder, E., Rewega, M., & Audrey, L.H. (2003). Syntactic frame and verb bias in aphasia: Plausibility judgments of undergoer-subject sentences. *Brain and Cognition, 53*(2), 223–228.

Gainotti, G., Miceli, G., Caltagirone, C., Silveri, C., & Masullo, C. (1981). Contiguity versus similarity of paraphasic substitutions in Broca's and in Wernicke's aphasia. *Journal of Communication Disorders, 14,* 1–9.

Gardner, H., & Zurif, E. (1975). *Bee* but not *be*: Oral reading of single words in aphasia and alexia. *Neuropsychologia, 13,* 181–190.

Garnham, A. (2010). Models of processing: Discourse. *Wiley Interdisciplinary Reviews: Cognitive Science, 1*(6), 845–853. doi:10.1002/wcs.69

Garrett, M.F. (1975). The analysis of sentence production. In G. Bower (Ed.), *Psychology of learning and motivation, Vol. 9.* New York: Academic Press.

Garrett, M.F. (1976). Syntactic processes in sentence production. In R.J. Wales & E.C.T. Walker (Eds.), *New approaches to language mechanisms* (pp. 231–256). Amsterdam: North Holland.

Garrett, M.F. (1980). Levels of processing in sentence production. In B. Butterworth (Ed.), *Language production.* London: Academic Press.

Garrett, M.F. (1982). Production of speech: Observations from normal and pathological language use. In A.W. Ellis (Ed.), *Normality and pathology of language functions.* London: Academic Press.

Garrett, M.F. (1988). Processes in language production. In N. Frederick (Ed.), *Linguistics: The Cambridge survey, Vol. 3.* Cambridge: Cambridge University Press.

Glaser, W.R. (1992). Picture naming. *Cognition, 42*(1–3), 61–105.

Glaser, W.R., & Dungelhoff, F.J. (1984). The time course of picture-word interference. *Journal of Experimental Psychology: Human Perception and Performance, 10,* 640–654.

Goldberg, A.E. (1995). *Constructions: A construction grammar approach to argument structure.* Chicago: University of Chicago Press.

Goldberg, A.E. (2003). Constructions: A new theoretical approach to language. *Trends in Cognitive Sciences, 7*(5), 219–224.

Goldman-Eisler, F. (1968). *Psycholinguistics: Experiments in spontaneous speech.* London and New York: Academic Press.

Goldrick, M., & Rapp, B. (2007). Lexical and post-lexical phonological representations in spoken production. *Cognition, 102,* 219–260.

Griffin, Z.M. (2001). Gaze durations during speech reflect word selection and phonological encoding. *Cognition, 82,* B1–B14.

Griffin, Z.M. (2004). Why look? Reasons for eye movements related to language production. In F. Ferreira & J.M. Henderson (Eds.), *The interface of language, vision, and action: Eye movements and the visual world* (pp. 213–247). New York: Psychology Press.

Griffin, Z.M., & Bock, K. (2000). What the eyes say about speaking. *Psychological Science, 11,* 274–279.

Griffin, Z.M., & Crew, C. (2012). Research in language production. In M. Spivey, M. Joinisse, & K. McRae (Eds.), *Cambridge handbook of psycholinguistics* (pp. 409–425). New York: Cambridge University Press.

Griffin, Z. M., & Mouzon, S. S. (2004). Can speakers order a sentence's arguments while saying it? Poster presented at the 17th Annual CUNY Sentence Processing Conference in College Park, Maryland.

Griffin, Z.M., & Spieler, D.H. (2006). Observing the what and when of language production for different age groups by monitoring speakers' eye movements. *Brain and Language, 99,* 272–288.

Grimshaw, J. (1990). *Argument structure.* Cambridge, MA: MIT Press.

Hashimoto, N., & Thompson, C.K. (2009). The use of the picture–word interference paradigm to examine naming abilities in aphasic individuals. *Aphasiology, 24*(5), 580–611. doi:10.1080/02687030902777567

Hatzidaki, A., Branigan, H.P., & Pickering, M.J. (2011). Co-activation of syntax in bilingual language production. *Cognitive Psychology, 62*(2), 123–150.

Janssen, N., & Caramazza, A. (2003). The selection of closed-class words in noun phrase production: The case of Dutch determiners. *Journal of Memory and Language, 48*(3), 635–652. doi:http://dx.doi.org/10.1016/S0749-596X(02)00531-4

Jescheniak, J.D., & Schriefers, E. (1998). Discrete serial versus cascaded processing in lexical access in speech production: Further evidence from coactivation of near-synonyms. *Journal of Experimental Psychology, 24,* 1256–1274.

Joanisse, M.F., & Seidenberg, M.S. (1999). Impairments in verb morphology after brain injury: A connectionist model. *Proceedings of the National Academy of Sciences, 96,* 7592–7597.

Kay, J., & Ellis, A. (1987). A cognitive neuropsychological case study of anomia: Implications for psychological models of word retrieval. *Brain, 110,* 613–629.

Kegl, J. (1995). Levels of representation and units of access relevant to agrammatism. *Brain and Language, 50,* 151–200.

Kemmerer, D., & Tranel, D. (2000). Verb retrieval in brain-damaged subjects: 1. Analysis of stimulus, lexical, and conceptual factors. *Brain and Language, 73*(3), 347–392.

Kempen, G., & Hoenkamp, E. (1987). An incremental procedural grammar for sentence formulation. *Cognitive Science, 11,* 201–258.

Kempen, G., & Huijbers, P. (1983). The lexicalization process in sentence production and naming: Indirect election of words. *Cognition, 14,* 185–209.

Kim, M., & Thompson, C.K. (2000). Verb retrieval in agrammatism. *Brain and Language, 74,* 1–25.

Kim, M., & Thompson, C.K. (2004). Verb deficits in Alzheimer's disease and agrammatism: Implications for lexical organization. *Brain and Language, 88,* 1–20.

Kiss, K. (2000). Effects of verb complexity on agrammatic aphasic's sentence production. In R. Bastiaanse & Y. Gordzinsky (Eds.), *Grammatical disorders in aphasia.* London: Whurr Publishers./

Kok, P., van Doorn, A., & Kolk, H. (2007). Inflection and computational load in agrammatic speech. *Brain and Language, 102*(3), 273–283.

Konopka, A.E. (2012). Planning ahead: How recent experience with structures and words changes the scope of linguistic planning. *Journal of Memory and Language, 66*(1), 143–162. doi:http://dx.doi.org/10.1016/j.jml.2011.08.003

Lane, L., & Ferreira, V.S. (2010). Abstract syntax in sentence production: Evidence from stem-exchange errors. *Journal of Memory and Language, 62,* 151–165.

LaPointe, S.G., & Dell, G.S. (1989). A synthesis of some recent work in sentence production. In N. Carlson & M.K. Tanenhaus (Eds.), *Linguistic structure in language processing.* Dordrecht: Kluwer Academic Publishers.

Lee, E.-K., Brown-Schmidt, S., & Watson, D.G. (2013). Ways of looking ahead: Hierarchical planning in language production. *Cognition, 129*(3), 544–562.

Lee, J., & Thompson, C.K. (2011a). Real-time production of unergative and unaccusative sentences in normal and agrammatic speakers: An eyetracking study. *Aphasiology, 25*(6–7), 813–825.

Lee, J., & Thompson, C.K. (2011b). Real-time production of arguments and adjuncts in normal and agrammatic speakers. *Language and Cognitive Processes, 26*(8), 985–1021.

Levelt, W. (1989). *Speaking: From intention to articulation.* Cambridge, MA: MIT Press.

Levelt, W. (1993). Language use in normal speakers and its disorders. In G. Blanken, J. Dittman, H. Grimm, J.C. Marshall, & C.-W. Wallesh (Eds.), *Linguistic disorders and pathologies.* Berlin: Walter de Gruyter.

Levelt, W. (1999). Producing spoken language: A blueprint of the speaker. In C.M. Brown & P. Hagoort (Eds.), *The neurocognition of language.* New York: Oxford University Press.

Lindsley, J.R. (1975). Producing simple utterances: How far ahead do we plan? *Cognitive Psychology, 7*(1), 1–19.

Lindsley, J.R. (1976). Producing simple utterances: Details of the planning process. *Journal of Psycholinguistic Research, 5*(4), 331–354.

Luzzatti, C., Raggi, R., Zonca, G., Pistarini, C., Contardi, A., & Pinna, G.-D. (2002). Verb-noun double dissociation in aphasic lexical impairments: The role of word frequency and imageability. *Brain and Language, 81*, 432–444.

Mack, J.E., Cho-Reyes, S., Kloet, J.D., Weintraub, S., Mesulam, M.M., & Thompson, C.K. (2013). Phonological facilitation of object naming in agrammatic and logopenic primary progressive aphasia (PPA). *Cognitive Neuropsychology, 30*(3), 172–193.

Marslen-Wilson, W.D., & Tyler, L.K. (1997). Dissociating types of mental computation. *Nature, 387*(6633), 592–594.

Martin, N., Dell, G.S., Saffran, E.M., & Schwartz, M.F. (1994). Origins of paraphasia in deep dysphasia: Testing the consequences of a decay impairment to an interactive spreading activation model of lexical retrieval. *Brain and Language, 47*, 609–660.

Martin, R.C., & Blossom-Stach, C. (1986). Evidence of syntactic deficits in a fluent aphasic. *Brain and Language, 28*(2), 196–234.

Mätzig, S., Druks, J., Masterson, J., & Vigliocco, G. (2009). Noun and verb differences in picture naming: Past s/tudies and new evidence. *Cortex, 45*(6), 738–758.

McDonald, J.L., Bock, K., & Kelly, M.H. (1993). Word and word order: Semantic, phonological, and metrical determinants of serial position. *Cognitive Psychology, 25*, 188–230.

McRae, K., Hare, M., Elman, J.L., & Ferretti, T. (2005). A basis for generating expectancies for verbs from nouns. *Memory and Cognition, 33*(7), 1174–1184.

Meyer, A. S. (1996). Lexical access in phrase and sentence production: results from picture-word interference experiments. *Journal of Memory and Language, 35*, 477–496.

Meyer, A.S., & Lethaus, F. (2004). The use of eye tracking in studies of sentence generation. In J.M. Henderson & F. Ferreira (Eds.), *The interface of language, vision, and action: Eye movements and the visual world* (pp. 191–211). New York: Psychology Press.

Miceli, G., Silveri, C., Romani, C., & Caramazza, A. (1989). Variation in the pattern of omissions and substitutions of grammatical morphemes in the spontaneous speech of so-called agrammatic patients. *Brain and Language, 36*, 447–492.

Murray, L.L., Holland, A.L., & Beeson, P.M. (1998). Spoken language of individuals under focused and divided attention conditions. *Journal of Speech, Language and Hearing Research, 41*, 213–227.

Nanousi, V., Masterson, J., Druks, J., & Atkinson, M. (2006). Interpretable vs. uninterpretable features: Evid/ence from six Greek-speaking agrammatic patients. *Journal of Neurolinguistics, 19*(3), 209–238.

Nespoulous, J.-L., Dordain, M., Perron, C., Ska, B., Bub, D., Caplan, D., Mehler, J., & Lecours, A.R. (1988). Agrammatism in sentence production without comprehension deficits: Reduced availability of syntactic structures and/or of grammatical morphemes? A case study. *Brain and Language, 33*, 273–295.

Nozari, N., Kittredge, A.K., Dell, G.S., & Schwartz, M.F. (2010). Naming and repetition in aphasia: Steps, routes, and frequency effects. *Journal of Memory and Language, 63*(4), 541–559. Do/i:10.1016/j.jml.2010.08.001

Petrie, H. (1987). The psycholinguistics of speaking. In J. Lyons, R. Coates, M. Deuchar, & G. Gazdar (Eds.), *New Horizons in Linguistics* (pp. 336–367). New York: Penguin.

Pickering, M.J. & Branigan, H.P. (1998). The representation of verbs: Evidence from syntactic priming in language production. *Journal of Memory and Language, 39*, 633–651.

Pinker, S. (1989). *Learnability and cognition: The acquisition of argument structure.* Cambridge: The MIT Press.

Pinker, S., & Prince, A. (1991). Regular and irregular morphology and the psychological status of rules of grammar. *Berkeley Linguistics Society, 17*, 230–251.

Poncelet, M., Majerus, S., Raman, I., Warginaire, S., & Weekes, B.S. (2007). Naming actions and objects in bilingual aphasia: A multiple case study. *Brain and Language, 103*, 158–159.

Potter, M.C., & Lombardi, L. (1998). Syntactic priming in immediate recall of sentences. *Journal of Memory and Language, 38*, 265–282.

Ramchand, G.C. (2008). *Verb meaning and the lexicon: A first phase syntax.* Cambridge: Cambridge University Press.

Rapp, B., & Goldrick, M. (2000). Discreteness and interactivity in spoken word production. *Psychological Review, 107,* 460–499.

Rochon, E., Saffran, E.M., Berndt, R.S., & Schwartz, M.F. (2000). Quantitative analysis of aphasic sentence production: Further developments and new data. *Brain and Language, 72,* 193–218.

Roelofs, A. (1992). A spreading-activation theory of lemma retrieval in speaking. *Cognition, 42*(1–3), 107–142.

Roelofs, A. (1997). The WEAVER model of word-form encoding in speech production. *Cognition, 64*(3), 249–284.

Rumelhart, D., & McClelland, J. (1986). On learning the past tenses of English verbs: Implicit rules or parallel distributed processing. In D. Rumelhart & J. McClelland (Eds.), *Parallel distribute processing: Explorations in the microstructure of cognition.* Cambridge, MA: MIT Press.

Saffran, E.M., Berndt, R.S., & Schwartz, M.F. (1989). The quantitative analysis of agrammatic production: Procedure and data. *Brain and Language, 37*(3), 440–479.

Saffran, E.M., Schwartz, M.F., & Marin, O.S.M. (1980). The word order problem in agrammatism II: Production. *Brain and Language, 10,* 263–280.

Schriefers, H. (1990). Syntactic processes in the production of noun phrases. *Journal of Experimental Psychology: Learning, Memory, and Cognition, 19*(4), 841–885.

Schriefers, H., Meyer, A.S., & Levelt, W.J.M. (1990). Exploring the time course of lexical access in speech production: Results from picture-word interference experiments. *Journal of Memory and Language, 29,* 86–102.

Schriefers, H., Teruel, E., & Meinshausen, R.M. (1998). Producing simple sentences: Results from picture–word interference experiments. *Journal of Memory and Language, 39*(4), 609–632. doi:http://dx.doi.org/10.1006/jmla.1998.2578

Schwartz, M.F. (1987). Patterns of speech production deficit within and across aphasia syndromes: Application of a psycholinguistic model. In M. Coltheart, G. Sartori, & R. Job (Eds.), *The cognitive neuropsychology of language.* Hillsdale, NJ: Lawrence Erlbaum.

Schwartz, M.F., D/ell, G.S., Martin, N., Gahl, S., & Sobel, P. (2006). A case-series test of the interactive two-step model of lexical access: evidence from picture naming. *Journal of Memory and Language, 54,* 228–264.

Shao, Z., Roelofs, A., & Meyer, A.S. (2012). Sources of individual differences in the speed of naming objects and actions: The contribution of executive control. *Quarterly Journal of Experimental Psychology, 65*(10), 1927–1944.

Shapiro, L. P., Gordon, B., Hack, N., & Killackey, J. (1993). Verb-argument structure processing in complex sentences in Broca's and Wernicke's aphasia. *Brain and Language, 45*(3), 423–447.

Shapiro, L., & Levine, B.A. (1990). Verb processing during sentence comprehension in aphasia. *Brain and Language, 38*(1), 21–47.

Shapiro, L., Zurif, E., & Grimshaw, J. (1987). Sentence processing and mental representation of verbs. *Brain and Language, 27,* 219–246.

Shattuck-Hufnagel, S. (1987). The role of word onset consonants in speech production planning: New evidence form speech error patterns. In E. Keller & M. Gopnik (Eds.), *Motor and sensory processing in language* (pp. 17–51). Hillsdale, NJ: Erlbaum.

Slevc, L.R. (2011). Saying what's on your mind: Working memory effects on sentence production. *Journal of Experimental Psychology. Learning, Memory, and Cognition, 37*(6), 6–37.

Smith, M., & Wheeldon, L. (1999). High level processing scope in spoken sentence production. *Cognition, 73,* 205–246.

Spalek, K., & Schriefers, H.J. (2005). Dominance affects determiner selection in language production. *Journal of Memory and Language, 52*(1), 103–119. doi:http://dx.doi.org/10.1016/j.jml.2004.09.001

Spieler, D.H., & Griffin, Z.M. (2006). The influence of age on the time course of word preparation in multiword utterances. *Language and Cognitive Processes, 21,* 291–321.

Stemberger, J.P. (1995). Phonological and lexical constraints on morphological processing. In L.B. Feldman (Ed.), *Morphological aspects of language processing.* Hillsdale, NJ: Lawrence Erlbaum.

Stemberger, J.P. (2004). Phonological priming and irregular past. *Journal of Memory and Language, 50*(1), 82–95.

Thompson, C.K. (2003). Unaccusative verb production in agrammatic aphasia: The argument structure complexity hypothesis. *Journal of Neurolinguistics, 16,* 151–167.

Thompson, C.K., Cho, S., Price, C., Wieneke, C., Bonakdarpour, B., Rogalski, E., . . . Mesulam, M.M. (2012). Semantic interference during object naming in agrammatic and logopenic primary progressive aphasia (PPA). *Brain and Language, 120,* 237–250.

Thompson, C.K., Fix, S., & Gitelman, D. (2002). Selective impairment of morphosyntactic production in a neurological patient. *Journal of Neurolinguistics, 15*, 189–207.

Thompson, C.K., & Lee, M. (2009). Psych verb production and comprehension in agrammatic Broca's aphasia. *Journal of Neurolinguistics, 22*(4), 354–369.

Thompson, C.K., Riley, E., den Ouden, D., Meltzer-Asscher, A., & Lukic, S. (2013). Training verb argument structure production in agrammatic aphasia: Behavioral and neural recovery patterns. *Cortex, 48*(9), 2358–2376.

Ullman, M.T., Corkin, S., Coppola, M., & Hickok, G. (1997). A neural dissociation within language: Evidence that the mental dictionary is part of declarative memory, and that grammatical rules are processed by the procedural system. *Journal of Cognitive Neuroscience, 9*, 266–276.

van de Velde, M., Meyer, A.S., & Konopka, A.E. (2014). Message formulation and structural assembly: Describing "easy" and "hard" events with preferred and dispreferred syntactic structures. *Journal of Memory and Language, 71*(1), 124–144

Vigliocco, G., Antonini, T., & Garrett, M.F. (1997). Grammatical gender is on the tip of Italian tongues. *Psychological Science, 8*, 314–317.

Vigliocco, G., & Nicol, J. (1998). Separating hierarchical relations and word order in language production: Is proximity concord syntactic or linear? *Cognition, 68*, B13–B29.

Wheeldon, L., Ohlson, N., Ashby, A., & Gator, S. (2013). Lexical availability and grammatical encoding scope during spoken sentence production. *Quarterly Journal of Experimental psychology: QJEP (Hove), 66*(8), 1653–1673.

Woollams, A.M., Joanisse, M., & Patterson, K. (2009). Past-tense generation from form versus meaning: Behavioural data and simulation evidence. *Journal of Memory and Language, 61*(1), 55–76.

18

THE NEURAL BASIS OF SYNTACTIC PROCESSING

A Critical Review

David Caplan

Sentences convey relationships between the meanings of words, such as who is accomplishing an action or receiving it. This "propositional content" of a sentence is crucial to many human intellectual functions. Without propositions, language would consist of designating items, actions, and properties of items and actions—a far less rich functional capacity than what language consists of because it includes propositions.

Syntax is a system of formal rules that allows sentences to convey relationships between words in a flexible manner that allows unlikely or impossible relationships to be expressed (Chomsky, 1965, 1981, 1986, 1995). Without such a capacity, sets of words would always be understood to refer to the most likely situation; for instance, the set of words "man, dog, bite" would always be associated with the proposition that a dog is biting a man. The ability to express and manipulate unlikely or counterfactual propositions—such as that a man is biting a dog—depends on syntax and is critical to much human thinking. For instance, it underlies the ability to reason hypothetically, which is the basis for science, estimating outcomes, and much planning in everyday life. Thus syntax is a critical human cognitive capacity.

There is near universal agreement that syntactic structures are constructed from semantic and pragmatic representations as part of the production of spoken, written, and signed language and from lexical, prosodic, and other perceptual cues in comprehension (for different models of the parsing process, see Frazier & Clifton, 1996; Just & Carpenter, 1992; MacDonald, Pearlmutter, & Seidenberg, 1994; for discussion of the process of constructing syntactic structures in speech production, see Levelt, 1989; Bock & Levelt, 1994). The neural basis for syntactic processing may differ in these different tasks. In this review, I shall deal with studies of comprehension, because it is the domain in which the most studies have been done.

The 13 years since the publication of the first edition of this book have seen a few studies of deficit-lesion correlations and a large number of fMRI and ERP studies of syntactic processing. It is not possible to review all the new important studies that have been published since 2002. In this chapter, I present and comment on what I consider to be some of the most important new themes in this work.

The Gross Functional Neuroanatomy of Syntactic Processing in Language Comprehension

There is good evidence that syntactic processing in sentence comprehension involves the perisylvian association cortex—the pars triangularis and opercularis of the inferior frontal gyrus

(Brodmann's areas [BA] 45 and 44: Broca's area), the angular gyrus (BA 39), the supramarginal gyrus (BA 40), and the superior temporal gyrus (BA 22: Wernicke's area)—in the dominant hemisphere. Data regarding the functional neuroanatomy of syntactic comprehension were originally derived from deficit-lesion correlations and, more recently, come from functional neuroimaging and electrophysiological studies in normal subjects. All these sources of data indicate that the perisylvian association cortex is involved in this function.

Patients with lesions in parts of this cortex have been described who have had long-lasting impairments of this function (Caramazza & Zurif, 1976). We have estimated that over 90 percent of patients with aphasic disorders who have lesions in this region have disturbances of syntactic comprehension (Caplan, 1987). Disorders affecting syntactic comprehension after perisylvian lesions have been described in all languages that have been studied, in patients of all ages, with written and spoken input, and after a variety of lesion types, indicating that this cortical region is involved in syntactic processing, independent of these factors (see Caplan, 1987, for review). Functional neuroimaging studies have documented increases in regional cerebral blood flow (rCBF) using positron emission tomography (PET) or blood oxygenation level dependent (BOLD) signal using functional magnetic resonance imaging (fMRI) in tasks in which subjects' processing of more versus less syntactically complex sentences was compared (Stromswold et al., 1996; Caplan et al., 1998, 1999, 2000; Just et al., 1996; Dapretto & Bookheimer, 1999; Stowe et al., 1998; others, see below). Event-related potentials (ERPs) whose sources are likely to be in this region (the left anterior negativity [LAN], see below) have been described in relation to a variety of syntactic processes, including responses to category and agreement violations, comprehension of complex relative clauses, and others (Kluender & Kutas, 1993a, 1993b; Neville, Nical, Barss, Forster, & Garret, 1991; others, see below). These data all converge on the conclusion that syntactic processing in comprehension is carried out in the dominant perisylvian cortex.

Caplan et al. (2007b) found that lesions in two regions outside the perisylvian association cortex—the left superior parietal lobe and the left anterior inferior temporal cortex—were associated with deficits in syntactic comprehension. Evidence for the involvement of nonperisylvian regions in syntactic processing also comes from functional neuroimaging and ERP studies. Mazoyer and colleagues (1993) found increased rCBF in the anterior left temporal lobe when subjects heard stories in French, in French with all the content words replaced with nonwords, or a French story in which every content word was replaced with a semantically unrelated word from the same grammatical category, compared to when they listened to stories in a language they did not know (Tamil) or to lists of words. Bavelier and colleagues (1997) found increased BOLD signal in anterior temporal, as well as perisylvian, cortex when subjects read sentences compared to reading word lists. More-controlled activation studies of syntactic processing have also activated nonperisylvian regions. The cingulate gyrus and nearby regions of medial frontal lobe have shown increased blood flow when subjects process syntactically more complex sentences (Caplan et al., 1998, 1999, 2000). In several studies (Caplan et al., 1998; Carpenter, Just, Keller, Eddy, & Thulborn, 1999), there has been activation in superior parietal lobe in syntactic tasks. The involvement of the superior parietal lobe in syntactic processing is supported by electrophysiological data (event-related potentials), to be discussed later. Noppeney and Price (2004) reported BOLD signal priming effects (priming-related deactivation) of sentence structure in a memory task in the left anterior inferior temporal lobe, and argued that syntactic processing took place in that area.

The nondominant hemisphere may also be involved in syntactic comprehension. We found that 14 patients with nondominant hemisphere lesions showed effects of syntactic complexity on performance in an enactment task, which were independent of sentence length (Caplan, Hildebrandt, & Makris, 1996). Just and colleagues (1996) reported activation results supporting a role for nondominant hemisphere homologues of Broca's and Wernicke's areas in syntactic comprehension; these areas increased their BOLD signal in response to processing syntactically complex sentences, though to a lesser extent than Broca's and Wernicke's areas themselves. Ben-Shachar et al. (2003) found activation in both left and right superior temporal gyrus in response to comprehension of sentences with syntactic movement. The nondominant hemisphere appears to support some aspect of syntactic comprehension.

Finally, it has been suggested that subcortical structures involved in laying down procedural memories for motor functions—in particular, the basal ganglia—are involved in "rule-based" processing in language (Ullman, Corkin, et al., 1997, Ullman, Bergida, et al., 1997). Data on the role of these structures in rule-based processes have come largely from studies of morphological processes. However, some fMRI studies have shown activation of basal ganglia in paradigms that highlight syntactic comprehension (e.g., Fiebach et al., 2004, at the level of a trend). Lesions in the cerebellum have been associated with expressive agrammatism (DeSmet et al., 2007), but not with syntactic comprehension deficits to my knowledge.

The Functional Organization of the Perisylvian Association Cortex for Syntactic Processing

A major focus of investigation has been how the perisylvian association cortex is organized to support syntactic comprehension. Different researchers endorse strongly localizationist models (Grodzinsky, 1990, 1995, 2000; Swinney & Zurif, 1995; Zurif, Swinney, Prather, Solomon, & Bushell, 1993), distributed net models (Damasio, 1992; Mesulam, 1990, 1998), and models that postulate individual variability in the neural substrate for this function (Caplan, 1987a, 1994; Caplan, Baker, & Dehaut, 1985, 1996). Localizationist models have focused on Broca's area as the locus of all or part of syntactic processing. Distributed models have argued that the entire perisylvian association cortex constitutes a neural net in which this function takes place, although some theorists who have developed these models have also maintained that, within this net, Broca's area plays a more important role than other regions (e.g., Mesulam, 1990, 1998). Researchers who postulate individual variability maintain that different individuals use different parts of this cortex to process syntax or different parts of syntax. Data from both deficit-lesion correlation and functional neuroimaging studies bear on these models.

Deficit-Lesion Correlation Studies

Deficits in syntactic comprehension are identified by a patient being able to understand sentences whose meanings correspond to the most likely combination of word meanings (e.g., 1), but not sentences whose meanings depend on the ability to assign syntactic structure (e.g., 2):

1. The apple the boy is eating is red.
2. The girl the boy is chasing is tall.

In most studies, patients with these deficits are able to understand simple syntactic structures (e.g., in English, ones in which thematic roles are assigned in a strictly linear ["canonical"] order, as in 3):

3. The boy is chasing the girl who is tall.

Several studies have reported correlations between lesions seen in radiological images and deficits in syntactic comprehension deficits in aphasic stroke victims.

Caplan et al. (1996) studied 18 patients with left hemisphere strokes. Five perisylvian regions of interest were defined on CT scans following the Rademacher et al. (1992) criteria: the pars triangularis and the pars opercularis of the third frontal convolution; the supramarginal gyrus;

the angular gyrus; and the first temporal gyrus, excluding the temporal tip and Heschl's gyrus. Syntactic comprehension was assessed using an object manipulation task presenting 12 examples of each of 25 sentence types. Neither overall accuracy on the 25 sentence types, nor a syntactic complexity score, nor 19 separate measures that correspond to particular syntactic operations differed in groups defined by lesion location. None of 168 correlations between overall accuracy on the entire set of 25 sentence types, overall syntactic complexity score, the 19 separate measures of particular syntactic operations and normalized lesion volume in the language zone, normalized lesion volume in each of the five regions of interest, and normalized lesion volume in the anterior and posterior regions of interest were significant. These correlations remained insignificant when the effect of overall lesion size was partialled out in stepwise regression analyses. The results all remained unchanged in 10 patients who were studied and scanned at about the same time relative to their lesions. Caplan et al. (1996) concluded that the syntactic operations examined in this study were not invariantly localized in one small area, but were either distributed or showed variability in localization.

Dronkers et al. (2004) studied 64 patients with left hemisphere strokes as well as 8 right hemisphere stroke cases and 15 controls. The patients were tested on the Western Aphasia Battery (WAB) and the Curtiss-Yamada Comprehensive Language Evaluation (CYCLE) for sentence comprehension. A voxel-based lesion-symptom mapping (VLSM) approach to analysis of the data was reported. The performance of patients with and without lesions in five areas of the left hemisphere—the middle temporal gyrus; the anterior superior temporal sulcus; the superior temporal sulcus; the angular gyrus, midfrontal cortex (said to be in Brodmann area 46); and Brodmann area 47—differed on the total CYCLE score. The authors suggested that the middle temporal gyrus was involved with lexical processing, the anterior superior temporal sulcus with comprehension of simple sentences, the superior temporal sulcus and the angular gyrus with short-term memory, and the left frontal cortex with working memory required for complex sentences. They concluded that neither Broca's area nor Wernicke's area contributes to sentence comprehension and that the apparent involvement of these regions in previous studies was due to the role that adjacent cortex plays in these processes. This study suffers the limitations that no indication was given of how regions of interest were defined; normals performed at ceiling on all subtests of the CYCLE, so all the lesions were associated with abnormal performance on all tests, and errors in which lexical foils were selected were not excluded from the analysis. The absence of an effect of lesions in Broca's and Wernicke's areas thus only shows that patients with lesions in these areas are not more affected on language comprehension than patients whose lesions spare these areas, not that patients with lesions in these areas are not impaired relative to normal individuals.

Caplan et al. (2007b) imaged 32 patients and 13 controls using MR and FDG PET scanning. Participants were tested for the ability to understand 10 examples of each of 11 sentence types using three tasks—sentence-picture matching, grammaticality judgment, and object manipulation, the first two with both spoken whole sentence and self-paced listening presentation. Accuracy, reaction time (RT), and listening times for words in critical positions served as measures of syntactic processing ability. The range of performance on five measures in patients with lesions within 0.25 SD of the mean lesion size in four regions—the entire left hemisphere; the left hemisphere cortex; the perisylvian association cortex; and the combination of the perisylvian association cortex, the inferior anterior temporal lobe, and the superior parietal lobe—was almost as great as in the entire aphasic group; for one measure, the entire range of performance was found. Conversely, the range of lesion sizes in these four regions in patients whose performance fell within 0.25 SD of the mean performance on these measures covered a wide portion of the range of percent of region lesioned in all cases. These results argue against models that maintain that syntactic operations are distributed across large contiguous brain areas, such as the left hemisphere cortex or the perisylvian association cortex. Regression analyses showed that percent lesion volume on MR and mean

PET counts/voxel in a variety of small regions accounted for a significant amount of variance in individual performance measures, after total lesion size was entered into stepwise regressions. For instance, percent MR lesion in the inferior parietal lobe, the anterior inferior temporal lobe, and the superior parietal lobe and PET counts/voxel in Broca's area accounted for a significant amount of variance in first factor scores for all tasks combined and for object manipulation, suggesting that several areas are necessary for processing the same syntactic structure. Some areas, such as the anterior inferior temporal region, were significant in several tasks, implying that some cortical areas are necessary for multiple functions.

Thothathiri et al. (2012) reported the results of voxel-based deficit-lesion mapping and a region of interest analysis of accuracy on a sentence-picture matching task with five examples of each of six syntactic structures in 79 aphasic patients. Performance on both sentences with canonical and noncanonical word order correlated with lesion extent in left temporoparietal cortex, and the effects remained significant after performance on rhyme probe recognition and nonword repetition were used as covariates (to control for short-term memory). The difference between sentences with the canonical and noncanonical word order correlated with lesion size in Brodmann area 39. The authors concluded that left temporoparietal cortex plays a critical role in comprehending semantically reversible sentences. The study is limited by the small number of sentences of each type that were presented. In contrast to Thothathiri et al. (2012), Tyler et al. (2010) found the lesion size in left Brodmann area 45/47 correlated with performance of 14 aphasic patients on a sentence-picture matching task with reversible sentences that could not be understood using heuristics.

To summarize these reports, there is evidence from deficit-lesion correlations that syntactically based comprehension is not widely distributed but relies on small areas within the left perisylvian association cortex, as well as some other brain regions, such as the left inferior anterior temporal lobe. The lesion-deficit correlation data also argue against narrow localizationist models. The fact that lesions throughout the perisylvian cortex are associated with particular syntactic processing deficits is incompatible with invariant localization of syntactic processing in all normal adults. The data are most compatible with an individual variability model, and constitute the main reason that we postulated such a model (Caplan, 1987a, 1994; Caplan et al., 1985, 1996).

The studies reviewed above have two important limitations: (1) the comprehension performances on which a deficit analysis is based only use one task and (2) they are end-of-sentence measures that may not reflect on-line comprehension operations. Though performance on a broader range of tasks and on-line measures has not yet been related to lesions in a large number of studies, recent studies reveal the importance of these observations to understanding the deficits in people with aphasia. Because accurate characterization of the deficit is required to correctly interpret deficit-lesion correlations, I shall review these psychological studies.

First, there is evidence that people with aphasia perform differently on the same sentence type in different tasks. Cupples and Inglis (1993) reported poor performance on passive sentences in a sentence-picture matching (SPM) task but good performance in an enactment (or "object manipulation" [OM]) task in one patient. Caplan et al. (1997) found that performance across SPM and OM tasks correlated at about the $r = 0.6$ level for 10 different sentence types in 17 aphasic patients—a level of correlation that indicates that many patients differed in their accuracy relative to one another on a given sentence type in the two tasks. Caplan et al. (2006, 2007a) studied 42 patients using SPM and OM. Participants were presented 10 examples of each sentence type in each of six baseline/experimental pairs. Caplan et al. (2006) found that instances of good (i.e., above chance or normal) performance on a baseline sentence and poor performance on the corresponding experimental sentence in individual patients almost always occurred in only one task. Caplan et al. (in press) reported performances of 61 people with aphasia on 20 examples of each of 11 sentence types on sentence-picture matching, sentence-picture matching with auditory moving window presentation, and object manipulation. No individual had deficits affecting a syntactic structure or construction in all three tasks. Newhart et al. (2011) reported task-independent dissociation of performance on syntactically complex and simple sentences in association with transient hypoperfusion of Broca's area, but the criterion for a dissociation of performance on different sentence types was too lax. To date, when strict (in my view, reasonable) criteria are applied, there are no examples of a person with aphasia whose performances on more than one task reveal a task-independent deficit affecting a particular syntactic item or operation.

The fact that patients demonstrate good performance on an experimental sentence type on one task indicates that their deficit cannot be a failure of the comprehension system to assign the structure of that type of sentence or to use that structure to determine sentence meaning. Caplan et al. (2006, in press), however, both found instances in which a person with aphasia had a selective deficit affecting a structure in one task. These results point to the interaction of task demands and parsing and interpretive abilities in the genesis of patient performance.

On-line studies also present a more complex picture of the nature of deficits in syntactic comprehension in people with aphasia than is obtained from end-of-sentence measures. Tyler (1985) reported normal word monitoring times in one agrammatic patient whose end-of-sentence anomaly detection was at chance, including normal prolongations of word monitoring times following syntactic and semantic anomalies. Shankweiller et al. (1989) reported normal on-line anomaly detection times in six agrammatic patients with abnormal end-of-sentence comprehension. The fact that the participants with Broca's aphasia in these studies were sensitive to abnormalities at the point at which they arose argued against a deficit in syntactic processing. Caplan and Waters (2003) reported similar results in grammatically well-formed, meaningful sentences in a self-paced listening (SPL) study with sentence-picture matching (SPM) in 28 people with aphasia with a variety of clinical diagnoses, including Broca's aphasia. These individuals showed the same increased SPL times for the relative clause verb of an object compared to subject relatives and clefts, as was seen in neurologically normal controls, both when the people with aphasia performed correctly on a sentence-picture matching task and when they made errors. Caplan and Waters (2003) interpreted this pattern as indicating that initial on-line processing was normal, and that errors arose because of late-occurring competition from alternative interpretations. Caplan et al. (2007a) reported SPL times in SPM and grammaticality judgment tasks. There were longer SPL times at the verbs of passive than active, cleft object than cleft subject, and object-extracted than subject-extracted relative sentences in both SPM and grammaticality judgment. This pattern did not differ across neurologically normal control participants and six participants with Broca's aphasia. Caplan et al. (2007a) concluded that "the finding of the same listening time effects in Broca's aphasics and controls in multiple locations at which the co-indexation of a trace occurs . . . is incompatible with the hypothesis that Broca's aphasics have a deficit in the co-indexation of traces" (p. 144).

Similar conclusions have been reached based on results using the visual world paradigm. In this paradigm, a participant listens to a sentence while viewing a display containing pictures of nouns referred to in the sentence and distracters, and his/her eye fixations are recorded. Looks towards pictures are interpreted as indications that the concept corresponding to the picture is active at the point of the fixation. Dickey et al. (2007) presented short passages in which the last sentence consisted of an object-extracted wh-question, an object cleft, or a yes/no question. In the wh-object questions, both the people with aphasia and matched controls showed an object fixation preference at the point of the verb of the wh-question, and not before. The object preference continued for both controls and people with aphasia throughout the following phrase, and reversed in the people with aphasia, but not controls, to a subject preference at the last words in the sentence. Examination of fixations in sentences to which people with aphasia responded correctly and incorrectly showed that the late subject preference in people with aphasia only occurred in association with incorrect responses. Dickey et al. (2007) took the results in wh-questions as evidence for automatic activation of the noun phrase object of the verb in this position in those with Broca's aphasia. Dickey and Thompson (2009) studied eight people with Broca's aphasia who listened to object-extracted relatives and passives in a carrier phrase (*Point to*) and pointed to one of the displayed pictures. A theme preference was found for the control participants and for the people with aphasia at the relative clause verb of object-extracted sentences that were associated with correct, but not incorrect, performance. Neither controls nor people with aphasia showed a theme preference at any point in passives (both groups showed an agent preference after the agent had been introduced in the *by* phrase). However, the aphasic participants showed a theme advantage after the *by* phrase in sentences to which they responded correctly. The authors argue that the results with object relatives indicated that individuals with Broca's aphasia "compute wh-movement dependencies on-line, as the sentence unfolds" (p. 576). Thompson and Choy (2009) reported similar results in sentences with reflexives and pronouns. In correct responses, eight participants with agrammatic aphasia showed equivalent increases in fixations on the target picture at the same temporal latency following the occurrence of a reflexive or a pronoun as controls. In errors, they showed abnormally high numbers of looks to a competitor at later points in the sentence. Dickey et al. (2007) suggested that individuals with Broca's aphasia had a deficit in "lexical integration"—the assignment of syntactic structure and thematic roles based on lexical properties of words.

Other on-line studies point to possible abnormalities in on-line syntactic comprehension in people with aphasia. Love et al. (2008) found delayed cross-model lexical priming in aphasic participants compared to controls and argued that delays in lexical access underlie syntactic comprehension deficits by forcing people with aphasia (in particular, those with Broca's aphasia) to devote attention to word recognition rather than to parsing and interpretation. A related, but different, view is that people with aphasia (in particular, those with Broca's aphasia) have slowed syntactic processing itself (Haarman & Kolk, 1991a, 1991b; Burkhardt et al., 2003). Dickey et al. (2007) argued that the immediacy of looks to the theme at the verb of wh-questions in their study was inconsistent with the delayed lexical activation or the slowed parsing theory. The arguments for of these theories depend in part on the speed with which sentences were presented (for discussion, see Love et al., 2008; Dickey et al., 2007; Dickey & Thompson, 2009). Our work with self-paced listening is relevant to these models, because a self-paced presentation rate allows a person to compensate for delays in either lexical access or parsing by delaying input. Unlike the results in prior studies, Caplan et al. (under review) found on-line abnormalities in self-paced listening with sentence-picture matching in people with aphasia at all levels of severity, including those whose accuracy was within normal limits and/or above chance. These results were obtained after corrections for word duration and frequency, suggesting that something more than delayed lexical access produced the delays in self-paced listening times. This result points to the existence of syntactic comprehension disorders that vary in severity—less severe disorders slow on-line processing but do not disrupt it to the point of leading to abnormally high numbers of errors or to chance performance, while more severe disorders—which may or may not be the same as less severe ones—affect on-line processing to a greater extent and also lead to more errors than are seen in normals or to chance performance.

These two lines of research indicate that taking end-of-sentence accuracy on a single task as a measure of an individual's parsing ability is likely to be highly misleading. The absence of task-invariant deficits undermines the use of a single task as a means of identifying deficits in parsing and interpretation to correlate with lesion factors, and on-line measures provide evidence for possible parsing/interpretation deficits that may not be seen in accuracy and suggest that different deficits may lead to similar levels of accuracy. There are very few deficit-lesion correlation studies of either on-line measures or task effects on syntactic comprehension. Caplan et al. (2007b) reported correlations of lesion size in several regions of interest and on-line measures and of these measures of lesions with syntactic deficits in different tasks. Dickerson et al. (2013) found that lesions in different areas affect the same types of sentences differently in different tasks. I suggest that the central question regarding neural organization for syntactic processing in comprehension that emerges from the last decade of work using deficit-lesion correlations is whether areas of the brain support the incremental interaction of syntactic operations and task-related operations. Much more work is required to answer this question.

Functional Neuroimaging Studies

Unlike lesion-deficit correlation studies, there are now many functional neuroimaging studies of syntactically based comprehension using PET, fMRI, ERPs, and MEG. The approach has generally been to contrast sentences that differ in their syntactic structures, in an effort to find neural correlates of processing particular syntactic structures or elements or correlates of increased syntactic processing load in normal individuals. In general, these studies tend to report activation in the same areas in which lesions produce impairments in syntactic comprehension—the left inferior frontal gyrus and the left temporoparietal area, as well as some nonperisylvian areas, such as the left anterior inferior temporal lobe (Noppeney & Price, 2004), and the left superior parietal lobe (Caplan et al., 1998). As with deficit-lesion correlation studies, results differ across studies. This may be because of differences in sentence types and tasks used in different studies (Caplan, 2010), differences in strategies that participants use to understand sentences, or, possibly, differences in the areas that support aspects of syntactic processing in different individuals. MEG studies have begun to provide information about localization of syntactic operations (Brennan & Pylkkänen, 2012) and have great potential to contribute to understanding of the neural basis of these processes because of their combination of excellent temporal resolution and good spatial resolution (see Gow & Caplan, 2012, for discussion of application of Granger causality analysis of EEG-MEG data to syntactic comprehension).

Just et al. (1996) and Stromswold et al. (1996) were among the first researchers to study this topic. Using PET, Stromswold et al. (1996) reported increased rCBF in pars opercularis of Broca's area in the contrast of sentences with object and subject relative clauses in a written plausibility judgment task. Just et al. (1996) found increases in BOLD signal in Broca's area and Wernicke's area and, to a lesser degree, in their right hemisphere homologues, in similar contrasts. The authors attributed the increased neurovascular activity to the increased demands made by parsing in the object than in the subject relative clauses.

One line of subsequent work has focused on the question of whether these areas, or specific parts of them, support particular parsing or interpretive operations. Grodzinsky and his colleagues have argued that Broca's area supports comprehension of one type of syntactic movement. Ben-Shachar et al. (2003) found increased BOLD signal in the left inferior frontal gyrus and the left ventral precentral sulcus in the comparison of embedded wh-questions against yes/no questions in a verification task, consistent with this hypothesis. However, increased activation was also found bilaterally in superior temporal gyrus (marginally on the right). In a second experiment, the authors found increased BOLD signal in left inferior frontal gyrus and bilateral superior temporal sulcus in the comparison of topicalized sentences with noun phrase movement compared to sentences with datives without such movement. They concluded that the left inferior frontal gyrus, the left ventral precentral sulcus, and the bilateral superior temporal gyrus are involved in processing sentences with moved noun phrases.

Other researchers have suggested that Broca's area supports the memory operations of the parser/interpreter. Fiebach et al. (2004) studied BOLD signal responses in high- and low-span subjects in a verification task using externally paced word-by-word visual presentation of sentences that varied in subject-object extraction and ambiguity of case markings. They argued that the subject-object contrast varied computational load and the ambiguous/unambiguous contrast varied storage load. They found no main effect of the subject-object contrast on BOLD signal in the cortex. There was a main effect of storage costs bilaterally in Brodmann area 44 and the intraparietal sulcus. There was greater BOLD signal for object than subject sentences with high storage costs in the superior portion of Brodmann area 44 bilaterally only in low-span subjects. Fiebach and his colleagues concluded that their results supported a narrow localizationist view of the working memory system that supported syntactic processing. In their view, neurovascular increases occur in superior par opercularis, Brodmann area 44, when storage demands are high.

Friederici has proposed that Broca's area supports the construction of structures that are unique to human language. She and her colleagues (e.g., Makuuchi et al., 2009) studied the ability to assign structures in which constituents are nested and structures in which they are not. Nested structures have the form $[A_1 [A_2 [A_3 B_3] B_2] B_1]$ (subscripts indicate elements that are related to one another) and non-nested (linear) sequences have the form $A_1 C C C C B_1$. There is evidence that only humans have languages that have nested structures. Participants read sentences with four types of dependencies—long nested: $[A_1 [A_2 [A_3 B_3] B_2] B_1]$; short nested: $A_1 [A_2 B_2] B_1] C C$; long linear: $A_1 C C C C B_1$; short linear: $A_1 C C B_1 C C$—and answered questions about them. BOLD signal increased in the left pars opercularis in the contrast of nested versus linear structures and in left inferior frontal gyrus in the contrast of long and short structures. There was no interaction of these factors. Effective connectivity analysis showed robust connections between pars opercularis and the inferior frontal gyrus. The authors argue that left pars opercularis processes hierarchical nested structures. However, the absence of a greater effect of length in the nested than in the linear stimuli on BOLD signal in pars opercularis is inconsistent with that region assigning dependencies based on hierarchical structure on-line, since the long nested strings involve these processes to a greater extent than the short nested strings do. Petersson et al. (2012) have also shown that Broca's area supports learning of nonhierarchical artificial grammars. Petersson et al. (2012) discuss the relation between different types of grammars, memory limitations, and possible ways the brain might be organized to support syntactic processing.

The studies above localize particular parsing and interpretive operations, primarily focusing on Broca's area. Some authors have argued that this area is not engaged in specifically linguistic operations, but rather in operations that apply to many types of representations. For instance, Hagoort and his colleagues have argued that Broca's area supports "unification" operations that relate items to one another to create novel structures. Baggio and Hagoort (2011) offer several pieces of evidence that unification involves Broca's area, including the finding that the left inferior frontal gyrus shows greater BOLD signal in response to incongruencies between animal sounds and pictures (Hein et al., 2007), to mismatches between gestures and words in speech (Willems et al., 2008), and to mismatches between speaker identity and content (Tesink et al., 2009). These results point to increased activity in this area when representations that are not normally coupled must be combined. The fact that some of these examples involve nonlanguage stimuli is the basis for the claim that unification in left inferior frontal gyrus is not a purely linguistic operation.

Whether areas of the brain that support syntactic processing also support operations in other domains that have some similarities to syntax is critical for understanding the specificity of the neural basis for language (and of language itself). A body of work shows overlap among such functions (see, for instance, Patel, 2003, and Patel et al., 2008, regarding music). Hagoort and his colleagues have argued that "syntactic natural-language processing . . . is in fact dependent on a functional network of interacting brain regions, none of which is uniquely and exclusively involved in syntactic processing" (Petersson et al., 2012, p. 90). However, analyses that identify language areas using a functional screen have shown that some of these reports of overlap are due to group averaging, and that, within individuals, there appear to be small areas activated by language and syntax and not other, similar functions (Nieto-Castañon & Fedorenko, 2012; Fedorenko et al., 2012a, 2012b).

A variety of methodological issues pertaining to design limit the interpretability of many studies (see Caplan, 2009, for discussion). Contrasts of ill-formed and well-formed sentences could lead to BOLD signal related to detection of the ungrammaticality or attempts to interpret a sentence despite the ungrammaticality, not BOLD signal related to the parsing that led to the ungrammaticality. Contrasts of experimental conditions against a low-level (often perceptual) baseline do not isolate syntactic operations. Contrasts of experimental conditions against qualitatively different baselines (as in Petersson et al., 2012) are in general not interpretable (Caplan, 2009). A very large number of fMRI studies use designs of this sort, calling their interpretation into question.

A final issue, that unites deficit-lesion correlation and functional neuroimaging work in our lab, is the importance of task effects in determining BOLD signal effects. Sentence-type effects seen in functional neuroimaging studies may reflect operations related to a task that are carried out to a greater degree in more complex sentences. For instance, an analysis of the time course of BOLD signal responses to sentences in verification showed that sentence-type effects arose during the TR interval associated with the time between the target sentence and the probe, not that associated with the presentation of the target sentence (Caplan et al., 2008). This suggests that maintaining a representation of the target sentence in memory, not initial parsing and interpretation, led to greater BOLD signal for more complex sentences. In other studies, we have shown that, even when syntactic processing is implicit, as when the task is nonword detection or font change detection, the task affects BOLD signal associated with sentence types, perhaps by setting up conditions under which different parsing and interpretive operations are used (Caplan, 2010; Caplan et al., 2008). Not using a task does not solve these problems—it simply leads to less control over (and less information about) how participants process stimuli.

To summarize, fMRI studies have begun to ask whether specific syntactic operations lead to increases in BOLD signal in particular brain regions. The results converge with those of deficit-lesion correlation studies in suggesting a localization model in which Broca's area, the left superior temporal gyrus, and a few other regions play important roles, but the details of the functions carried out in particular regions remain unclear. There is no evidence from these studies for a distributed model, but it should be born in mind that analysis of BOLD signal is geared towards finding large differences between experimental conditions in small areas of the brain and is less likely to find small differences between experimental conditions that are distributed over large areas of the brain.

Electrophysiological Studies of Syntactic Processing

Event-related potentials (ERPs) are electrophysiological responses to sensory, motor, and cognitive events, averaged over trials and usually over individuals. ERPs are of positive or negative polarity, have millisecond-level temporal resolution, and can be recorded from electrodes over all the scalp. These features allow for the differentiation of ERPs on the basis of their polarity, time course, and spatial localization, which has allowed researchers to identify "components" of ERPs. The temporal resolution of ERPs allows them to be used to study on-line processes. ERPs can occur without subjects' overtly responding to a linguistic stimulus, and thus are capable of providing information relevant to the unconscious processes involved in language processing without the superimposition of a laboratory task upon such processing (though at the cost of not having behavioral information that could help understand the details of the psychological processes that underlie an ERP). Though spatial distribution of ERPs is relevant to their differentiation, the location of the source of an ERP is difficult to determine. Therefore, although spatial scalp distribution is an important aspect of defining components of ERPs, ERPs have less localizing specificity than

BOLD signal or MEG. The study of the relationship between different components of ERPs and particular aspects of sentence processing has led to models of the psychological determinants of these components.

To my knowledge, the first study that related an ERP component to a sentence-level process was Kutas and Hillyard (1983), which identified the N400 wave that is associated with the occurrence of a semantically anomalous word in a sentence (e.g., "I take my coffee with cream and cement"). This negative wave with a maximum in the mid-to-posterior scalp regions, often lateralized to the right scalp, has been extensively investigated. It was originally thought to reflect the integration of new lexical material into a developing semantic or conceptual context; more recent work has considerably altered this view, but it captures some of the causes of the N400. Kutas and Hillyard (1983) also described a second negative wave, distinguishable from the N400 by its slightly earlier occurrence but mostly because of its distribution over the left anterior scalp electrodes, that arose when subjects were presented with sentences that contained errors in noun number, verb number, and verb tense. This wave—subsequently called the left anterior negativity (LAN)—and a related earlier negative wave—known as the early left anterior negativity (ELAN)—have been described by a host of researchers in response to various syntactic violations (Neville et al., 1991; Friederici, Steinhauer, Mecklinger, & Meyer, 1998; Kluender & Kutas, 1993a, 1993b; Munte, Heinze, & Mangun, 1993; Rosler, Putz, Friederici, & Hahne, 1993) and are candidates for electrophysiological correlates of syntactic processing.

Osterhout and Holcomb (1992) described a second wave that has been associated with syntactic processing—the P600, or syntactic positive shift (SPS) (Hagoort, Brown, & Groothusen, 1993). The P600/SPS is a later, positive wave, arising about 500 msec or more after certain syntactic violations, with a centro-posterior scalp distribution, that is often maximal over the right hemisphere electrodes. Osterhout and Holcomb found that this wave occurred after violations of subcategory restrictions on verbal complements, as in "The man persuaded to eat" contrasted with "The man hoped to eat." Hagoort and colleagues (1993) found that it occurred after violations of subject-verb number agreement and violations of category sequences (which they called "phrase structure" violations). The P600/SPS has also been described and explored in numerous studies (Gunter, Stowe, & Mulder, 1997; McKinnon & Osterhout, 1996; Osterhout & Holcomb, 1992, 1993, 1995; Rosler et al., 1993).

In the previous version of this chapter, I reviewed a number of problems I saw with much of the ERP literature. It remains my view that many of the concerns I had derived from basic aspects of research using ERPs, and apply very generally, including to modern work, and I will therefore briefly restate the ones I consider most important.

One issue is that ERP components were originally identified visually and have continued to be distinguished subjectively. This leads to questions about their classification. For instance, the LAN has been noted over left anterior electrodes in many studies but has been found to be maximal over other left hemisphere sites in others. Neville and colleagues (1991) found that phrase structure violations (e.g., "The scientist criticized of proof the theorem") produced a negative left hemisphere wave beginning around 300 msec that was maximal over left temporal and parietal sites. Munte, Matzke, and Johannes (1997) found a left negativity from about 280 to 800 msec with a very broad distribution ranging from left anterior through midline parietal electrodes when subjects read sentences with pseudowords in which there were or were not subject-verb number agreement violations, and a negativity seen only in central and parietal electrodes, and only from 280 to 500 msec, when the same subjects performed a grammaticality judgment task. Discrepancies in the exact location of the P600/SPS have also been described. Coulson, King, and Kutas (1998a) review the location (and temporal course) of the P600/SPS waves that have been described in relation to five different types of syntactic violations, pointing out that, in response to phrase structure violations, this wave's location ranges from the right anterior electrodes (Osterhout & Holcomb, 1992) through the occipital leads (Neville et al., 1991), to a broad distribution (Hagoort et al., 1993). The distribution of these waves leads to interpretive problems. For instance, which two of the three waves associated with semantic violations, phrase structure violations, and specificity violations in Neville and colleagues' (1991) figure 2 are most similar is not obvious to my visual inspection, yet the second and third of these waves are taken as examples of the LAN and the first as an instance of the semantically driven N400. Researchers have deemphasized the importance of either the ELAN (Brown & Hagoort, 2000) or the P600/SPS (Coulson et al., 1998a, 1998b) as reflections of syntactic processing on the grounds of the inconsistency in scalp topography and temporal course of these waves in different studies.

A second broad issue is that not all studies have found waves that are expected, and the reason for the absence of waves in some studies is not clear. A common explanation has been that they are obscured by superimposed waves of opposite polarity. For instance, we noted above that Osterhout and Holcomb (1992) described a P600 after violations of subcategory restrictions such as "The man persuaded to eat." Hagoort and colleagues (1993), however, did not find this wave after a different type of subcategory violation—the presence of a direct object after an intransitive verb (e.g., "The son of the rich industrialist boasts the car"; note that, in Dutch, the sentential complement continuation ["... was a limited edition"] is impossible). Hagoort and colleagues explain the absence of this expected P600/SPS by saying that it was obscured by a concurrent N400. In a similar vein, Munte and colleagues (1997) found an LAN in a grammaticality judgment task with subject-verb agreement violations in pseudoword prose but not in a similar task with real words. They attributed the lack of an LAN to the overlap of the LAN with an earlier-than-usual positive wave associated with these violations. The principles that underlie deciding when waves superimpose and cancel one another out are not clear; we must ask if these failures to find expected waves are indications of different effects of particular stimuli, tasks, or subjects on ERPs associated with these types of ungrammatical sentences, and what this implies about the nature of these waves.

These and other concerns have not stopped researchers from developing models of the role of the ELAN and P600/SPS in syntactic processing. Probably the most encompassing theory has been developed by Friederici and her colleagues. Friederici (2002) presented a model of sentence comprehension based upon the interpretation of the ELAN, the LAN, and the P66/SPS that has been very widely quoted. The model is based upon the view that the ELAN has been found following lexical category violations (Neville et al., 1991; Friederici, Pfeifer, & Hahne, 1993; Friederici, Hahne, & Mecklinger, 1996) and the LAN has occurred after inflectional agreement and verb argument structure violations (Munte et al., 1993, 1997; Munte & Heinze, 1994; Osterhout & Mobley, 1995; Gunter et al., 1997; Coulson et al., 1998a, 1998b). This has suggested to Friederici (1999, 2002) that the ELAN reflects the assignment of phrase structure based on syntactic category membership and the LAN reflects the assignment of agreement and lexically specified subcategorization information. The LAN persists in sentences with pseudowords (Munte et al., 1997) and is not affected by the probability of occurrence of a syntactic violation in a stimulus set (Hahne & Friederici, 1999; Gunter et al., 1999). Because of their insensitivity to meaningfulness and the probability of a violation in the stimulus set, Friederici (1995, 1999, 2002) has suggested that the LAN and the ELAN reflect automatic processes. Friederici et al. (1999) found that the N400 did not occur in "double violations," where there were both syntactic category and semantic violations, as in 4:

4.   *Der Priester wurder vom gebaut. (The priest was by the built.)

Friederici (2002) took this to indicate that, in the absence of building a phrase marker, thematic roles are not assigned, and therefore not appreciated to be anomalous. This implies that parsing and interpretation is syntax-first, as claimed in modular models (Frazier & Clifton, 1996), not an interactive constraint satisfaction process, as claimed by most modern theorists (MacDonald et al., 1994).

The P600/SPS has been detected at the point at which violations of syntactic structure can be identified (Gunter et al., 1997; McKinnon & Osterhout, 1996; Osterhout & Holcomb, 1992, 1993, 1995; Rosler et al., 1993). Unlike the ELAN, it has also occurred when a less likely syntactic structure occurs (Gunter at al., 1997). The P600/SPS is sensitive to the probability of occurrence of a syntactic violation in the stimulus set (Coulson et al., 1998a; Hahne & Friederici, 1999). Because of this, Friederici (2002; Hahne and Friederici, 1999) argued that the P600/SPS is associated with controlled syntactic processing. The P600/SPS does not occur in sentences with pseudowords (Munte et al., 1997) and does occur in syntactically ambiguous sentences at the point at which they are disambiguated toward their less preferred reading (Mecklinger, Schriefers, Steinhauer, & Friederici, 1995). Because of these features, Friederici (1999, 2002) has suggested that the P600/SPS reflects making revisions to structures that have been created ("second-pass" parsing).

Friederici's model encounters many problems. An excellent, detailed, review of the ELAN can be found in Steinhauer and Drury (2012). Among the points these authors make are the following. The evidence for an ELAN with written presentation is very weak. In the auditory modality, the evidence for an ELAN comes from paradigms in which the critical word is held constant and the context is varied. Detailed analyses of the waves in published studies shows that the early negativity sometimes occurs before the onset of critical word, implying that it is sometimes due to the context, not to a failure to assign phrase structure on the basis of the critical word. One possible source of the ELAN is the prosodic abnormality associated with cross-splicing words; other ELANS and LANs are likely to be artifacts due to measuring deviations from a normalized pre-critical-word baseline. Early negativities are often sustained for long periods of times (> 600 msec), and temporally limited early negativities (the ELAN and LAN) only occur when there is a P600. This suggests that they are in fact sustained negativities upon which a positive wave is superimposed for a critical period (see discussion above about superimposition of waves). A similar point was made by Osterhout et al. (2004), who argued that the superposition of N400s and P600s may result in what are taken to be LAN-like components. These features of the literature, and others, raise the question of whether the ELAN exists.

If the ELAN does exist, Steinhauer and Drury (2012) point out that its behavior does not conform to that described by Friederici (2002). In many cases, the word that triggered an ELAN is actually grammatically possible in the "ungrammatical" context, albeit in rare constructions. This implies that the ELAN results from top-down expectations about the frequency of structures in a language, not from failure to apply structure-building rules in a bottom-up fashion. This is more in keeping with modern interactive activation models that with syntax-first models. N400 blocking, which appears to be a more robust finding, is, in their view, the strongest evidence in favor of aspects of Friederici's model, but it is still not convincing. N400 blocking can occur without an ELAN (Friederici et al., 1999), and appears to be task-specific (Hahne and Friederici, 2002, exp 2). Gunter and Friederici (1999) reported an N400 following the preposition *vom* and not other prepositions that led to ELANs. They argued that, unlike the other prepositions in that study, *vom* assigns thematic roles, but, within the Friederici model, this implies that thematic role assignment can occur despite the failure to construct phrase structure, an obvious contradiction.

There are also problems with Friederici's theories about the P600/SPS. The P600/SPS occurs in sentences in which all content words are randomly selected, so that the resulting material is syntactically well formed but semantically incoherent (Brown & Hagoort, 2000), making the hypothesis that it is triggered by reanalysis in the service of semantic integration unlikely. An early positive wave is sometimes seen without the late one (Mecklinger et al., 1995), while other experiments have yielded a late positive wave without an early one (Friederici et al., 1998). It is hard to see how either of these patterns could arise in subjects who understand syntactically ambiguous sentences with unpreferred meanings correctly, if these late positive waves are associated with detection and revision processes, respectively. Friederici's view that the P600/SPS reflects controlled processing also encounters problems. Hahne and Friederici (1999) found that the P600/SPS occurred when ungrammatical sentences made up 20 percent of the stimuli in a set, but not when they made up 80 percent of the stimuli. Coulson and colleagues (1998b) found that it occurred in grammatical sentences at a point at which they differed from ungrammatical sentences (e.g., "Ray fell down and skinned his/he knee") when the grammatical sentences made up a small proportion (20 percent) of the stimuli. Controlled processes are more likely to be engaged by a high proportion of relevant stimuli (Posner & Snyder, 1975). This speaks against Friederici's suggestion that the P600/SPS results from controlled processing. The P600/SPS does not appear to be specific for syntactic processing: Munte, Heinze, Matzke, Wieringa, and Johannes (1998) had subjects read short passages in which target nouns were replaced by semantically incorrect nouns, morphologically incorrect nouns, or orthographically incorrect nouns and found that all these stimuli elicited similar P600s. If the P600/SPS is best considered a part of the P300 complex (Coulson et al., 1998a, 1998b), this wave would not be a correlate of reanalysis processes specifically related to syntactic structures per se (for an opposing view, see Osterhout, McKinnon, Bersick, & Corey, 1996; Osterhout & Hagoort, 1999).

I will conclude this part of this brief review by noting that, while currently accepted views of ERP correlates of syntactic processing recognize two (potentially divisible) possible syntactic waves—an early left negativity and a late centro-parietal positivity—all possible variants of positivity and negativity crossed by early and late temporal occurrence characterize the ERPs that have been associated with this function. The early left negativity and the late centro-parietal positivity are documented above. An early positivity, at about 350 msec, roughly the time period at which the LAN arises, was described by Mecklinger and colleagues (1995) at a point that signals the presence of an unpreferred syntactic structure—the auxiliary in previously ambiguous object relative sentences. A (somewhat) late negativity, at around 400 to 600 msec, arose in association with an earlier disambiguation toward the same less preferred structure—the first NP in the relative clause—in a study by Friederici and colleagues (1998). Until the specific aspects of syntactic processing that drive these different waves are better understood, these different types of ERPs, with their presumably different cerebral generators, are all candidates for correlates of what may be, at least in part, the same aspects of syntactic processing.

I have focused on Friederici's model because it is so widely cited. Steinhauer and Drury, (2012) estimated that the 2002 paper has been cited once a week since its publication. However, it is not the only model of what drives ERP components and what they tell us about parsing and interpretation. Steinhauer and Drury (2012), for instance, argue that early negative waves, which they say are always prolonged, reflect working memory demands of parsing and interpretation. They argue that the presence of these waves in studies with auditory but not visual presentation is due to spoken language automatically entering a phonological short-term store. Bornkessel and Schlesewsky (2006) present a model of parsing/interpretation based upon mapping of features to meanings, in which, among other things, they place considerable emphasis upon a fronto-central negativity between approximately 300 and 500 msec post argument onset whose spatial distribution lies between that of the N400 and the LAN, that was associated with in clause-medial word order variations in German ("scrambling"). They interpreted this "scrambling negativity" as a result of the parser/interpreter having to process an argument whose prominence status is not compatible with previously established phrase structure representations. Kuperberg (see Kuperberg, in press, for review) has developed a model in which the LAN and P600 arise because of discrepancies between expectations and incoming input (prediction errors). In my view, these models also have loose ends. For instance, the view that negativities that appear early and are sustained are due to the use of short-term working memory by the parser/interpreter is inconsistent with modern views of short-term memory (see Caplan et al., 2012, for review) and with the view that skilled parsing and interpretation rely on a form of procedural memory devoted to cognitive functions (long-term working memory; see Caplan and Waters, 2013). Whether Bornkessel and Schlesewsky's scrambling negativity differs from the ELAN is not clear.

Overall, the ERP literature has developed theories of the relationship of different waves to different syntactic processes. These models have been related to important features of models of parsing and interpretation, but the relationships of these components to psycholinguistic processes remain to be firmly established. The implications of these studies for the neuroanatomical structures that support parsing are limited because the exact neural structures that generate different ERP components are hard to identify. New technologies, such as magnetoencephalography, that can be coupled with electrophysiological techniques are very likely to yield much more information on this subject.

Overview

I closed the previous version of this chapter with the view that many brain regions had been implicated in syntactic processing in comprehension, and that available evidence pointed to significant individual variability in the localization of aspects of this process. The evidence for this is far from overwhelming, and, arguably, less highly valued relative to evidence for other models, but since no model of the neural basis for syntactic processing receives very strong support from any empirical data, and this "variation" model raises interesting issues, I will include that discussion here. Accepting variability of localization as a point of departure, the next question to ask is whether there is any systematicity to the pattern of individual differences in the localization of syntactic operations. Factors that could affect localization can be grouped into different classes: endogenous, biologically determined factors, such as sex, handedness, and age; exogenous, socially determined factors, such as language spoken; and factors that cannot be clearly assigned to either of these categories uniquely but may reflect both, such as verbal working memory capacity and language processing proficiency. It is possible that any of these factors, or others, determine localization; that is, that women differ systematically from men, or left-handers from right-handers, or highly proficient language users from less proficient language users, with respect to what neural areas within the perisylvian association cortex support aspects of syntactic processing. The effects of these factors could be absolute or relative; that is, these factors might *determine* localization or *constrain variability* in localization. The latter mechanism is clearly at work in patterns of lateralization, with handedness constraining variability in the pattern of which hemisphere is dominant for representing and processing language.

The hypothesis that there is significant individual variability in the localization of syntactic processing in sentence comprehension would superficially suggest that the organization of the perisylvian cortex for syntactic processing differs from the functional neuroanatomy of other brain regions for other functions, in which such individual variability is minimal, if it exists at all. However, on closer inspection, these better-understood function-structure relationships are limited to early aspects of perception and late aspects of motor planning and execution. Very little is known about the details of localization of higher functions within a general region. Exactly what region of the dorsolateral prefrontal cortex is involved in functions such as shifting attention, for instance, and is this region the same in all individuals? The notion of individual variability for syntactic processing within perisylvian cortex may not be an entirely iconoclastic suggestion within cognitive neuropsychology.

Nonetheless, the theme of this version of this chapter is that this hypothesis, as all others, is grossly underdetermined by available data. Many aspects of methodology and methods will have to be clarified, and much more data gathered, to answer the question of how the brain is organized to support this function. The encouraging feature of current research is that the investigative techniques now available in both psychology and neuroimaging offer unparalleled opportunities to make progress in this domain.

Acknowledgment

Aspects of the research reported here was supported by NIDCD grant DC00942 to David Caplan.

References

Baggio, G., & Hagoort, P. (2011). The balance between memory and unification in semantics: A dynamic account of the N400. *Language and Cognitive Processes, 26,* 1338–1367.

Bavelier, D., Corina, D., Jezzard, P., Padmanabhan, S., Clark, V.P., Karni, A., Prinster, A., Braun, A., Lalwani, A., Rauschecker, J.P., Turner, R., & Neville, H. (1997). Sentence reading: A functional MRI study at 4 Tesla. *Journal of Cognitive Neuroscience, 9,* 664–686.

Ben-Shachar, M., Hendler, T., Kahn, I., Ben-Bashat, D., & Grodzinsky, Y. (2003). The neural reality of syntactic transformations: Evidence from functional magnetic resonance imaging. *Psychological Science, 14,* 433–440.

Bock, K., & Levelt, P. (1994). Language production: Grammatical encoding. In M. Gernsbacher (Ed.), *Handbook of psycholinguistics.* New York: Academic Press.

Bornkessel, I., & Schlesewsky, M. (2006). The role of contrast in the local licensing of scrambling in German: Evidence from online comprehension. *Journal of Germanic Linguistics, 18,* 1–43.

Brennan, J., & Pylkkänen, L. (2012). The time-course and spatial distribution of brain activity associated with sentence processing. *Neuroimage, 60*(2), 1139–1148.

Brown, C., & Hagoort, P. (2000). On the electrophysiology of language comprehension: Implications for the human language system. In M.P. Matthew, W. Crocker, & C. Clifton, Jr. (Eds.), *Architectures and mechanisms for language processing.* Cambridge: Cambridge University Press.

Burkhardt, P., Piñango, M.M., & Wong, K. (2003). The role of the anterior left hemisphere in real-time sentence comprehension: evidence from split intransitivity. *Brain and Language, 86*(1), 9–22.

Caplan, D. (1987a). Discrimination of normal and aphasic subjects on a test of syntactic comprehension. *Neuropsychologia, 25,* 173–184.

Caplan, D. (1987b). *Neurolinguistics and linguistic aphasiology.* Cambridge: Cambridge University Press.

Caplan, D. (1994). Language and the brain. In M. Gernsbacher (Ed.), *Handbook of psycholinguistics.* New York: Academic Press.

Caplan, D. (2009). Experimental design and interpretation of functional neuroimaging studies of cognitive processes. *Human Brain Mapping, 30,* 59–77.

Caplan, D. (2010). Task effects on BOLD signal correlates of implicit syntactic processing. *Language and Cognitive Processes, 25,* 866–901.

Caplan, D., Alpert, N., & Waters, G.S. (1998). Effects of syntactic structure and propositional number on patterns of regional cerebral blood flow. *Journal of Cognitive Neuroscience, 10,* 541–552.

Caplan, D, Albert, N., & Waters, G.S. (1999). PET Studies of sentence processing with auditory sentence presentation. *NeuroImage, 9,* 343–351.

Caplan, D., Alpert, N., Waters, G., & Olivieri, A. (2000). Activation of Broca's area by syntactic processing under conditions of concurrent articulation. *Human Brain Mapping, 9,* 65–71.

Caplan, D., Baker, C., & Dehaut, F. (1985). Syntactic determinants of sentence comprehension in aphasia. *Cognition, 21,* 117–175.

Caplan, D., Chen, E., Waters, G. (2008). Task-dependent and task-independent neurovascular responses to syntactic processing. *Cortex, 44,* 257–275.

Caplan, D., DeDe, G., & Michaud, J. (2006). Task-independent and task-specific syntactic deficits in aphasic comprehension, *Aphasiology, 20,* 893–920.

Caplan, D., Hildebrandt, N., & Makris, N. (1996). Location of lesions in stroke patients with deficits in syntactic processing in sentence comprehension. *Brain, 119,* 933–949.

Caplan, D., Michaud, J., & Hufford, R. (in press). Dissociations and associations of performance in syntactic comprehension in aphasia and their implications for the nature of aphasic deficits. *Brain and Language.*

Caplan, D., Michaud, J., & Hufford, R. (under review). Effects of syntactic structure on self-paced listening in aphasia.

Caplan, D., & Waters, G.S. (2003). On-line syntactic processing in aphasia: Studies with auditory moving windows presentation. *Brain and Language, 84*(2), 222–249.

Caplan, D., & Waters, G. (2013). Memory mechanisms supporting syntactic comprehension. *Psychonomic Bulletin Review, 20*(2), 243–268.

Caplan, D., Waters, G.S., DeDe, G., Michaud, J., & Reddy, A. (2007a). A study of syntactic processing in aphasia I: Behavioral (psycholinguistic) aspects. *Brain and Language, 101*(2), 103–150.

Caplan, D., Waters, G., & Hildebrandt, N. (1997). Determinants of sentence comprehension in aphasic patients in sentence-picture matching tasks. *Journal of Speech and Hearing Research, 40*, 542–555.

Caplan, D., Waters, G.S., Kennedy, D., Alpert, N., Makris, N., DeDe, G., Michaud, J., & Reddy, A. (2007b). A study of syntactic processing in aphasia II: Neurological aspects. *Brain and Language, 101*, 151–177.

Caplan, D., Waters, G.S., & Howard, D. (2012). Slave systems in verbal short-term memory. *Aphasiology, 26*, 279–316.

Caramazza, A., & Zurif, E. B. (1976). Dissociation of algorithmic and heuristic processes in language comprehension: Evidence from aphasia. *Brain and Language, 3*, 572–582.

Carpenter, P.A., Just, M.A., Keller, T.A., Eddy, W.F., & Thulborn, K.R. (1999). Time course of fMRI-activation in language and spatial networks during sentence comprehension. *Neuroimage, 10*, 216–224

Chomsky, N. (1965). *Aspects of the theory of syntax.* Cambridge, MA: MIT Press.

Chomsky, N. (1981). *Lectures on government and binding.* Dordrecht: Foris.

Chomsky, N. (1986). *Knowledge of language.* New York: Praeger.

Chomsky, N. (1995). *Barriers.* Cambridge, MA: MIT Press.

Coulson, S., King, J.W., & Kutas, M. (1998a). Expect the unexpected: Event-related brain potentials to morphosyntactic violations. *Language and Cognitive Processes, 13*, 21–58.

Coulson, S., King, J.W., & Kutas, M. (1998b). ERPs and domain specificity: Beating a straw horse. *Language and Cognitive Processes, 13*, 653–672.

Cupples, L., & Inglis, A.L. (1993). When task demands induce "asyntactic" sentence comprehension: A study of sentence interpretation in aphasia. *Cognitive Neuropsychology, 10*, 201–234.

Damasio, A.R. (1992). Aphasia. *New England Journal of Medicine, 326*, 531–539.

Dapretto, M., & Bookheimer, S.Y. (1999). Form and content: Dissociating syntax and semantics in sentence comprehension. *Neuron, 24*, 427–432.

De Smet, H.J., Baillieux, H., De Deyn, P.P., Mariën, P., & Paquier, P. (2007). The cerebellum and language: the story so far. *Folia phoniatrica et logopaedica, 59*(4), 165–170.

Dickerson, B., Caplan, D., Michaud, J., Hufford, J., & Makris, N. (2013). Deficit lesion correlation for syntactic comprehension differs as a function of task. *Academy of Aphasia*, Lucerne.

Dickey, M.W., Choy, J., & Thompson, C.K. (2007). Real time comprehension of wh- movement in aphasia: Evidence from eyetracking, while listening. *Brain and Language, 100*, 1–22.

Dickey, M.W., & Thompson, C.K. (2007). The relation between syntactic and morphological recovery in agrammatic aphasia: A case study. *Aphasiology, 21*(6–8), 604–616.

Dickey, M.W., & Thompson, C.K. (2009). Automatic processing of wh- and NP-movement in agrammatic aphasia: Evidence from eyetracking. *Journal of Neurolinguistics, 22*(6), 563–583.

Dronkers, N.F., Wilkins, D.P., Van Valin, R.D., Redfern, B.B., & Jaeger, J.J. (2004). Lesion analysis of the brain areas involved in language comprehension. *Cognition, 92*(1–2), 145–177.

Fedorenko, E., Duncan, J., & Kanwisher, N. (2012a). Language-selective and domain-general regions lie side by side within Broca's area. *Current Biology, 22*, 2059–2062.

Fedorenko, E., McDermott, J., Norman-Haignere, S. & Kanwisher, N. (2012b). Sensitivity to musical structure in the human brain. *Journal of Neurophysiology, 108*, 3289–3300.

Fiebach, C.J., Vos, S.H., & Friederici, A.D. (2004). Neural correlates of syntactic ambiguity in sentence comprehension for low and high span readers. *Journal of Cognitive Neuroscience, 16*, 1562–1575.

Frazier, L., & Clifton, C. (1996). *Construal.* Cambridge, MA: MIT Press.

Friederici, A.D. (1995). The time course of syntactic activation during language processing: A model based on neuropsychological and neurophysiological data. *Brain and Language, 49*, 259–281

Friederici, A.D. (1999). Diagnosis and reanalysis: Two processing aspects the brain may differentiate. In J.D. Fodor & F. Ferreira (Eds.), *Reanalysis in sentence processing.* New York: Kluver.

Friederici, A.D. (2002). Towards a neural basis of auditory sentence processing. *Trends in Cognitive Sciences, 6*(2), 78–84.

Friederici, A.D., Hahne, A., & Mecklinger, A. (1996). Temporal structure of syntactic parsing: Early and late event-related brain potentials effects. *Journal of Experimental Psychology: Learning, Memory, and Cognition, 22*, 1219–1248.

Friederici, A.D., Pfeifer, E., & Hahne, A. (1993). Event-related brain potentials during natural speech processing: Effects of semantic, morphological, and syntactic violations. *Cognitive Brain Research, 1*, 183–192.

Friederici, A.D., Steinhauer, K., Mecklinger, A., & Meyer, M. (1998). Working memory constraints on syntactic ambiguity resolution as revealed by electrical brain responses. *Biological Psychology, 47*, 193–221.

Gow, D.W. Jr., & Caplan, D. (2012). New levels of language processing complexity and organization revealed by Granger causation. *Frontiers in Psychology, 3*, 506.

Grodzinsky, Y. (1990). *Theoretical perspectives on language deficits.* Cambridge, MA: MIT Press.

Grodzinsky, Y. (1995). A restrictive theory of agrammatic comprehension. *Brain and Language, 50*, 27–51.

Grodzinsky, Y. (2000). The neurology of syntax: Language use without Broca'a area. *Behavioral and Brain Sciences, 23*, 47–117.

Gunter, T.C., & Friederici, A.D. (1999). Concerning the automaticity of syntactic processing. *Psychophysiology, 36*, 126–137.

Gunter, T.C., Stowe, L.A., & Mulder, G. (1997). When syntax meets semantics. *Psychophysiology, 34*, 660–676.

Gunter, T.C., Vos, S. H., & Friederici, A.D. (1999). Memory or aging? That's the question: An electrophysiological perspective on language. In S. Kemper & R. Kliegel (Eds.), *Constraints on language: Aging, grammar and memory* (pp. 249–282). Boston: Kluwer.

Haarmann, H.J., & Kolk, H.H.J. (1991a). A computer model of the temporal course of agrammatic sentence understanding: The effects of variation in severity and sentence complexity. *Cognitive Science, 15*, 49–87.

Haarmann, H.J., & Kolk, H.H.J. (1991b). Syntactic priming in Broca's aphasia: Evidence for a slow activation. *Aphasiology, 5*, 1–36.

Hagoort, P., Brown, C., & Groothusen, J. (1993). The syntactic positive shift (SPS) as an ERP measure of syntactic processing. *Language and Cognitive Processes, 8*, 485–532.

Hahne, A., & Friederici, A.D. (1999). Electrophysiological evidence for two steps in syntactic analysis: Early automatic and late controlled processes. *Journal of Cognitive Neuroscience, 11*, 194–205.

Hahne, A., & Friederici, A.D. (2002). Differential task effects on semantic and syntactic processes as revealed by ERPs. *Cognitive Brain Research, 13*(3), 339–356.

Hein, G., Doehrmann, O., Muller, N.G., Kaiser, J., Muckli, L., & Naumer, M.J. (2007). Object familiarity and semantic congruency modulate responses in cortical audiovisual integration areas. *Journal of Neuroscience, 27*(30), 7881–7887.

Just, M. A., & Carpenter, P.A. (1992). A capacity theory of comprehension: Individual differences in working memory. *Psychological Review, 99*(1), 122–149.

Just, M. A., Carpenter, P.A., Keller, T.A., Eddy, W.F., & Thulborn, K.R. (1996). Brain activation modulated by sentence comprehension. *Science, 274*, 114–116.

Kluender, R., & Kutas, M. (1993a). Bridging the gap: Evidence from ERPs on the processing of unbounded dependencies. *Journal of Cognitive Neuroscience, 5*, 196–214.

Kluender, R., & Kutas, M. (1993b). Subjacency as a processing phenomenon. *Language and Cognitive Processes, 8*, 573–633.

Kuperberg, G.R. (in press). The proactive comprehender: What event-related potentials tell us about the dynamics of reading comprehension. In B. Miller, L. Cutting, & P. McCardle (Eds.), *Unraveling the behavioral, neurobiological, and genetic components of reading comprehension*. Baltimore: Paul Brookes Publishing.

Kutas, M., & Hillyard, S.A. (1983). Event-related potentials to grammatical errors and semantic anomalies. *Memory and Cognition, 11*, 539–50.

Levelt, W.J.M. (1989). *Speaking: From intention to articulation.* Cambridge, MA: MIT Press.

Love, T., Swinney, D., Walenski, M., & Zurif, E. (2008). How left inferior frontal cortex participates in syntactic processing: Evidence from aphasia. *Brain and Language, 107*(3), 203–219.

MacDonald, M.G., Pearlmutter, N.J., & Seidenberg, M.S. (1994). Lexical nature of syntactic ambiguity resolution. *Psychological Review, 101*, 676–703.

Makuuchi, M., Bahlmann, J., Anwander, A., & Friederici, A.D. (2009). Segregating the core computational faculty of human language from working memory. *Proceedings of the National Academy of Sciences of the USA, 106*(20), 8362–8367.

Mazoyer, B., Tzourio, N., Frak, V., Syrota, A., Murayama, N., Levrier, O., & Salamon, G. (1993). The cortical representation of speech. *Journal of Cognitive Neuroscience, 5*, 467–479.

McKinnon, R., & Osterhout, L. (1996). Constraints on movement phenomena in sentence processing: Evidence from event-related brain potentials. *Language and Cognitive Processes, 11*(5), 495–523.

Mecklinger, A., Schriefers, E., Steinhauer, K., & Friederici, A.D. (1995). Processing relative clauses varying on syntactic and semantic dimensions: An analysis with event-related potentials. *Memory and Cognition, 23*, 477–494.

Mesulam, M-M. (1990). Large-scale neurocognitive networks and distributed processing for attention, language, and memory. *Annals of Neurology, 28*(5), 597–613.

Mesulam, M-M. (1998). From sensation to cognition. *Brain, 121*(6), 1013–1052.

Munte, T.F., & Heinze, H. (1994). ERP negativities during syntactic processing of written words. In H.J. Heinze, T.F. Munte, & G.R. Mangun (Eds.), *Cognitive Electrophysiology*. La Jolla, CA: Birkhauser Boston.

Munte, T.F., Heinze, H., & Mangun, G.R. (1993). Dissociation of brain activity related to syntactic and semantic aspects of language. *Journal of Cognitive Neuroscience, 5*, 335–344.

Munte, T.F., Heinze, H., Matzke, M., Wieringa, B. M., & Johannes, S. (1998). Brain potentials and syntactic violations revisited: No evidence for specificity of the syntactic positive shift. *Neuropsychologia, 36*, 217–226.

Munte, T.F., Matzke, M., & Johannes, S. (1997). Brain activity associated with syntactic incongruities in words and pseudo-words. *Journal of Cognitive Neuroscience, 9*, 318–329.

Neville, H., Nicol, J.L., Barss, A., Forster, K. I., & Garret, M.F. (1991). Syntactically based sentence processing classes: Evidence from event-related brain potentials. *Journal of Cognitive Neuroscience, 2*, 151–165.

Newhart, M., Trupe, L.A., Gomez, Y., Cloutman, L., Molitoris, J.J., Davis, C., Leigh, R., et al. (2011). Asyntactic comprehension, working memory, and acute ischemia in Broca's area versus angular gyrus. *Cortex, 48*(10), 1288–1297.

Nieto-Castañon, A., & Fedorenko, E. (2012). Subject-specific functional localizers increase sensitivity and functional resolution of multi-subject analyses. *Neuroimage, 63*, 1646–1669.

Noppeney, U., & Price, C.J. (2004). An fMRI study of syntactic adaptation. *Journal of Cognitive Neuroscience, 16*, 702–713.

Osterhout, L., & Hagoort, P. (1999). A superficial resemblance doesn't necessarily mean that you're part of a family: Counter-arguments to Coulson, King, and Kutas (1998) in the P600/SPS-P300 debate. *Language and Cognitive Processes, 14*(1), 1–14.

Osterhout, L., & Holcomb, P. (1992). Event-related brain potentials elicited by syntactic anomaly. *Journal of Memory and Language, 31*, 785–806.

Osterhout, L., & Holcomb, P. (1993). Event-related potentials and syntactic anomaly: Evidence of anomaly detection during the perception of continuous speech. *Language and Cognitive Processes, 8*, 413–437.

Osterhout, L., & Holcomb, P.J. (1995). Event-related brain potentials and language comprehension. In M. Rugg & M. Coles (Eds.), *Electrophysiological studies of human cognitive function*. Oxford: Oxford University Press.

Osterhout, L., McKinnon, R., Bersick, M., & Corey, V. (1996). On the language specificity of the brain response to syntactic anomalies: Is the syntactic positive shift a member of the P300 family? *Journal of Cognitive Neuroscience, 8*, 507–526.

Osterhout, L., McLaughlin, J., Kim, A., Greenwald, R., & Inoue, K. (2004). Sentences in the brain: Event-related potentials as real-time reflections of sentence comprehension and language learning. In M. Carreiras & C. Clifton, Jr. (Eds.), *The on-line study of sentence comprehension: Eyetracking, ERP, and beyond*. New York: Psychology Press.

Osterhout, L., & Mobley, L.A. (1995). Event-related brain potentials elicited by failure to agree. *Journal of Memory and Language, 34*, 739–773.

Patel, A.D. (2003). Language, music, syntax and the brain. *Nature Neuroscience, 6*, 674–681.

Patel, A.D., Iversen, J., Wassenaar, M., & Hagoort, P. (2008). Musical syntactic processing in agrammatic Broca's aphasia. *Aphasiology, 22*, 776–789.

Petersson, K.M., Folia, V., & Hagoort, P. (2012). What artificial grammar learning reveals about the neurobiology of syntax. *Brain and Language, 120*, 83–95.

Posner, M.I., & Snyder, C.R. (1975). Attention and cognitive control. In R.L. Solso (Ed.), *Information processing and cognition*. New York: Lawrence Erlbaum.

Rademacher, J., Galaburda, A.M., Kennedy, D.N., Filipek, P.A., & Caviness, V.S. (1992). Human cerebral cortex: Localization, parcellation, and morphometry with magnetic resonance imaging. *Journal of Cognitive Neuroscience, 4*(4), 352–374.

Rosler, F., Putz, P., Friederici, A., & Hahne, A. (1993). Event-related potentials while encountering semantic and syntactic constraint violations. *Journal of Cognitive Neuroscience, 5*, 345–362.

Shankweiler, D., Crain, S., Gorrell, P., & Tuller, B. (1989). Reception of language in Broca's aphasia. *Language & Cognitive Processes, 4*(1), 1–33.

Steinhauer, K., & Drury, J.E. (2012). On the early left-anterior negativity (ELAN) in syntax studies. *Brain and Language, 120*(2), 135–162.

Stowe, L.A., Broere, C.A.J., Paans, A. M., Wijers, A. A., Mulder, G., Vaalbur, W., & Zwarts, F. (1998). Localizing components of a complex task: Sentence processing and working memory. *Neuroreport, 9*, 2995–2999.

Stromswold, K., Caplan, D., Alpert, N., & Rosch, S. (1996). Localization of syntactic comprehension by positron emission tomography. *Brain and Language, 52*, 452–473.

Swinney, D., & Zurif, E. (1995). Syntactic processing in aphasia. *Brain and Language, 50*, 225–239.

Tesink, C.M., Petersson, K.M., Van Berkum, J. J., Van Den Brink, D., Buitelaar, J.K., & Hagoort, P. (2009). Unification of speaker and meaning in language comprehension: An FMRI study. *Journal of Cognitive Neuroscience, 21*(11), 2085–2099.

Thompson, C.K., & Choy, J. (2009). Pronominal resolution and gap-filling in agrammatic aphasia: Evidence from eyetracking. *Journal of Psycholinguistic Research, 38*, 255–283.

Thothathiri, M., Kimberg, D.Y., & Schwartz, M.F. (2012). The neural basis of reversible sentence comprehension: Evidence from voxel-based lesion symptom mapping in aphasia. *Journal of Cognitive Neuroscience, 24*(1), 212–222.

Tyler, L.K. (1985). Real-time comprehension processes in agrammatism: A case study. *Brain and Language, 26*, 259–275.

Tyler, L.K., Wright, P., Randall, B., Marslen-Wilson, W.D., & Stamatakis, E.A. (2010). Reorganization of syntactic processing following left-hemisphere brain damage: Does right-hemisphere activity preserve function? *Brain: A Journal of Neurology, 133*(11), 3396–3408.

Ullman, M.T., Bergida, R., & O'Craven, K.M. (1997). Distinct fMRI activation patterns for regular and irregular past tense. *Neuroimage, 5*, S549.

Ullman, M.T., Corkin, S., Coppola, M., Hickok, G., Growdon, J., Koroshetz, W., & Pinker, S. (1997). A neural dissociation within language: Evidence that the mental dictionary is part of declarative memory and grammatical rules are processed by the procedural system. *Journal of Cognitive Neuroscience, 9*, 289–299.

Willems, R.M., Ozyürek, A., & Hagoort, P. (2008). Seeing and hearing meaning: ERP and fMRI evidence of word versus picture integration into a sentence context. *Journal of Cognitive Neuroscience, 20*(7), 1235–1249.

Zurif, E., Swinney, D., Prather, P., Solomon, J., & Bushell, C. (1993). An on-line analysis of syntactic processing in Broca's and Wernicke's aphasia. *Brain and Language, 45*, 448–464.

19

ASSESSMENT AND TREATMENT OF SENTENCE PROCESSING DISORDERS

Jane Marshall

Introduction

Many people with aphasia can produce and understand single words, but not sentences. Clinically this problem demands attention, mainly because it severely limits the range of meanings that the person can convey and comprehend.

Typical production problems are illustrated by the samples of aphasic speech in Table 19.1. The first four speakers all have difficulties conveying events, although the reasons for their difficulties vary. SW has limited verb access, a problem shared by many aphasic people (e.g., Berndt, Haendiges, Mitchum, & Sandson, 1997a; Breedin, Saffran, & Schwartz, 1998; Bastiaanse & Jonkers, 1998; Druks, 2002; Luzzatti et al., 2002; Marshall, 2003; Matzig et al., 2009). BG accesses a useful verb, but fails to combine it with sentence structure. PB also has structural difficulties, although of a different kind. His speech is not agrammatic and contains syntactic structures that are generally compatible with the subcategorization of the verb. Yet he cannot map the nouns appropriately onto those structures. The last speaker, VB, has more success communicating events and states, mainly because she can compose verb argument structure. Her problem seems specific to function

---

Table 19.1 Samples of Aphasic Speech

SW (talking about her daughter)
I would get Saffron and I would have to . . . because warm hair, got to . . .
(unpublished data)

BG (written description of a picture in which a man buys flowers for his girlfriend)
Interflora . . . love . . . aah . . . telephone . . . paid . . . wallet
(unpublished data)

PB (describing a picture in which a man buys a cat from a woman)
One woman and a cat is buying the man and paying the money the till
(Marshall, Chait, & Pring, 1997)

VB (description of a friend)
Valerie is big . . . fat round hip . . . she quite tall . . . she work British Telecom . . . she always borrow pattern and not bring back
(Marshall et al., 1999)

---

words and inflections. Yet, this is not without semantic consequences. For example, it is difficult for her to convey subtleties of time, aspect, and focus.

Some (but not all) of these speakers have parallel difficulties in comprehension. They understand nouns well, but fail when verbs or sentences are tested. Structures expressing reversible relations are particularly problematic. An example would be, "The man chases the woman," where a woman chasing a man is equally plausible. Functionally, this leads to problems whenever meaning cannot be inferred from context or pragmatic cues.

Clinicians have developed numerous assessment and therapy techniques in response to sentence-level problems. This chapter will provide an overview of these techniques. The first section will cover assessment, initially of production and then of comprehension, and will conclude with a discussion about diagnosis. The second section will summarize a range of therapy approaches for different types of sentence impairments and discuss technological innovations. The final discussion will briefly appraise a number of clinical issues, such as generalization of effects, the mechanism by which therapy achieves change, and possible goals for sentence-level therapies.

Assessment of Sentence Production

Sampling and Analyzing Spontaneous Speech

Generating a hypothesis about an individual's sentence processing impairment usually requires a sample of connected speech. There are various methods of sampling, each with its own advantages and disadvantages. Samples of conversation arguably offer the most authentic illustration of a person's output. However, evaluating such samples is problematic. Conversation is subject to multiple variables; for example, relating to the topic, setting, and contribution of the conversation partner. It is therefore difficult to know whether a sample is typical of the speaker, and difficult to compare samples across time. Analyzing errors is similarly problematic, particularly if the topic is unknown.

Beeke and her colleagues (Beeke, Wilkinson, & Maxim, 2007; Beeke, Maxim, Best, & Cooper, 2011) argue that Conversation Analysis (CA) circumvents many of these problems. This qualitative technique is rarely used to identify the nature of the processing impairment. Rather, it can illuminate how interactions proceed despite such impairments. To give an example, Beeke et al. (2007) use CA to show that formal grammatical structures may be "replaced" with the systematic conjunction of elements (such as nouns, adjectives, temporal terms, reported speech, and mime) in order to convey relational meanings. The application of CA in the clinical context is supported by two published clinical tools based on the approach (the Conversation Analysis Profile for People with Aphasia by Whitworth, Perkins, & Lesser, 1997; Supporting Partners of People with Aphasia in Relationships and Conversation, by Lock, Wilkinson, & Bryan, 2001).

Conversation data can also be analyzed using the POWERS (Profile of Word Errors and Retrieval in Speech; Herbert, Best, Hickin, & Howard, 2013). This quantifies the production of nouns and other content words in a speech sample, but does not address structural and morphological aspects.

In order to identify grammatical impairments, narrative samples may be preferred to conversation (e.g., because the topic is known and production can be compared to data from healthy controls). A typical technique involves retelling a familiar story, such as Cinderella. If this approach is deemed inappropriate, alternative stimuli, such as silent videos, can be used.

There are published procedures for analyzing narratives (e.g., Thompson, Shapiro, Tait, Jacobs, & Schneider, 1996; Berndt, Wayland, Rochon, Saffran, & Schwartz, 2000). These generate a range of lexical, morphological, and structural indices and can stimulate hypotheses about where processing is breaking down. For example, an abnormal verb-to-noun ratio suggests that a lexical impairment with verbs is contributing to the problem, whereas depressed morphological measures may indicate that processing function words and inflections is a site of particular difficulty.

Narrative samples cannot meet all needs. Some people with aphasia find such an unconstrained task difficult and require more cues to generate output. Storytelling is culturally specific, and may have been rarely undertaken by the person with aphasia even before their stroke. Narratives also cannot be used to elicit particular sentence forms.

Elicitation of Target Structures

Clinicians may be interested in whether a person with aphasia can produce particular structures, or in whether structural variables influence success. These questions can be addressed through picture description tasks; for example, to elicit different verb argument structures (e.g., Marshall, Chiat, & Pring, 1997) or active and passive sentences (e.g., Mitchum, Haendiges, & Berndt, 1995; Thompson & Lee, 2009). The latter is achieved by showing the person a picture of an event and then asking them to begin either with the agent noun (for actives) or the theme (for passives). Question and other moved argument forms have also been elicited; for example, through lead-in dialogues (Springer, Willmes, & Haag, 1993) or by combining modelling and pictures (Thompson et al., 1996; Ballard & Thompson, 1999). The Verb and Sentence Test (VAST; Bastiaanse, Edwards, & Rispins, 2002) includes a picture description task that targets different verb and sentence types.

None of these techniques is trouble free. It is difficult to develop event pictures that reliably target particular structures. For example, a picture in which a man feeds hay to a horse may elicit the target (three-argument) structure or any number of alternatives, such as "the horse is eating" or "the man wants the horse to eat." Imposing constraints, in the hope of eliciting particular structures, can render the task atypical. As a result, even if the person succeeds, it may be difficult to conclude that he or she could access the same structures spontaneously.

Investigating Lexical Aspects of Production

Many people with aphasia access verbs less successfully than nouns (see reviews in Druks, 2002; Marshall, 2003), and this difficulty is strongly associated with sentence production problems (e.g., Berndt et al., 1997b; Luzzatti et al., 2002, Matzig et al., 2009). Furthermore, people showing the inverse pattern (where nouns are more impaired than verbs) typically preserve sentence production skills (e.g., Marshall, Pring, Chiat, & Robson, 1996). Verb naming also seems sensitive to grammatical factors, in that verbs with complex argument structures are particularly vulnerable (Thompson, 2003).

Such findings suggest that sentence impairments may originate with a lexical difficulty with verbs and motivate assessments of verb production. This can be achieved through picture naming assessments, such as the Object and Action Naming Battery (Druks & Masterson, 2000). This provides verb and noun sets that are matched on a range of variables, including word frequency, age of acquisition, and imageabilty. Another resource is the VAST (Bastiaanse et al., 2002), which contains a verb naming test (see also Raymer, chapter 9, this volume, for additional suggestions). Some studies have explored whether sentence production is facilitated when lexical production is cued; for example, by providing the verb (see Marshall, Pring, & Chait, 1998, as well as the therapy section of this chapter). Such cueing effects support the view that the sentence impairment is at least partly attributable to lexical difficulties.

Lexical aspects of sentence production are explored rather differently by the TRIP test (Thematic Roles in Production; Whitworth, 1996). Whitworth argues that lexical retrieval in sentences and in isolation are fundamentally different. The TRIP test enables the clinician to compare naming of the same nouns in response to single item and event pictures. Evidence of successful naming in isolation, but poor naming in sentences suggests that the person is unable to access nouns as part of a thematic structure.

Competence versus Performance

It has been argued that competence may outstrip performance in agrammatism, or individuals have concealed grammatical knowledge that is not evident from their spontaneous speech. Their syntax is thought to be preserved, but difficult to activate or subject to decay (Kolk, 2006, 2008).

An early indicator of this was the finding that agrammatic speakers could carry out grammaticality judgment tasks or spot grammatical violations in spoken sentences (Linebarger, Schwartz, & Saffran, 1983). It was also revealed by priming studies. Hartsuiker and Kolk (1998) asked people with agrammatism to describe pictures, both with and without the aid of a prime. In the primed condition, they first repeated a sentence, such as "The speaker was interrupted by the noise"[1] and then described a picture (e.g., showing a golfer being struck by lightning). The primes elicited complex structures, such as passives, that were not evident in spontaneous speech or unaided picture description. It seemed that these speakers retained surprising syntactic skills that were only revealed in certain test conditions.

Sentence anagram tasks, which require the person to construct a sentence from given written phrases, may also reveal submerged skills with sentences; that is, here the person may show an awareness of word order because the burden of speech has been removed. The VAST (Bastiaanse et al., 2002) includes such a task. Marshall and colleagues (1997) developed a variant involving four fragments, where three had to be ordered into a sentence and one discarded; for example:

> the water (direct object)
> the glass (distracter)
> pours (verb)
> the man (subject)

Success on this task not only indicates sentence ordering skills, but also requires subtle knowledge of the verb's assignment rules. For example, the person has to know that "pour" maps the theme of the event, rather than the goal, onto the direct object.

Assessment of Sentence Comprehension

Identification of a sentence comprehension impairment is typically achieved via sentence-to-picture matching tasks. Here the person hears or reads a sentence and has to match it to one of a number of pictures, with distracters bearing various relationships to the target. Tasks can explore a range of structures and different types of predicate; for example, see examples in the VAST (Bastiaanse et al., 2002) and PALPA (Kay et al., 1992).

It is well established that many people with aphasia fail sentence-to-picture matching tasks whenever sentences express plausibly reversible meaning relations, and when one of the distracters represents the reversal of the target. While reversal errors can occur with subject-verb-object (SVO) structures, they are most frequent with moved argument forms such as passives and object clefts (e.g., Caramazza & Zurif, 1976; Saffran, Schwartz, & Marin, 1980; Black, Nickels, & Byng, 1992; Druks & Marshall, 1995; Berndt, Mitchum, & Wayland, 1997). The pattern is observed across languages, and even when case marking provides an additional cue to the meaning relations of a sentence (e.g., Friedmann, Reznick, Dolinski-Nuger, & Soboleva, 2010; Yarbay Duman, Altınok, Özgirgin, & Bastiaanse, 2011).

Although the occurrence of reversible errors in sentence comprehension is widely acknowledged, the source of such errors is controversial (e.g., see Schwartz et al., 1987; Miyake, Carpenter, & Just, 1994, Grodzinsky, 1995, Berndt, Mitchum, & Wayland, 1997; Bastiaanse & van Zonneveld, 2006; Yarbay et al., 2011; see also chapters 16 and 18 in this volume). In terms of clinical diagnosis, it is likely that different people fail the sentence comprehension task for different reasons. Therefore, further tasks are needed to help the clinician pin down the level of deficit.

Grammaticality Judgment Tasks

One explanation for poor sentence comprehension may be an inability to parse the syntactic structure of sentences. This hypothesis would be supported by evidence that comprehension declines as a factor of syntactic complexity. Further corroboration might be sought from tests of grammaticality judgment, in which the person is asked to judge whether heard sentences are syntactically correct or not. Stimuli can violate a range of syntactic rules, such as constituent order ("pours the water the man") and the use of auxiliaries ("is the boy is having a good time").

There is evidence that many people who fail tests of reversible sentence comprehension can nevertheless carry out grammaticality judgments (e.g., Linebarger et al., 1983; Berndt, Salasoo, Mitchum, & Sandson, 1988; Schwartz, Saffran, Fink, Myers, & Martin, 1994; Marshall et al., 1997). This led to the proposal that sentence comprehension impairments, at least for some individuals, may have a semantic rather than syntactic origin. It was argued that aphasic people could not interpret the product of the parse or determine which phrase was performing which role with respect to the verb. One explanation for such "mapping impairments" could be inadequate verb information, and particularly an inability to retrieve the grammatically relevant properties of verbs.

Tests of Verb Knowledge

Tests of verb knowledge can employ a variety of formats, including verb-to-picture matching, odd-one-out tasks, or matching verbs to video scenes of events (e.g., see examples in Byng, 1988; Marshall et al., 1993, 1996, 1997; Breedin et al., 1994). Such tasks can be used to explore different dimensions of verb meaning, particularly with respect to grammatical relevance.

Theories of verb semantics draw a distinction between the properties of verbs that do and do not carry grammatical relevance (e.g., Pinker, 1989). For example, verbs can encode information about the manner ("drip," "dribble," "smear") or direction ("spin," "roll," "fall," "rise") of movement. Such perceptual features are part of the core meaning of the verb, in that they delineate the nature of the event it describes. However, they do not play a role in specifying the structures that are, or are not, licensed by the verb. In contrast, information about the number of entities involved in an event does have grammatical relevance, in that this determines the number of arguments carried in the verb phrase. There are further, grammatically relevant distinctions of focus. For example, some verbs focus on the movement of a theme (such as "pour"), while others focus on the effect on a goal (such as "fill"). This distinction underpins the different grammatical behaviors of the verbs, particularly with respect to the thematic role that can be mapped onto the direct object:

Ben poured water into the glass
*Ben filled water into the glass
*Ben poured the glass with water
Ben filled the glass with water.

Kemmerer (2000) developed a number of tasks that explored comprehension of such grammatically irrelevant and relevant features of verb meaning. The former was tested in a verb to picture matching task (e.g., where a picture of a man coiling ribbon around a pole had to be matched to "coil," rather than "spin" and "roll"). The latter involved judging sentences that violated the relationship between verb meaning and structure. For example, one presented "coil" (a theme-focused verb) in a goal object sentence: "Sam is coiling the pole with the ribbon." These tasks showed that verb knowledge may be differentially impaired in aphasia. Two of the participants performed well on the grammatically irrelevant task, indicating retained knowledge about perceptual features of verb meaning, but were impaired when grammatically relevant knowledge was required.

Alternative approaches for exploring verb knowledge, and particularly thematic verb knowledge, have been described in the literature. Breedin and colleagues (1994) used a verb odd-one-out paradigm in which some stimuli required core meaning judgments (e.g., "harvest," "reap," "plant") and others required thematic judgments (e.g., "buy," "sell," "purchase"). Marshall and colleagues (1997) used a picture pointing task. Here the person was shown a picture of an interactive event, such as a woman giving a boat to a boy, and asked to point to one of the participants in response to a verb. So, for the given example, on one occasion the experimenter asked, "Who is giving?" and on another, "Who is taking?" PB, the person in the study, was at chance on this, despite being able to distinguish related verbs (such as "eat" and "drink") in another verb-to-picture matching task.

As suggested above, tests such as these have shown that many people cannot access the grammatically relevant properties of verbs, even though core meaning may be retained. Such difficulties may underpin, or contribute to, sentence comprehension impairments. Importantly, not all people with aphasia show this pattern, and there are at least two documented cases where participants performed best when tasks tapped grammatically relevant aspects of verb meaning (Breedin et al., 1994; Marshall, Chiat, Pring, & Robson, 1996). Such double dissociations suggest that different aspects of verbs may be vulnerable to different types of brain damage. Clinically, these findings argue for assessments that can uncover different skills and weaknesses with verbs and provide a basis for individually tailored therapy.

Assessment of Working Memory

Sentence comprehension may be compromised by difficulties in storing and manipulating linguistic information; that is, because of a working memory deficit (Just & Carpenter, 1992; Miyake et al., 1994; Harrmann, Just, & Carpenter, 1997; Friedmann & Gvion, 2003).

Assessing working memory in aphasia is challenging. Tests of digit span may be impaired by production deficits, or, in the case of backward tasks, by difficulties in comprehending instructions. Other tasks may be too linguistically demanding. For example Daneman and Carpenter's Reading Span test (Daneman & Carpenter, 1980) requires the person to read sentences while retaining the final words in their original order. Given such challenges, studies often employ manipulated versions of tests (e.g., where responses require recognition rather than recall; see Wright and Shisler, 2005, for review).

Wright and colleagues (2007) argue that N Back tasks offer a good methodology. In this task, the person hears a list of words or sentences and has to respond (by pressing a button) whenever an item is the same as the one immediately preceding it or one that was two back; for example:

apple . . . peach . . . *peach* (1 back)
plum . . . apple . . . *plum* (2 back)

This task can manipulate the type of linguistic information that has to be processed: phonological, semantic, or syntactic. Phonological items involve rhyming words (e.g., where the stimuli all end in "at"). Semantic items involve stimuli from the same semantic category, such as fruit. Syntactic items require participants to detect active ("The doctor kissed the banker") or passive ("The banker was kissed by the doctor") sentences that match previous stimuli.

Wright et al. (2007) showed that people with aphasia could comply with this task, with a similar pattern of performance to healthy controls. In several of the individuals, performance was affected by the nature of the stimuli, with phonological and syntactic items being the most impaired. Furthermore, there seemed to be a relationship between syntactic working memory and sentence comprehension (e.g., those who were impaired on the syntactic memory items also had impaired comprehension).

Some case studies have manipulated test stimuli in order to explore memory effects. For example, Mitchum and colleagues (1995) explored the effect of length in a sentence-to-picture matching test. They found that their subject, ML, performed worse when sentences were padded with (irrelevant) adjectives and adverbs; for example, "The *friendly* man is *gently* pushing the *stubborn* woman." He was also poor at repeating such sentences. Interestingly, material within the verb phrase was often omitted in the padded condition.

Byng and colleagues (1994) developed a number of tasks to explore sentence retention. In one, subjects were shown three character pictures—for example, of a nun, a cowboy, and an astronaut. They then heard an SVO sentence involving two of the characters and had to point to the relevant pictures in their order of mention. In another task, the person heard two sentences and had to judge whether or not they were identical. Different sentences had reversed word order; for example, "the nun splashes the queen" versus "the queen splashes the nun."

There is considerable debate about the role of working memory in sentence comprehension (see Wright & Shisler, 2005; chapter 16, this volume). One possibility is that memory impairments interact with other deficits (e.g., because they limit the resources available for linguistic computation). This seemed to be the case for ML above (Mitchum et al., 1995). He displayed evidence of poor verb processing. So, when memory capacity was exceeded, as in the padded sentence repetition task, verb information was particularly vulnerable to omission. It seems that clinicians need to be alert to the memory limitations of their clients, not necessarily as an explanation for the comprehension deficit, but as a possible contributor.

On-Line Procedures

All the above assessment techniques are off-line. They require the person to carry out a conscious task, such as pointing to a picture, in response to a given stimulus. It is assumed that processing of the stimulus is complete before the task is executed.

A number of studies use alternative on-line techniques (e.g., Shapiro & Levine, 1990; Tyler, 1992; Zurif, Swinney, Prather, Solomon, & Bushell, 1993; Tyler, Ostriu, Cooke, & Moss, 1995; Dickey, Choy, & Thompson, 2007; Dickey & Thompson, 2009; DeDe, 2012; Mack, Ji, & Thompson, 2013). Here, the skills or knowledge being tested are exposed to less conscious manipulation. The procedures also tap processing as it takes place, and so provide insights into its time course.

One on-line procedure uses lexical decision, where the probe word is presented within different linguistic contexts. Of interest is how these contexts affect judgment times. Such tasks can expose interesting skills in aphasic people, which might be missed by more conventional testing. For example, Shapiro and colleagues (1990, 1993) presented lexical decision probes within a variety of sentences. The verbs used in the sentences had various argument structures. Some allowed for just one structure, such as "put," which takes an obligatory three-place structure, while others allowed for multiple structures, such as "send," which can be used either with two arguments or with three. Previous testing with nonaphasic people had shown that the complexity of a verb's argument structures affected latencies on the lexical decision task, in that verbs with multiple argument structures delayed decision times (Shapiro, Zurif, & Grimshaw, 1987). These findings were replicated with a group of people with Broca's aphasia. It seemed that the participants with Broca's aphasia, like controls, were retrieving all the argument options of a verb during sentence processing, even in sentences that they could not comprehend.

An alternative on-line methodology employs eye tracking, where the participant's gaze is monitored during sentence comprehension. Dickey et al. (2007) used this methodology to explore the comprehension of noncanonical wh-sentences, such as, "Who did the boy kiss that day at school?" Participants first heard a story. They then listened to the questions while their eye movements were monitored over an array of pictures showing figures from the story. Eye movements of healthy controls were found to fixate on the picture representing the moved element (e.g., the person who was kissed) at the point of the verb. Crucially, this pattern was also revealed by the participants with agrammatic aphasia. It seemed that both groups were processing phrase movement, even those with aphasia who had poor off-line comprehension of moved argument forms.

On-line findings have interesting clinical potential. For at least some participants they offer further evidence that competence may exceed performance (e.g., they reveal latent verb and sentence processing skills that are not fully exploited in sentence comprehension). Therapy could aim to bring such skills more to a level of consciousness.

Tests of Event Knowledge

Events and states do not automatically map onto language. Rather, speakers express a particular idealization or construal of events. As noted by Pinker (1989):

> The meaning of a sentence ... is a highly schematic construal of an event or state, an austere idealization into a structure built of foundational notions such as causation, motion and change. The same situation, even the same state of knowledge about a situation, must first be mapped onto one of the many possible idealizations of it before it can be described in words.
>
> (p. 360)

Pinker argues for a level of cognitive processing that acts as a mediator between our general ideas and the production of language (and see similar arguments in Pinker, 2007). Furthermore, this thinking is linguistically driven. In other words, we have to adopt idealizations over events that can be mapped onto the words and structures available in our language. Slobin (1996), in a similar discussion, refers to this as "thinking for speaking."

"Thinking for speaking" might be illustrated via the event in Figure 19.1. Even a simple event like this presents the speaker with a number of options. English allows us to focus on the manner in which the sand is moved (in which case we might select a verb like "shovel") or on the effect on the wheelbarrow (in which case we might select "fill"). Such idealizations do not merely affect verb selection, but also the mapping of arguments around the verb. So, if we construe the event as having an effect on the barrow, we might opt for sentence (1) below, whereas if our focus is more on the sand we might opt for (2):

1. The man is loading the wheelbarrow with sand.
2. The man is loading sand into the wheelbarrow.

It has been suggested that some people with aphasia may struggle to formulate language-appropriate idealizations of events, and that this may underpin their difficulties with sentences (e.g., Marshall, Pring, & Chiat, 1993; Byng et al., 1994; Dipper, 1999, Black & Chiat,

Figure 19.1   Shovel/fill/load event

2000; Marshall & Cairns, 2005; Cairns, Marshall, & Dipper, 2007; Marshall 2009). Exploring this proposal is not easy, as it requires investigation of the thinking that takes place just before speech.

A number of assessments have focused on event knowledge. Dipper (1999) used a video task to investigate whether subjects were aware that an event was taking place. Twenty scenes were presented, half of which depicted events (e.g., someone washing up) and half states (e.g., washing up on a draining board). Participants had to indicate whether or not something was happening. To exclude the possibility that decisions were based purely on the detection of motion, Dipper introduced the illusion of movement when filming the states; for example, by using camera panning (for a similar task using pictures see Byng et al., 1994).

Other tasks explore whether or not subjects can categorize events. In the Event Perception Test the person has to match two representations of the same verb, in the presence of a distracter (Marshall et al., 1999), and in Dipper's Event Photograph Task subjects are asked to identify the odd one out from three photos; for example, where two represent "have" states and one an "act" event (Dipper, 1999). The Kissing and Dancing Test (Bak & Hodges, 2003) also probes semantic knowledge of actions. This presents triplets of action pictures, two of which have to be associated on the basis of their semantic relationship.

The Role Video (Marshall et al., 1993) investigates whether the person can identify the role structure of events. In this task, the person is shown a video clip of an event, such as a man ironing a shirt. The person is then provided with three photographs and asked to pick the one that shows the outcome of the event. One distracter retains the theme, but shows an outcome from a different type of event; for example, a picture of a torn shirt. The other shows an outcome from the same type of event, but with a different theme; for example, a picture of ironed trousers. Half the stimuli involve interactive events, such as a woman punching a man. Here, one of the distracters shows the outcome of the role reversal; for example, a picture of a woman with a bandaged eye. Thus, in this task the person has to judge both what type of event has taken place, and who was performing which role.

Cairns and colleagues (2007) used naming as a window on thinking. Participants were shown pictures of events and asked not to describe them but to name the entities involved. All the events involved a person acting on either an object or another person with an instrument. Controls showed an interesting pattern. They typically named only the three main entities and adopted a sentence-like order in their naming; that is, they usually named the agent first, then the theme, and finally the goal. Two people with agrammatic aphasia were tested. One showed the typical pattern of controls. This pattern suggested that she retained knowledge of the role structure of events, despite her agrammatism. The other did not. He named many peripheral items in the pictures in addition to the main entities, and his order of naming was less driven by the argument structure of the event. It seemed that this participant was not fully analyzing the role structure of the depicted events. In line with this, he was impaired on nonverbal tests of event knowledge, such as the Role Video and the Kissing and Dancing Test.

On-line techniques might offer further insights into "thinking for speaking." Thompson and colleagues (Thompson, Dickey, Cho, Lee, & Griffin, 2007) asked participants to describe two- and three-argument pictures, while tracking their eye movements. Controls showed anticipatory fixations on entities in the pictures that corresponded with the upcoming arguments in the sentences. This pattern was revealed by the participants with aphasia, but only for two-argument items. The authors relate this finding to the argument structure complexity hypothesis, which states that verb production in agrammatic aphasia reflects argument structure. It might also point to difficulties in event analysis, particularly when multiple arguments are involved in the event.

The above tasks may illuminate whether or not the person can make language-relevant judgments about events. However, findings are rarely conclusive. For example, judgments in picture tasks may be based on idiosyncratic features of the stimuli, and the naming behaviors revealed by Cairns et al. (2007) may have reflected factors that were unconnected to the hypothesis being tested. Nevertheless, such tasks might point to "early" difficulties in event processing that at least contribute to a problem with sentences.

Diagnosis

This section has described numerous assessment tools and techniques, only some of which are widely available. This raises the question of what constitutes a clinically viable assessment regime. Given the constraints on clinical time the following could offer a core assessment of sentence skills:

- A test of reversible sentence comprehension, ideally involving a range of verb types and structures.
- A test of verb comprehension, ideally exploring both core and thematic meaning.
- An analysis of connected speech; for example, from a narrative sample or picture description.
- A test of noun and verb naming.

The reversible sentence comprehension test can be used to identify a comprehension impairment and to generate hypotheses about the sources of that impairment. For example, performance may be affected by sentence length or complexity. This may signal a difficulty in parsing or in working memory. Evidence of improved performance in the written modality might signal the latter. Alternatively, it may emerge that errors are most related to predicate type. For example, sentences with agentive predicates (like "splash") may be understood, whereas sentences with nonagentive predicates (like "admire") are not. This might suggest that sentence difficulties originate with a semantic problem with verbs, in which case the verb comprehension test may provide corroborating evidence. This should also indicate which verb properties are most accessible. For example, the person may cope well with core meaning distinctions but not thematic distinctions. On the production side, the regime should highlight diagnostic patterns, such as verb omission, reduced production of closed-class words, and structural poverty. Of course, in individual cases this basic regime could be supplemented by further assessments, such as tests of working memory, grammaticality judgments, or explorations of event knowledge.

Sentence processing impairments are complex and difficult to explore. It is not, therefore, realistic to expect clinicians to arrive at cast-iron diagnoses of their patients' difficulties. Rather, they need assessments that help to formulate a rationale for therapy; for example, by identifying aspects of processing that are at least contributing to the problem and likely to make a difference if improved. A number of studies have demonstrated that it is possible to develop a therapy hypothesis from an economical assessment regime (e.g., see Webster, Morris, & Franklin, 2005) and within routine clinical settings (e.g., see Swinburn, 1999; Perkins & Hinshelwood, 2007). These studies may not have fully diagnosed the individual's sentence processing impairments. However, in all cases it seemed that the impairment was sufficiently understood for successful therapy to commence.

Therapy

Therapy Working at the Level of the Event

It has been argued that sentence production depends upon the ability to compose focused and constrained conceptual representations of events, and that this may be difficult for some people with aphasia (Marshall, 2009). If this is the case, therapy might target this level.

This was the approach taken with MM (Marshall et al., 1993; Marshall & Cairns, 2005). MM had a range of verb and sentence impairments. Production was nonfluent, with few verbs and no verb argument structures. Reversal errors occurred in comprehension, even with simple SVO sentences. Verb comprehension was poor, particularly in tasks requiring thematic knowledge. In addition to these difficulties, MM made errors on nonverbal event processing tasks. For example, with the Role Video she could select outcomes for nonreversible events, but not reversible ones. With the latter, she tended to select the role distracter. So, when shown an event in which a man sells a camera to a woman, she chose an outcome picture in which the man holds the camera.

From these findings, the authors hypothesized that MM's difficulties with verbs, and verb argument structures were underpinned by a failure to conceptualize the role structure of events. Therapy targeted this level. The task required her to make a number of decisions about events presented on video. These decisions were supported by photographs illustrating the various event participants. So, for example, MM was required to identify the agent and theme of the event by picking the relevant photos. She also had to specify the nature of the action by selecting an appropriate outcome photograph (so for an event in which a man ironed a shirt, she selected a picture of an ironed shirt as opposed to a torn shirt). Therapy was made more complex by increasing the number of photographs from which MM had to select and by progressing from nonreversible to reversible events.

Therapy was almost entirely confined to such event tasks: it involved no production or comprehension of sentences. Despite this, after therapy MM produced more verbs and verb argument structures on a picture description task. The authors account for this by arguing that therapy helped MM to develop language-appropriate event construals, which mapped more readily onto verbs and verb structures.

Therapy conducted with EM (Marshall, 1999; Marshall & Cairns, 2005) also engaged event analysis. EM had agrammatic speech with reduced structure and limited verb production. Her first therapy program targeted verb access (see below). Although this improved both verb and sentence production, gains were limited to picture description tasks. When asked to retell a story, without the aid of pictures, EM's difficulties remained.

These results invited a reappraisal of EM's deficit. It seemed that production was dependent on the conceptual demands of the task. When her thinking was directed by a picture, EM could access the treated verbs. In more open tasks, where no such scaffolding was available, she could not.

A second program of therapy aimed to help EM to formulate constrained messages that could be mapped onto simple verb argument structures. The main task involved recounting clips of commercial videos (one film used in therapy was *Ruthless People*). EM was provided with a number of strategies to assist narrative production; for example, think of one event at a time, act out each event, and then try to describe your gesture. She was also familiarized with 10 general verbs (such as "put" and "go") that might be used to describe a wide range of events. There was evidence during therapy that these strategies effectively cued EM's production:

> EM Oh dear . . . no
>
> JM OK. He's got to the door. Think about what he does next. Just the first thing. Try acting it out.

EM (mimes putting something on the floor) put the bag on the ground . . . (mimes opening it) open the bag . . . (mimes reaching in) pick up the credit card . . . oh no

JM (mimes inserting the card in the door)

EM put the card in the . . . crack

Such gains were also observed in post-therapy measures of narrative production, in that there was an increase in verb and verb argument production and less dependence on single noun phrases. Marshall (1999) hypothesized that therapy changed EM's conceptual preparations for language (see also Marshall & Cairns, 2005). It helped EM to formulate highly focused idealizations that could be more readily mapped onto the verbs and verb argument structures available to her.

Event-level therapy might be attempted if there are signs that conceptual difficulties are contributing to the problem with sentences. For example, the person may be impaired on nonverbal tasks, such as the Kissing and Dancing Test (Bak & Hodges, 2003). Picture description tasks may also be informative. These may reveal an inability to focus on the key features of the event (e.g. with the naming of peripheral elements in place of the argument nouns). Alternatively, such tasks might elicit verb argument structures that are not available in spontaneous speech or narrative. As with EM, this might suggest that the person needs help to organize their focus on events.

Therapies Based on the Mapping Hypothesis

In the 1980s, Schwartz and colleagues published a series of influential papers arguing that people with Broca's aphasia can process syntactic information—for example, in carrying out grammaticality judgments—but cannot relate that information to meaning. It was claimed that their difficulties reflected an inability to map thematic roles onto sentence positions, either because they could not access thematic information from verbs, or because they lacked assignment procedures (e.g., Saffran et al., 1980; Schwartz, Saffran, & Marin, 1980; Linebarger et al., 1983; Schwartz, Linebarger, & Saffran, 1985; Schwartz et al., 1987).

The mapping hypothesis had clear implications for therapy. Rather than training surface sentence forms, therapy should aim to clarify connections between meaning and structure. Numerous therapy studies were influenced by the hypothesis (e.g., Jones, 1986; Byng, 1988; Nickels, Byng, & Black, 1991; Le Dorze, Jacob, & Coderre, 1991; Byng, Nickels, & Black, 1994; Schwartz et al., 1994; Mitchum et al., 1995; Haendiges, Berndt, & Mitchum, 1996; Crerar, Ellis, & Dean, 1996; Marshall et al., 1997; Mitchum, Greenwald, & Berndt, 1997; Berndt & Mitchum, 1998; Rochon, Laird, Bose, & Schofield 2005; and see reviews in Marshall, 1995; Mitchum, Greenwald, & Berndt, 2000).

Various techniques are employed in mapping therapy. One approach, developed by Jones (1986), involves the metalinguistic analysis of verb argument structure (see also Le Dorze et al., 1991; Schwartz et al., 1994). Therapy stimuli take the form of written sentences. The person is first asked to segment each sentence into syntactic phrases and find and mark the verb. Then the patient or theme is identified (e.g., "What is s/he V-ing?"); followed by the agent (e.g., "Who is V-ing?"). These roles are marked with relevant wh-words or underlined in different colors. Therapy progresses from simple to more complex, moved argument sentences. Schwartz and colleagues (1994) also manipulated predicate type, in that one group of sentences involved verbs that assign the role of stimulus/experiencer (such as "love").

Jones's therapy requires certain skills on the part of the aphasic person. They need to comprehend wh-questions, since these feature prominently in the task, and be able to read (although Le Dorze and colleagues bypassed this problem by using "pictorial sentences"). The treatment also assumes that the person can identify phrase boundaries, although this is consistent with the mapping hypothesis.

Other treatments impose less stringent demands. Mitchum and colleagues (1995) used variants of a sentence-to-picture matching task. These included verification, in which the person had to confirm whether or not a spoken sentence matched a picture, and forced choice, in which the person had to match a spoken sentence to one of two pictures. Feedback either confirmed a correct judgment or identified errors while repeating the target (see also Haendiges, Berndt, & Mitchum, 1996; Berndt & Mitchum, 1998).

Word order tasks also feature in mapping therapy. Byng (1988) and Nickels and colleagues (1991) asked participants to describe pictures by ordering sentence fragments. Pictures were presented in related pairs; for example, one might show a monk writing a letter and the other a robber writing a letter. The person had to select one picture and compose a description using given sentence fragments. When this was accomplished, they were asked to change the sentence so that it described the other picture; for example, by swapping the first noun phrase.

From these brief descriptions, it is clear that mapping therapies encompass a wide range of techniques and strategies. Further approaches have been developed; for example, to exploit language-specific markers of thematic role assignment (Santamaria, Munoz, Atkins, Hobbs, & O'Donald, 2013) or to treat a range of sentence forms (Rochon et al., 2005). Perhaps the most unusual therapy was developed by Byrne and Varley (2011). Their participant retained striking skills in mathematics, despite severe agrammatic aphasia. Treatment called upon his math skills in order to bootstrap his understanding of grammar. So, for example, reversible mathematical expressions (such as $10 - 2$ vs. $2 - 10$) were used to illuminate reversible linguistic expressions (such as "the cat chases the monster" vs. "the monster chases the cat").

Although varying, mapping treatments are united by a common aim—that is, to clarify how sentence structure expresses meaning. Thus they all emphasize where event participants are mapped in relation to the verb. Many of the therapies also engage a level of conscious reflection on the part of the aphasic person. For example, Nickels and colleagues (1991) did not immediately correct the production errors made by their participant, AER, preferring to promote self-judgment and correction. In this way therapy aims to develop an underlying linguistic skill, rather than simply drilling sentences (see Byng & Black, 1995, for similar arguments).

Although positive, outcomes from mapping therapy have been variable. The two seminal studies (Jones, 1986; Byng, 1988) suggested that treatment could significantly (and in the case of Byng, rapidly) improve sentence skills. There were also intriguing signs of generalization. Both studies indicated that input therapy could benefit production, and Byng (1988) showed that therapy focusing on just one predicate type (prepositions) could bring about improved production and comprehension of others. Such findings led to the proposal that one mapping mechanism might be common to production and comprehension, and with procedures shared by different predicates.

Subsequent studies, however, qualified these early claims. Many failed to achieve generalization from comprehension to production (e.g., see Mitchum et al., 1995; Rochon et al., 2005), and improvements were often confined to the treated predicate type. For example, PB received therapy focusing on three-argument structures. After treatment, descriptions of three-argument events improved, but not descriptions of two-argument events (Marshall et al., 1997). Conversely, AER (Nickels et al., 1991) only improved with two-argument, agentive sentences, which were the treated type. Studies have also reported participants who either failed to benefit at all or only very minimally (e.g., see Schwartz et al., 1994; Byng et al., 1994).

These different outcomes almost certainly reflect a number of factors. In some cases progress may be hindered by additional deficits, such as limitations in working memory (e.g., see Mitchum et al., 1995), or problems with event conceptualization (e.g., Byng et al., 1994). Mitchum and colleagues (1995) also suggest that early claims for input to output generalization may have been overstated, in that post-therapy production may have simply contained more verb arguments, rather than improved mapping per se. They also argue that therapy may have included a production element, even if this was not specifically focused in the task. Nevertheless, the various approaches to mapping therapy have improved either sentence comprehension or production, with most of the people involved. Furthermore, most studies achieve a degree of generalization, if only with untreated examples of the target sentence type. Such generalization suggests that therapy has not simply drilled sentences, but has restored competence in mapping arguments of at least the target predicate types.

Selection of a mapping approach is encouraged by evidence of a mapping impairment. Typical signs of mapping impairment are poor comprehension of reversible sentences, verb omissions, and reduced verb argument structure in output. People with pure mapping impairments should be able to carry out grammaticality judgments or detect syntactic errors in sentences. A further indicant may be poor verb comprehension, particularly with tasks that require access to thematic information. Interestingly, mapping impairments are not confined to agrammatic speakers but can also occur in fluent forms of aphasia (Mitchum et al., 1995; Marshall et al., 1997).

Therapy Aiming to Improve Verb Retrieval

The prevalence of verb impairments in aphasia has made them a particular focus for therapy (see Conroy et al., 2006; Webster and Whitworth, 2012, for reviews). Many of the treatments used techniques drawn from the anomia therapy literature, such as repeated semantic and/or phonological cueing (Raymer & Ellsworth, 2002; Raymer, Ciampitti, Holliway, et al., 2007; Wamburgh, Doyle, Martinez, & Kalinyak-Fliszar, 2002) and semantic feature analysis (Wambaugh & Ferguson, 2007). In some cases single word tasks are combined with sentence closure cues (e.g., Edwards & Tucker, 2006; McCann & Doleman, 2011). Gesture has also been explored as a facilitator of verb production based on the hypothesis that this may act as a semantic cue (e.g., Pashek 1998; Rodriguez, Raymer, & Gonzalez-Rothi, 2006; Rose & Sussmilch, 2008; Boo & Rose, 2011). Conroy and colleagues have carried out a series of verb therapy experiments comparing different approaches, such as errorless versus errorful learning (Conroy, Sage, & Lambon Ralph, 2009a), sentence versus single word cues (Conroy et al., 2009b), and increasing versus decreasing cues (Conroy et al., 2009c).

These studies show that therapy can significantly enhance verb production (e.g., as assessed on picture naming tasks). However, benefits are typically confined to the words that have featured in therapy, with little or no generalization to untreated verbs. Comparisons of therapy techniques have also failed to identify the most effective approach. For example, including gesture in therapy was no more effective than using verbal tasks alone (Rodriguez et al., 2006, Rose & Sussmilch, 2008), and benefits from semantic cueing, phonological cueing, and mere repetition were the same (Raymer & Ellsworth, 2002). Conroy et al. (2009a, 2009b, 2009c) found no effect of cue type, and no difference between errorless and errorful learning. Given such equivocal findings, Webster and Whitworth (2012) suggest that all therapy tasks, regardless of format, may work in rather similar ways (i.e., by strengthening the connections between semantics and phonology for target verbs).

Verb deficits are particularly, although not exclusively, associated with difficulties in sentence production (e.g. Berndt et al., 1997; Luzzatti et al., 2002, Matzig et al., 2009). This is, perhaps, not surprising, as verbs are thought to encode information that is crucial for sentence generation, such as the number of arguments that can be combined in the verb phrase. Therapies that restore verb access might, therefore, bring about associated gains in sentence production.

Therapy conducted with EM (Marshall et al., 1998; Marshall 1999) supported this view. EM's speech was typically agrammatic, with virtually no sentence structure and few verbs. Verb naming was poor, regardless of the task and despite considerable success with nouns.

EM retained many skills with verbs. She comprehended verbs well and could read them aloud (regardless of regularity) and write them, for example, in naming tasks. These findings suggested that semantic representations of verbs were preserved, together with their phonological and orthographic forms. Her problems were confined to spoken naming, and were therefore attributed to a deficit in accessing phonology from semantics.

One final assessment suggested that EM's difficulties with sentence production were strongly related to her verb retrieval problem. EM was asked to generate spoken sentences from 64 provided nouns and (uninflected) verbs, which were matched for frequency. EM responded very positively to the verb cues. She generated 27 correct sentences from them, compared to just 11 with the nouns, and her responses included some complex structures; for example, "The girl was drowned in the pool" (cued with "drown"). It seemed that merely providing the phonology of the verb all but eliminated EM's agrammatism. This was a positive prognosticator for therapy. If therapy could recover spontaneous access to verbs, improved sentence production should follow.

Therapy included word-to-picture matching tasks with verbs, odd-one-out judgments, and producing verbs from given scenarios. Many tasks provided written options for selection. Given EM's good ability to read aloud, this ensured that she was able to access phonology while also processing the meaning of the target verbs. EM was also encouraged to cue herself by writing verbs and then reading them aloud.

After therapy, EM's ability to access the treated verbs in a picture description task improved significantly. Encouragingly, there was a corresponding improvement in her sentence production with these verbs. Thus, with EM, verb retrieval therapy not only improved verb production, but also stimulated more sentences.

Webster and Whitworth (2012) show that the results achieved with EM were not exceptional. Their review of 26 verb therapy studies identified 6 that brought about gains in sentence production purely from single word treatment tasks. Seven further studies reported sentence gains. But these engaged sentence-level activities in therapy (e.g., by using sentence completion cues). Less positively, there were a number of individuals, across all studies, who failed to benefit at the sentence level, and half the reviewed studies (12) did not assess sentence-level gains.

An approach that specifically targets generalization to sentence contexts is Verb Network Strengthening Treatment (VNeST; Edmonds, Nadeau, & Kiran, 2009; Edmonds & Babb, 2011). VNeST is based on the hypothesis that verbs activate thematic networks, including agents and patients who typically participate in the activity. So the verb "measure" might activate "chef," "carpenter" and "seamstress" together with "flour," "wood," and "fabric." In line with this hypothesis, VNeST does not work with verbs in isolation. Rather, it encourages the participant to associate target verbs with typical argument nouns. Tasks include generating agents and patients for given verbs, judging sentences with appropriate and inappropriate thematic role pairings ("The designer measures the room" vs. "The infant measures the lumber") and asking questions about who or what can play different roles with respect to a verb. VNeST was tested with six aphasic participants, across two studies, with promising results (Edmonds et al., 2009; Edmonds & Babb, 2011). All showed improved production of agents, verbs and patients when describing pictures with trained verbs. Most (five of the six) achieved similar results when describing pictures of semantically related, but untreated, stimuli. There were also generalizations to tests of verb and noun naming, sentence generation, and discourse, although not with all participants.

In summary, research has shown that therapy can improve access to verbs through a variety of cued naming tasks. As effects are often, although not always, confined to verbs that appear in therapy, targets should be carefully chosen based on their relevance to the person being treated. Gains in sentence production may follow verb therapy, but cannot be assumed. Such generalization may be promoted by tasks that associate verbs with other sentence components.

Selecting verb retrieval therapy is encouraged by evidence of reduced verb access, particularly in relation to nouns. However, this is a common aphasic symptom, which often accompanies other sentence-level deficits. Furthermore, other therapies, such as mapping treatments, can have a positive impact on verb production (e.g., see Byng, 1988; Schwartz et al., 1994; Marshall et al., 1993).

The clinician might focus therapy purely on verb access if there is evidence that the verb deficit is the main contributor to the output problem, as seemed to be the case for EM. Verb therapy might also be attempted if other treatments have been unhelpful, or if there is a residual verb problem, even after the successful application of another approach.

Treatment for Verb Morphology

Difficulties with freestanding and affixed grammatical morphology are common in aphasia. Verb morphology is often disproportionately impaired (e.g., Faroqi-Shah & Thompson, 2004), with tense being a particular site of difficulty (Arabatzi & Edwards, 2002; Stavrakaki & Kouvava, 2003). Druks and Carroll (2005) argue that tense impairments may have wide-reaching consequences. They describe DOR, who had poor sentence and verb production coupled with a tense impairment. For example, when a verb was produced it was typically stripped of its tense marker: "maybe two or three weeks time go abroad." The authors argue that DOR's tense impairment underpinned his verb and sentence difficulties. Without tense, verbs had lost their grammatical status. They were simply labelling actions, rather than providing the building blocks for verb argument structure.

Similar proposals were put forward by Mitchum and her colleagues (Mitchum et al., 1993; Mitchum & Berndt, 1994). They provided verb retrieval therapy to two individuals, which improved verb access, but with limited generalization to sentence production. The authors hypothesized that there was an additional impairment in recovering the morphosyntactic elements of the verb phrase, and that without these elements sentence production could not proceed.

This impairment was targeted in a second therapy program, aiming to facilitate the production of verb phrases inflected for future, present, and past tense. Therapy was based on 14 sets of sequential pictures, showing an action about to happen, the action being carried out, and the action just completed. The task involved ordering and describing these pictures. Tense markers were cued by specific verbal instructions; for example, the present was triggered by the instruction that the action was happening "right now." Further cues provided the uninflected verb and increasing portions of the sentence.

This therapy improved the sentence production of both participants, with several important generalizations. First, verb morphology improved even with untreated verbs. Second, the effects generalized to tasks that differed from those used in therapy (although not to open narrative). Finally, there were cross-modality effects. So, one participant, whose treatment was confined to written tasks, nevertheless achieved better spoken production after therapy. These generalizations suggested that the participants had acquired a general competence in building the target grammatical frames. Furthermore, this competence seemed modality free, which suggested that tense representations are abstract in nature, rather than phonologically or orthographically specified.

Faroqi-Shah (2008) compared the effects of two therapies for tense. One was termed morphosyntactic treatment. This involved repeated practice with tensed forms, but with little emphasis on meaning. Tasks included auditory discrimination of tensed verb forms (e.g., "Do these words sound the same 'washes' . . . 'washed'?"), lexical decision with legal and illegal tensed verbs ("washed" vs. "digged"), the generation of tensed verbs from given verb roots, and transformation tasks (e.g., where a verb in the past tense had to be expressed in the present tense). The contrastive therapy was termed morphosematic treatment. As the name implies, this involved tasks that engaged meaning. For example, participants had to detect tense anomalies, such as "yesterday the boy will wash his hands," and then carry out sentence-to-picture matching tasks that required a grasp of tense. Production tasks involved the completion and ordering of tensed sentences to describe pictures.

Four participants were randomly assigned to the treatment conditions. Results from the first were disappointing, as assessed by picture description and narrative tasks. Although more tensed verbs were produced, they were often anomalous: "tomorrow . . . the . . . he peeled. She is peeling" (target: "the lady will peel the potatoes"). Those who received the morphosemantic treatment achieved much better outcomes, with the production of more correctly tensed verbs. Interpreting these findings, Faroqi-Shah (2008) argues that aphasic tense impairments reflect an inability to map conceptual temporal information onto the required verb form (see similar arguments in Faroqi-Shah & Thompson, 2007). Therefore therapy must engage such semantic mapping in order to be effective.

A replication of this study (Faroqi-Shah, 2013) addressed a further theoretical question: that is, the processing of regular and irregular tense forms. A number of accounts suggest that verbs with regular tenses are processed via a default rule (verb + past = verbed), while tense for irregular verbs is encoded in the lexicon (give + past = gave) (e.g., Ullman, Pancheva, Love, Yee, Swinney, & Hickok, 2005). Faroqi-Shah further argues that a blocking mechanism prevents the inappropriate application of the regular rule. So when tensing "give" the illegal form "gived" is generated, but then blocked and replaced by the lexically specified "gave." Thus irregular verbs excite the regular rule, even though the product of the rule is subsequently eliminated.

According to this account treatment with irregular verbs might achieve generalization to regular forms, while the inverse would not be anticipated. Faroqi-Shah (2013) tested this prediction in her therapy study. Six individuals with agrammatic aphasia took part. All received morphosemantic therapy, three with regular stimuli (such as "play/played") and three with irregular stimuli (such as "sit/sat"). Results were consistent with the prediction. All participants made gains with the treated verbs (i.e., they were much more able to describe tensed pictures using the verbs). Generalization to untreated regular verbs was also achieved, regardless of whether regular or irregular verbs were used in therapy. Conversely, generalization to untrained irregular verbs was inconsistent, even if this verb type had been trained.

Therapy for tense might be attempted if tense markers are omitted or used in error. Where there are multiple symptoms (e.g. affecting verb retrieval, sentence structure, and morphology), other therapies might be attempted first, such as mapping or verb retrieval therapy. However, studies suggest that even when these therapies are successful deficits in morphology may remain and require intervention.

Treatment for Complex Structures

Sentences in which arguments have been moved from their canonical positions pose particular difficulties for people with aphasia, possibly because of a difficulty in processing traces and co-indexes. So, for example, sentence (1) below is more likely to be understood or produced than sentences (2) and (3).

1. The soldier is pushing the woman in the street.
2. It is the woman *i* who the soldier is pushing *trace i* in the street.
3. Who *i* is the soldier pushing *trace i* in the street?

Thomson and colleagues have developed a treatment protocol that aims to restore skills in processing phrase movement, now termed Treatment of Underlying forms (TUF; Thompson 2008; and see Thompson, Shapiro, & Roberts, 1993; Thompson & Shapiro, 1995; Thompson, Shapiro, Tait, Jacobs, & Schneider, 1996; Thompson, Shapiro, Ballard, Jacobs, Schneider, & Tait, 1997; Ballard & Thompson, 1999; Jacobs and Thompson, 2000).

In a typical TUF treatment task, participants first hear models of the target sentence structure, such as wh-questions like (3) above. They are then provided with a written canonical sentence, which they have to transform into the target structure. The sentence elements are written on separate cards, to permit movement, and the person is given relevant wh-word and question mark cards. In the first therapy step, the verb and its thematic roles are identified. So, for example, the therapist might point to the verb and say: "This is *pushing*; it is the action of the sentence" and then point to the object noun phrase, saying: "This is the *woman*; she is the person being pushed." When all roles have been identified, the object NP is replaced by the relevant wh-card (who) and the question mark added to the end of the sentence. The aphasic person is now asked to produce the modified sentence: "The soldier is pushing *who* in the street?" After this, the therapist demonstrates subject/auxiliary verb inversion. Finally, the wh-word is moved to the beginning of the sentence, and the aphasic person is asked to produce the resultant question form. All steps are then repeated, with less input from the therapist. These therapy stages aim to clarify the verb argument relations of the sentence and demonstrate how they are expressed in the noncanonical structure.

A number of evaluations have shown that TUF brings about improved production of the target sentence forms, with generalizations to untreated exemplars. Generalizations to untreated sentence types have also been demonstrated. Crucially, such generalizations occur only when sentences share the same type of argument movement. So, for example, Thompson and colleagues (1997) found that training wh-movement with object clefts improved other wh-movement structures, such as wh-questions, but not syntactically unrelated forms, such as passives (and see Ballard & Thompson, 1999). There is also evidence that generalization is most likely to occur when complex sentences are trained. So training complex object relative clause structures (such as "Pete saw the man who the woman saved") benefits simpler wh-questions (such as "who did the woman save"), but not vice versa (Thompson & Shapiro, 2007; and see similar arguments in Stadie, Schroder, Postler, Lorenz, Swoboda-Moll, Burchert, & De Bleser, 2008). Some studies have suggested that improvements are not confined to the treatment task, but extend to open narrative (e.g., Thompson et al., 1996; Thompson & Shapiro, 2007), although findings here have been variable (see Ballard & Thompson, 1999).

Selecting TUF as a treatment approach might be determined by a number of factors. The therapy is based on a theory of agrammatism, which presumably excludes people with other forms of sentence impairment. Candidates should also show particular difficulties with moved argument, noncanonical forms; for example, in sentence comprehension. There is some evidence that this approach may have rather limited success with people who have severe impairments (see Ballard & Thompson, 1999). Given that the treatment focuses on the production of complex forms this is perhaps not surprising.

A further question concerns functional relevance. Although many people with aphasia struggle with the structures targeted by TUF, they may nevertheless express the meanings carried by such structures. For example, many people can communicate questions despite severe problems with wh-forms. The value of training grammatically correct question production might therefore be challenged. Here the evidence of generalization seems critical. Such generalization suggests that TUF can establish linguistic principles that are applicable to a number of related structures. In other words, the benefits of therapy are not simply in training target structures, but in restoring aphasic peoples' command over a grammatical feature of their language. There is evidence that such enhanced grammatical competence *does* have functional benefits. For example, JD (Thompson, 1998) showed post-therapy gains in narrative production and in his scores on the ASHA FACS (American Speech-Language-Hearing Association Functional Assessment of Communication Skills for Adults; Frattali, Thompson, Holland, Wohl, & Ferketic, 1995).

Engaging Technology

Many of the treatments described in this chapter call for relatively high therapy doses, which may not be available in some clinical settings. For example, TUF requires up to 20 therapy sessions. One response to this problem is to develop a computerized version of the therapy that can be self-administered. Thompson and colleagues have taken this approach by creating Sentactics, an interactive computer program that delivers TUF (Thompson, Choy, Holland, & Cole, 2010). A trial involving six people with agrammatic aphasia showed that Sentactics successfully trained production and comprehension of the target structure (object relatives) with some generalization to untrained, but linguistically related structures (object clefts and object wh-questions). There was also evidence of generalized improvements to connected speech, as assessed by a narrative task. Importantly, the participants treated with Sentactics achieved very similar gains to previous participants who had received clinician-administered TUF, and there was no difference in the amount of therapy needed to reach criterion between those who received computer therapy and those who were treated face-to-face.

A rather different computer tool is SentenceShaper (Linebarger, Schwartz, Romania, Kohn, & Stephens, 2000). The developers of this programme were influenced by the evidence of submerged grammatical competence in aphasia (see the assessment section of this chapter). SentenceShaper aims to reveal that competence, mainly by removing all time pressure from speech production. It enables people whose spontaneous speech may be limited to single words or phrases to compose much more elaborated and connected output. This is achieved not by training specific forms, but by enabling the person largely to draw on their own resources. Use of the program involves a number of steps:

- First the user records snippets of speech. Each snippet is marked by an icon on the screen, and is replayed whenever that icon is clicked. Snippets can thus be retained, discarded, or replaced.
- The user orders the retained snippets into sentence units by dragging the icons into a given frame. Once sentences are assembled they can be further ordered into narrative-like structures.
- The aid provides lexical support in the form of side buttons. When clicked, these play prerecorded words, such as verbs or prepositions. These are selected by the user (e.g., because they are particularly difficult to access spontaneously).

There is a good evidence base for SentenceShaper. The first study (Linebarger et al., 2000) showed that approximately 15 hours of practice with SentenceShaper enabled six people with agrammatism to improve narrative output when supported with the aid. A subsequent study (Linebarger, Schwartz, & Kohn, 2001) involving two participants showed that practice with SentenceShaper even benefited unaided production, and encouragingly, much of the practice in this study was independent (i.e., not therapist led). Such treatment effects, where there is carryover to spontaneous speech, were replicated in further studies (e.g., Linebarger, McCall, Virata, & Berndt, 2007; McCall, Virata, Linebarger, & Berndt, 2009). The latter study also showed that the aid can be used successfully to target specific grammatical structures, in this case subordinate clauses. Finally, studies have reported positive benefits from a portable version of the aid: SentenceShaper To Go (Bartlett, Schwartz, Fink, Lowery, Linebarger, & Schwartz, 2007; Linebarger, Romania, Fink, Bartlett, & Schwartz, 2008). Here, utterances created on SentenceShaper are downloaded onto a handheld computer and are used to support a range of communication encounters, such as going to the doctor or giving a speech.

Another software response to the problem of aphasic sentence generation is AphasiaScripts (Cherney, Halper, Holland, & Cole, 2008). Users of this program practice personalized scripts with the aid of a virtual therapist. Scripts can take the form of a conversation or a monologue; examples include talking to a grandchild, ordering food in a restaurant, or recounting personal information. They are developed collaboratively by the therapist and person with aphasia. After training in the use of the program, users undertake self-directed practice on each of their scripts. Initially maximum support is provided by the program; that is, each turn is spoken by the virtual therapist, who appears as an avatar with realistic mouth movements, and is presented simultaneously in written form. The user can then reduce or remove the cues; for example, by eliminating the sound, then the view of the avatar's articulators, and finally the written words. Other hierarchical manipulations involve increasing the length of the script or giving the user more responsibility for initiating the conversation.

Studies have shown that this software improves performance on the practiced scripts (e.g., in terms of the production of target words and grammatical morphology; Cherney et al., 2008). Gains are related to dose, with better outcomes achieved by those who practiced the most (Lee, Kaye, & Cherney, 2009). Evidence of improvements beyond the practiced material is marginal, although two of the three participants in the first study made gains of more than 5 points on the Western Aphasia Battery, and all reported generalizations to everyday communication (Cherney et al., 2008).

Technological aids are likely to become increasingly prominent in aphasia therapy. They offer a cost-effective means of raising the therapy dose, while giving a high degree of autonomy to the user. Programs can be designed that are accessible and acceptable to people with aphasia, even when there has been minimal premorbid computer use. Programs like Sentactics, SentenceShaper, and AphasiaScripts show that technology can address problems with connected speech, rather than just single words. Technology can also be used to mimic authentic communication, addressing the problem of generalizing therapy gains to everyday language. A current project at City University London is piloting a virtual communication environment, called Eva Park, which enables people with aphasia to communicate with each other and with support workers in a range of simulated settings, including a home, a restaurant, a health center, and a night club. Preliminary observations suggest that the environment stimulates creative and extended interactions that may be difficult to engender in the speech and language therapy clinic.

Discussion

Generalization of Therapy Effects

The reviewed treatment approaches demonstrate that aphasic sentence processing skills can respond positively to therapy. In virtually all cases, experimental design enables us to locate the source of change to the content of treatment, rather than nonspecific effects. Furthermore, studies have included people with severe and chronic aphasia. Despite these positive findings, the degree of change varies from study to study, particularly in terms of generalization. This is a crucial issue. Clinically, evidence of generalization enhances the claim that therapy is of functional benefit. Theoretically, generalization can help to identify processing changes that may have occurred as a result of our intervention.

In many of the reviewed studies, generalizations are limited to the target treatment structure (e.g., Nickels et al., 1991; Marshall et al., 1997). So, for example, therapy involving SVO sentences may improve the production or comprehension of this form, with generalization to untreated exemplars, but with no generalization to untreated sentence types. Such within-type generalizations suggest that the person has learned just one grammatical frame, even though he or she can employ that frame with a degree of creativity.

Some studies achieve generalizations to untreated sentence types (e.g., Stadie et al., 2008). This argues for the acquisition of a general grammatical procedure that can be applied to different structures, with implications for models of language processing. For example, Thompson and colleagues argue that the language system includes procedures for processing phrase movement, which are shared by linguistically related structures. Thus training in one structure achieves generalization, but only to other structures that employ the treated processing. They further argue that such generalization is promoted by treatment targeting complex forms (Thompson & Shapiro, 2007).

Another issue concerns cross-modality effects, or generalization from input to output and vice versa. Such generalization is potentially important, since it indicates that production and comprehension may share processing components. In particular, we might envisage that production and comprehension share a central semantic processor; for example, dealing with the verb and its arguments. In this case, therapies targeting such semantic features should have the best prognosis for cross-modality generalization. Yet, results here are contradictory, with some studies achieving generalization (e.g., Jones, 1986; Schwartz et al., 1994; Jacobs & Thompson, 2000) and others not (e.g., Mitchum et al., 1995; Rochon et al., 2005). Of course, many studies cannot contribute to this debate, since therapy involved both production and comprehension (e.g., Nickels et al., 1991; Marshall et al., 1997). Even when therapy is confined to one modality, it is difficult to ensure that elements of the other do not sneak in. For example, the person may read aloud or repeat sentences provided for comprehension, thus introducing output to an input task. Overall, it is very difficult to draw any firm conclusions about this aspect of generalization.

Perhaps the key question is whether treatment effects generalize to spontaneous speech. Evaluating this is problematic. As discussed at the start of this chapter, sampling techniques may be subject to multiple variables, which mask treatment effects. Yet attempts to control these variables (e.g., by increasing constraints on the task), may result in a sample that is unrepresentative of the person's normal production. Therefore it is often difficult to be confident that generalization has (or has not) occurred.

Despite these difficulties, some studies have addressed this question. Results are mixed, with both positive (e.g., Schwartz et al., 1994; Thompson, 1998; Webster et al., 2005), and negative (Marshall et al., 1993; Mitchum et al., 1993) findings. It is disappointing that few studies explicitly target generalization to everyday speech in treatment; for example, by incorporating tasks that at least mimic authentic communication. It was suggested above that current and future technologies may help clinicians to achieve this aim.

Mechanisms of Change

It has been repeatedly stated that we do not understand how therapy affects the working of the language processing system (see arguments in Hillis, 1993, and Marshall, 2008, for example). We can gather clues from the behavioral effects of therapy and patterns of generalization, but it is difficult to determine the underlying changes that led to such effects.

Many of the therapy studies described in this chapter take a computational view of language processing. Rule-based models of sentence production, or comprehension, are assumed, with treatment aiming to restore or augment a level of processing within such models. Exemplar-based models encourage a rather different view. According to these models, syntax is computed not from abstract linguistic rules, but by drawing analogies with stored tokens or exemplars (e.g., Gahl & Yu, 2006; Bod, 2006). These models would argue for a different mechanism of change. Rather than restoring a linguistic process, treatment may affect the store of representations; for example, by increasing the number of exemplars or making them more available for production.

Regardless of our theoretical stance, it would be particularly interesting to know whether therapy recovers on-line access to linguistic processes and representations, or whether it develops alternative strategies and devices. The limited effects of therapy may suggest the latter. For example, the person may be able to apply painstaking strategies within constrained tasks, but not in open and spontaneous narrative. A means of probing this would be to compare on- and off-line evaluations. Evidence of improvement only on off-line tasks would argue for strategic gains, whereas gains on both would argue for more automatic, on-line gains.

The nature of change is functionally important. If therapy builds conscious strategies we can only reasonably expect the intermittent use of such strategies. So, the person may choose to apply his or her enhanced sentence skills in some contexts, but not in others. Indeed, part of our therapy might help the person make such decisions to best effect. For example, we might encourage them to apply the skills whenever meaning cannot be inferred from context alone. If, on the other hand, therapy restores automatic access to linguistic skills, much more widespread and generalized use of the skills can be expected.

Goals of Sentence Therapy

This chapter began by stating that aphasic sentence disorders matter because they limit the meanings that can be conveyed or comprehended. Therapy, therefore, should aim to expand these meanings. This may not equate to grammatically perfect language. So, for example, we may decide that therapy goals have been met even if the person is producing truncated or telegrammatic forms, providing they are expressing more meaning than they were before. Indeed, one therapy program specifically targets such a strategic approach to production (Springer, Huber, Schlenk, & Schlenk, 2000). This encourages us to expand our therapy goals. We may target conventional devices for conveying sentential meanings, such as word order and grammatical morphology. But we might equally target strategies that can replace such devices, such as the sequenced use of nouns or gestures (Beeke et al., 2007). Above all, we should aim to achieve change that is functionally meaningful, and show that it occurs not just on clinical tasks, but in the hurly-burly of everyday language.

Note

1 This is the English equivalent of one of the German stimuli used in the study.

References

Arabatzi, M., & Edwards, S. (2002). Tense and syntactic processes in agrammatic speech. *Brain and Language, 80*, 314–327.

Bak, T.H., & Hodges, J.R. (2003). Kissing and dancing—a test to distinguish the lexical and conceptual contributions to noun/verb and action/object dissociation. Preliminary results in patients with frontotemporal dementia. *Journal of Neurolinguistics, 16*(2–3), 169–181.

Ballard, K., & Thompson, C. (1999). Treatment and generalisation of complex sentence production in agrammatism. *Journal of Speech, Language and Hearing Research, 42*, 690–707.

Bartlett, M.R., Fink, R.B., Schwartz, M.F., & Linebarger, M.C. (2007). Informativeness ratings of messages created on an AAC processing prosthesis. *Aphasiology, 21*(5), 475–498.

Bastiaanse, R., & Jonkers, R. (1998). Verb retrieval in action naming and spontaneous speech in agrammatic and anomic aphasia. *Aphasiology, 12*, 951–969.

Bastiaanse, R., Edwards, S., & Rispens, J. (2002). *The verb and sentence test.* Bury St. Edmunds: Thames Valley Test Company.

Bastiaanse, R., & van Zonneveld, R. (2006). Comprehension of passives in Broca's aphasia. *Brain and Language, 96*, 135–142.

Beeke, S., Wilkinson, R., & Maxim, J. (2007). Individual variation in agrammatism: A single case study of the influence of interaction. *International Journal of Language and Communication Disorders, 42*(6), 629–647.

Beeke S., Maxim J., Best W., & Cooper F. (2011). Redesigning therapy for agrammatism: Initial findings from the ongoing evaluation of a conversation-based intervention study. *Journal of Neurolinguistics, 24*, 222–236.

Berndt, R.S., Haendiges, A., Mitchum, C., & Sandson, J. (1997a). Verb retrieval in aphasia 1: Characterising single word impairments. *Brain and Language, 56*, 107–137.

Berndt, R.S., Haendiges, A., Mitchum, C., & Sandson, J. (1997b). Verb retrieval in aphasia 2: Relationship to sentence processing. *Brain and Language, 56*, 68–106.

Berndt, R.S., & Mitchum, C. (1998). An experimental treatment of sentence comprehension. In N. Helm-Estabrooks & A. Holland (Eds.), *Approaches to the treatment of aphasia*. San Diego, CA: Singular Publishing.

Berndt, R.S., Mitchum, C., & Wayland, S. (1997). Patterns of sentence comprehension in aphasia: A consideration of three hypotheses. *Brain and Language, 60*, 197–221.

Berndt, R.S., Salasoo, A., Mitchum, C., & Blumstein, S. (1988). The role of intonation cues in aphasic patients' performance on the grammaticality task. *Brain and Language, 34*, 65–97.

Berndt, R., Wayland, S., Rochon, E., Saffran, E., & Schwartz, M. (2000). *Quantitative production analysis*. Hove: Psychology Press.

Black, M., & Chiat, S. (2000). Putting thoughts into verbs: Developmental and acquired impairments. In W. Best, K. Bryan, & J. Maxim (Eds.), *Semantic processing: Theory and practice* (pp. 52–79). London: Whurr Publishers.

Black, M., Nickels, L., & Byng, S. (1992). Patterns of sentence processing deficit: Processing simple sentences can be a complex matter. *Journal of Neurolinguistics, 6*, 79–101.

Bod, R. (2006) Exemplar-based syntax: How to get productivity from examples. *The Linguistic Review, 23*, 291–320.

Boo, M., & Rose, M. (2011). The efficacy of repetition, semantic, and gesture treatments for verb retrieval and use in Broca's aphasia. *Aphasiology, 25*(2), 154–175.

Breedin, S., Saffran, E., & Coslett, H. (1994). Reversal of the concreteness effect in a patient with semantic dementia. *Cognitive Neuropsychology, 11*, 617–660.

Breedin, S., Saffran, E., & Schwartz, M. (1998). Semantic factors in verb retrieval: An effect of complexity. *Brain and Language, 63*, 1–31.

Byng, S. (1988). Sentence processing deficits: Theory and therapy. *Cognitive Neuropsychology, 5*, 629–676.

Byng, S., & Black, M. (1995). What makes a therapy? Some parameters of therapeutic intervention in aphasia. *European Journal of Disorders of Communication, 30*, 303–316.

Byng, S., Nickels, L., & Black, M. (1994). Replicating therapy for mapping deficits in agrammatism: Remapping the deficit? *Aphasiology, 8*, 315–341.

Byrne, C., & Varley, R. (2011). From mathematics to language: A novel intervention for sentence comprehension difficulties in aphasia. *Journal of Neurolinguistics, 24*, 173–182.

Cairns, D., Marshall, J., Cairns, P., & Dipper, L. (2007). Event processing through naming: Investigating event focus in two people with aphasia. *Language and Cognitive Processes, 22*(2), 201–233.

Caramazza, A., & Zurif, E. (1976). Dissociation of algorithmic and heuristic processes in language comprehension: Evidence from aphasia. *Brain and Language, 3*, 572–582.

Cherney, L.R., Halper, A.S., Holland, A.L., & Cole, R. (2008). Computerized script training for aphasia: Preliminary results. *American Journal of Speech Language Pathology, 17*, 19–34.

Conroy, P., Sage, K., & Lambon Ralph, M.A. (2006). Towards theory-driven therapies for aphasic verb impairments: A review of current theory and practice. *Aphasiology, 2*, 1159–1185.

Conroy, P., Sage, K.E., Lambon Ralph, M.A. (2009a). Errorless and errorful therapy for verb and noun naming in aphasia. *Aphasiology, 23*(11), 1311–1337.

Conroy, P., Sage, K., & Lambon Ralph, M. (2009b). A comparison of word versus sentence cues as therapy for verb naming in aphasia. *Aphasiology, 23*(4), 462–482.

Conroy, P., Sage, K., & Lambon Ralph, M. (2009c). The effects of decreasing and increasing cue therapy on improving naming speed and accuracy for verbs and nouns in aphasia. *Aphasiology, 23*(6), 707–730.

Crerar, A., Ellis, A., & Dean, L. (1996). Remediation of sentence processing deficits in aphasia using a computer based microworld. *Brain and Language, 52*, 229–275.

Daneman, M., & Carpenter, P. (1980). Individual differences in working memory and reading. *Journal of Verbal Learning and Verbal Behavior, 19*, 450–466.

DeDe, G. (2012). Lexical and prosodic effects on syntactic ambiguity resolution in aphasia. *Journal of Psycholinguistic Research, 41*(5), 387–408.

Dickey, M., Choy, J., & Thompson, C. (2007). Real-time comprehension of wh- movement in aphasia: Evidence from eyetracking while listening. *Brain and Language, 100*(1), 1–22.

Dickey, M., & Thompson, C. (2009). Automatic processing of wh- and NP-movement in agrammatic aphasia: Evidence from eyetracking. *Journal of Neurolinguistics, 22*(6), 563–583.

Dipper, L. (1999). Event processing for language: An investigation of the relationship between events, sentences, and verbs, using data from 6 people with non-fluent aphasia. Unpublished Ph.D. thesis, University College, London.

Druks, J. (2002). Verbs and nouns—a review of the literature. *Journal of Neurolinguistics, 15*(3–5), 289–315.

Druks, J., & Carroll, E. (2005). The crucial role of tense for verb production. *Brain and Language, 94,* 1–18.

Druks, J., & Marshall, J.C. (1995). When passives are easier than actives: Two case studies of aphasic comprehension. *Cognition, 55,* 311–331.

Druks, J., & Masterson, J. (2000). An object and action naming battery. Hove: Psychology Press.

Edmonds, L., & Babb, M. (2011). Effect of verb network strengthening treatment in moderate-to-severe aphasia. *American Journal of Speech Language Pathology, 20,* 131–145.

Edmonds, L., Nadeau, S., & Kiran, S. (2009). Effect of Verb Network Strengthening Treatment (VNeST) on lexical retrieval of content words in sentences in persons with aphasia. *Aphasiology, 23,* 402–424.

Edwards, S., & Tucker, K. (2006). Verb retrieval in fluent aphasia: A clinical study. *Aphasiology, 20*(7), 644–675.

Faroqi-Shah, Y. (2008). A comparison of two theoretically driven treatments of verb inflection deficits in aphasia. *Neuropsychologia, 46,* 3088–3100.

Faroqi-Shah, Y. (2013). Selective treatment of regular versus irregular verbs in agrammatic aphasia: Efficacy data. *Aphasiology, 27*(6).

Faroqi-Shah, Y., & Thompson, C.K. (2004). Semantic, lexical, and phonological influences on the production of verb inflections in agrammatic aphasia. *Brain and Language, 89,* 484–498.

Faroqi-Shah, Y., & Thompson, C. (2007). Verb inflections in agrammatic aphasia: Encoding of tense features. *Journal and Memory and Language, 56,* 129–151.

Frattali, C., Thompson, C., Holland, A., Wohl, C., & Ferketic, M. (1995). *American Speech-Language-Hearing Association functional assessment of communication skills for adults.* Rockville, MD: ASHA.

Friedmann, N., & Gvion, A. (2003). Sentence comprehension and working memory limitation in aphasia: A dissociation between semantic-syntactic and phonological reactivation. *Brain and Language, 86,* 23–39.

Friedmann, N., Reznick, J., Dolinski-Nuger, D., & Soboleva, K. (2010). Comprehension and production of movement-derived sentences by Russian speakers with agrammatic aphasia. *Journal of Neurolinguistics, 23,* 44–65

Gahl, S., & Yu, A. (2006). Introduction to the special issue on exemplar-based models in linguistics. *The Linguistic Review, 23,* 213–216.

Grodzinsky, Y. (1995). A restrictive theory of trace deletion in agrammatism. *Brain and Language, 50,* 27–51.

Haarman, H., Just, M., & Carpenter, P. (1997). Aphasic sentence comprehension as a resource deficit: A computational approach. *Brain and Language, 59,* 76–120.

Haendiges, A., Berndt, R.S., & Mitchum, C.C. (1996). Assessing the elements contributing to a mapping deficit: A targeted treatment study. *Brain and Language, 52,* 276–302.

Hartsuiker, R., & Kolk, H. (1998). Syntactic facilitation in agrammatic sentence production. *Brain and Language, 62,* 221–254.

Herbert, R., Best, W., Hickin, J., Howard, D., & Osborne, F. (2013). *Profile of word errors and retrieval in speech (POWERS).* North Guilford: J&R Press.

Hillis, A. (1993). The role of models of language processing in rehabilitation of language impairments. *Aphasiology, 7,* 5–26.

Jacobs, B., & Thompson, C. (2000). Cross-modal generalization effects of training noncanonical sentence comprehension and production in agrammatic aphasia. *Journal of Speech Language and Hearing Research, 43, 1,* 5–20.

Jones, E. (1986). Building the foundations for sentence production in a non-fluent aphasic. *British Journal of Disorders of Communication, 21,* 63–82.

Just, M., & Carpenter, P. (1992). A capacity theory of comprehension: Individual differences in working memory. *Psychological Review, 99,* 122–149.

Kay, J., Lesser, R., & Coltheart, M. (1992). *Psycholinguistic assessment of language processing in aphasia.* Hove: Lawrence Erlbaum.

Kemmerer, D. (2000). Grammatically relevant and grammatically irrelevant features of verb meaning can be independently impaired. *Aphasiology, 14*(10), 997–1020.

Kolk, H.H.J. (2006). How language adapts to the brain. In L. Progovac, K. Paesani, E. Casielles, & E. Barton (Eds.), *The syntax of nonsententials: Multi-disciplinary perspectives* (pp. 229–258). Amsterdam/Philadelphia: John Benjamins Publishing.

Kolk, H.H.J. (2008). Time in agrammatic aphasia. Commentary on Wearden. *Language and Learning, 58*(Suppl 1), 173–177.

Le Dorze, G., Boulay, N., Gaudreau, J., & Brassard, C. (1994). The contrasting effects of a semantic versus a formal-semantic technique for the facilitation of naming in a case of anomia. *Aphasiology, 8,* 127–141.

Le Dorze, G., Jacob, A., & Coderre, L. (1991). Aphasia rehabilitation with a case of agrammatism: A partial replication. *Aphasiology, 5,* 63–85.

Lee, J., Kaye, R., & Cherney, L. (2009) Conversational script performance in adults with non-fluent aphasia: Treatment intensity and aphasia severity. *Aphasiology, 23*(7–8), 885–897.

Linebarger, M.C., McCall, D., Virata, T., & Berndt, R.S. (2007). Widening the temporal window: Processing support in the treatment of aphasic language production. *Brain and Language, 100*, 53–68.

Linebarger, M.C., Romania, J.R., Fink, R.B., Bartlett, M., & Schwartz, M.F. (2008) Building on residual speech: A portable processing prosthesis for aphasia. *Journal of Rehabilitation Research and Development, 45*(9), 1401–1414.

Linebarger, M.C., Schwartz, M.F., & Kohn, S.E. (2001). Computer-based training of language production: An exploratory study. *Neuropsychological Rehabilitation, 11*(1), 57–96.

Linebarger, M.C., Schwartz, M.F., Romania, J.F., Kohn, S.E., & Stephens, D.L. (2000). Grammatical encoding in aphasia: Evidence from a "processing prosthesis." *Brain and Language, 75*, 416–427.

Linebarger, M.C., Schwartz, M., & Saffran, E. (1983). Sensitivity to grammatical structure in so-called agrammatic aphasics. *Cognition, 13*, 361–392.

Lock, S., Wilkinson, R., & Bryan, K. (2001). *SPPARC (Supporting Partners of People with Aphasia in Relationships and Conversation): A resource pack.* Bicester: Speechmark.

Luzzatti, C., Raggi, R., Zonca, G., Pistarini, C., Contardi, A., & Pinna, D. (2002). Verb-noun double dissociation in aphasic lexical impairments: The role of word frequency and imageability. *Brain and Language, 81*, 432–444.

Mack, J., Ji, W., & Thompson, C. (2013). Effects of verb meaning on lexical integration in agrammatic aphasia: Evidence from eyetracking. *Journal of Neurolinguistics, 26*(6), 619–636.

Marshall, J. (1995). The mapping hypothesis and aphasia therapy. *Aphasiology, 9*, 517–539.

Marshall, J. (1999). Doing something about a verb impairment: Two therapy approaches. In S. Byng, K. Swinburn, & C. Pound (Eds.), *The aphasia therapy file.* Hove: Psychology Press.

Marshall, J. (2003). Noun-verb dissociations: Evidence from acquisition and developmental and acquired disorders. *Journal of Neurolinguistics, 16*, 67–84.

Marshall, J. (2008). Aphasia therapy and cognitive neuropsychology: A promise still to be fulfilled? In V. Joffe, M. Cruice, & S. Chiat (Eds.), *Language disorders in children and adults: New issues in research and practice.* London: Wiley.

Marshall, J. (2009). Framing ideas in aphasia: The need for thinking therapy. *International Journal of Language and Communication Disorders, 44*(1), 1–14.

Marshall, J., & Cairns, D. (2005). Therapy for sentence processing problems in aphasia: Working on thinking for speaking. *Aphasiology, 19*(10/11), 1009–1020.

Marshall, J., Chiat, S., & Pring, T. (1997). An impairment in processing verbs' thematic roles: A therapy study. *Aphasiology, 11*, 855–876.

Marshall, J., Chiat, S., & Pring, T. (1999). *The event perception test.* Telford: Winslow Press.

Marshall, J., Chiat, S., Pring, T., & Robson, J. (1996). An investigation of semantic jargon. Part 2: Verbs. *Journal of Neurolinguistics, 9*, 251–260.

Marshall, J., Pring, T., & Chiat, S. (1993). Sentence processing therapy: Working at the level of the event. *Aphasiology, 7*, 177–199.

Marshall, J., Pring, T., & Chiat, S. (1998). Verb retrieval and sentence production in aphasia. *Brain and Language, 63*, 159–188.

Matzig, S., Druks, J., Masterson, J., & Vigliocco, G. (2009). Noun and verb differences in picture naming: Past studies and new evidence. *Cortex, 45*(6), 738–758.

McCall, D., Virata, T., Linebarger, M., & Berndt, R.S. (2009). Integrating technology and targeted treatment to improve narrative production in aphasia: A case study. *Aphasiology, 23*(4), 438–461.

McCann, C., & Doleman, J. (2011). Verb retrieval in nonfluent aphasia: A replication of Edwards & Tucker, 2006. *Journal of Neurolinguistics, 24*, 237–248.

Mitchum, C., & Berndt, R.S. (1994). Verb retrieval and sentence construction: Effects of targeted intervention. In M. Riddoch & G. Humphreys (Eds.), *Cognitive neuropsychology and cognitive rehabilitation.* Hove: Lawrence Erlbaum.

Mitchum, C., Greenwald, M., & Berndt, R.S. (1997). Production specific thematic mapping impairment: A treatment study. *Brain and Language, 60*, 121–123.

Mitchum, C., Haendiges, A., & Berndt, R.S. (1993). Model-guided treatment to improve written sentence production: A case study. *Aphasiology, 7*, 71–109.

Mitchum, C., Haendiges, A., & Berndt, R.S. (1995). Treatment of thematic mapping in sentence comprehension: Implications for normal processing. *Cognitive Neuropsychology, 12*, 503–547.

Mitchum, C., Greenwald, M., & Berndt, R. (2000). Cognitive treatments of sentence processing disorders: What have we learned? *Neuropsychological Rehabilitation, 10*(3), 311–336.

Miyake, A., Carpenter, P., & Just, M. (1994). A capacity approach to syntactic comprehension disorders: Making normal adults perform like aphasic patients. *Cognitive Neuropsychology, 11*, 671–717.

Nickels, L., Byng, S., & Black, M. (1991). Sentence processing deficits: A replication of therapy. *British Journal of Disorders of Communication, 26*, 175–201.

Pashek, G. (1998). Gestural facilitation of noun and verb retrieval in aphasia: A case study. *Brain and Language, 65*, 177–180.

Perkins, L., & Hinshelwood, F. (2007). Symptom-based versus theoretically motivated therapy for anomia: A case study. In S. Byng, J. Felson Duchan, & C. Pound (Eds.), *The Aphasia Therapy File*, vol. 2. Hove: Psychology Press.

Pinker, S. (1989). *Learnability and cognition: The acquisition of argument structure*. Cambridge MA: MIT Press.

Pinker, S. (2007). *The stuff of thought: Language as a window into human nature*. London: Penguin.

Raymer, A., Ciampitti, M., Holliway, B., Singletary, F., Blonder, L., Ketterson, T., Anderson, S., Lehnen, J., Heilman, K., & Rothi, L. (2007). Semantic-phonologic treatment for noun and verb retrieval impairments in aphasia. *Neuropsychological Rehabilitation, 17*(2), 244–270.

Raymer, A., & Ellsworth, T. (2002). Response to contrasting verb retrieval treatments: A case study. *Aphasiology, 16* (10/11), 1031–1045.

Rochon, E., Laird, L., Bose, A., & Scofield, J. (2005). Mapping therapy for sentence production impairments in nonfluent aphasia. *Neuropsychological Rehabilitation, 15*(1), 1–36.

Rodriguez, A.D., Raymer A.M., & Gonzalez Rothi, L.J. (2006). Effects of gesture + verbal and semantic-phonologic treatments for verb retrieval in aphasia. *Aphasiology, 20*, 286–297.

Rose, M., & Sussmilch, G. (2008). The effects of semantic and gesture treatments on verb retrieval and verb use in aphasia. *Aphasiology, 22*, 691–706.

Saffran, E., Schwartz, M., & Marin, O. (1980). The word order problem in agrammatism 2: Production. *Brain and Language, 10*, 263–280.

Santamaria, K., Munoz, M., Atkins, J., Hobbs, D., & O'Donald, K. (2013). A preliminary investigation into the application of processing instruction as a therapy for aphasia in Spanish speakers. *Journal of Communication Disorders, 46*, 338–350.

Schwartz, M., Linebarger, M., & Saffran, E. (1985). The status of the syntactic deficit theory of agrammatism. In M.-L. Kean (Ed.), *Agrammatism*. Orlando: Academic Press.

Schwartz, M., Linebarger, M., Saffran, E., & Pate, D. (1987). Syntactic transparency and sentence interpretation in aphasia. *Language and Cognitive Processes, 2*, 85–113.

Schwartz, M., Saffran, E., Fink, R., Myers, J., & Martin, N. (1994). Mapping therapy: A treatment programme for agrammatism. *Aphasiology, 8*, 19–54.

Schwartz, M., Saffran, E., & Marin, O. (1980). The word order problem in agrammatism 1: Comprehension. *Brain and Language, 10*, 249–262.

Shapiro, L., Gordon, B., Hack, N., & Killackey, J. (1993). Verb argument structure processing in complex sentences in Broca's and Wernicke's aphasia. *Brain and Language, 45*, 423–447.

Shapiro, L., & Levine, B. (1990). Verb processing during sentence comprehension in aphasia. *Brain and Language, 38*, 21–47.

Shapiro, L., Zurif, E., & Grimshaw, J. (1987). Sentence processing and the mental representation of verbs. *Cognition, 27*, 219–246.

Slobin, D. (1996). From "thought and language" to "thinking for speaking." In J. Gumperz & S. Levinson (Eds.), *Rethinking linguistic relativity*. Cambridge: Cambridge University Press.

Springer, L., Willmes, K., & Haag, E. (1993). Training in the use of wh-questions and prepositions in dialogues: A comparison of two different approaches in aphasia therapy. *Aphasiology, 7*, 251–270.

Springer, L., Huber, W., Scnhlenck, K-J., & Schlenck, C. (2000). Agrammatism: Deficit or compensation? Consequences for aphasia therapy. *Neuropsychological Rehabilitation, 10*(3), 279–309.

Stadie, N., Schroder, A., Postler, J., Lorenz, A., Swoboda-Moll, M. Burchert, F. & De Bleser, R. (2008). Unambiguous generalization effects after treatment of non-canonical sentence production in German agrammatism. *Brain and Language, 104*, 211–229.

Stavrakaki, S., & Kouvava, S. (2003). Functional categories in agrammatism: Evidence from Greek. *Brain and Language, 86*(1), 129–141.

Swinburn, K. (1999). An information example of a successful therapy for a sentence processing deficit. In S. Byng, K. Swinburn, & C. Pound (Eds.), *The aphasia therapy file*. Hove: Psychology Press.

Thompson, C. (1998). Treating sentence production in agrammatic aphasia. In N. Helm-Estabrooks & A. Holland (Eds.), *Approaches to the treatment of aphasia*. San Diego, CA: Singular.

Thompson, C. (2003). Unaccusative verb production in agrammatic aphasia: The argument structure complexity hypothesis. *Journal of Neurolinguistics, 16*, 151–161.

Thompson, C. (2008). Treatment of syntactic and morphological deficits in agrammatic aphasia: Treatment of underlying forms. In R. Chapey (Ed.), *Language intervention strategies in aphasia and related neurogenic communication disorders* (5th ed.). Baltimore: Lippincott, Williams and Wilkins.

Thompson, C., Choy, J., Holland, A., & Cole, R. (2010). Sentactics®: Computer-Automated Treatment of Underlying Forms. *Aphasiology, 24*(10), 1242–1266.

Thompson, C., Dickey, M., Cho, S., Lee, J., & Griffin, Z. (2007). Verb argument structure encoding during sentence production in agrammatic aphasic speakers: An eye-tracking study. *Brain and Language, 103*, 8–249.

Thompson, C., & Lee, M. (2009). Psych verb production and comprehension in agrammatic Broca's aphasia. *Journal of Neurolinguistics, 22*(4), 354–369.

Thompson, C., & Shapiro, L. (1995). Training sentence production in agrammatism: Implications for normal and disordered language. *Brain and Language, 50*, 201–224.

Thompson, C., & Shapiro, L. (2007). Complexity in treatment of syntactic deficits. *American Journal of Speech-Language Pathology, 16*, 30–42.

Thompson, C., Shapiro, L., Ballard, K., Jacobs, B., Schneider S., & Tait, M. (1997). Training and generalized production of wh- and NP- movement structures in agrammatic aphasia. *Journal of Speech, Language, and Hearing Research, 40*, 228–244.

Thompson, C., Shapiro, L., & Roberts, M. (1993). Treatment of sentence production deficits in aphasia, a linguistic specific approach to wh-interrogative training and generalization. *Aphasiology, 7*, 111–133.

Thompson, C., Shapiro, L., Tait, M., Jacobs, B., & Schneider, S. (1996). Training wh-question production in agrammatic aphasia: Analysis of argument and adjunct movement. *Brain and Language, 52*, 175–228.

Tyler, L. (1992). *Spoken language comprehension: An experimental approach to disordered and normal processing.* Cambridge MA: MIT Press.

Tyler, L., Ostrin, R., Cooke, M., & Moss, H. (1995). Automatic access to lexical information in Broca's aphasics: Against the automaticity hypothesis. *Brain and Language, 48*, 131–162.

Ullman, M., Pancheva, R., Love, T., Yee, E., Swinney, D., & Hickok, G. (2005). Neural correlates of lexicon and grammar: Evidence from the production, reading, and judgment of inflection in aphasia. *Brain and Language, 93*(2), 185–238.

Wambaugh, J., Doyle, P., Martinez, A., & Kalinyak-Fliszar, M. (2002). Effects of two lexical retrieval cueing treatments on action naming in aphasia. *Journal of Rehabilitation Research and Development, 39*(4), 455–466.

Wambaugh, J., & Ferguson, M. (2007). Application of semantic feature analysis to retrieval of action names in aphasia. *Journal of Rehabilitation Research and Development, 44*, 381–394.

Webster, J., Morris, J., & Franklin, S. (2005). Effects of therapy targeted at verb retrieval and the realisation of the predicate argument structure: A case study. *Aphasiology, 19*(8), 748–764.

Webster, J., & Whitworth, A. (2012). Treating verbs in aphasia: exploring the impact of therapy at the single word and sentence levels. *International Journal of Language & Communication Disorders, 47*, 619–636.

Whitworth, A. (1996). *Thematic roles in production.* London: Whurr Publishers.

Whitworth, A., Perkins, L., & Lesser, R. (1997). *Conversation Analysis Profile for People with Aphasia (CAPPA).* London: Whurr Publishers.

Wright, H.H., & Shisler, R. (2005). Working memory in aphasia: Theory, measures, and clinical implications. *American Journal of Speech-Language Pathology, 14*, 107–118.

Wright, H.H., Downey, R.A., Gravier, M., Love, T., & Shapiro, L.P. (2007). Processing distinct linguistic information types in working memory in aphasia. *Aphasiology, 21*(6/7/8), 802–813.

Yarbay Duman, T., Altınok, N., Özgirgin, N., & Bastiaanse, R. (2011). Sentence comprehension in Turkish Broca's aphasia: An integration problem. *Aphasiology, 25*(8), 908–926.

Zurif, E., Swinney, D., Prather, P., Solomon, J., & Bushell, C. (1993). An on-line analysis of syntactic processing in Broca's and Wernicke's aphasia. *Brain and Language, 45*, 448–464.

PART 7

Other Types of Models and Treatment Approaches

20

HOW CAN CONNECTIONIST COGNITIVE MODELS OF LANGUAGE INFORM MODELS OF LANGUAGE REHABILITATION?

Nadine Martin, Matti Laine, and Trevor A. Harley

Introduction

Cognitive models of language theories have served well as frameworks within which to evaluate acquired language impairments. This is because brain damage does not result in a random malfunctioning of language abilities, but leads to systematic patterns of behavioral breakdown that respect the underlying regularities and rules of the language processing system. The practice of interpreting aphasic deficits within a cognitive-linguistic (or psycholinguistic) model has been extended to include recommendations for therapy approaches based on a subject's cognitive-linguistic profile. This endeavor began with great enthusiasm but was met almost immediately with many difficult challenges. It became increasingly clear that the issues to be addressed in rehabilitation theory and practice are complex and require an understanding of mental processing that is not yet fully realized in cognitive models. In this chapter, we aim to acquaint the reader with some of the issues that need to be addressed in order to understand the cognitive underpinnings of rehabilitation and how scientists have used cognitive-linguistic models to approach these issues. With this background, we will discuss the emergence of connectionist cognitive-linguistic models that characterize dynamic aspects of language processing and their role in the development of theories of rehabilitation. In the last section of this chapter, we provide examples of treatment approaches that have been motivated by principles of connectionist models of cognition and language. The approaches we will describe represent two areas in which connectionist models can inform language rehabilitation: (1) choice of treatment stimuli that will maximize access to mental representations of words and sentences and generalization of treatment effects to untrained stimuli and (2) strengthening non-linguistic cognitive processes that support language processing (e.g., short-term working memory).

There are two broad classes of cognitive cognitive-linguistic models, and each type is well suited to characterize particular aspects of the language system. Functional models have been around in one form or another since the 1950s. These models (also known as "box and arrow" models; e.g., Caplan, 1992; Howard & Franklin, 1988; Morton, 1982) are intended to identify the mental components of the language system (the information processing units that map input to stored linguistic representations) and their functional roles in encoding and decoding language. Connectionist models are a more recent development, but their use has increased dramatically in the last two decades. These models provide an additional means to investigate the properties of processing mechanisms of the language system (e.g., Dell, 1986; Harley, 1993; Hinton & Shallice, 1991; Plaut & Shallice, 1993).

By the middle of the 1980s, there was little disagreement about the general mental structure of the language system (e.g., Caplan, 1992; Ellis, 1985; Morton, 1982). Moreover, it was a well-established practice in aphasia research to use cognitive-linguistic models to interpret effects of brain damage on language (e.g., Caplan, 1992) and in turn, to use aphasic language performance as tests of those models (e.g., Caramazza, 1984). This interplay between functional cognitive-linguistic models and language deficits greatly increased our understanding of the cognitive components of the language system. Diagnostically, the taxonomy of impairments to various cognitive structures and functions has proven invaluable. Unfortunately, this knowledge has not readily advanced our understanding of mechanisms underlying recovery from language impairment or the influences of treatment on impaired language abilities. This is because recovery from aphasia and treatment of language depend on the integrity of processes that encode and decode language, as well as those processes that mediate learning and relearning of language. Functional models are not intended to provide descriptions of these processes and, consequently, cannot adequately address questions concerning cognitive and behavioral changes that accompany recovery and treatment. Connectionist models, on the other hand, are meant to account for dynamic processes of language and memory, and it is this potential that makes them particularly relevant to rehabilitation science.

The advent of "connectionism" led to much anticipation that connectionist models will advance our understanding of dynamic aspects of language processing. Although this may well be the case someday, despite major strides, we are a long way from addressing some important rehabilitation issues. There are at least two reasons for this. First, the cognitive mechanisms underlying recovery and treatment are likely to be very complex. There may be multiple alternative cognitive adaptations and strategies that underlie mechanisms of recovery and treatment. Moreover, it is likely that these cognitive mechanisms are influenced by a variety of "human" factors that cannot be addressed in connectionist models (e.g., age, education, intelligence, motivation). Second, rehabilitation science presents many difficult questions. It is important at the outset to identify and prioritize general and specific issues to be addressed. On the broadest level, for example, we want to know how the cognitive system recovers. Does it reorganize? Does it adapt to use unimpaired systems when possible? Are parallel structures and processes in the contralesional hemisphere engaged as part of recovery or treatment? There are a host of specific questions as well. How do our therapy techniques affect language processing—normal and impaired? How do such techniques make representations accessible? Can we learn to predict what techniques will improve effects of therapy? How do we facilitate processing of words and under what conditions? How can we promote generalization of training to untrained items? How can we increase the speed of learning? How can we ensure that what is learned (or relearned) remains accessible after training is completed?

To answer these and other related questions, we need to understand the processing dynamics of the language system. That is, we need to identify the principles that govern access, retrieval, and storage of information as well as learning new linguistic information. Given the enormity of this task and the relative newness of the science, it is no surprise that we still have much to learn. And yet, because connectionist modeling has great potential to further our understanding of cognitive processes relevant to rehabilitation, it is important to periodically take stock of this approach as it is applied to rehabilitation issues. It is our goal in this chapter to provide such a report and evaluate the progress of connectionist cognitive models toward fulfilling that goal. The rest of the chapter is organized as follows. The following section clarifies some basic definitions and issues that pertain to connectionist cognitive models. Next, we discuss questions and issues that need to be addressed in a theory of rehabilitation; then we review past and current efforts of connectionist cognitive-linguistic models to address these questions. Last, we provide illustrations of treatment approaches that have been advanced in the last decade and that are based on principles of connectionist models of language processing.

Connectionist Cognitive Models of Language: Some Clarifications and Definitions

The use of connectionist models to study language has increased dramatically in a relatively short period. Moreover, these models are fairly complex compared to the functional descriptive models that dominated cognitive neuropsychology for a number of years. It is useful, therefore, to review some fundamental questions about connectionist models and cognitive models in general.

How Does a Cognitive Model of Language Represent Language Theory?

When evaluating the validity and usefulness of a connectionist model (or any cognitive model), it is important to keep in mind that models are not theories themselves, but rather are representations of a theory. As such, they sometimes make simplifying assumptions because the questions being investigated do not require certain theoretical detail. In this way, simplifying assumptions makes it easier to investigate a particular behavior. Ideally, simplifying assumptions should not gloss over operations or variables that will clearly affect the behavior being examined. This may be unavoidable, however, because it is no easy task to characterize in a model every variable that will affect a particular language behavior. For example, the seemingly simple process of word production is carried out over several stages of representation, including a conceptual stage that initiates the process. Many models of word production do not detail the complex stage of conceptual activation (a modeling task in and of itself!), but do assume that it has some general influences (e.g., imageability effects) on word retrieval that are evident in empirical studies. These influences may be built into the model with the understanding that a model more capable of providing these details will be developed in the future.

A final point to be made about the use of models to represent theories is that no model or simulation can ensure that it has reached the ultimate truth about phenomena with 100 percent certainty. Models can only be falsified. A successful simulation shows but one way in which a phenomenon could happen, and there are always other possible ways. Thus, models and model simulations should be evaluated in conjunction with empirical data. If there are no other discriminating data available between two or more models of a phenomenon, the principle of Occam's razor is typically used; that is, the simplest solution is deemed to be the best.

What Is a Computational Model?

Computational modeling is a method for studying cognitive processes underlying language and other behaviors. This tool is particularly important to connectionist models because they formulate hypotheses about the parameters of dynamic processes. It has been argued by some (e.g., Forster, 1994; McCloskey, 1991) that computational simulations of phenomena do not constitute explanations of those phenomena. This depends on what is meant by explanation. The computational implementation of a model is a tool that is used to test a theory's hypotheses about processing dynamics and their role in language use. As such, it can demonstrate the theory's account (or explanation) of a particular phenomenon.

As our theories advance to include postulations of complex and dynamic cognitive phenomena, it will become increasingly difficult to predict from a theory how certain processes will fare in a given context (e.g., a specific kind of functional deficit). Although guesses can be made, it is useful to have a computational model of the theory that can be used to simulate a process under specific conditions. When a theoretical model is implemented on the computer, it can be used to generate predictions about dynamic processes that are not intuitively obvious. However, as noted above, some additional assumptions are always necessary when using models to evaluate a particular aspect of a theory. This is especially true when models are computationally implemented. There are many linguistic processes and operations that have not yet been simulated in any detailed fashion on a computer, even if they are articulated in a theoretical model. Consequently, some simplifying assumptions are made to accommodate the limitations of the implemented version of the model. For example, the word production model of Dell (1986; Dell & O'Seaghdha, 1991) used a small lexicon (five words), and the words had only three phonemes. Obviously, this does not represent the actual size and content of the mental lexicon. However, this "mini-lexicon" enables the theorist to examine characteristics of processing (e.g., effects of semantic and phonological similarity among words in the lexicon on word retrieval) without the complications of implementing a larger lexicon with words of varying lengths and syllable structure. As computational studies address the problems of representing phonemic and syllable structure of words, simulated lexicons can be elaborated accordingly, and features of word retrieval can be examined in a more realistic simulation of the lexical network.

How Do Connectionist Models Differ from Other Models of Cognition?

Grainger and Jacobs (1999) provide a comprehensive analysis of cognitive model types and their relations to each other. Within their scheme, connectionist models are first identified as quantitative models. This differentiates them from "box and arrow"—type functional models (e.g., Caplan, 1992). Additionally, functional models postulate the existence of functional operations (e.g., retrieval) in the language system, but unlike connectionist models, they do not detail the processes that mediate those operations (e.g., spreading activation, competitive learning), although the theories they represent might do so.

Although our definition of connectionist models seems clear enough thus far, there remain a few misconceptions. First, it is not unusual for connectionist models to be falsely equated with distributed network models (Bechtel & Abrahamsen, 1991). Although distributed (PDP) models certainly are prime examples of connectionist models, not all connectionist models have distributed representations. Connectionist models are further divided into two types depending on whether they have localist or distributed representations. Whereas localist models are used to simulate performance of an already developed system, distributed models are capable of learning and therefore can be applied to problems that involve acquisition of new information. More will be said about these two types of connectionist models in the next section.

Norris (1993) made the point that connectionist models are sometimes falsely equated with interactive theories of processing. This misconception has been fueled by the prevalence of connectionist theories that assume interaction. Norris views connectionism as a tool to simulate processing characteristics of language regardless of what that theory of processing is. Network models were used, for example, in Norris's (1993) demonstration of a bottom-up feedforward theory of word recognition and in Laine, Tikkala, and Juhola's (1998) simulation of modular stages of word production. These models used network architectures to simulate language generation as a dynamic process, but they are actually hybrid models that combine "box and arrow" models with connectionist tools to simulate the functioning of the model. The existence of hybrid models suggests that any given functional model can be easily translated directly into a connectionist model, but this is not entirely true. Such a transformation requires the modeler to make more assumptions than the original "box and arrow" model did. Even so, once those assumptions are made, the new model can retain some basic features of the original architecture; for example, Laine and colleagues' (1998) simulation included the seriality and discreteness assumptions of Levelt's (1989) model of word production.

In sum, the core description of a connectionist model is that it is a computationally implemented network architecture with localist or distributed representations that are massively interconnected and processed via activation and/or learning algorithms. The networks of a connectionist model are composed of elementary units that can be activated to some degree and are connected to each other such that active units excite or inhibit other units. The system is dynamic in that it spreads excitatory and inhibitory activation among its units. Although this unique set of features defines connectionist models, the number of variant models that incorporate only some aspects of that ideal continues to expand.

What Are Localist and Distributed Connectionist Models?

A localist connectionist model of language combines representations of single linguistic units (e.g., phonemes or words) with dynamic processes that serve to retrieve those representations over the course of language generation and comprehension. Localist representations are used in models that have built-in parameters and are capable of performing a task at the outset. These models are used to examine performance by the language system in its fully developed state, either intact or lesioned in some way to simulate impairment. Figure 20.1 shows one example of a localist connectionist model of word production (adapted from Dell & O'Seaghdha, 1991). Numerous similar models of word production have been developed by a number of researchers (e.g., Harley, 1984, 1993; MacKay, 1987; Schade & Berg, 1992; Stemberger, 1985). Grainger and Jacobs (1999) note that localist connectionist models differ from the early spreading activation networks, such as those used by Collins and Loftus (1975). Whereas the connections in a localist model represent

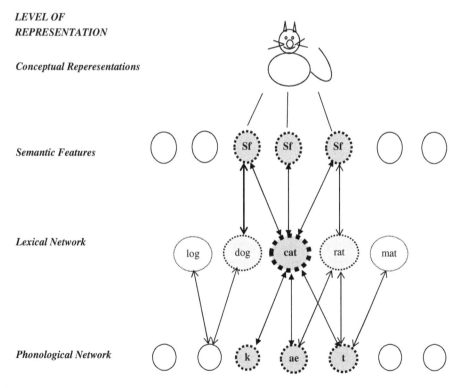

Figure 20.1 An interactive activation model of word production (adapted from Dell & O'Seaghdha, 1991). Activation spreads forward and feeds back across three layers of representational nodes: semantic, lexical, and phonological.

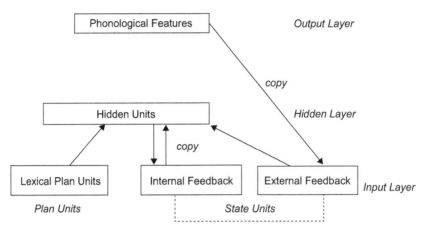

Figure 20.2 An adaptation of the PDP architecture used by Dell, Juliano, and Govindjee (1993). There are three layers (input, output, hidden). Each rectangle within a layer represents a set of units (phonological, hidden, lexical, internal context, and external context).

simple causal relations between two representations (e.g., the word *dog* and its semantic features), the connections in the Collins and Loftus network represent information about the relationship of the connected representations (e.g., a dog has fur).

In distributed connectionist models, representations are not single units, but rather are patterns of activity over many units. It is the strength of these activated units that determines the extent to which the patterns act as conceptual units. An example of a distributed model is shown in Figure 20.2. This figure shows a representation of the PDP architecture used by Dell, Juliano, and Govindjee (1993) in their study of phonological speech errors in word production. This is one of many distributed models that have been developed to investigate written or spoken-word processing (e.g., Hinton & Shallice, 1991; Plaut, 1996; Seidenberg & McClelland, 1989). Distributed models are learning models and therefore can be used to examine issues that revolve around learning and relearning. While there are some issues in cognition that can be addressed by either type of model, there are other issues that are best handled by one type or the other. These are discussed below.

What Are Some Uses of a Localist Connectionist Model?

Localist connectionist models are relatively easy to understand and have been viewed by some as a useful bridge between functional models and more complex connectionist models (Grainger & Jacobs, 1999). They have several useful applications. Localist models can be used to explore effects of "fixed" variables on processing of language. By "fixed," we mean those variables that are relatively constant once a language is learned; for example, a word's frequency, its imageability, or its relation to other words in the network. Of course, even a seemingly fixed variable (e.g., word frequency) is subject to changes in the relative strength of its effect on word processing. Such alterations would be temporary and due to competing effects of other variables. It is also likely that the relative strength of a fixed variable varies depending on the task. For example, in picture naming, the words being retrieved are all imageable, but vary in frequency. Thus, in this task, word frequency would have a prominent influence on word retrieval. In a word repetition task, both imageability and frequency of the words can be manipulated, allowing both variables to influence performance. Understanding the effects of fixed variables on word processing has relevance to both diagnostic and therapeutic aspects of rehabilitation. Diagnostically, effects of variables such as imageability, frequency, and familiarity have been associated with the integrity of specific stages of word representation. With respect to rehabilitation issues, these variables are reflected in the choice of materials used in therapy (e.g., the concreteness or abstractness of words). Awareness of the influences of these variables on language function enables a therapist to maximize or minimize their effects by choosing therapy materials and activities appropriate to the severity and type of impairment.

Another area in which localist models have proved particularly useful is the investigation of speech error phenomena in both normal and aphasic speakers. Much of our understanding of how the language processing system is organized comes from the study of speech errors. This research has yielded a set of constraints on error occurrence that is presumed to derive from the underlying organization of language production. A fundamental mechanism of word retrieval in localist models is a process of competitive activation and (in some models) inhibition among activated nodes in the lexical network. When a word is activated, that activation spreads to other related word nodes in what is termed its "lexical neighborhood." These nodes all compete for activation and either the target word is selected or, in error, a close "neighbor." This mechanism plays an important role in word recognition (see Frauenfelder & Peters, 1999), word production (e.g., Dell, 1986; Schade & Berg, 1992), and error production (Dell & Reich, 1981; Harley, 1984). The competition among lexical nodes is affected by their linguistic relationships (e.g., semantic, phonological) to each other, effects of variables such as frequency and imageability, and the parameters of processing mechanisms (e.g., activation strength) in the model. Although it is possible that the representations of linguistic concepts are distributed, a localist version of that distribution is useful when examining the behavior of representations within a neighborhood of other activated representations. This is because it is easier to see how the characteristics of those representations affect characteristics of the output. Distributed models also can be used to simulate language performance, but the layers of hidden units in a distributed network, where much of the "learning" takes place, make it difficult to understand how various representations and processing assumptions influenced the output of the network (e.g., McCloskey, 1991; Forster, 1994).

What Are Some Uses of a Distributed Connectionist Model?

Like localist models, distributed models are able to simulate effects of relatively stable variables on word processing. Although, as noted above, it is more difficult to understand how those effects take place in a distributed model, there are techniques for analyzing the activity of the hidden units that have helped to address this concern. Distributed connectionist models add something more to the arsenal of tools available to study language processing. Because they are learning models, distributed models can be used to examine questions about cognitive processes involved in learning and relearning. Moreover, they can be used to examine interactions between learning and fixed variables such as frequency of words to be learned. A distributed model also would be used if we want to identify underlying regularities of a phenomenon that could be captured by interactions between the elements of a distributed representation. In semantics, for example, the features that presumably comprise semantic representations of an object are the subunits that make one semantic representation similar to another. When features of two objects are shared, they are connected. This connection contributes to processes of learning and generalization of learning. These are certainly concepts that are important to rehabilitation.

Computer simulations using distributed networks can reveal interesting emergent properties that are not readily apparent in the model. In very complex systems, which the language system surely is, we might not be able to deduce or intuit all of the implications for recovery that will emerge from a model before that modeling is carried out. This ability of connectionist models to

411

reveal emergent properties not immediately apparent in a theory will be very important to the future of research in cognitive rehabilitation. Throughout the literature on model-based therapy programs there are instances in which a therapy program designed on the apparent logic of a model did not work as planned (e.g., Nettleton & Lesser, 1991). Moreover, there are likely many instances of failed model-based therapies that are never reported. There are many possible reasons for an unpredicted outcome, but one of them is that the logic of the model was misunderstood. Complex dynamic systems do not always behave in intuitively predictable ways. A computational instantiation of such a system enables the generation of predictions about its behavior. This feature will be discussed further in our review of connectionist investigations of recovery and treatment.

Is It Better to Use a Localist or Distributed Model?

Localist and distributed models each have features that are well suited to the investigation of different phenomena. Dell and Juliano (1996) compared the abilities of two models of phonological encoding (a localist and a distributed model) to account for some constraints associated with phonological speech errors. The first constraint, phonotactic regularity, holds that speech errors rarely result in sound sequences that are not already present in a language. The second constraint, the consonant-vowel category effect, states that in single sound substitutions consonants replace consonants and vowels replace vowels. The third constraint, known as the syllable constituent effect, refers to instances when adjacent vowel and consonants are replaced. This occurs more often with rhyme (final vowel-consonant, VC) constituents than with initial consonant-vowels (CV). Finally, there is the initialness effect; initial consonants are more likely to engage in slip errors than noninitial consonants.

Dell and Juliano (1996) found that although both models could account for most of these phenomena fairly well, the PDP model was unable to produce movement errors (e.g., the phoneme exchange error: left *h*emisphere → *h*eft *l*emisphere), thus preventing it from accounting for some very important phenomena in speech production. Despite this, Dell and Juliano conclude that each model has some unique advantages that are suitable to the study of speech error phenomena. They note that the localist interactive activation model is better able to account for more phenomena in speech production than the distributed model, and that it is better integrated with linguistic theory. On the other hand, a virtue of the PDP model is that its account of error effects is simple and straightforward: they emerge as products of a massed influence of the vocabulary. Also, because the PDP model can learn, it can be used to study phenomena of change as a function of experience (e.g., short-term training effects and long-term developmental changes).

The foregoing illustration is but one example of a comparison between applications of PDP and localist connectionist models to a particular theoretical question. There should be more instances of this kind of comparison in future studies. As a general rule, it should be kept in mind that cognitive models of all types are *tools*. As such, their value is best weighed according to their suitability for investigating a particular processing issue.

Issues Relevant to the Development of a Cognitive Theory of Rehabilitation

A complete theory of rehabilitation requires both neurophysiological and cognitive accounts of the fundamental mechanisms underlying cognitive changes associated with recovery and rehabilitation. Nonetheless, there are some specific aspects of recovery and treatment that can be addressed in the context of cognitive-behavioral dynamics independently of the underlying neural mechanisms. Information from this line of investigation should have immediate application to methodologies used in cognitive rehabilitation. In this section, we will identify questions that need to be

LIVERPOOL JOHN MOORES UNIVERSITY

answered to develop ideal programs of treatment for word retrieval and other language disorders and discuss the contributions of connectionist models to those efforts.

What Skills Should Be Targeted in Treatment?

There are two parts to this question. First, we need to identify the language deficit. Diagnosis of a deficit needs to be accurate and described at a level of detail that will be useful to the clinician. Once a diagnosis is made, there is a second question: Do we treat the deficit directly or focus therapy on the remaining strengths of communication ability? In one sense, this question goes back to the early days of rehabilitation medicine when it was uncertain whether treatment would improve damaged abilities. If there was hope that brain functions could be restored or reconstituted, then direct treatment seemed warranted. If no such hope existed, it seemed more appropriate to focus therapy on promoting functional communication. Although this controversy remains unresolved, the question of treating a deficit directly is raised in a slightly different way with respect to therapy approaches that aim to restore the damaged function. As our models of cognition have become more sophisticated, it is increasingly apparent that even when the goal is to restore a functional system, there are circumstances in which one would not approach the impaired subsystem head on. Rather, depending on the deficit, it might be advisable to work on the strengths of the damaged system in hopes of stimulating activity in the impaired subsystem. These options will be discussed later in this chapter.

How Do Our Therapy Techniques Affect Language Processing—Normal and Impaired?

This is one of the most important and challenging questions of rehabilitation theory. To answer this question, we need a greater understanding of how brain damage affects both the representations and processes of language. Most cognitive models distinguish between linguistic representations and the processes that access and retrieve those representations. Presumably, brain damage can affect either or both of these components. For example, difficulty in understanding semantic aspects of language could be due to impaired semantic representations or to impairment of processes that access and retrieve those representations. Although these two aspects of language function have long been recognized, treatment research has focused primarily on the remedial effects of linguistic content and less on the dynamic components of the task itself. Therapy tasks are often chosen on the basis of a match between their linguistic content and the representations that are impaired or inaccessible (e.g., semantic tasks for semantic impairment).

As our cognitive models become more explicit about processes involved in accessing and retrieving linguistic representations, there can be more speculation about how impairments to those processes might affect language. For example, one model (Dell, Martin, & Schwartz, 2007; Dell, Schwartz, Martin, Saffran, & Gagnon, 1997; Schwartz, Dell, Martin, Gahl, & Sobel, 2006) attributes word production disorders to impairment of processing parameters that regulate access to word representations: reduced rate of activation spread or increased rate of decay of activated representations. To the extent that such processing deficits are shown to be real, it will be important to consider how these deficits are treated in therapy. It may not be sufficient to say that an individual's word processing impairment is due to a deficit in accessing semantics. Rather, the access deficit could be defined further with respect to the underlying processing impairment that is impeding access (e.g., weak activation or too-fast decay). Moreover, these two kinds of impairments (or others postulated by other models) might respond differently to different kinds of tasks depending on the extent to which those tasks promote activation of the target and competing representations (Abel, Wilmes, & Huber, 2007; Martin, Dell, Saffran, & Schwartz, 1994; Martin, Saffran, & Dell, 1996).

Another issue to consider in choosing therapy tasks is how stimulation of one level of representation (e.g., semantic) affects processing at another level of representation (e.g., phonological). In cascading and interactive activation models it is postulated that impairment at later stages of encoding can be influenced by tasks that strengthen activation at earlier stages. Presumably, an effect of therapy would be to strengthen activation transmission to subsequent stages. If this is the case, it might be advisable, for example, to treat a phonologically based word retrieval deficit with semantically stimulating materials and activities.

These are but a few examples of the kinds of "treatment" questions that could be posed given a theory of language *processing*. Some of these questions have been addressed in the last few decades (e.g., Laine & Martin, 1996; Martin et al., 2004; Martin et al., 2006; Nettleton & Lesser, 1991; Renvall, Laine, & Martin, 2007). If brain damage affects processing (and consequently activation of representations), a therapy plan should consider the characteristics of the content (words, pictures, and other stimuli) as well as those of the tasks used in therapy. Moreover, the choice of task should be made with an understanding of the process that has gone wrong, how it has gone wrong, and how the dynamics of the therapy task will affect the impaired process. These issues will be discussed further later in this chapter.

What Techniques Facilitate Processing and Under What Conditions?

This question is directly related to the previous question. Rehabilitation science currently lacks an understanding of the dynamic influences of the therapy tasks. This knowledge would help us to determine what tasks facilitate or impede improvement. Most speech therapy tasks that are used to improve comprehension or production involve one or both of two fundamental phenomena: *priming* and *contextual* effects. Priming is the concept of one event (e.g., hearing a word) affecting another (saying the same or another word). When a word is activated and/or retrieved, its residual activation can influence processing of subsequent words for a period of time. Also, the activation of one-word representation spreads to other related word representations, increasing their level of activation. Spreading activation is one mechanism that is presumed to mediate priming. Additionally, processes that are under the subject's strategic control can be invoked; these include postlexical semantic matching and expectancy-based processing (e.g., Neely, 1991).

Priming takes a number of forms. The target word can be primed directly by presenting the word itself or a task that elicits that word. Semantic priming occurs when facilitation cues that are semantically related to the target word are presented. Examples of semantic cues include the definition of a word, words that are in the same category (*banana* → *apple*), or a phrase cue that includes semantic information about the target ("You pound nails with a _____"). Any activity that probes semantic information about the target word or related concepts will prime the target and related word representations. Phonological priming involves providing part of the word's phonological form (e.g., initial phoneme and the rime). For instance, /ba/ will prime phonological representations of numerous words, including *Bob, bottle, bog*, and *bomb*. Once a word representation has been primed, it is presumed that its activation is raised for a period of time, making it temporarily more accessible.

A second factor that affects word retrieval is the linguistic context in which a word is retrieved. In the process of word retrieval, linguistic context is formed as part of the natural course of spreading activation; when representations of a word to be spoken are activated, related representations are also "primed" to some degree, creating a context in which the target word will be activated. We will call this *internal priming*. Context is also created by *external priming*. External priming can create different contexts for word retrieval. A prime word that is semantically or phonologically related to the target word creates a related context. Unrelated primes do not create related contexts, although semantic and phonological neighboring word representations would be activated somewhat by internal priming from spreading activation. Priming and context are two interdependent phenomena: priming creates the context, and in turn, context adds to the priming.

There are number of important issues about priming and contextual effects. How do they affect normal and impaired processing? Research to date indicates that priming and context can be facilitative or disruptive to naming performance in normal (e.g., Martin & Laine, 2000; Martin, Weisberg, & Saffran, 1989) and impaired speakers depending, in part, on the nature of their naming impairment (Laine & Martin, 1996). When does priming facilitate processing and when does it interfere? Therapy tasks typically employ external priming and context quite liberally. In some cases, priming and context are used to directly facilitate retrieval of the target word (e.g., phonemic and semantic cues). In other tasks, priming directly activates both the target and competitors and thus presents a more challenging situation for the subject. This sort of priming may or may not be facilitative. For example, in the synonymy judgment and yes/no questions (e.g., "Is an apple yellow?" "Do birds have feathers?"), the task is to judge what could be conflicting or overlapping information and to choose between words that are related. These and other tasks (e.g., word-to-picture matching) activate words that overlap in features and thus can make the task of retrieving the target word more difficult. It would be a worthwhile enterprise to describe therapy tasks in terms of whether the priming and context effects they promote are facilitative (prompt target retrieval directly), challenging (priming competitor representations as well as the target word), or both. Once treatment tasks were analyzed in this way, we could determine circumstances in which one approach would be better than another for promoting immediate and long-lasting improvements in retrieval.

Priming and context effects are products of language processing. This means that impaired language processes will alter these effects in different ways. It is for this reason that we need to have a clear understanding of processes that access and transmit linguistic representations and what goes wrong with them when they are impaired. Connectionist models should be able to determine parameters of priming and contextual effects via simulation, and this basic research should serve as a foundation to investigate the effects of therapy techniques on impaired and healthy language processes.

What Factors Promote Generalization of Learning from Trained to Untrained Items?

The question of how generalization works has long been an issue in rehabilitation research. Understanding the mechanisms underlying generalization of learning from trained to untrained items is very important to the overall efficacy of a treatment program. Otherwise, training would have to be item specific. A related issue is whether training generalizes across modalities; for example, from input tasks to output abilities. In naming treatments, this generalization is only observed some of the time, and we are not yet certain of the factors that promote this generalization. Some factors thought to affect generalization of training include linguistic relatedness among items being trained (priming and context effects), prototypicality of items in a category being trained, and set size of items being trained. Additionally, the type of learning that a particular treatment approach is triggering may be important. Should treatment approaches use explicit or implicit learning methods? Interest in this question and others related to learning and relearning (e.g., intensity of treatment) has increased in the last decade and has led to some exploration of the effects of these factors on treatment efficacy (e.g., Schuchard & Thompson, 2014). Connectionist models are equipped to explore mechanisms of spreading activation and learning that presumably mediate generalization and can be used as frameworks for such studies because they can generate and test hypotheses about how these factors influence generalization under normal conditions and under conditions of impairment (e.g., Plaut, 1996).

What Factors Contribute to Learning and the Endurance of Treatment Effects?

There are a number of issues about the nature of learning that need to be addressed in order to tackle more specific questions about the endurance of treatment effects. We need to understand the differences and similarities between learning new information and the "relearning" of information after a stroke (Laine, 2000). These may or may not involve the same processes. Recent studies are identifying cognitive-linguistic factors that can adversely affect learning of new information (Martin & Saffran, 1999; Tuomiranta, Rautakoski, Rinne, Martin, & Laine 2012), including the integrity of short-term memory, the lexical system, and access to semantic representations. It is likely that effective treatments will require both relearning and new learning. Thus, to address specific questions about the effectiveness of treatment, we will need to gain further understanding of the fundamentals of verbal learning. There has recently been an increase in empirical studies of new word learning in aphasia, and these data will hopefully be modeled with distributed connectionist models that enable the exploration of the dynamics of learning in the normal and damaged brain. This line of investigation is in its early stages, but holds promise in its potential to increase our understanding of the learning processes that support recovery and treatment effects in aphasia.

Contributions of Connectionist Models to Rehabilitation: Progress and Potential

In theory, connectionist models can describe the dynamics of cognitive systems, and herein lies their potential contribution to rehabilitation. The investigation of some issues requires distributed models that learn, while other questions could be addressed using either localist or distributed connectionist models. Of the questions relevant to rehabilitation science that were noted earlier, functional models were able to adequately address the question of what deficit should be treated. They also provided some insight into the kinds of therapy materials and activities to use for a specific deficit. Connectionist models can add to this effort, but also can address many of the other questions. Below, we discuss preliminary efforts of connectionist models to address some of these questions.

How Does the Damaged Language System Repair Itself?

A complete answer to this question will require investigations of both behavioral and neurophysiological changes that occur with recovery. For example, it is important to know whether physical systems are restored or whether other physical structures (e.g., tissue surrounding a lesion site or structures in the intact hemisphere) assume function. Cognitive models can explore behavioral changes that would be expected to accompany recovery or relearning. Such changes may or may not parallel measurable physiological changes.

One important question about the nature of recovery is whether the impaired language system recovers in a way that returns the system to its premorbid state or whether new patterns of functioning (physical and cognitive) emerge. Cognitive theories can address the behavioral side of this question. Martin, Dell, Saffran, and Schwartz (1994) and Martin, Saffran, and Dell (1996) studied the patterns of language recovery of a person with aphasia, NC, whose naming and repetition were seriously compromised. They documented the kinds of speech errors that NC produced early in the course of his recovery and again after a year or so of recovery. NC's error patterns were noteworthy because they included semantic errors in repetition and form-related word errors (formal paraphasias) in naming. This error pattern was difficult to account for in a functional model without multiple lesion sites (e.g., Howard & Franklin, 1988). Another challenge to an account of this error pattern is that it is unlike typical error patterns of normal speakers. Although normal speakers produce formal paraphasias in production (termed "malapropisms"), the predominant error type is semantic (Dell et al., 1997; Harley & MacAndrew, 2001). In repetition, healthy individuals make few errors, and so a true record of what kind of error would predominate is unavailable. However, the simulation of an interactive activation model used by Martin and colleagues (1994), based on Dell and O'Seaghdha's (1991) model (see Figure 20.1) indicates that semantic errors would be extremely unlikely. Indeed, they are very rare in cases of repetition impairment. The comparison of normal speech error patterns with this subject's error pattern is an important one to the issue of recovery. Martin and colleagues wanted to know whether NC's "abnormal" speech error pattern would resolve back to a more normal error pattern, or whether some new pattern of error would emerge with recovery. If the former recovery pattern were observed, it would provide evidence that recovery involves, at least in part, some return to premorbid behavioral patterns.

The first step in studying this problem was to account for NC's "abnormal" error pattern in acute stages. This step was examined within the framework of Dell and O'Seaghdha's (1991) inter-active spreading activation model. This model assumes that activation processes that mediate lexical retrieval are regulated by two parameters, connection strength (the rate of activation spread) and decay rate (the rate of activation decline toward resting level). Noise and the number of time steps to production are additional parameters. Martin and Saffran (1992) and Martin, Shelton, and Yaffee (1994) hypothesized that NC's error pattern resulted from a pathologically rapid decay of primed nodes in the semantic-lexical-phonological network. This prediction was partly intuitive, based on NC's severely impaired short-term memory and his complaint that words spoken to him would "disappear" before he could grasp what they were. Martin and colleagues (1994) confirmed in a computer simulation that the model also made this prediction. In a series of simulations, the model reproduced NC's error pattern in both naming and repetition, with the same functional lesion to the model. In a second part of this same study, Martin and colleagues (1994) examined NC's error pattern after some recovery. At that time, NC no longer made semantic errors in repetition of single words or formal paraphasias in naming. They compared this pattern to the model's simulation of naming and repetition performance after the decay rate was reduced from 0.8 (abnormally high) to a lower rate that was closer to normal. The simulation again produced an error pattern comparable to NC's (no semantic errors in repetition, no formal paraphasias in naming).

Dell and colleagues (1997) used a version of the model described above to account for the error patterns of 18 aphasic subjects by increasing the normal decay rate (increasing it) and/or reducing the normal connection weight. In this same study, they investigated the recovery patterns of a subset of those 18 subjects (those who were available) and showed that the changes in their error patterns could be simulated by altering the impaired parameters back toward their normal levels (i.e., lowered decay rate, increased connection weight). These two studies of recovery (Dell et al., 1997; Martin et al., 1994) provide evidence that the path of recovery for impaired cognitive mechanisms underlying speech production follows a trajectory toward their normal premorbid state.

In another study of patient NC, Martin and colleagues (1996) examined his recovery of word processing abilities in conjunction with recovery of a severe auditory-verbal short-term memory (STM) impairment that was also present in his profile. They found that as NC recovered, his performance on auditory-verbal STM tasks improved (span increased to two items), and his pattern of error in word repetition changed as well (fewer semantic errors, more formal paraphasias and neologisms). Other features of his span performance resembled patterns associated with STM-based repetition impairments (reduced recency effects and reduced word length effects). In a series of computer simulation and empirical studies, Martin and colleagues (1996) showed that NC's repetition performance could be accounted for by varying two parameters of the interactive activation model of repetition adapted from Dell and O'Seaghdha's (1991) model of production: decay rate and temporal interval. In their previous study of NC's recovery, the model demonstrated that such a reduction would result in greater accuracy and fewer semantic errors in immediate repetition of single words (Martin et al., 1994), a pattern that simulated NC's performance as he recovered. Martin and colleagues (1996) confirmed a further prediction of the model regarding NC's repetition error pattern: semantic errors would emerge in the repetition error pattern even after the decay rate had recovered somewhat, *if* the amount of time between input and output in a repetition task was increased. This was demonstrated in two tasks: repetition of two words and repetition of a single word after a delay. In each of these tasks, semantic errors reemerged as predicted. These results provide support for the view that auditory-verbal STM and lexical processing are related. NC's changes in recovery also support the view that deep dysphasia and STM-based repetition disorders are quantitative variants of the same underlying disturbance.

Accounting for Naming and Repetition in the Context of Dell's Interactive Activation Model of Word Processing

The studies of Martin and colleagues demonstrate how a connectionist model (in this case a localist connectionist model) can account for the complexities of behavioral changes that accompany recovery. These studies were based on a large-scale project aimed at accounting for the processing impairments leading to word retrieval deficits in aphasia (Dell et al., 1997; Dell, Martin, & Schwartz, 2007; Martin & Dell, 2007; Schwartz et al., 2006; Schwartz, Saffran, Bloch, & Dell, 1994). Schwartz et al. (2006) extended the studies of Dell et al. (1997) and developed two processing accounts of naming and repetition in 96 individuals with aphasia, the weight and decay account and the semantic and phonological weight account. As noted earlier, Dell's interactive activation model postulates two processing parameters that regulate access to and retrieval of semantic and phonological representations of words, connection weight and decay weight. In the 1997 and 2006 models, naming and repetition error patterns were mapped to the model as disturbances of connection weight (reduced strength of activation) and/or decay rate (too fast decay of activated representations). In the Schwartz et al. (2006) computational modeling studies, a second account was introduced that accounted for individual naming and repetition error patterns as reduced connection weight of semantic representations and/or reduced connection weight of phonological representations. Although it is beyond the scope of this chapter to provide details of these two studies, familiarity with this body of work is highly recommended, as it provides a foundation for the new pathways to treatment that focus on processes of language.

Also, they show that apparently distinct disturbances (short-term memory and word processing) are at least functionally related. The studies discussed so far are examples of how computational simulations can provide accounts of phenomena that are not easily explained. Martin and colleagues postulated a relationship between lexical retrieval and temporal components of word processing. While this hypothesis was supported by the data, the computational simulation revealed the interactive activation model's account of this relationship. This series of studies is an excellent example of how connectionist modeling and experimental investigations of patients can interact to produce a more comprehensive study of cognitive neuropsychological issues. There are undoubtedly many other such puzzles in cognitive neuropsychology that involve complex behaviors and that would benefit from a study that combines empirical computational methods of analysis.

How Do Therapy Techniques Affect Normal and Impaired Processes?

At present, there have been few studies that explore directly the effects of therapy techniques on normal and impaired processes. We shall describe one of these below and also some empirical studies that explore this question. A major goal of cognitive neuropsychological research has been to determine how representations and processes are affected by brain damage. We certainly need theories of normal and impaired processing before we can explore the dynamics of therapy techniques and their interactions with those processes. There are a number of studies using localist and distributed connectionist models that have explored effects of damage to linguistic representations and processes on language output (e.g., Dell et al., 1997; Foygel & Dell, 2000; Hinton & Shallice, 1991; Plaut, 1996; Plaut & Shallice, 1993; Rapp & Goldrick, 2000). Models such as these can serve as frameworks in future studies to examine more complex questions concerning the interaction of external stimuli and inner processes of the language system.

Damage and Retraining in a Distributed Connectionist Model: The Effects of Site of Functional Lesion

One question that is important to understanding effects of treatment is whether those effects vary depending on where the site of a functional lesion is located within a cognitive-linguistic model. Are deficits affecting semantic processes and representations more or less amenable to treatment than those affecting phonological or orthographic processing? The answer to this question could depend on what kind of treatment is being administered. However, there also could be an effect of site of functional lesion on relearning that is independent of the treatment being administered. In the first study we discuss below, Plaut (1996) explored the issue of whether relearning is differentially affected by the site of functional lesion using a distributed network model of reading.

In Plaut's (1996) model of reading, there are three levels of representation: orthographic, intermediate, and semantic. There are also clean-up units connected to the semantic representations that serve to refine the semantic representation as learning proceeds. Functional lesions are simulated by removing connections between the following representations: (1) orthographic and intermediate, (2) intermediate and semantic, and (3) semantic and clean-up units. Plaut explored the effectiveness of retraining in relation to the site of functional lesion. Retraining in this model involved presenting a set of words that had been learned by the model before it was lesioned. Of this set of words, the now-lesioned model recognized only half. Because retraining was the same for each site of a functional lesion, this study provides no insight into differential effects on relearning related to task differences or how such task differences might interact with a functional lesion site. Thus, Plaut's study is more a simulation of recovery in response to general language stimulation rather than an examination of specific treatment effects. Nevertheless, it provides important information about recovery of semantic versus orthographic lesions (and in the auditory modality, phonological lesions).

Plaut demonstrated that relearning and generalization varied depending on the site of functional lesion and that more relearning occurred in the case of semantic-to-clean-up lesions than in lesions affecting earlier stages of processing (orthographic-to-intermediate units and intermediate units-to-semantic units). The network model demonstrates this as a function of the degree of structure in the subtasks performed by each part of the network. Mapping of orthographic representations onto partially organized semantic representations (the intermediate representations) is not very structured. More structure is observed in the mapping of the intermediate representations onto the semantic representations, and finally, the interactions of the semantic representations and the clean-up units have the greatest amount of structure.

Although Plaut's analysis of the network's behavior is logical, the conclusion, that greater improvement and generalization would be observed following lesions to the semantic level than to the orthographic (or phonological) lesions, is counterintuitive. First, it is inconsistent with much of what we know about top-down contextual effects on word processing. For example, semantic representations that are processed later in the course of word comprehension influence processing of earlier-stage phonological representations (Marslen-Wilson & Welsh, 1988; McClelland & Rumelhart, 1981; Tanenhaus, Dell, & Carlson, 1987). Extending this idea to impairments of word processing, when phonological input processing is impaired, top-down influences are available to facilitate comprehension. When the incoming spoken word is degraded by phonological impairment, presumably several semantic representations would be activated. This semantic information would be used to disambiguate the input and help the listener determine what words were actually spoken. When semantic processes are impaired, phonological input would provide no information about semantic structure and therefore would do little to facilitate semantic processing. At the same time, knowing the phonological form of the word is insufficient to achieve comprehension of that word. It is difficult to reconcile this pattern of interactive influences during input processing with the notion that semantic lesions recover more quickly than phonological lesions.

A second reason to question the prediction of Plaut's model is that there are no empirical data to support this pattern of recovery. In fact, it was challenged in a study by Weekes and Coltheart (1996) that investigated the effects of a treatment program for surface dyslexia. Their patient showed significant generalization of training effects despite the fact that his impairment was orthographic and not semantic. Although Plaut argues that this patient's functional lesion may have involved semantic deficits as well as orthographic deficits, the fact remains that this counterintuitive prediction about prognosis needs to be verified with empirical data.

What do we know about prognosis for recovery of language in relation to cognitive-linguistic impairment? Kertesz and McCabe (1977) examined recovery patterns associated with the classical aphasia syndromes (e.g., Wernicke's, Broca's). They found that the least amount of recovery was observed in global aphasia and Wernicke's aphasia, and the greatest amount in Broca's aphasia. This latter group demonstrates impaired phonological processing, particularly in output, but semantic processing and comprehension are relatively spared. Those individuals with conduction aphasia, in which semantic processing is relatively spared and phonological processing is impaired, also showed a relatively high rate of recovery. Global and Wernicke's aphasia are associated with both phonological and semantic deficits. The robust recovery of people with Broca's or conduction aphasia, who demonstrate good semantic processing and relatively impaired phonological processing, suggests a pattern that is inconsistent with the predictions of Plaut's (1996) model.

A proper test of Plaut's predictions requires a recovery study that isolates the lesions of the cognitive components of language (e.g., semantic impairment) comparable to those postulated in Plaut's model. A study by Schwartz and Brecher (2000) provides some relevant data. They used Dell and colleagues' (1997) model as theoretical framework and examined recovery of naming abilities from the perspective of changes in error pattern in relation to severity. They observed that the rate of phonological errors increased with severity and that the rate of semantic errors did not. This finding was consistent with the model's predictions that phonological errors are severity-sensitive and that semantic errors are severity-insensitive. On the basis of these findings, Schwartz and Brecher predicted that with partial recovery, error patterns would show a greater decrease in the rate of phonological errors than in the rate of semantic errors. Their study of the partial recovery of seven subjects confirmed this prediction. This finding, that phonological errors, characteristic of phonological lesions, were more likely to resolve with recovery than semantic errors (characteristic of some types of semantic lesions and some types of phonological output deficits; e.g., Caramazza & Hillis, 1990), fails to provide support for the predictions of Plaut's model. Although data to support the predictions generated by Plaut's (1996) model are lacking, they remain plausible and should be investigated further. Plaut's study is another example of the way in which connectionist models (with or without a distributed network) can lead to interesting emergent properties of complex systems that might not be apparent before modeling. These predictions cannot be taken as fact, however, until verified by empirical data. Combined computational and empirical studies should prove to be a very effective approach to solving many of the intricate puzzles in language theory and rehabilitation.

Interactions of Treatment and Site of Functional Lesion: Exploring Differential Effects of Semantic and Phonological Context on Word Retrieval

As described earlier, Martin and colleagues (1994) and Dell and colleagues (1997) used a localist connectionist model to characterize the picture naming abilities of people with aphasia and also to examine dynamics of their recovery (Martin et al., 1996; Schwartz & Brecher, 2000). Patterns of word production in aphasia were described in terms of two processing impairments: a weakened connection weight that affects the strength of information transmission and an increased decay rate that affects the integrity of activated representations. These studies attempted to define what could go wrong with processing and what the consequences of those impairments are for speech output. A potential next step would be to explore the interaction of the fundamental components of therapy techniques (e.g., priming and context) with impairments to each of these processing parameters. This line of research would be similar to that of the many studies that examined the effects of therapy tasks on semantic versus phonological impairments, except that the focus would be on decay rate versus connection weight impairments. Ultimately, it should be possible to vary both the processing parameters and the locus of a functional lesion to define aphasic impairment (see Foygel & Dell, 2000, for relevant steps toward this goal).

Laine and Martin (1996) and Martin and Laine (2000) investigated the interaction of treatment (priming) with the site of a functional lesion, using the Dell model as a theoretical framework. They employed a paradigm that exploits both priming and context through massed repetition priming of picture names that are linguistically (semantically or phonologically) related. One goal of studies using this paradigm was to determine whether a subject's naming ability was facilitated or impeded by the priming context. Specifically, would priming type (semantic or phonological) interact with the linguistic impairment (semantic and/or phonological) that underlies the naming deficit? Laine and colleagues demonstrated that some patients improve when the words being trained are semantically (categorically) related (Kiviniemi, Laine, Tarkiainen, Järvensivu, Martin, & Salmelin, 2000; Laine & Martin, 1996), while others improve when the words being trained are phonologically related (Martin & Laine, 2000). Following the work of Laine and Martin, several studies used the contextual priming procedure to further understand the effects of priming type in relation to type of language impairment (Martin, Fink, Laine, & Ayala, 2004a; Martin, Fink, & Laine, 2004b; Martin & Laine, 2000; Martin, Fink, Renvall, & Laine, 2006; Renvall, Laine, Laakso, & Martin, 2003; Renvall, Laine, & Martin, 2005; Renvall, Laine, & Martin, 2007). Some of these studies are described below.

Martin et al. (2004a) examined effects of repetition priming combined with three contexts (semantic, phonological, unrelated) on naming. Eleven participants with different types of language impairment were included in the study. One aim of the study was to determine if different patterns of performance related to sensitivity of context and site of language breakdown would emerge. A second aim was to determine if a match between training context (semantic or phonological relatedness of training set) and source of naming impairment (semantic or phonological) would be facilitative or interfering with word retrieval.

Martin et al. (2004a) found different patterns of performance during the contextual priming session and in the post-test following the session. During the priming session, three participants with primarily semantic impairments showed evidence of interference in the semantic context (more contextual errors and/or fewer correct) and three of the four participants classified as having primarily phonological deficits showed evidence of interference in the phonological context. Six of these seven participants also showed short-term facilitation of naming in all contexts at the end of the treatment session. A similar observation was made in a contextual priming treatment study reported by Renvall, Laine, and Martin (2005). The participant in their study, PH, demonstrated good input access to semantics, but difficulty activating word forms from semantics.

They found that although short-term interference was evident in rates of contextual errors that occurred during treatment, short-term improvement was evident in post-treatment naming tests. These outcomes suggest that immediate interference during training does not preclude short-term improvement of naming.

Outcomes of several naming treatment studies that used contextual priming treatment suggested that intact access to semantics was a strong predictor of improved naming. Renvall et al. (2003) reported a single case treatment study, YK, who also presented with postsemantic deficits in production, affecting activation of lexical phonological forms, phoneme assembly and articulatory difficulties. They found that YK's naming performance improved in semantic and phonological training contexts but that generalization to untrained items occurred only in the semantic context.

Martin et al. (2004b) used the contextual priming procedure in a treatment study with two participants with contrasting patterns of language impairment. LP demonstrated intact semantic processing abilities, but a marked deficit in phonological processing. AS demonstrated a primary impairment in accessing semantics coupled with a mild phonological processing difficulty. LP's naming ability benefited from all three contexts. AS demonstrated greater difficulty with naming of pictures in the semantic context than other contexts. He produced high rates of contextual errors and made only short-term gains in accuracy of naming. Martin et al. (2006) studied two individuals, BM and BQ, with semantically based production impairments who also had input processing deficits affecting access to semantics from the lexicon. BM showed some evidence of improvement only in the phonological condition. BQ did not benefit from any context, and at most showed short-term gains that were not maintained at follow-up.

These treatment studies suggested that individuals with impaired access to semantic representations of words showed only modest short-term effects of treatment. To address this issue, Renvall et al. (2007) developed a modified version of the contextual priming treatment, which included additional semantic (word-to-picture matching) and phonological (rhyming syllable identification) tasks. These tasks were intended to "boost" stimulation of connections between semantics and the lexicon. There were two participants in the study, LV, with a primarily semantic deficit affecting input and output processing, and JP, with primarily a phoneme sequencing deficit. Both participants demonstrated short-term facilitation of naming in all treatment contexts. LV's post-treatment tests indicated significant improvement of naming in the semantic condition only when extra semantic and phonological tasks were incorporated into training. JP's post-treatment tests indicated significant improvement in the semantic context (with extra semantic tasks) and unrelated context (with extra semantic and phonological task conditions).

From these case studies, some patterns have emerged. The importance of good access to semantics on input became increasingly evident as more case studies were reported. The observation that two cases with primarily only phonological impairment performed well in all context conditions is consistent with this hypothesis, as both participants had intact semantic processing. Priming in a linguistic context that directly matches with the main source of naming impairment was sometimes beneficial, but also increased the level of interference during training (increased rates of errors and fewer correct responses during training). This suggests that some additional factor needs to be considered beyond matching locus of deficit in a cognitive-linguistic model (semantic, phonological) with the type of context (semantic or phonological). That additional factor could be the type of processing deficit as postulated in Dell et al.'s (1997) modeling study (see also Schwartz et al., 2006), slowed connection weight or too fast decay of activated representations. This possibility requires investigation, but is an appropriate direction for this research to take.

Future investigations using this paradigm could focus on the possible interaction of processing impairment with tasks that promote priming of a neighborhood of related representations. Within the framework of Dell and colleagues' (1997) model, this would involve identifying differential effects of priming on naming impairments attributed to connection weight impairments (slowed activation) and decay rate impairments (premature decay of activated representations). Connection weight lesions lead to reduced activation of the target and competing representations. Therefore, priming should boost the activation of these representations toward a normal state and facilitate activation of the target word. In contrast, deficits caused by too rapid decay of activated representations do not reduce activation, but rather upset the balance between activation of the target word and competing neighborhood representations. In this case, it is conceivable that priming would be disruptive to naming because too many related and competing representations would be activated. Although the hypothesis has not yet been tested computationally, it is consistent with general performance features of Dell and colleagues' (1997) model. But how does one determine what kind of processing problem is present? Computer simulations are useful for addressing this kind of question. Again, using Dell and colleagues' (1997) modeling study as an example, simulations of connection weight and decay rate impairments yielded distinctive error patterns associated with each type and severity of lesion. Each subject's error profile was then matched to the model's predicted error patterns, enabling classification of the subject's processing impairment within the framework of the model. This method could be used in future studies requiring such a classification.

The Dell model is but one framework within which we can try to understand the effects of therapy tasks on normal and impaired processing. It is noteworthy because it has sparked an interest in processing impairments in aphasia. Recent studies have investigated the ability of other models to account for the error patterns that were modeled in the Dell et al. (1997) study as well as data that could not be fit to that model (e.g., Foygel & Dell, 2000; Rapp & Goldrick, 2000; Ruml & Caramazza, 2000). These models are taking the initial assumptions of the Dell et al. model and modifying them in several important ways. For example, an important aspect of the simulations of impaired language using the Dell et al. model was that the parameter impairments were set globally throughout the lexical network. That is, it was assumed that the processing deficit (increased decay rate or reduced connection weight) affected semantic, lexical, and phonological processing equally. This characterization of aphasic impairment seemed at odds with neuropsychological data indicating the existence of cases with clear dissociations of semantic and phonological stages of naming. The global "weight-decay" model shows that the interaction of the global processing deficit and the temporal course of processing from semantic to lexical and then to phonological representations yields error patterns that appear to selectively involve one or another level of representation to some extent. Nonetheless, there remain cases with patterns of error on naming and other tasks that indicate a clear dissociation between semantic and phonological abilities. For this reason, other models that capture the possibility of such dissociations are being tested against the naming data from Dell and colleagues (1997) and other patients reported in the literature (e.g., Foygel & Dell, 2000; Rapp & Goldrick, 2000; Ruml & Caramazza, 2000).

The studies discussed above are meant to illustrate the very first steps that connectionism is taking toward an eventual contribution to rehabilitation of naming deficits. These and other models that attempt to characterize naming and object specification (e.g., Schade & Eikmeyer, 1999) indicate that the time is ripe to begin thinking about how training techniques might affect those same processing parameters, whether they are impaired or not. Future efforts by connectionist models should be able to determine parameters of these contextual effects via simulation by exploring, for example, effects of linguistic relatedness or neighborhood size on word access.

How Do We Promote Generalization of Training to Untrained Items?

Generalization of treatment effects from a set of trained items to other untrained items is one of the more important issues in rehabilitation. Connectionist models, both localist and distributed, have mechanisms that would mediate such generalization.

Generalization in a Localist Model

In localist connectionist models, spreading activation is the means by which generalization effects would occur. Training on one item would presumably cause spreading activation to other related words. In this model, both semantic and phonological spreading activation should contribute to the effect. Some evidence for this notion comes from the contextual priming studies of Laine and Martin (1996; Martin & Laine, 2000), in which sets of related and unrelated items were trained with a repetition priming procedure. In those studies, they examined the effects of context on rates of correct responses as well as on rates of contextual and noncontextual errors. Contextual errors are those errors that came from within the set of items being trained and would be an example of external priming. Noncontextual errors are those errors that are not items in the set. They are presumed to result from internal priming and as evidence of spreading activation to related items. These same processes, according to Martin and Laine, play a role in generalization of learning.

A Study of Generalization in a Distributed Model

In distributed models, generalization is mediated by overlapping semantic features among items being trained. Plaut (1996) demonstrated in a computational study of reading that relearning is strongly influenced by the regularity of structure in mapping one representation onto another. In the network he used, the mapping between orthography and semantics was determined by the semantic organization of the words. This suggested that if a set of words to be trained was representative of the semantic structure of the entire set of words, generalization to untrained words in the set could be expected. Plaut proposed that the typicality of a concept (i.e., the proximity to the central tendency of a category) is a variable that would affect the estimate of the semantic structure. His experiments showed that generalization was greater when the network was retrained on both typical and atypical members of the category. Plaut attributes this effect to the probability that atypical members of a category include more information about the structure and central tendency of that category than do more typical members. At first glance, this prediction of Plaut's model could appear to be counterintuitive. In therapy, the general inclination is to train the most typical and familiar objects of a category. This practice might result in improvement of specific items, but not much generalization to untrained items. Plaut's model provides an insight that suggests that more generalization will occur if a wider representation of the category is trained. In the final section, we describe a treatment studies that use this study as their theoretical framework and directly test the predictions of Plaut's simulation.

Other Learning Issues Relevant to Rehabilitation: Models That Link Language, Short-Term Memory, and Learning

The connectionist models we have discussed thus far address automatic aspects of language processing. Controlled strategic processes that are important to the formation of compensatory strategies are currently outside the scope of these models and may be for some time to come. However, there is another realm of investigation and a host of connectionist models that ultimately should provide some information relevant to our understanding of controlled processing and its role in rehabilitation. Studies of short- and long-term memory, verbal learning, and the connections of these systems with language processing aim to understand the processes involved in learning and factors that affect those processes. Empirical data from a variety of populations (e.g., developmental, normal and impaired adults, and bilinguals) bear on these issues, and there are an increasing number of models designed to account for some of these findings (e.g., Baddeley, 1986; Burgess & Hitch, 1992; Gupta & MacWhinney, 1997; Hartley & Houghton, 1996; Page & Norris, 1998).

Ultimately, this line of research should reveal factors that affect speed and longevity of learning (and relearning) and other issues of learning that are relevant to rehabilitation.

A full account of this line of research is beyond the scope of this chapter. However, the work of Gupta and MacWhinney (1997) provides a good example of a model that attempts to link verbal STM and vocabulary acquisition. The model employs connectionist processing elements and learning algorithms, and provides an explicit account of lexical access and retrieval. The model also offers an account of word learning, nonword repetition, and immediate serial recall, and relates these three phenomena to each other and to the lexical processing system. Importantly, Gupta (1996) demonstrated that all three abilities depend crucially on the strength of long-term phonological knowledge in the system. Word learning and immediate serial recall also depend on the strength of long-term semantic knowledge. This model is very promising as an account of links between verbal STM, verbal learning, and language processing. Moreover, its potential extends to accounts of the language, memory, and learning problems observed in aphasia. This and other similar models should serve well as frameworks within which to explore the breakdown of the interactions of STM, language, and learning in brain damage. Clearly, such studies should have implications for treatment of language impairment.

Application of Connectionist Models to Treatment of Aphasia: Progress in the Last Decade

Here we discuss two areas of language rehabilitation that have benefited from connectionist modeling. The first group of studies pertains to the choice of stimuli or procedures based on predictions of connectionist models that would maximize access to semantic or phonological representations of words. These studies go beyond matching characteristics of and the type of linguistic impairment (e.g., category matching tasks for semantic impairment) and address ways to vary stimuli choices or procedures to improve access to words or maximize generalization of treatment effects to untreated items. A second group of studies are motivated by connectionist models that postulate a role of verbal STM in word processing impairments.

The reader will note that most of the evidence to date comes from single or multiple case studies. This was also true of the studies of contextual priming treatment and new word learning studies discussed earlier in this chapter. Single case studies represent the early stages of the process of establishing evidence of a treatment's efficacy. They are quite valuable when the line of inquiry is not well charted and variables need to be identified that will be useful in future studies of a particular treatment paradigm.

Studies that Manipulate Stimuli Characteristics and Procedures to Maximize Access to Words and Promote Generalization to Untrained Items

(1)   Semantic Feature Analysis (e.g., Boyle 2004; Boyle & Coelho, 1995)

This treatment approach has become one of the more widely used theoretically driven treatment approaches for naming. It capitalizes on the hypothesized network of associations among semantic features of concepts that have been postulated in several word processing models, including Dell's connectionist model of word production (Dell, 1986; Dell & O'Seaghdha, 1992). The treatment involves collaboration of the client with aphasia and the clinician. Together, they build a chart of semantic attributes of a particular concept that is associated with a word. Reviewing the features of the concept is intended to facilitate retrieval of the word associated with that concept. The clinician provides questions or sentence cues to help elicit these features. To help elicit features, the clinician poses questions or provides partial sentences to be completed by the client. These questions probe for information such as semantic category membership functions of the object and so on. This treatment approach has proved to be somewhat successful in improving the ability to retrieve words that are directly treated as well as untreated items that were probed during and after training. Some generalization to discourse production has also been observed (Boyle, 2004).

(2) Maximizing Generalization of Training Effects from Treated to Untreated Items within a Semantic Category

Earlier in this chapter, we discussed an extensive computational simulation study by Plaut (1996) that examined a number of issues relating to effects of processing variables in normal and impaired language systems on recovery from brain damage and relearning after brain damage. One such issue had to do with relearning a semantic category after brain damage and what approach should be used in rehabilitation of naming deficits in aphasia. Plaut's study showed that a connectionist model of word processing predicted that relearning was better when training included both typical and atypical category members compared to just training typical members. For example, if one is trying to relearn the names of birds, it is better for training sets to include typical (*robin, sparrow*) and atypical (*ostrich, flamingo*) birds. This prediction was borne out in a treatment study by Kiran and Thompson (2003) in which they showed that training on atypical members of a category resulted in learning both atypical and typical members of a category, but training on typical members did not generalize to learning of atypical members. The logic behind this principle is that by including a broad range of category membership, all features of the category are learned. When only typical members are trained, the range of semantic features learned is more limited.

(3) Manipulating Characteristics of Stimuli to Improve Access to Semantics

One of the cardinal features of deep dysphasia is an imageability effect, manifested as extreme difficulty in repeating or recognizing abstract words. This along with semantic errors in single word repetition and difficulty in repeating nonwords define the syndrome of deep dysphasia. Milder cases, now termed phonological dysphasia, include all the symptoms of deep dysphasia except that semantic errors occur when repeating multiple word utterances. These two patterns of deep and phonological dysphasia were evident in the longitudinal case study of NC, discussed earlier in this chapter. There have been numerous case studies of deep dysphasia reported in the last several decades, and these have been instrumental in informing our models of language and verbal STM. The interactive activation model of Dell and colleagues has provided a comprehensive account of this disorder, as reviewed earlier. Little has been done, however, to improve our treatment approaches. Recently, McCarthy, Kohen, Kalinyak-Fliszar, and Martin (2014) reported a treatment approach that aimed to improve access to abstract words by a person, LT, whose language profile fit the deep phonological dysphasia continuum. Motivated by the idea that activation of word forms is stronger for highly imageable words than low-imageable (abstract) words, McCarthy et al. (2014) constructed a treatment protocol that trained abstract words in pairs that were more imageable than each of the two words. For example, whereas the words *joyous* and *occasion* on their own are not easy to image, the phrase *joyous occasion* calls to mind a more imageable concept. In the context of a treatment study, McCarthy et al. (2014) demonstrated that repetition of the individual abstract words improved after training in the semantically cohesive phrases, but not after training in phrases that were only syntactically cohesive (e.g., *long agility*). This improvement was still present 15 weeks after treatment was ended.

These studies suggest development of treatments for aphasia should consider the concept of cognitive plasticity. Manipulation of stimulus characteristics can be carried out to match the linguistic component of language that is impaired, but can also be used to improve access to representations and generalization of improvements in a network of concepts.

(4) Cueing Hierarchies: Vanishing Cues or Increasing Cues?

The IA model of Dell and colleagues (Dell et al., 1997; Schwartz et al., 2006) has also been used to make specific predictions about the outcome of a naming treatment procedure (Abel, Willmes, & Huber, 2007; Abel, Dell, & Huber, 2009). Based on the hypothesis that some naming impairments stem from reduced connection strength and others from too fast decay of activated representations, Abel et al. (2007) made specific predictions about two cueing hierarchy treatments for word retrieval disorders: the vanishing cue method and the increasingly facilitative cueing hierarchy. They postulated that the vanishing cue method would be more effective with connection weight lesions because naming with this kind of impairment would require maximal assistance to access the word's representations. For decay lesions, they postulated that it would be more effective to use increasing cues because the target is accessed but decays too quickly. Four participants were diagnosed in the context of the IA model as having processing impairments that involved either slowed connection weight or too fast decay rate. The vanishing cue method is an errorless training approach and was more effective for those whose processing impairment was characterized as slowed connection weight. In contrast, the increasing cueing method was more beneficial to those with decay lesions. Abel et al. (2007) also examined the effectiveness of the cueing hierarchies of several individuals whose naming impairments were defined as a connection weight lesion affecting semantic activation or phonological activation. They found that the phonological lesions were more responsive to the vanishing cue method.

In a recent study, Abel, Weber, Huber, and Willmes (2014) examined changes in naming ability of 14 individuals with aphasia who received the increasing cue version of the cueing hierarchy. These individuals were modeled on the version of interactive activation model (Schwartz et al., 2006) that modeled impairments of naming as either weakened semantic connection strength or weakened phonological connection strength. They included an imaging study that was intended to identify regions of cortex in each of these impairment groups that changed after treatment. They found that individuals with reduced semantic connection weight lesions who were trained with the increasing cues method demonstrated increased reliance on right frontal areas the inferior frontal gyrus and pars triangularis. For those whose naming impairment was modeled as having weakened phonological connection weights, changes in neural activity were noted in the left inferior frontal gyrus, pars opercularis. This study is remarkable as one of the first to link effects of treatment on groups defined by constructs of a computational model with areas of cortex showing a response to the treatment.

Studies That Manipulate Short-Term Working Memory Load in Language Treatment Tasks in Order to Improve Access to and Maintenance of Word Representations

This approach to treatment is motivated by connectionist models that postulate a role of STM in word processing. The relationship of verbal STM and word processing has been a subject of study in cognitive psychology and cognitive neuropsychology for many years. Numerous studies of verbal STM in normal speakers provide strong evidence for a close relationship between language processing and storage of verbal information. In typical speakers, verbal span varies depending on the characteristics of the items to be recalled (e.g., digit span > word, word span > nonword span; Hulme, Maughan, & Brown, 1991). Span capacity also is influenced by phonological similarity (Conrad & Hull, 1964), word frequency (Hulme, Roodenrys, Schweickert, Brown, Martin, & Stuart, 1997; Watkins & Watkins, 1977), and semantic similarity (Brooks & Watkins, 1990; Crowder, 1979; Poirier & Saint Aubin, 1995; Shulman, 1971).

Observations of an almost invariable co-occurrence of verbal STM and word processing impairments in aphasia has prompted a considerable body of research to determine the role of

STM in language processing (e.g., Saffran, 1990; Saffran & Martin, 1990). Martin and Gupta (2004) proposed an extension of the IA model that characterized the interactive activation of semantic-lexical-phonological representations for multiword utterances. An important principle in their model of word processing and verbal STM is that the verbal *processing* component of verbal STM has a temporal course of its own and therefore requires short-term maintenance of activated word representations. A processing impairment can compromise access to *and maintenance of* semantic and/or phonological representations of single or multiple words, depending on the severity of impairment. In turn, this affects performance on measures of verbal STM and accounts for the co-occurrence of word processing and verbal STM deficits in aphasia.

Earlier in this chapter, we discussed the longitudinal case study of NC (Martin et al., 1996) documenting the tandem recovery of word repetition accuracy and increased verbal span, suggesting a close relationship of these two abilities. Since that case study, considerable empirical support for this model has been established from associations observed between verbal STM capacity and word processing impairments in speakers with aphasia. Severity of word processing impairment (naming, lexical decision) is directly related to severity of span impairment (Martin & Ayala, 2004). Patterns of serial position effects in verbal span performance are consistent with impaired access to semantic or phonological impairment (Martin & Saffran, 1997): semantic deficits are associated with loss of primacy (initial items in a sequence) and phonological impairment is associated with loss of recency (final items in the sequence). Performance on verbal span measures varies depending on characteristics (e.g., imageability, frequency, lexicality) of the items to be recalled (Martin & Ayala, 2004; Martin & Saffran, 1997). Span capacity also varies depending on the pathways through the word processing network (phonological, lexical, semantic) that are used in the span task (*Martin & Ayala, 2004*). To complete a pointing span task, for example, one hears a sequence of words and points to the corresponding pictures in an array of nine pictures. This task engages input phonological, lexical, and semantic processes, and, accordingly, it has been found that performance on the pointing span task correlates with lexical and semantic ability. To complete a repetition span task, one hears a sequence of words and repeats them in the same order they were presented. This task requires only the use of input and output phonological processes. Accordingly, it has been found that performance on this task correlates positively with measures of phonological ability but not semantic ability (Martin & Ayala, 2004).

In the last decade, researchers have begun to develop treatments that consider the role of verbal STM in word processing and that incorporate some form of increased STM load in language tasks in order to improve language function. The underlying principle of these treatments is that word processing takes place over time and therefore must involve some form of STM. Treating the ability to maintain activation of a word's semantic and phonological representations is essential to improve word processing. Below is a summary of the recent studies of word processing treatment that include manipulations of memory load in the training.

Majerus et al. (2005) treated an individual with phonological STM deficit using a task that involved delayed repetition of word pairs. Improvements were observed in digit and nonword span, nonword repetition, and rhyme judgment. Additionally, the client reported improved comprehension in conversational contexts. Francis et al. (2003) treated the STM deficit of a person with impaired comprehension. They observed improvement on the Token Test (McNeil & Prescott, 1978), but comprehension of sentences with reversible semantic roles did not improve. Fridriksson and colleagues (Fridriksson, 2005; Morrow & Fridriksson, 2006) treated three cases of anomia using a spaced-retrieval paradigm. This treatment varies interval time between presentations of a picture to be named (more when named correctly and less when named incorrectly). Compared to another treatment (cueing hierarchy; Linebaugh & Lerner, 1977) this treatment showed more lasting improvements in follow-up testing. Koenig-Bruhin, and Studer-Eichenberger (2007) used a treatment task that involved sentence repetition after a delay to improve short-term maintenance of verbal information in a case of conduction aphasia. They observed increased accuracy of sentence repetition as well as an increase in digit and word spans. Kalinyak-Fliszar et al. (2011) reported a treatment case study of a person, FS, with conduction aphasia and impaired phonological processing. The treatment involved repeating words and nonwords after 5-second unfilled and filler intervals and was intended to improve FS's ability to maintain activation of these representations in the context of a language task (repetition). Following this treatment, improvements were noted in repetition of treated stimuli and other language and verbal STM measures: rhyming and synonymy judgments, word pair repetition, and seven verbal span tasks (of 11 administered). Salis (2012) reported a treatment study to improve sentence comprehension. Training involved use of listening span training tasks that required serial word recognition. Improvements in verbal span and sentence comprehension were observed.

These studies indicate that incorporating tasks that engage verbal STM processes into language treatments can improve language function (in one study, more than without a STM component). As this direction of research continues, it will be important to establish conditions under which adding memory load to a language task contributes to improved language function. Recalling the parameters of Dell et al.'s (1997) model that were hypothesized to affect word processing, increased decay rate and reduced connection weight will affect word processing differently under conditions of increased memory load. In the case of an increase in decay rate, this should make processing more difficult. In the case of a reduced connection strength, however, it is conceivable that imposing a delay before a response in a repetition task could allow the increased processing needed to repeat the utterance. Additionally, as with many of the treatment tasks we have discussed in this chapter, it will be important to determine if impairments of semantic processing are affected differently from phonological impairments when memory load is added to language tasks.

Conclusions: What Are Some Future Directions of Connectionist Modeling of Rehabilitation?

In recent years, there has been an increase in the use of cognitive-linguistic theories to guide treatment of language disorders. This practice presupposes that both clinical and theoretical enterprises will benefit from this alliance. This mutual benefit is possible as long as theories can address the issues that are pertinent to treatment. In order to do this, theories must afford detailed descriptions of dynamic aspects of processing, the effects of brain damage on those processes, and the effects of specific treatment procedures on healthy and impaired processes (Harley, 1996; Hillis & Caramazza, 1994; Plaut, 1996). In this chapter, we have reviewed the history of the practice of using cognitive models to guide therapy and provided a review of recent treatment studies that reflect efforts to apply principles of connectionist models of language to the procedures and stimuli used in treatment. This line of research has been challenging and filled with controversy. Progress has been made, and yet much more needs to be done.

Functional models of language advanced the practice of model-based treatment and essentially rekindled a conviction of the value of therapy for neurogenic language impairments. The most important contribution of these models has been the framework they provide for diagnosing linguistic impairments associated with aphasia. Eventually, their shortcomings as complete frameworks for treatment became apparent, and yet, this so-called failing was actually an important contribution. The realization that treatment research required a theory of process came about, in part, because functional models of language proved insufficient to address issues pertaining to the dynamics of recovery and treatment.

The emergence of connectionist models provides new tools that can help theories of rehabilitation begin to address the dynamics of treatment methods (Harley, 1996). Although it is clear from this review that there are only a few studies that directly apply connectionist models to treatment issues, we should not be discouraged about their potential contribution to rehabilitation science. There is an active use of connectionist models to address more fundamental issues of processing characteristics, short- and long-term memory, and learning. In the last decade, we have witnessed some efforts to apply these fundamental processes to treatment. In the next decade, we anticipate even greater advances in developing treatment approaches that link directly with the dynamics of normal and impaired processing of language.

Acknowledgments

This chapter was written with the support of a grant from the National Institutes of Health (NIDCD grants R01 DC01924-07, R21 DC008782-02, and R01DC013196) awarded to Temple University (PI: Nadine Martin), a grant from the James S. McDonnell Foundation (98-25 CEH-QUA.109) awarded to Matti Laine and Nadine Martin, and grants from the Academy of Finland (43301, 260276, 135688) awarded to Matti Laine. We gratefully acknowledge this support.

References

Abel, S., Huber, W., & Dell, G.S. (2009). Connectionist diagnosis of lexical disorders in aphasia. *Aphasiology, 23*(11), 1353–1378.

Abel, S., Weiller, C., Huber, W., & Willmes, K. (2014). Neural underpinnings for model-oriented therapy of aphasic word production. *Neuropsychologia, 57*, 154–165.

Abel, S., Willmes, K., &Huber, W. (2007). Model-oriented naming therapy. Testing predictions of a connectionist model. *Aphasiology, 21*(5), 411–447.

Baddeley, A.D. (1986). *Working memory.* Oxford, England: Clarendon Press.

Bechtel, W., & Abrahamsen, A.A. (1991). Connectionism and the mind: An introduction to parallel processing in networks. Oxford: Basil Blackwell.

Boyle, M. (2004). Semantic feature analysis treatment for anomia in two fluent aphasia syndromes. *American Journal of Speech-Language Pathology, 13*, 236–249.

Boyle, M., & Coelho, C. (1995). Application of semantic feature analysis as a treatment for aphasic dysnomia. *American Journal of Speech and Language Pathology, 4*(4), 94–98.

Brooks III, J.O., & Watkins, M.J. (1990). Further evidence of the intricacy of memory span. *Journal of Experimental Psychology: Learning, Memory and Cognition, 16*(6), 1134–1141.

Burgess, N., & Hitch, G.J. (1992). Toward a network model of the articulatory loop. *Journal of Memory and Language, 31*, 429–460.

Caplan, D. (1992). *Language: Structure, processing, and disorders.* Cambridge, MA: MIT Press.

Caramazza, A. (1984). The logic of neuropsychological research and the problem of patient classification in aphasia. *Brain and Language, 21*, 9–20.

Caramazza, A., & Hillis, A.E. (1990). Where do semantic errors come from? *Cortex, 26*, 95–122.

Collins, A.M., & Loftus, E.F.A. (1975). A spreading activation theory of semantic processing. *Psychological Review, 82*, 407–428.

Conrad, R., & Hull, A.J. (1964). Information, acoustic confusion and memory span. *British Journal of Psychology, 55*, 429–432.

Crowder, R.G. (1979). Similarity and order in memory. In G.H. Bower (Ed.), *The psychology of learning and motivation: Advances in research and theory*. Vol. 13 (pp. 319–353). New York: Academic Press.

Dell, G.S. (1986). A spreading activation theory of retrieval in language production. *Psychological Review, 93*, 283–321.

Dell, G.S., & Juliano, C. (1996). Computational models of phonological encoding. In T. Dijkstra & K. DeSmedt (Eds.), *Computational psycholinguistics.* London: Taylor and Francis.

Dell, G.S., Juliano, C., & Govindjee, A. (1993). Structure and content in language production: A theory of frame constraints in phonological speech errors. *Cognitive Science, 17*, 149–195.

Dell, G.S., Martin, N., & Schwartz, M.F. (2007). A case-series test of the interactive two-step model of lexical access: Predicting word repetition from picture naming. *Journal of Memory and Language, 56*, 490–520.

Dell, G.S., & O'Seaghdha, P.G. (1991). Stages in lexical access in language production. *Cognition, 42*, 287–314.

Dell, G.S., & O'Seaghdha, P.G. (1992). Stages in lexical access in language production. *Cognition, 42*, 287–314.

Dell, G.S., & Reich, P. (1981). Stages in sentence production: An analysis of speech error data. *Journal of Verbal Learning and Verbal Behavior, 29,* 611–629.

Dell, G.S., Schwartz, M.F., Martin, N., Saffran, E. M., & Gagnon, D. A. (1997). Lexical access in aphasic and non-aphasic speakers. *Psychological Review, 104*(4), 801–838.

Ellis, A. (1985). The production of spoken words: A cognitive neuropsychological perspective. In A.W. Ellis (Ed.), *Progress in the psychology of language,* Vol. 2. London: Lawrence Erlbaum.

Foygel, D., & Dell, G.S. (2000). Models of impaired lexical access in speech production. *Journal of Memory and Language, 43,* 182–216.

Forster, K. (1994). Computational modeling and elementary process analysis in visual word recognition. *Journal of Experimental Psychology: Human Perception and Performance, 20,* 1292–1310.

Francis, D.R., Clark, N., & Humphreys, G.W. (2003). The treatment of an auditory working memory deficit and the implications for sentence comprehension abilities in mild "receptive" aphasia. *Aphasiology, 17,* 723–750.

Frauenfelder, U.H., & Peters, G. (1999). Simulating the time course of spoken word recognition: An analysis of lexical competition in TRACE. In J. Grainger & A.M. Jacobs (Eds.), *Localist connectionist approaches to human cognition.* Mahwah, NJ, and London: Lawrence Erlbaum.

Fridriksson, J., Holland, A.L., Beeson, P., & Morrow, L. (2005). Spaced retrieval treatment of anomia. *Aphasiology, 19,* 99–109.

Grainger, J., & Jacobs, A.M. (1999). On localist connectionism and psychological science. In J. Grainger & A.M. Jacobs (Eds.), *Localist connectionist approaches to human cognition.* Mahwah, NJ, and London: Lawrence Erlbaum.

Gupta, P. (1996). Word learning and verbal short-term memory: A computational account. In *Proceedings of the eighteenth annual conference of the Cognitive Science Society.* Hillsdale, NJ: Lawrence Erlbaum.

Gupta, P., & MacWhinney, B. (1997). Vocabulary acquisition and verbal short-term memory: Computational and neural bases. *Brain and Language, 59,* 267–333.

Harley, T.A. (1984). A critique of top-down independent levels models of speech production: Evidence from non-plan internal speech errors. *Cognitive Science, 8,* 191–219.

Harley, T.A. (1993). Phonological activation of semantic competitors during lexical access in speech production. *Language and Cognitive Processes, 8,* 291–309.

Harley, T. A. (1996). Connectionist modeling of the recovery of language functions following brain damage. *Brain and Language, 52,* 7–24.

Harley, T. A., & MacAndrew, S.B., G. (2001). Constraints upon word substitution speech errors. *Journal of Psycholinguistic Research, 30,* 395–418

Hartley, T., & Houghton, G. (1996). A linguistically constrained model of short-term memory for nonwords. *Journal of Memory and Language, 35,* 1–31.

Hillis, A.E., & Caramazza, A. (1994). Theories of lexical processing and rehabilitation of lexical deficits. In M.J. Riddoch & G.W. Humphreys (Eds.), *Cognitive neuropsychology and cognitive rehabilitation.* Hove, England: Lawrence Erlbaum.

Hinton, G.E., & Shallice, T. (1991). Lesioning an attractor network: Investigations of acquired dyslexia. *Psychological Review, 99,* 74–95.

Howard, D., & Franklin, S. (1988). *Missing the meaning? A cognitive neuropsychological study of processing words by an aphasic patient.* Cambridge MA: MIT Press.

Hulme, C., Maughan, S., & Brown, G. (1991). Memory for familiar and unfamiliar words: Evidence for a long-term memory contribution to short-term span. *Journal of Memory and Language, 30,* 685–701.

Hulme, C., Roodenrys, S., Schweickert, R., Brown, G.D., Martin, A., & Stuart, G. (1997). Word frequency effects on short-term memory tasks: Evidence for redintegration process in immediate serial recall. *Journal of Experimental Psychology: Learning, Memory and Cognition, 23,* 1217–1232.

Kalinyak-Fliszar, M., Kohen, F.P., & Martin, N. (2011). Remediation of language processing in aphasia: Improving activation and maintenance of linguistic representations in (verbal) short-term memory. *Aphasiology, 25*(10), 1095–1131.

Kertesz, A., & McCabe, P. (1977). Recovery patterns and prognosis in aphasia. *Brain, 100,* 1–18.

Kiran, S., & Thompson, C. (2003). The role of semantic complexity in the treatment of naming deficits: Training semantic categories in fluent aphasia by controlling exemplar typicality. *Journal of Speech, Language and Hearing Research, 46,* 773–787.

Kiviniemi, K., Laine, M., Tarkiainen, A., Järvensivu, T., Martin, N., & Salmelin, R. (2000). Anomia treatment modifies naming-related cortical activation: Evidence from an MEG study. *Brain and Language, 74,* 433–435.

Koenig-Bruhin, M., & Studer-Eichenberger, F. (2007). Therapy of verbal short-term memory disorders in fluent aphasia: A single case study. *Aphasiology, 21*(5), 1–11.

Laine, M. (2000). The learning brain. *Brain and Language, 71,* 132–134.

Laine, M., & Martin, N. (1996). Lexical retrieval deficit in picture naming: Implications for word production models. *Brain and Language, 53,* 283–314.

Laine, M., Tikkala, A., & Juhola, M. (1998). Modelling anomia by the discrete two-stage word production architecture. *Journal of Neurolinguistics, 10*(2), 139–158.

Levelt, W.J.M. (1989). *Speaking: From intention to articulation.* Cambridge, MA: MIT Press.

Linebaugh, C.W., & Lehner, L.H. (1977). Cueing hierarchies and word retrieval: A therapy program. In R.H. Brookshire (Ed.), *Clinical aphasiology conference proceedings.* Minneapolis, MN: BRK Publishers.

MacKay, D.G. (1987). *The organization of perception and action: A theory for language and other cognitive skills.* New York: Springer-Verlag.

Majerus, S., Van der Kaa, M.A., Renard, C., Van der Linden, M., & Poncelet, P. (2005). Treating verbal short-term memory deficits by increasing the duration of temporary phonological representations: A case study. *Brain and Language, 95*(1), 174–175.

Marslen-Wilson, W.D., & Welsh, A. (1988). Processing interactions and lexical access during word recognition in continuous speech. *Cognitive Psychology, 10,* 29–63.

Martin, N., & Ayala, J. (2004). Measurements of auditory-verbal STM in aphasia: Effects of task, item and word processing impairment. *Brain and Language, 89,* 464–483.

Martin, N., & Dell, G.S. (2007). Common mechanisms underlying perseverative and non-perseverative speech errors. *Aphasiology, 21,* 1002–1017.

Martin, N., Dell, G.S., Saffran, E.M., & Schwartz, M.F. (1994). Origins of paraphasias in deep dysphasia: Testing the consequences of a decay impairment to an interactive spreading activation model of language. *Brain and Language, 47,* 609–660.

Martin, N., Fink, R., & Laine, M. (2004b). Treatment of word retrieval with contextual priming. *Aphasiology, 18,* 457–471.

Martin, N., Fink, R., Laine, M., & Ayala, J. (2004a). Immediate and short-term effects of contextual priming on word retrieval. *Aphasiology, 18,* 867–898.

Martin, N., Fink, R., Renvall, K., & Laine, M. (2006). Effectiveness of contextual repetition priming treatments for anomia depends on intact access to semantics. *Journal of International Neuropsychological Society, 12,* 1–14.

Martin, N., & Gupta, P. (2004). Exploring the relationship between word processing and verbal STM: Evidence from associations and dissociations. *Cognitive Neuropsychology, 21,* 213–228.

Martin, N., & Laine, M. (2000). Effects of contextual priming on word retrieval in anomia. *Aphasiology, 14*(1), 53–70.

Martin, N., & Saffran, E. M. (1992). A computational account of deep dysphasia: Evidence from a single case study. *Brain and Language, 43,* 240–274.

Martin, N., & Saffran, E. M. (1999). Effects of word processing and short-term memory deficits on verbal learning: Evidence from aphasia. *International Journal of Psychology, 34*(5/6), 339–346.

Martin, N., & Saffran, E.M. (1997). Language and auditory-verbal short-term memory impairments: Evidence for common underlying processes. *Cognitive Neuropsychology, 14*(5), 641–682.

Martin, N., Saffran, E.M., & Dell G.S. (1996). Recovery in deep dysphasia: Evidence for a relation between auditory-verbal STM and lexical errors in repetition. *Brain and Language, 52,* 83–113.

Martin, R.C., Shelton, J., & Yaffee, L. (1994). Language processing and working memory: Neuropsychological evidence for separate phonological and semantic capacities. *Journal of Memory and Language, 33,* 83–111.

Martin, N., Weisberg, R.W., & Saffran, E. M. (1989). Variables influencing the occurrence of naming errors: Implications for models of lexical retrieval. *Journal of Memory and Language, 28,* 462–485.

McCarthy, L.M., Kohen, F.P., Kalinyak-Fliszar, M., & Martin, N. (2014). Improving auditory access to low imageability words by embedding them in imageable semantic-syntactic contexts in a case of deep-phonological dysphasia. Paper presented at the Clinical Aphasiology Conference, St. Simon's Island, GA, May 27–June 1.

McClelland, J.L., & Rumelhart, D.E. (1981). An interactive activation model of context effects in letter perception, part I: An account of the basic findings. *Psychological Review, 88,* 375–407.

McCloskey, M. (1991). Networks and theories: The place of connectionism in cognitive science. *Psychological Science, 6,* 387–395.

McNeil, M.R., & Prescott, T. E. (1978). *The revised token test.* Baltimore, MD: University Park Press.

Morrow, K.L., & Fridriksson, J. (2006). Comparing fixed- and randomized-interval spaced retrieval in anomia treatment *Journal of Communication Disorders, 39,* 2–11.

Morton, J. (1982). Disintegrating the lexicon: An information processing approach. In J. Mehler, E.C.T. Walker, & M.F. Garrett (Eds.), *Perspectives on mental representation: Experimental and theoretical studies of cognitive processes and capacities.* Hillsdale, NJ: Lawrence Erlbaum.

Neely, J.H. (1991). Semantic priming effects in visual word recognition: A selective review of current findings and theory. In D. Besner & G.W. Humphreys (Eds.), *Basic processes in reading: Visual word recognition.* Hillsdale, NJ: Lawrence Erlbaum.

Nettleton, J., & Lesser, R. (1991). Therapy for naming difficulties in aphasia: Application of a cognitive neuropsychological model. *Journal of Neurolinguistics, 6,* 139–157.

Norris, D. (1993). Bottom-up connectionist models of interaction. In G.T.M. Altmann & R. Shillcock (Eds.), *Cognitive models of speech processing: The second Sperlonga meeting.* Hillsdale, NJ: Lawrence Erlbaum.

Page, M., & Norris, D. (1998). Modeling immediate serial recall with a localist implementation of the primacy model. In J. Grainger & A.M. Jacobs (Eds.), *Localist connectionist approaches to human cognition.* Mahwah, NJ, and London: Lawrence Erlbaum.

Plaut, D. (1996). Relearning after damage in connectionist networks: Toward a theory of rehabilitation. *Brain and Language, 52,* 25–82.

Plaut, D., & Shallice, T. (1993). Deep dyslexia: A case study of connectionist neuropsychology. *Cognitive Neuropsychology, 10*(5), 377–500.

Poirier, M., & Saint Aubin, J. (1995). Memory for related and unrelated words: Further evidence on the influence of semantic factors immediate serial recall. *Quarterly Journal of Experimental Psychology A, 48*(2), 384–404.

Rapp, B., & Goldrick, M. (2000). Discreteness and interactivity in spoken word production, *Psychological Review, 107,* 460–499.

Renvall, K., Laine, M., Laakso, M., & Martin, N. (2003). Anomia rehabilitation with contextual priming: A case study. *Aphasiology, 17,* 305–308.

Renvall, K., Laine, M., & Martin, N. (2005). Contextual priming in semantic anomia: A case study. *Brain and Language, 95,* 327–341.

Renvall, K., Laine, M., & Martin, N. (2007). Treatment of anomia with contextual priming: Exploration of a modified procedure with additional semantic and phonological tasks. *Aphasiology, 21,* 499–527.

Ruml, W., & Caramazza, A. (2000). An evaluation of a computational model of lexical access. *Psychological Review, 107,* 609–634.

Saffran, E.M. (1990). Short-term memory and language impairment. In A. Caramazza (Ed.), *Cognitive neuropsychology and neurolinguistics: Advances in models of cognitive function and impairment* (pp. 135–168). Hillsdale, NJ: Lawrence Erlbaum.

Saffran, E.M., & Martin, N. (1990). Neuropsychological evidence for lexical involvement in short-term memory. In G. Vallar and T. Shallice (Eds.), *Neuropsychological impairments of short-term memory* (pp. 145–166). Cambridge: Cambridge University Press.

Salis, C. (2012). Short-term memory treatment: Patterns of learning and generalisation to sentence comprehension in a person with aphasia. *Neuropsychological Rehabilitation, 22*(3), 428–448.

Schade, U., & Berg, T. (1992). The role of inhibition in a spreading activation model of language production, part 2: The simulational perspective. *Journal of Psycholinguistic Research, 22,* 435–462.

Schade, U., & Eikmeyer, H.-J. (1999). Modeling the production of object specifications. In J. Grainger & A.M. Jacobs (Eds.), *Localist connectionist approaches to human cognition.* Mahwah, NJ, and London: Lawrence Erlbaum Associates.

Schuchard, J., & Thompson, C.K. (2014). Implicit and explicit learning in individuals with agrammatic aphasia. *Journal of Psycholinguistic Research, 43,* 209–224.

Schwartz, M.F., & Brecher, A. (2000). A model-driven analysis of severity, response characteristics, and partial recovery in aphasics' picture naming. *Brain and Language, 73,* 62–91.

Schwartz, M.F., Dell, G.S., Martin, N., Gahl, S., & Sobel, P. (2006). A case series test of the two-step interactive model of lexical access: Evidence from picture naming. *Journal of Memory and Language, 54,* 228–264.

Schwartz, M.F., Saffran, E.M., Bloch, D.E., & Dell, G.S. (1994). Disordered speech production in aphasic and normal speakers. *Brain and Language, 47,* 52–88.

Seidenberg, M.S., & McClelland, J.L. (1989). A distributed, developmental model of word recognition and naming. *Psychological Review, 96,* 523–568.

Shulman, H.G. (1971). Similarity effects in short-term memory. *Psychological Bulletin, 75,* 399–415.

Stemberger, J.P. (1985). An interactive model of language production. In A.W. Ellis (Ed.), *Progress in the psychology of language,* vol. 1. Hillsdale, NJ: Lawrence Erlbaum.

Tanenhaus, M.K., Dell, G.S., & Carlson, G. (1987). Context effects in lexical processing: A connectionist approach to modularity. In J.L. Garfield, *Modularity in knowledge representation and natural-language understanding.* Cambridge, MA: MIT Press.

Tuomiranta, L., Rautakoski, P., Rinne, J.O., Martin, N., & Laine, M. (2012). Long-term maintenance of novel vocabulary in persons with chronic aphasia. *Aphasiology, 26*(8), 1053–1073.

Watkins, O.C., & Watkins, M.J. (1977). Serial recall and the modality effect. *Journal of Experimental Psychology: Human Learning and Memory, 3,* 712–718.

Weekes, B., & Coltheart, M. (1996). Surface dyslexia and surface dysgraphia: Treatment studies and their theoretical implications. *Cognitive Neuropsychology, 13*(2), 277–315.

21

BIOLOGICAL APPROACHES TO TREATMENT OF APHASIA

Daniel A. Llano and Steven L. Small

A typical consultation for the neurology service:

A 72-year-old right-handed man presents to the emergency department with difficulty speaking, right arm weakness and a right-sided facial droop. On exam, he has a Broca-type aphasia and a right hemiparesis. Imaging reveals a moderate-sized infarct in the left hemisphere, centered on the inferior frontal gyrus and the white matter underlying this region. His family has many questions for you. Will he recover his language function? What therapies might be helpful? Are there any drugs or other treatments that can help?

This scenario plays out commonly in hospitals around the world, and clinicians are often faced with the daunting challenge of answering these questions and facilitating the rehabilitation of such patients. This chapter is focused on the last question posed above: Are there pharmacotherapeutic or other biological approaches that can facilitate his recovery from aphasia? Herein, we will summarize the known literature on these topics and offer recommendations for clinicians.

Etiological Considerations

Any acute lesion in the frontal, temporal, or parietal cortices has the potential to cause language deficits (aphasia), with those in the dominant hemisphere causing the most apparent deficits. In clinical practice, the most commonly encountered cause of aphasia is acute stroke. Approximately 10–30% of all strokes produce a long-lasting aphasia (Wade et al. 1986; Pedersen et al. 1995; Bersano et al. 2009), and these are etiologically heterogeneous. Common mechanisms for aphasia-producing stroke include cardioembolic events, *in situ* thrombosis of large vessels such as the middle cerebral artery, or lobar hemorrhage. Small vessel strokes or deep hemorrhages may also lead to aphasia based on their effects on the basal ganglia and thalamus (Booth et al. 2007; Crosson 2012). Outside of stroke, aphasia may be seen in the setting of brain tumors, neurodegenerative disease, traumatic brain injury and other brain lesions, each with their own natural histories. It is likely that the efficacy and optimal implementation of therapies based on restoration or replacement of neuronal connections will depend on the underlying cause of the neuronal insult. Further, aphasia can manifest itself in a variety of ways, with many different types of language problems, and this variability may have therapeutic implications. For example, aphasic patients with poor fluency often retain significant insight into their deficits, and may be more motivated to participate in therapy, which will, as will be described below, influence the likelihood that particular interventions will have an impact. Therefore, therapeutic interventions described in the literature for one type of aphasia of a particular etiology may not be effective for other types and other etiologies. All of these factors need to be taken into consideration when adopting any of the potentially therapeutic interventions described in this chapter.

General Approach to Biological Treatments for Aphasia

There is a substantial body of work documenting the natural history and the impact of pharmacological modulation of stroke recovery in animal models. Most of this research has involved lesions of the motor cortex and has used motor performance as the primary outcome measure. Once a small area of cortex is lost, a host of short- and long-range mechanisms are engaged to facilitate reorganization of cortical function (Murphy and Corbett 2009; Hermann and Chopp 2012). These mechanisms are activity dependent, and include axonal sprouting (Dancause et al. 2005; Overman et al. 2012), which can extend distances of as much as 1 cm (or more) across the adult primate cortex, elaboration of dendritic spines (Brown and Murphy 2008; Ueno et al. 2012), migration of subventricular stem cells to the infarction zone (Lichtenwalner and Parent 2005; Danilov, Kokaia and Lindvall 2012; Kahle and Bix 2013) and modulation of the strength or excitability of existing synapses (Yao et al. 2005; Di Filippo et al. 2008; Jaenisch, Witte and Frahm 2010). Since such mechanisms are likely to be differentially sensitive to pharmacological manipulation, one might postulate that different etiological mechanisms of infarction would require different forms of intervention. It is also possible that some forms of modulation of synaptic strength could be *maladaptive* (Di Filippo et al. 2008; Costigan, Scholz and Woolf 2009) and therapeutic modalities, appropriately targeted and timed, could be used to interfere with such forms of pathological plasticity. An example here is the potential maladaptive involvement of the uninjured hemisphere in recovery from aphasia, and will be discussed further under *Cortical Modulation Techniques*.

Several concepts have arisen from the animal literature on stroke recovery (and brain lesion recovery more generally) that may inform our review of the literature on drug therapy for aphasia. First, it is clear that maximal benefit is derived not from drugs or rehabilitation approaches on their own, but with *combination therapy*. There is a rich history of studies supporting the idea that synaptic plasticity, which is presumed to be the dominant mechanism underlying stroke recovery, is highly stimulus dependent and facilitated by manipulations of several neuromodulators (Kilgard and Merzenich 1998; Bao, Chan and Merzenich 2001; Schultz 2002). Further, many of the classes of drugs discussed in this review have been explicitly hypothesized to help support and strengthen neural networks that are modified by behavioral training (Korchounov and Ziemann 2011), such that their efficacy in the absence of behavioral training may be greatly reduced. Taken further, one might even speculate that drugs supporting synaptic plasticity, when used in the absence of targeted behavioral therapy, could actually reinforce maladaptive patterns of neuronal activity. In addition, it is of high clinical relevance that the cerebral cortex undergoes plastic changes for at least *months* following stroke, and that these adaptive changes occur not only in the tissue immediately surrounding the lesion, but also in areas remote from the site of injury (Jenkins and Merzenich 1987; Nudo et al. 1996; Nudo and Friel 1998; Xerri et al. 1998). Finally, the animal studies suggest that certain classes of drugs that are commonly used in clinical practice, particularly drugs used to treat hypertension (such as thiazides or alpha blockers), drugs used to treat anxiety and seizures (such as benzodiazepines) and drugs used to treat gastrointestinal or behavioral issues (such as dopamine antagonists), can impede the reorganization of brain networks after injury (Goldstein 2000; Larson and Zollman 2010). Given the emerging recognition of the importance of post-stroke depression and anxiety on stroke recovery (Aben et al. 2003; Barker-Collo 2007; Robinson et al. 2008; Mikami et al. 2011; Mikami et al. 2013) and the relatively high incidence of seizures after stroke (Olsen 2001; Lossius et al. 2002), both of which may be treated with benzodiazepines, these data indicate that non-sedating alternatives may be more appropriate to avoid interference with post-stroke recovery mechanisms. Thus, clinical interventions for aphasia may involve a combination of adding new drugs and removing others.

Speech and Language Therapy

Although this chapter is focused on biological treatments, some comments on Speech and Language Therapy (SLT) are warranted. SLT is the gold standard for the recovery of language function in aphasia (Bhogal, Teasell and Speechley 2003; Brady et al. 2012), and in fact is the only generally accepted treatment for aphasia. Typically in modern medical practice, SLT is often provided as a therapy separate from a physician's care. As will be described below, biological therapeutic interventions, which in general are designed to strengthen or restore neuronal connections, will find their maximal utility when *combined* in a rational way with SLT. For example, drugs whose main putative mechanism of action is to enhance training-induced plastic effects (such as drugs that potentiate the actions of dopamine or norepinephrine) are likely to be most beneficial when taken prior to SLT, so that their drug levels can be maximal at the time that synaptic connections are being strengthened by behavioral training. Conversely, the assumption that biological therapies can strengthen neuronal connections also suggests that their use in the absence of appropriate behavioral therapies could strengthen *maladaptive* neuronal connections, worsening long-term outcomes. These ideas suggest that biological therapies should be prescribed in conjunction with SLT, which implies a closer level of cooperation between physicians and therapists than is typically found in contemporary care scenarios.

Drug Therapy

No drugs are currently approved for the treatment of aphasia. However, a number of drugs approved for other indications, such as attention-deficit hyperactivity disorder, Parkinson's disease and Alzheimer's disease, have been studied for their benefits in aphasia, and are potentially available to the clinician. Most of the drugs that have been tested for aphasia are drugs that elevate synaptic norepinephrine, dopamine or acetylcholine levels. The clinical trials that have been performed with these agents have been motivated by many animal studies demonstrating their efficacy, primarily in models of motor stroke, and their generally good safety profile. Unfortunately, the clinical literature on this topic is riddled with very small, uncontrolled trials with poor design, yielding a very low level of evidence for the efficacy of these therapies. Ideally, to demonstrate that a drug helps the brain to reorganize to support language function after aphasic stroke, one would like to see a double-blind placebo-controlled, parallel-designed trial with assessments focused on a primary language outcome measured after drug washout, to exclude temporary arousal-based efficacy. In addition, this trial should be powered sufficiently to assess both risks and benefits of the therapeutic intervention. There have been very few studies meeting these criteria, and none have been independently replicated (as would be demanded for a new drug approval). Therefore, we are left to evaluate a literature dominated by low-grade clinical evidence to look for potential therapies. Below, we describe what has been learned from these studies, with a focus on those that have the potential to impact clinical practice. In addition, those drugs used in clinical practice to treat stroke comorbidities or consequences of stroke, such as hypertension, seizures and anxiety, that can interfere with recovery of language function post-stroke, are also reviewed below. Finally, an often neglected component of post-stroke care is the surveillance for, and treatment of, post-stroke depression and anxiety, which are common, treatable (Aben et al. 2003; Barker-Collo 2007; Robinson et al. 2008; Mikami et al. 2011; Mikami et al. 2013) and may directly impact language function and diminish the likelihood that patients will participate in SLT.

Sympathomimetics

Historically, the drugs that have been most studied for the treatment of aphasia are those that elevate brain catecholamine levels (the sympathomimetics). The notion that catecholamine augmentation can facilitate stroke recovery is derived from early work demonstrating (1) decreases in brainstem and cortical catecholamine levels after stroke (Brown et al. 1974; Cohen, Waltz and Jacobson 1975; Robinson et al. 1975; Robinson, Shoemaker and Schlumpf 1980), and (2) that interference with catecholamine receptors can delay recovery (Feeney and Westerberg 1990; Goldstein and Bullman 1997). In addition, a highly influential study by Feeney et al. demonstrated that a single dose of dextroamphetamine, which causes the release of presynaptic norepinephrine and dopamine, facilitated the recovery of rats walking on a beam after a lesion of the motor cortex, while haloperidol, which primarily blocks D2 dopamine receptors, interfered with recovery (Feeney, Gonzalez and Law 1982).

The mechanism(s) by which catecholamines can facilitate brain reorganization are not known. However, a number of studies have shown that norepinephrine and dopamine modulate multiple forms of synaptic plasticity, including long-term potentiation, long-term depression and spike timing–dependent plasticity (Gu 2002; Wolf, Mangiavacchi and Sun 2003; Dommett et al. 2008; Carey and Regehr 2009; Edelmann and Lessmann 2013; Clem and Huganir 2013; Ghanbarian and Motamedi 2013). All of these forms of synaptic plasticity are highly dependent on specific patterns of synaptic activity, suggesting that the efficacy of drugs that enhance catecholamine levels would also be highly dependent on behavioral training regimes that are coupled to the use of these drugs. In fact, this has been highly borne out in the literature, such that virtually all studies demonstrating the efficacy of sympathomimetic drugs after brain lesions have shown enhancement of recovery by combining these drugs with physical training (Ramic et al. 2006; Rasmussen et al. 2006; Barbay et al. 2006; Papadopoulos et al. 2009; Beltran et al. 2010). Other possible mechanisms for the efficacy of sympathomimetics include axonal sprouting (Papadopoulos et al. 2009) and the enhancement of neural regeneration via neural stem cells (Hiramoto, Ihara and Watanabe 2006; Spiegel et al. 2007; Lloyd et al. 2010). These data suggest that sympathomimetic drugs may function to alter neuronal plasticity on several different temporal and spatial scales. This may ultimately inform the most appropriate way to use these drugs clinically.

Although at least four trials have examined the potential for dextroamphetamine to enhance recovery after stroke, three of these were quite small or used crossover designs and will not be discussed further here (Darley, Keith and Sasanuma 1977; McNeil et al. 1997; Whiting et al. 2007). The largest study on dextroamphetamine was conducted by Walker-Batson et al. (Walker-Batson et al. 2001). In this study, subjects with subacute stroke were treated with dextroamphetamine or placebo, and treatment was coupled to traditional speech therapy over a 5-week period. A greater percentage of dextroamphetamine subjects demonstrated improvement on the Porch Index of Communicative Ability scale than their placebo counterparts at the 6-week time point (83% vs. 22%), which was assessed 1 week after last dose of drug. There was no statistically significant benefit at 6 months ($p = 0.0482$, not significant after correction for multiple comparisons). This study was confounded by differences in age (dextroamphetamine patients were 9.5 years younger), the amount of therapy received (dextroamphetamine patients received 21% more therapy time) and the absence of screening for post-stroke depression, which may have been partially treated with amphetamine, therefore affecting the outcomes. The authors found that significant differences were maintained after adjusting for baseline age, but unfortunately there was no adjustment for therapy time. In this context, it is worth noting that dextroamphetamine has been studied in large, well-controlled studies after motor stroke, with no efficacy for motor recovery (Platz et al. 2005; Gladstone et al. 2006; Sprigg et al. 2007; Sonde and Lökk 2007). Note that dextroamphetamine had shown promise for motor stroke in earlier, smaller studies, thus tempering enthusiasm for this drug for aphasia recovery.

Another approach within the sympathomimetic class of drugs has been to enhance dopaminergic signaling, typically via the use of either levodopa or a dopamine agonist, such as bromocriptine. These drugs have a lower abuse potential than dextroamphetamine and are commonly used to treat Parkinson's disease, and are therefore established to be relatively safe in a population similar in age to most stroke patients. Similar to the dextroamphetamine literature, there have been several trials for aphasia, but most were small or had crossover designs (Gupta et al. 1995; Sabe et al. 1995; Bragoni et al. 2000; Leemann et al. 2011). Here, we review the two largest studies, both of which were double-blind, placebo-controlled, parallel cohort studies.

Seniów et al. studied the impact of levodopa on language recovery after subacute stroke (Seniów et al. 2009). Thirty-nine subjects completed the study. All aphasic subtypes were included, and roughly similar numbers had "anterior" lesions versus "posterior" lesions. The study had a parallel design, with 20 subjects receiving 100 mg of levodopa and 19 subjects receiving placebo, and the administration of drug or placebo was timed to precede SLT by 30 minutes. SLT was given five times a week for 45 minutes per day for 3 weeks. The primary outcome measure was performance on subtests of the Boston Diagnostic Aphasia Examination (BDAE). The authors found improvement with levodopa on all subtests, but this was statistically significant only for verbal fluency ($p = 0.011$), repetition of phrases and sentences ($p = 0.028$). Note that no correction was done for multiple comparisons and that washout performance was not assessed. Levodopa patients were younger than placebo subjects by 6.3 years, potentially confounding the analysis, but the investigators found that age was not associated with BDAE outcome. In an additional study, Ashtary et al. (Ashtary et al. 2006) examined the impact of bromocriptine, 10 mg daily, started during the acute phase after stroke and continued for 4 months. Nineteen active and 19 placebo patients with non-fluent aphasia were enrolled. SLT was not required during this study, and it is not clear if any of the subjects received SLT. All subjects (placebo and drug treated) showed statistically significant improvement relative to baseline, but the investigators did not find any benefit to the addition of bromocriptine compared to placebo on a standardized Persian Language Test.

It is notable that the only study that demonstrated efficacy for dopamine therapy explicitly coupled dopamine therapy to SLT (Seniów et al. 2009), while the study that did not show efficacy had no requirement for SLT (Ashtary et al. 2006). These findings are also consistent with much of the data on human motor recovery, where levodopa, when coupled with physical therapy, has improved motor outcomes (Scheidtmann et al. 2001; Rösser et al. 2008). It is also possible that levodopa and dopamine agonists may work differently, such that levodopa may better preserve endogenous patterns of synaptic activity in dopaminergic systems in the brain via its presynaptic effect. As recently noted (Gill and Leff 2013), a relatively narrow range of dopaminergic agents and doses has thus far been explored in these studies.

Cholinergic Drugs

Many studies in animal models demonstrate the potential for the manipulation of synaptic acetylcholine levels to facilitate rewiring of neural circuits (Bear and Singer 1986; Kilgard and Merzenich 1998; Rasmusson 2000; Froemke, Merzenich and Schreiner 2007). For example, in the auditory cortex, experience-dependent alterations of sensory maps was greatly enhanced when sensory stimulation was coupled with stimulation of cholinergic fibers from the basal forebrain (Kilgard and Merzenich 1998). Notably, map reorganization parameters were directly related to the specific training stimuli used, emphasizing the importance of understanding the interactions between specific speech and language therapies with pharmacologic intervention.

Clinically, there is significant experience with cholinergic potentiators because of their use for the treatment of Alzheimer's disease, where three drugs are in common clinical use: donepezil, galantamine and rivastigmine. These drugs are well tolerated in elderly patients, with age ranges similar to many stroke patients. Several open-label pilot studies have suggested that potentiation of acetylcholine can improve language performance in aphasia (Tanaka, Miyazaki and Albert 1997; Tsz-Ming and Kaufer 2001; Pashek and Bachman 2003; Berthier et al. 2003; Hong et al. 2012), including a case study that involved a patient with a small subcortical lacunar infarction, where improvement was noted with donepezil, but not dopamine agonist therapy (Hughes, Jacobs and Heilman 2000).

One randomized controlled trial has examined the utility of cholinesterase inhibitor therapy for treatment of stroke-related aphasia. Berthier et al. (Berthier et al. 2006) studied the effect of 16 weeks of donepezil (up to 10 mg daily) in patients at least 1 year from aphasic stroke, and included subjects with all types of aphasia (Berthier et al. 2006). This parallel study design included 13 patients receiving donepezil and 13 receiving placebo, with all patients receiving standard SLT. Primary outcome measures were the Aphasia Quotient of the Western Aphasia Battery and performance on the Communicative Activity Log, which records daily functional language use. Subjects taking donepezil showed significant improvement on both measures, as well as the picture naming subtest of the Psycholinguistic Assessment of Language Processing in Aphasia Test, which was a secondary measure. Interestingly, the improvements noted at the end of drug administration at week 16 were not present at the washout point of week 20, suggesting that the benefits of donepezil were transient and potentially not related to neural reorganization. The lack of persistent benefit of donepezil is similar to what has been seen with respect to memory improvements in Alzheimer's disease (Rogers et al. 1998). Given this, it would have been interesting to assess if the aphasic patients in Berthier's study showed a more general improvement in cognitive function, characteristic of donepezil, and whether this generalized cognitive enhancement may have contributed to language improvements. If so, this might imply that the donepezil benefit may not rely on SLT and may rely on the improvement in other cognitive domains to improve language performance. This may be significant, because of a substantial number of patients who do not have access to SLT or cannot afford SLT, but may have access to drug therapy.

Piracetam

Piracetam has been the subject of much interest over the years because of several studies suggesting that it can act as a cognitive enhancer (Malykh and Sadaie 2010). Piracetam chemically resembles gamma-aminobutyric acid (GABA) and facilitates cholinergic and excitatory amine neurotransmission (Giurgea, Greindl and Preat 1983; Vernon and Sorkin 1991), increases regional cerebral blood flow (Jordaan et al. 1996) and alters neuronal membrane properties (Müller, Eckert and Eckert 1999). It has been claimed that this agent improves learning and memory, but it is not clear which of its biological effects (e.g., neuroprotective, circulatory or others) may be responsible for the purported cognitive benefit. Piracetam is currently available in the U.S. as a nutritional supplement and is approved for the treatment of myoclonus in Europe.

Piracetam was studied in a relatively large study (n = 50 completers) of aphasic patients (stroke and non-stroke) by Huber et al. (Huber et al. 1997). Both fluent and non-fluent patients enrolled in this study. They found that after 6 weeks of piracetam + SLT, there was no significant improvement on the Aachen Aphasia Test. They reported a significant benefit in a written language subtest, but this was not an a priori outcome measure. In a randomized study of piracetam in general stroke recovery, a subgroup of 67 subacute patients with aphasia was selected out of 137 total stroke patients who received either piracetam or placebo (Enderby et al. 1994). In the analysis of the aphasia subgroup, a significant improvement was observed on a multivariate analysis of Aachen Aphasia subtest scores relative to baseline in favor of piracetam ($p = 0.02$) at 12 weeks. This effect was no longer present at the washout point of 24 weeks. An important consideration is that this study is based on a subgroup analysis and that certain baseline characteristics were not matched (e.g., the piracetam group was 4.7 years younger, on average, than the control group), limiting the interpretability of the study. A large multicenter study ($n = 927$) treated all stroke patients with piracetam within 12 hours and used a variety of outcome measures, including an assessment of aphasia (De Deyn et al. 1997). This study only showed benefits when using post-hoc analysis and will not be further considered (Orgogozo 1999; Huber 1999).

Kessler and colleagues integrated blood flow imaging measures into a treatment trial of patients with subacute stroke and aphasia ($n = 12$ per group; Kessler et al. 2000). They observed an increase in task-related blood flow in left hemisphere regions generally associated with language over the course of the treatment period, which was greater in the piracetam group than the placebo group. The piracetam group improved on six language measures, the placebo group on three, though there were no direct statistical comparisons reported between drug versus placebo groups. Finally, a recent single-blind study found only marginal benefit of 6 months piracetam after aphasic stroke on a secondary outcome measure (Güngör, Terzi and Onar 2011). Thus, none of the studies of piracetam showed benefits on any of the primary outcome measures that were examined.

Memantine

Memantine is commonly used for the treatment of Alzheimer's disease and has a mechanism of action that is not fully understood. The drug is generally thought of as a non-competitive antagonist at the N-methyl-D-aspartate (NMDA) receptor, though other mechanisms have been postulated, such as actions on serotonin receptors and dopamine receptors and diminishment of excitotoxicity (Johnson and Kotermanski 2006; Lipton 2006). There are animal data suggesting that memantine can both offer acute neuroprotection after ischemia and may facilitate the reorganization of brain circuits in the chronic post-ischemic state (Volbracht et al. 2006).

One trial has examined the efficacy of memantine in chronic stroke-related aphasia in 27 patients with various types of stroke (Berthier et al. 2009). Patients were given 20 mg of memantine daily for 16 weeks initially *without* SLT. This intervention produced significant improvement on the Western Aphasia Battery (WAB; $p = 0.002$ for the Aphasia Quotient). Incorporation of constraint-induced aphasia therapy for 2 weeks produced further separation of the memantine group from the placebo group. After a 4-week washout, the memantine group's WAB performance declined substantially, but remained slightly better than the placebo group ($p = 0.041$). This study is suggestive of an effect of memantine in the absence of SLT, although evidence for a synergistic relationship between constraint-induced aphasia therapy (CIAT) and memantine is weakened by the differences in WAB scores at the onset of CIAT. Significant improvement on the Communicative Activity Log occurred after the implementation of CIAT. Similar to the donepezil study (Berthier et al. 2006), based on these data, one cannot exclude that the benefits of memantine were related to more general cognitive improvements. Given the good efficacy and tolerability profile of combination use of donepezil and memantine for Alzheimer's disease (Tariot et al. 2004), and the positive studies for both drugs and aphasia described here, it would be interesting to examine the effects of combination therapy on aphasia recovery.

Other Drugs: Zolpidem and Vasopressin

Zolpidem and vasopressin have both been postulated to be effective for aphasia (as well as other cognitive disorders), though the evidence of their efficacy at this point remains relatively thin. Given the widespread interest in these compounds, they will be briefly reviewed here. Zolpidem potentiates GABA at those receptors that contain the alpha-1 subunit. Although the evidence supporting zolpidem has been low grade (case reports), the reported benefits have been dramatic. For example, an open-label case study reported the improvement in language function in an aphasic patient with a single dose of zolpidem (Cohen, Chaaban and Habert 2004). In this case report, an individual with a non-fluent aphasia and a lesion in the left insula, putamen and superior temporal gyrus had a mild insomnia and was prescribed zolpidem, which led to sudden and unexpected improvement in her speech and naming ability. This remitted when the zolpidem wore off, and was reproducible. An electroencephalogram failed to show any changes after zolpidem administration. Technetium-99 single-photon emission computed tomography (SPECT) scanning demonstrated an increase in blood flow to Broca's area, left middle frontal gyrus, left supramarginal gyrus and the bilateral orbitofrontal and mesial frontal cortices. Similarly dramatic case reports have been published for patients with disorders in arousal or awareness (Thomas et al. 1997; Clauss et al. 2000; Brefel-Courbon et al. 2007). It has been speculated that the paradoxical increase in arousal seen with zolpidem is related to zolpidem-induced suppression of globus pallidus interna, which is likely disinhibited in various forms of brain injury, suppressing output from the central thalamus (Schiff 2010). An important consideration is that the reports of significant improvements with zolpidem are not dissimilar to very early reports with other sedating drugs, such as amobarbital (Linn 1947), which ultimately proved not to be effective (see Small 1994 for further history).

Vasopressin is thought to be important in mediating social behavior (Donaldson and Young 2008) and has been examined by Tsikunov and Belokoskova (Tsikunov and Belokoskova 2007) for the treatment of chronic aphasia. They examined the effects of intranasal desmopressin (a V2-receptor agonist) in 26 patients with chronic stroke-related aphasia in a single-cohort crossover design. They observed "good" responses (improvements on at least 3 out of 10 language tests) in 13 of 26 subjects. SLT was not incorporated into this trial. Given the speculation of the role of vasopressin in social behavior, it would be interesting to determine the degree to which the improvements in language function correlate with indices of social functioning in these patients. If vasopressin-based recovery has a different mechanism of action than "traditional" neurotransmitter-based therapy, this approach holds promise in being a non-redundant form of pharmacotherapy for subjects receiving one of the above-mentioned classes of drugs.

Quality of Evidence and Recommendations

We have compiled a table of drug trials for aphasia recovery that have met the following criteria: (1) they were randomized, double-blind and placebo-controlled; (2) they were primarily designed to assess the impact of a drug on language and used a language battery as a primary outcome measure; (3) they were parallel designed (to avoid period effects) and (4) they enrolled at least 10 aphasic subjects. When these criteria are applied, a total of six studies were found. These studies examined the following drugs or mechanisms: dextroamphetamine (Walker-Batson et al. 2001), dopamine enhancement (Ashtary et al. 2006; Seniów et al. 2009), piracetam (Huber et al. 1997), donepezil (Berthier et al. 2006) and memantine (Berthier et al. 2009). In our estimation, of these six clinical trials, three of them (Walker-Batson et al. 2001; Berthier et al. 2006; Berthier et al. 2009) convincingly demonstrated efficacy in a primary outcome measure, and one of them demonstrated efficacy not only on laboratory testing but also on functional daily language function (Berthier et al. 2009). Unfortunately, all three of these studies are all quite small, and none of these studies has been replicated, thus making it not possible to consider any of three to be a class A recommendation for use in aphasic subjects (Harris et al. 2001). In addition, some of these drugs have not been shown to be efficacious for aphasia in other contexts. For example, despite the apparent superiority of memantine over the other drugs in aphasic stroke shown in Table 21.1, when memantine has been studied to treat aphasia in dementia, it has had a mixed track record of efficacy (Pomara et al. 2007; Saxton et al. 2012; Boxer et al. 2013). Therefore, these results await independent confirmation before clear treatment recommendations can be provided.

Table 21.1 Summary of Studies of Drug Therapy for Aphasia (Criteria for inclusion in the table outlined in the text.)

Study	Drug	Subjects	Design	Results	Merits of study design or results	Potential deficiencies
Huber et al. 1997	Piracetam 1.6 g three times daily	Subacute chronic aphasia from any type of brain lesion. N = 32 piracetam (24 completers) N = 30 placebo (26 completers)	Parallel. Treated for 6 weeks. Aachen Aphasia Test given at baseline and at 6 weeks. All subjects received SLT, but not timed to drug.	Overall score performance not provided. When correcting for baseline, efficacy seen on one subtest (written language) with $p = 0.05$. No benefit on other five subtests.	Relatively large study.	No significant improvement on primary outcome measure, and benefits on subtests were modest.
Walker-Batson et al. 2001	Dextro-amphetamine 10 mg daily	Subacute ischemic stroke N = 12 dextro-amphetamine N = 9 placebo	Parallel. Treated for 5 weeks. Drug given just prior to SLT. Porch Index of Communicative Ability was assessed at baseline, at 6 weeks and 6 months.	Improvement seen in overall score at 6 weeks ($p = 0.015$) and trend seen at 6 months ($p = 0.048$).	Long-term follow-up data are suggestive of sustained benefits.	Age and amount of therapy differed between groups. No control for post-stroke depression.
Seniów et al. 2009	Levodopa 100 mg + benserazide 25 mg daily	Subacute stroke N = 20 levodopa + benserazide N = 19 placebo	Parallel. Treated for 3 weeks. Drug given just prior to SLT. Boston Diagnostic Aphasia Examination was primary outcome measure.	Overall score performance not provided. Improvements seen on animal naming ($p = 0.011$), word repetition ($p = 0.05$), high-frequency repetition ($p = 0.028$). No significance on other subtests.	Drugs given just prior to SLT, maximizing the likelihood that drug may have potentiated circuitry that was involved in SLT.	Benefits only seen in subtests of BDAE. No correction for multiple comparisons.
Ashtary et al. 2006	Bromocriptine 10 mg daily	Non-fluent acute-subacute stroke N = 19 bromocriptine N = 19 placebo	Parallel. Treated for 4 months. No requirement for SLT. Persian Language Test given at 0, 8 and 16 weeks.	No significant differences seen between drug and placebo groups.	Long duration of therapy.	No requirement for SLT.

(Continued)

Table 21.1 (Continued)

Study	Drug	Subjects	Design	Results	Merits of study design or results	Potential deficiencies
Berthier et al. 2006	Donepezil 10 mg daily	Chronic stroke N = 13 donepezil N = 14 placebo	Parallel. Treated for 12 weeks. SLT given to all subjects, but not timed to drug. Western Aphasia Battery and Communicative Activity Log at 0, 4, 16 and 20 weeks.	Overall aphasia quotient at 16 weeks was better in donepezil group ($p = 0.037$). Trends for improvement in Communicative Activity Log when comparing doses. No benefit at washout.	Language performance measured at washout.	Relatively small study.
Berthier et al. 2009	Memantine 20 mg daily	Chronic stroke N = 14 memantine N = 13 placebo	Parallel. Treated without SLT for 16 weeks, then given constraint-induced aphasia therapy for 2 weeks. Western Aphasia Battery and Communicative Activity Log at multiple time points.	Improvement seen on Western Aphasia Battery-Aphasia Quotient during study pre- and post-SLT ($p < 0.001$) and at washout ($p = 0.041$). Improvement in Communicative Activity Log after SLT ($p = 0.04$).	Benefits seen even in the absence of SLT. Benefits seen on functional measures. Benefits seen at washout.	Relatively small study.

Drugs to Avoid

One practical intervention for physicians caring for aphasic patients is to ensure that they are not being treated with drugs that can interfere with neurologic recovery. In general, drugs that suppress synaptic transmission, such as the anticonvulsant drugs, are likely to interfere with synaptic activity-based mechanisms of neuronal reorganization and therefore may suppress recovery of language function. Seizures are seen in approximately 5–10% of chronic stroke patients (So et al. 1996; Bladin et al. 2000), and thus it would not be uncommon to have a post-stroke aphasic patient taking an anticonvulsant. However, benzodiazepines, phenytoin or phenobarbital have all been associated with worse motor outcomes after stroke (Goldstein 1995). In addition, newer anticonvulsants, such as vigabatrin and topiramate, potentially cause significant cognitive impairment, including worsening language performance (Gil and Neau 1995; Jambaqué et al. 1998; Wong and Lhatoo 2000). Topiramate is particularly notable for its potential to worsen cognitive deficits, particularly language disorders. For example, Mula et al. (Mula et al. 2003) observed word-finding difficulty in 7.2% of over 400 patients with epilepsy taking topiramate, and a case report demonstrated reversible focal left frontal hypoperfusion and motor aphasia in a seizure patient taking topiramate (Cappa et al. 2007). Language disturbances have been observed in a substantial proportion of migraine patients who use topiramate for headache prophylaxis (Coppola et al. 2008). These studies do not specifically address the ability of topiramate or other anticonvulsants to alter the recovery from a lesion in the language network. Given the importance of SLT on language recovery, it is likely that topiramate would interfere with the ability of patients to participate optimally in SLT, and should therefore be avoided if possible.

Other drugs can potentially suppress recovery after a stroke. For example, the animal data described above suggest that cholinergic, dopaminergic and noradrenergic potentiation may enhance activity-dependent synaptic plasticity and therefore facilitate stroke recovery. Therefore, it is probable that drugs that block these neurotransmitters can impede stroke recovery. Several investigators examined this issue. For example, Goldstein found that stroke patients taking an alpha-2 agonist (e.g., clonidine), and alpha-1 antagonist (e.g., prazosin), a dopamine receptor antagonist (e.g., an antipsychotic), a benzodiazepine, a barbiturate or phenytoin, had delayed motor recovery after stroke (Goldstein 1995; Goldstein 1998). In addition, use of thiazide diuretics have been associated with worse language outcome after stroke (Porch and Feeney 1986). Given the frequency of the use of antihypertensives, antipsychotics and drugs with anticholinergic mechanisms, it is prudent to weigh the potential impact of these drugs on synaptic reorganization when prescribing these drugs, especially when alternatives may be available. See Table 21.2 for a list of drugs that are potentially deleterious to aphasia rehabilitation.

Table 21.2 Drugs Potentially Deleterious for Aphasia Recovery

Drug	Mechanism	Indication
Haloperidol	D2 blocker	Psychosis, agitation
Prazosin, phenoxybenzamine	Alpha-1 blocker	Hypertension
Clonidine	Alpha-2 agonist	Hypertension
Labetalol	Alpha-1 and beta-blocker	Hypertension
Hydrochlorothiazide	Thiazide diuretic	Hypertension
Barbiturates	Positive allosteric modulator at GABA receptors	Seizures
Benzodiazepines	Positive allosteric modulator at GABA receptors	Seizures, anxiety
Phenytoin	Sodium channel blocker	Seizures
Topiramate	Effects on glutamate and GABA receptors	Seizures, migraine
Vigabatrin	Blocks GABA transaminase, elevating GABA levels	Seizures

Treating Depression

An important consideration for the treatment of post-stroke aphasia is the treatment of depression. Untreated depression can interfere with language performance and motivation to engage in SLT (Gabaldón et al. 2007; Skidmore et al. 2010). Post-stroke depression is highly prevalent, with estimates ranging from 30–60% (Starkstein and Robinson 1989; van de Weg, Kuik and Lankhorst 1999; Aben et al. 2003; Barker-Collo 2007; Robinson et al. 2008). Post-stroke depression is also highly under-diagnosed (Robinson 1998), since not all patients with post-stroke depression fit into the classic DSM criteria of major depression. Nevertheless, these individuals with symptoms of "minor depression" may have significant dysfunction. Depression can be particularly difficult to detect in aphasic subjects because of their difficulty in expressing emotions and the possible misattribution of social withdrawal to language deficits. Aphasic patients may be more prone to post-stroke depression than their nonaphasic counterparts (Laska et al. 2007), and have a greater compromise to their quality of life (Hilari and Byng 2009). In addition, patients with depression have more cognitive impairment than patients with comparable lesions but no depression (Morris, Raphael and Robinson 1992; Downhill and Robinson 1994). Some data suggest that depression is more common in patients with left hemisphere stroke than right (Starkstein et al. 1991; Morris et al. 1996; Rajashekaran et al. 2013), which would be of major importance for aphasia rehabilitation, though this relationship has not been seen in all studies (Iacoboni et al. 1995; Aben et al. 2006). Finally, a recent update to a Cochrane analysis concluded that pharmacotherapy produced a small, but significant, reduction in depressive symptoms in patients with post-stroke depression (Hackett et al. 2008; Hackett et al. 2009). One complicating factor in the interpretation of all of these data is that aphasic patients are routinely excluded from clinical trials that assess the efficacy of post-stroke depression pharmacotherapy. Though tools currently exist to evaluate depression in aphasic patients (Benaim et al. 2004; Cobley et al. 2012), we are not aware of any randomized controlled trial that examined this issue specifically.

Treatment with antidepressants, particularly those that elevate synaptic norepinephrine or serotonin levels, may also have a direct impact on neural reorganization and cognitive function. Serotonin regulates some forms of cortical map reorganization (Gu and Singer 1995; Jitsuki et al. 2011; Vetencourt et al. 2011), as well as adult neurogenesis in the hippocampus (Li et al. 2009; Daszuta 2011), and may drive the production of brain-derived neurotrophic factor (BDNF; Martinowich and Lu 2007, see below) and therefore may facilitate post-stroke recovery beyond its effects on depression. For example, Jorge et al. found that escitalopram given prophylactically in the subacute period after stroke improved overall performance on the Repeatable Battery for the Assessment of Neuropsychological Status (RBANS). Notably, the improvement on the RBANS was independent of escitalopram's effect on depression (Jorge et al. 2010). Several other studies have observed positive results in terms of language outcomes with the use of antidepressants after stroke (Kimura, Robinson and Kosier 2000; Narushima et al. 2003; Tanaka et al. 2004), though at least one study showed no benefit with antidepressant intervention (Laska et al. 2005). Therefore, given the high prevalence of post-stroke depression and its negative impacts on language, combined with the generally positive data regarding treatment with modern antidepressants, treatment of depression should be considered a fundamental part of any aphasia rehabilitation program.

Other Biological Interventions

Non-pharmacological approaches to the treatment of chronic aphasia after stroke or other brain lesions are beginning to show promise. As described above, the efficacy of drug therapies at this point appear to be modest. In addition, by their nature, drug therapies are limited in their ability to target specific brain networks in the absence behavioral training. Other therapies, such as cortical modulation techniques or cellular transplantation strategies, have the potential to target specific diseased brain networks. To date, none of these techniques is in broad clinical practice, but given their promise for the future, they will be discussed here.

Cortical Modulation Techniques

Stroke induces a broad range of changes in the functional network architecture of the brain. This implies that brain structures remote from the brain lesion may serve as targets of focal therapeutic interventions, which may either increase or decrease their excitability. In addition, given the strong dependence of synaptic plasticity on underlying neuronal activity patterns, it is likely that therapeutic modulation of neuronal excitability can alter the efficacy of behavioral interventions, such as SLT. These facts have led to substantial excitement in the aphasia community about brain stimulation techniques. The hope is that these tools may ultimately play a role in the treatment of aphasia and much has been written recently about this topic (Hamilton, Chrysikou and Coslett 2011; Monti et al. 2012; Cherney et al. 2013).

Multiple approaches exist for the modulation of cortical excitability. Direct cortical modulation techniques, such as epidural stimulation, allow for highly focal stimulation to be applied to targeted cortical areas. This approach is more invasive than surface-level modulation described below, but has shown some promise for aphasia rehabilitation in a very preliminary pilot study (Cherney et al. 2012). It should be noted in this context that initial small trials in motor stroke showed similar promise, but when studied carefully in a large controlled study (Plow et al. 2009) the initial promise did not lead to an efficacious intervention. Other less invasive techniques include repetitive transcranial magnetic (rTMS) and direct current (tDCS) electrical stimulation. Though both techniques are relatively safe and show some efficacy (see below and chapter 22, this volume), tDCS has found favor recently because of its ease of use. Both techniques are applied to the scalp, and are thought to alter neuronal excitability in directional ways. For example, anodal tDCS is thought to provide depolarizing bias to underlying cortical neurons, while cathodal tDCS provides hyperpolarizing bias (Monti et al. 2012). The approach is couched in a theory that during aphasia, certain brain regions may be hypoactive (e.g., peri-infarct zones) and others may be maladaptively hyperactive (e.g., contralesional regions; Heiss et al. 1997; Karbe et al. 1998; Thiel et al. 2006) and that upregulation of hypoactive and downregulation of maladaptively hyperactive zones may provide benefit. It is worth noting, however, that providing biasing current to particular cortical brain regions provides very little insight into the impact of brain stimulation on the activity of that brain region. For example, electrical stimulation may affect excitatory and inhibitory neurons, and it may do so differentially. In addition, changes in membrane potential can produce paradoxical effects, such as depolarizing block or hyperpolarization-induced rebound firing, and damaged neuronal tissue may respond in ways that are different than healthy tissue. Therefore, it is quite difficult to predict the consequences of any of these brain stimulation techniques, and we must rely on empirical data, which are still relatively sparse.

Most studies examining the efficacy of TMS or tDCS on aphasia rehabilitation are small (fewer than five subjects), uncontrolled, of short duration and/or without examination of any potential long-term effects. We limit our discussion here to studies that are larger (at least 10 subjects) and have sham controls. Five studies focused on the impact of *right-sided* rTMS or tDCS on language performance. Three of these five studies found that presumably suppressive actions (either through rTMS or cathodal tDCS) on the right-sided homologs of either Broca's or Wernicke's area improved language performance (You et al. 2011; Barwood et al. 2011; Kang et al. 2011). One group found no impact (Waldowski et al. 2012) and one group found enhancements with anodal, presumably excitatory, stimulation on the right superior temporal gyrus (Flöel et al. 2011). One study that examined the impact of left-sided modulation (Baker, Rorden and Fridriksson 2010) found that anodal tDCS over a region of the left frontal cortex that showed high BOLD signal on an overt naming task improved naming performance. They also found that the magnitude of the improvement depended on the relationship between the stimulating electrode and lesion site (closer = better). All of these studies were relatively short in duration (1–3 weeks) and the longest post-stimulation time that a benefit was seen was 2 weeks (Flöel et al. 2011). Chapter 22, this volume, provides a more detailed review of the use of tDCS in aphasia rehabilitation.

Cell- and Tissue-Based Therapies

The previous discussions of pharmacological agents and electrical stimulation for treatment of aphasia were based on the assumption that recovery of language function after stroke was due to re-wiring of synaptic connections between existing neurons. An emerging treatment modality within the clinical neurosciences is the use of biological agents to induce the growth of new neurons or to replace lost cells with exogenously supplied precursors. A wealth of animal studies now suggests that approaches involving the use of embryonic, fetal or adult stem cells, or the use of agents that facilitate endogenous recovery processes in the brain, can enhance functional recovery after brain injury (reviewed in Smith and Gavins 2012; Lees et al. 2012). Though no stem cell therapies for stroke have yet come to fruition for humans, there is an intense interest in this, pushing this field further, as evidenced by the 30+ actively recruiting clinical trials found on clinicaltrials. gov (as of October 2013) studying the use of stem cells to treat stroke patients.

In addition to direct cellular therapy, several forms of non-stem cell pharmacological therapy may promote tissue regeneration. For example, stroke induces the expression of a number of extracellular molecules that are potentially hostile to axonal outgrowth that may serve as suitable drug targets. These include myelin-associated extracellular molecules, such as Nogo-A, myelin-associated glycoprotein and oligodendrocyte-myelin glycoprotein and extracellular matrix proteins, such as tenascin and chondroitin sulfate proteoglycans (Carmichael 2006). Among these, the Nogo-A system has been the best characterized, and inhibitors of this system have moved forward into clinical trials for spinal cord injury, and are under consideration for stroke. In animal models of motor cortical stroke, inhibition of Nogo-A activity via passive immunization resulted in enhanced recovery of motor function in several studies in both subacute and chronic states (Tsai et al. 2007; Brenneman et al. 2008; Tsai et al. 2011). Although most work in animal models of stroke has focused on motor recovery, a few have focused on recovery of cognitive deficits. For example, intraventricular administration of anti-Nogo antibodies promotes recovery in a rodent model of hemispatial neglect (Brenneman et al. 2008) and post-stroke spatial memory deficits (Gillani et al. 2010). Since the studies referenced above have not demonstrated any alteration in infarct size after anti-Nogo therapy, anti-Nogo therapy may promote neural reorganization, rather than neuronal protection, suggesting that anti-Nogo therapy represents a feasible path forward for studies of chronic stroke patients.

One potential concern with either the anti-Nogo approach or with the use of rat as a model for human stroke recovery is that the benefits of anti-Nogo therapy in both motor stroke studies (Tsai et al. 2007) and at least one of the "cognitive" stroke studies (Brenneman et al. 2008) were in large part mediated by activation of *contralesional* structures. These data suggest that anti-Nogo therapy may promote sprouting of long-range axons of contralesional origin rather than remaining ipsilateral axons. Since recovery in human motor stroke (Fridman et al. 2004), aphasia (Heiss et al. 1997; Karbe et al. 1998; Beharelle et al. 2010; Szaflarski et al. 2013) and neglect (Corbetta et al. 2005) is likely optimally mediated by ipsilesional structures, promotion of sprouting of contralesional axons may not be an optimal recovery strategy.

Another approach involves the use of growth factors to enhance recovery from brain injury. In this regard, a great deal of attention has been paid to BDNF. For example, rodent studies have shown (1) that BDNF increases both locally and remotely after stroke onset (Béjot et al. 2011), (2) that providing exogenous BDNF can enhance recovery (Schäbitz et al. 2007; Chang et al. 2012) and (3) that inhibition of BDNF using antisense oligonucleotides impairs functional recovery from motor cortex stroke (Ploughman et al. 2009). The latter study also revealed a synergistic interaction between physical therapy and BDNF expression. Despite the suggestive findings regarding BDNF and stroke, a major hurdle to the translation of this therapy to the clinic is delivery of such a large molecule to the CNS, particularly in the chronic phase of stroke when the blood-brain barrier has reconstituted. This provides an opportunity to drive BDNF expression indirectly via serotonin augmentation (e.g., through the use of selective serotonin reuptake inhibitors, SSRIs; Martinowich and Lu 2007).

As described above, there have been few completed studies utilizing cell- or growth factor–based therapy for stroke, and none of these studies have looked at aphasic patients. It is likely that the next several years will bring new data regarding the potential to stimulate the regeneration of lost circuits via cell- or growth factor–based therapy. Unfortunately, none of the ongoing studies are recruiting subjects in the chronic phases of stroke. It bears pointing out that the biological issues during the acute and chronic phases of stroke are quite different, and it should not be assumed that the efficacy, or lack thereof, in the current cohort of studies will necessarily be predictive of efficacy for chronic stroke patients. As with pharmacotherapy and electrical stimulation, cell- and tissue-based methods also entail the basic requirement that biological interventions be accompanied by behavioral practice.

Conclusions

In this chapter, we have adopted a *medical model* for the treatment of aphasia. That is, rather than focusing rehabilitation strategies that develop compensatory behaviors to increase functionality of aphasic patients, we assume that major goals of therapy should be (1) to promote means of synaptic plasticity that lead to improved language behavior and (2) to remove factors (e.g., drugs) that impede synaptic plasticity. There are several drugs that appear to hold promise for aphasia: cholinesterase inhibitors, memantine and sympathomimetics. However, none has been tested to a high level of evidence, and even some of the best-implemented trials have included fewer than 50 subjects and have not been independently replicated. Further, combinations of drugs with different mechanisms, which are commonly and effectively used in other disorders such as Parkinson's disease and Alzheimer's disease, have not been tested for aphasia. The situation is similar for cortical modulation techniques. Most of the early data are promising, but there has only been a small number of randomized trials, and the trials themselves have been quite small, and only show modest benefits. Given the relative safety of cortical modulation techniques and the use of already-approved drugs, we are likely to see more of these studies in the coming years, which will hopefully add some clarity to their utility. Further, as network imaging approaches continue to develop, it will be possible to gain a better understanding of the impact of these drugs and cortical modulation techniques on the behavior of large-scale neural networks, which will inform our understanding of these treatment modalities.

Currently, from a practical perspective, there are a number of interventions recommended for aphasic patients. First is to ensure that secondary prevention measures have been put in place to prevent a recurrent stroke. Second is to review the medication lists of post-stroke aphasic patients for potentially deleterious drugs. It is common for patients to take several antihypertensive drugs as well as anticonvulsant or antipsychotic drugs. Given what is known about the potential for some of these drugs to interfere with recovery from aphasia (see Table 21.2), it is prudent to review these drugs and to carefully remove or replace certain drugs. Third, post-stroke depression is common, treatable and interferes with language recovery, and should be screened for and treated in post-stroke aphasia. Fourth, the gold standard for treatment of aphasia is SLT, and all efforts should be made to ensure that post-stroke aphasic patients receive appropriate SLT. Finally, whether or not to use currently available drugs in an off-label fashion for the treatment of aphasia will be up to the individual prescriber. However, such drugs should only be used in conjunction with active SLT and ideally should be used in the context of a clinical trial so that the broader community of providers can gain more knowledge about these interventions.

References

Aben, I., J. Lodder, A. Honig, R. Lousberg, A. Boreas and F. Verhey (2006). "Focal or generalized vascular brain damage and vulnerability to depression after stroke: a 1-year prospective follow-up study." *International Psychogeriatrics 18*(1): 19–35.

Aben, I., F. Verhey, J. Strik, R. Lousberg, J. Lodder and A. Honig (2003). "A comparative study into the one year cumulative incidence of depression after stroke and myocardial infarction." *Journal of Neurology, Neurosurgery & Psychiatry 74*(5): 581–585.

Ashtary, F., M. Janghorbani, A. Chitsaz, M. Reisi and A. Bahrami (2006). "A randomized, double-blind trial of bromocriptine efficacy in nonfluent aphasia after stroke." *Neurology 66*(6): 914–916.

Baker, J.M., C. Rorden and J. Fridriksson (2010). "Using transcranial direct-current stimulation to treat stroke patients with aphasia." *Stroke 41*(6): 1229–1236.

Bao, S., V.T. Chan and M.M. Merzenich (2001). "Cortical remodelling induced by activity of ventral tegmental dopamine neurons." *Nature 412*(6842): 79–83.

Barbay, S., E.V. Zoubina, N. Dancause, S.B. Frost, I. Eisner-Janowicz, A. M. Stowe, E.J. Plautz and R.J. Nudo (2006). "A single injection of d-amphetamine facilitates improvements in motor training following a focal cortical infarct in squirrel monkeys." *Neurorehabilitation and Neural Repair 20*(4): 455–458.

Barker-Collo, S.L. (2007). "Depression and anxiety 3 months post stroke: Prevalence and correlates." *Archives of Clinical Neuropsychology 22*(4): 519–531.

Barwood, C., B. Murdoch, B.M. Whelan, D. Lloyd, S. Riek, J. O'Sullivan, A. Coulthard and A. Wong (2011). "Improved language performance subsequent to low-frequency rTMS in patients with chronic nonfluent aphasia post-stroke." *European Journal of Neurology 18*(7): 935–943.

Bear, M.F., and W. Singer (1986). "Modulation of visual cortical plasticity by acetylcholine and noradrenaline." *Nature 320*(6058): 172–176.

Beharelle, A.R., A.S. Dick, G. Josse, A. Solodkin, P.R. Huttenlocher, S.C. Levine and S.L. Small (2010). "Left hemisphere regions are critical for language in the face of early left focal brain injury." *Brain 133*(6): 1707–1716.

Béjot, Y., A. Prigent-Tessier, C. Cachia, M. Giroud, C. Mossiat, N. Bertrand, P. Garnier and C. Marie (2011). "Time-dependent contribution of non neuronal cells to BDNF production after ischemic stroke in rats." *Neurochemistry International 58*(1): 102–111.

Beltran, E.J., C.M. Papadopoulos, S.-Y. Tsai, G.L. Kartje and W.A. Wolf (2010). "Long-term motor improvement after stroke is enhanced by short-term treatment with the alpha-2 antagonist, atipamezole." *Brain Research 1346*(0): 174–182.

Benaim, C., B. Cailly, D. Perennou and J. Pelissier (2004). "Validation of the Aphasic Depression Rating Scale." *Stroke 35*(7): 1692–1696.

Bersano, A., F. Burgio, M. Gattinoni, L. Candelise on behalf of the PROSIT Study Group (2009). "Aphasia burden to hospitalised acute stroke patients: Need for an early rehabilitation programme." *International Journal of Stroke 4*(6): 443–447.

Berthier, M., C. Green, C. Higueras, I. Fernandez, J. Hinojosa and M. Martin (2006). "A randomized, placebo-controlled study of donepezil in poststroke aphasia." *Neurology 67*(9): 1687–1689.

Berthier, M.L., C. Green, J.P. Lara, C. Higueras, M.A. Barbancho, G. Dávila and F. Pulvermüller (2009). "Memantine and constraint-induced aphasia therapy in chronic poststroke aphasia." *Annals of Neurology 65*(5): 577–585.

Berthier, M.L., J. Hinojosa, M. del Carmen Martín and I. Fernández (2003). "Open-label study of donepezil in chronic poststroke aphasia." *Neurology 60*(7): 1218–1219.

Bhogal, S.K., R. Teasell and M. Speechley (2003). "Intensity of Aphasia Therapy, Impact on Recovery." *Stroke 34*(4): 987–993.

Bladin, C.F., A.V. Alexandrov, A. Bellavance, N. Bornstein, B. Chambers, R. Cote, L. Lebrun, A. Pirisi and J.W. Norris (2000). "Seizures after stroke: A prospective multicenter study." *Archives of Neurology 57*(11): 1617–1622.

Booth, J.R., L. Wood, D. Lu, J.C. Houk and T. Bitan (2007). "The role of the basal ganglia and cerebellum in language processing." *Brain Research 1133*: 136–144.

Boxer, A.L., D.S. Knopman, D.I. Kaufer, M. Grossman, C. Onyike, N. Graf-Radford, M. Mendez, D. Kerwin, A. Lerner, C.-K. Wu, M. Koestler, J. Shapira, K. Sullivan, K. Klepac, K. Lipowski, J. Ullah, S. Fields, J.H. Kramer, J. Merrilees, J. Neuhaus, M.M. Mesulam and B.L. Miller (2013). "Memantine in patients with frontotemporal lobar degeneration: A multicentre, randomised, double-blind, placebo-controlled trial." *The Lancet Neurology 12*(2): 149–156.

Brady, M.C., H. Kelly, J. Godwin and P. Enderby (2012). "Speech and language therapy for aphasia following stroke." *Cochrane Database of Systematic Reviews 5*: CD000425.

Bragoni, M., M. Altieri, V. Di Piero, A. Padovani, C. Mostardini and G. Lenzi (2000). "Bromocriptine and speech therapy in non-fluent chronic aphasia after stroke." *Neurological Sciences 21*(1): 19–22.

Brefel-Courbon, C., P. Payoux, F. Ory, A. Sommet, T. Slaoui, G. Raboyeau, B. Lemesle, M. Puel, J.L. Montastruc and J.F. Demonet (2007). "Clinical and imaging evidence of zolpidem effect in hypoxic encephalopathy." *Annals of Neurology 62*(1): 102–105.

Brenneman, M.M., S.J. Wagner, J.L. Cheatwood, S.A. Heldt, J.V. Corwin, R.L. Reep, G.L. Kartje, A.K. Mir and M.E. Schwab (2008). "Nogo-A inhibition induces recovery from neglect in rats." *Behavioural Brain Research 187*(2): 262–272.

Brown, C.E. and T.H. Murphy (2008). "Livin' on the edge: imaging dendritic spine turnover in the peri-infarct zone during ischemic stroke and recovery." *The Neuroscientist 14*(2): 139–146.

Brown, R.M., A. Carlson, B. Ljunggren, B.K. Siesjö and S.R. Snider (1974). "Effect of ischemia on monoamine metabolism in the brain." *Acta Physiologica Scandinavica 90*(4): 789–791.

Cappa, S., P. Ortelli, V. Garibotto and M. Zamboni (2007). "Reversible nonfluent aphasia and left frontal hypoperfusion during topiramate treatment." *Epilepsy & Behavior 10*(1): 192–194.

Carey, M.R. and W.G. Regehr (2009). "Noradrenergic control of associative synaptic plasticity by selective modulation of instructive signals." *Neuron 62*(1): 112–122.

Carmichael, S.T. (2006). "Cellular and molecular mechanisms of neural repair after stroke: making waves." *Annals of Neurology 59*(5): 735–742.

Chang, D., N. Lee, C. Choi, I. Jeon, S. Oh, D. Shin, T. Hwang, H. Lee, S. Kim and H. Moon (2012). "Therapeutic effect of BDNF-overexpressing human neural stem cells (HB1. F3. BDNF) in a rodent model of middle cerebral artery occlusion." *Cell Transplantation 22*(8): 1441–1452.

Cherney, L., E. Babbitt, R. Hurwitz, L. Rogers, J. Stinear, X. Wang, R. Harvey and T. Parrish (2013). "Transcranial direct current stimulation and aphasia: The case of Mr. C." *Topics in Stroke Rehabilitation 20*(1): 5–21.

Cherney, L.R., R.L. Harvey, E.M. Babbitt, R. Hurwitz, R.C. Kaye, J.B. Lee and S.L. Small (2012). "Epidural cortical stimulation and aphasia therapy." *Aphasiology 26*(9): 1192–1217.

Clauss, R., W. Güldenpfennig, H. Nel, M. Sathekge and R. Venkannagari (2000). "Extraordinary arousal from semi-comatose state on zolpidem: A case report." *South African Medical Journal 90*(1): 68–72.

Clem, R.L. and R.L. Huganir (2013). "Norepinephrine enhances a discrete form of long-term depression during fear memory storage." *The Journal of Neuroscience 33*(29): 11825–11832.

Cobley, C.S., S.A. Thomas, N.B. Lincoln and M.F. Walker (2012). "The assessment of low mood in stroke patients with aphasia: reliability and validity of the 10-item Hospital version of the Stroke Aphasic Depression Questionnaire (SADQH-10)." *Clinical Rehabilitation 26*(4): 372–381.

Cohen, H.P., A.G. Waltz and R.L. Jacobson (1975). "Catecholamine content of cerebral tissue after occlusion or manipulation of middle cerebral artery in cats." *Journal of Neurosurgery 43*(1): 32–36.

Cohen, L., B. Chaaban and M.-O. Habert (2004). "Transient improvement of aphasia with zolpidem." *New England Journal of Medicine 350*(9): 949–950.

Coppola, F., C. Rossi, M.L. Mancini, I. Corbelli, K. Nardi, P. Sarchielli and P. Calabresi (2008). "Language disturbances as a side effect of prophylactic treatment of migraine." *Headache: The Journal of Head and Face Pain 48*(1): 86–94.

Corbetta, M., M.J. Kincade, C. Lewis, A.Z. Snyder and A. Sapir (2005). "Neural basis and recovery of spatial attention deficits in spatial neglect." *Nature Neuroscience 8*(11): 1603–1610.

Costigan, M., J. Scholz and C.J. Woolf (2009). "Neuropathic pain: A maladaptive response of the nervous system to damage." *Annual Review of Neuroscience 32*: 1.

Crosson, B. (2012). "Thalamic mechanisms in language: A reconsideration based on recent findings and concepts." *Brain and Language 126*(1): 73–88.

Dancause, N., S. Barbay, S.B. Frost, E.J. Plautz, D. Chen, E.V. Zoubina, A.M. Stowe and R.J. Nudo (2005). "Extensive cortical rewiring after brain injury." *The Journal of Neuroscience 25*(44): 10167–10179.

Danilov, A.I., Z. Kokaia and O. Lindvall (2012). "Ectopic ependymal cells in striatum accompany neurogenesis in a rat model of stroke." *Neuroscience 214*(0): 159–170.

Darley, F.L., R.L. Keith and S. Sasanuma (1977). "The effect of alerting and tranquilizing drugs upon the performance of aphasic patients." In *Clinical aphasiology: Proceedings of the conference* (pp. 91–97). Minneapolis, MN: BRK Publishers.

Daszuta, A. (2011). "Serotonergic control of adult neurogenesis: Focus on 5-HT2C receptors. In G. Di Giovanni, E. Esposito and V. Di Matteo (Eds.), *5-HT2C receptors in the pathophysiology of CNS disease* (pp. 169–185). New York: Springer.

De Deyn, P.P., J. De Reuck, W. Deberdt, R. Vlietinck and J.-M. Orgogozo (1997). "Treatment of acute ischemic stroke with piracetam." *Stroke 28*(12): 2347–2352.

Di Filippo, M., A. Tozzi, C. Costa, V. Belcastro, M. Tantucci, B. Picconi and P. Calabresi (2008). "Plasticity and repair in the post-ischemic brain." *Neuropharmacology 55*(3): 353–362.

Dommett, E.J., E.L. Henderson, M.S. Westwell and S.A. Greenfield (2008). "Methylphenidate amplifies long-term plasticity in the hippocampus via noradrenergic mechanisms." *Learning and Memory 15*(8): 580–586.

Donaldson, Z.R. and L.J. Young (2008). "Oxytocin, vasopressin, and the neurogenetics of sociality." *Science 322*(5903): 900–904.

Downhill, J.R., Jr. and R.G. Robinson (1994). "Longitudinal assessment of depression and cognitive impairment following stroke." *Journal of Nervous and Mental Disease 182*(8): 425–431.

Edelmann, E. and V. Lessmann (2013). "Dopamine regulates intrinsic excitability thereby gating successful induction of spike timing-dependent plasticity in CA1 of the hippocampus." *Frontiers in Neuroscience 7*(25).

Enderby, P., J. Broeckx, W. Hospers, F. Schildermans and W. Deberdt (1994). "Effect of piracetam on recovery and rehabilitation after stroke: a double-blind, placebo-controlled study." *Clinical Neuropharmacology 17*(4): 320–331.

Feeney, D.M., A. Gonzalez and W.A. Law (1982). "Amphetamine, haloperidol, and experience interact to affect rate of recovery after motor cortex injury." *Science 217*(4562): 855–857.

Feeney, D.M. and V.S. Westerberg (1990). "Norepinephrine and brain damage: Alpha noradrenergic pharmacology alters functional recovery after cortical trauma." *Canadian Journal of Psychology / Revue canadienne de psychologie 44*(2): 233.

Flöel, A., M. Meinzer, R. Kirstein, S. Nijhof, M. Deppe, S. Knecht and C. Breitenstein (2011). "Short-term anomia training and electrical brain stimulation." *Stroke 42*(7): 2065–2067.

Fridman, E.A., T. Hanakawa, M. Chung, F. Hummel, R.C. Leiguarda and L.G. Cohen (2004). "Reorganization of the human ipsilesional premotor cortex after stroke." *Brain 127*(4): 747–758.

Froemke, R.C., M.M. Merzenich and C.E. Schreiner (2007). "A synaptic memory trace for cortical receptive field plasticity." *Nature 450*(7168): 425–429.

Gabaldón, L., B. Fuentes, A. Frank-García and E. Díez-Tejedor (2007). "Poststroke depression: importance of its detection and treatment." *Cerebrovascular Diseases 24*(Suppl 1): 181–188.

Ghanbarian, E. and F. Motamedi (2013). "Ventral tegmental area inactivation suppresses the expression of CA1 long term potentiation in anesthetized rat." *PLoS One 8*(3): e58844.

Gil, R. and J. Neau (1995). "Rapid aggravation of aphasia by vigabatrin." *Journal of Neurology 242*(4): 251–252.

Gill, S.K. and A.P. Leff (2013). "Dopaminergic therapy in aphasia." *Aphasiology 28*(2): 155–170.

Gillani, R.L., S.-Y. Tsai, D.G. Wallace, T.E. O'Brien, E. Arhebamen, M. Tole, M.E. Schwab and G.L. Kartje (2010). "Cognitive recovery in the aged rat after stroke and anti-Nogo-A immunotherapy." *Behavioural Brain Research 208*(2): 415–424.

Giurgea, C., M.-G. Greindl and S. Preat (1983). "Nootropic drugs and aging." *Acta Psychiatrica Belgica*.

Gladstone, D.J., C.J. Danells, A. Armesto, W.E. McIlroy, W.R. Staines, S.J. Graham, N. Herrmann, J.P. Szalai, S.E. Black, for the Subacute Therapy with Amphetamine Rehabilitation for Stroke Study Investigators (2006). "Physiotherapy coupled with dextroamphetamine for rehabilitation after hemiparetic stroke: A randomized, double-blind, placebo-controlled trial." *Stroke 37*(1): 179–185.

Goldstein, L.B. (1995). "Common drugs may influence motor recovery after stroke." *Neurology 45*(5): 865–871.

Goldstein, L.B. (1998). "Potential effects of common drugs on stroke recovery." *Archives of Neurology 55*(4): 454.

Goldstein, L.B. (2000). "Effects of amphetamines and small related molecules on recovery after stroke in animals and man." *Neuropharmacology 39*(5): 852–859.

Goldstein, L.B. and S. Bullman (1997). "Effects of dorsal noradrenergic bundle lesions on recovery after sensorimotor cortex injury." *Pharmacology Biochemistry and Behavior 58*(4): 1151–1157.

Gu, Q. (2002). "Neuromodulatory transmitter systems in the cortex and their role in cortical plasticity." *Neuroscience 111*(4): 815–835.

Gu, Q. and W. Singer (1995). "Involvement of serotonin in developmental plasticity of kitten visual cortex." *European Journal of Neuroscience 7*(6): 1146–1153.

Güngör, L., M. Terzi and M.K. Onar (2011). "Does long term use of piracetam improve speech disturbances due to ischemic cerebrovascular diseases?" *Brain and Language 117*(1): 23–27.

Gupta, S.R., A.G. Mlcoch, C. Scolaro and T. Moritz (1995). "Bromocriptine treatment of nonfluent aphasia." *Neurology 45*(12): 2170–2173.

Hackett, M.L., C.S. Anderson, A. House and J. Xia (2008). "Interventions for treating depression after stroke." *Cochrane Database of Systematic Reviews 4.*

Hackett, M.L., C.S. Anderson, A.O. House and J. Xia (2009). "Interventions for treating depression after stroke." *Stroke 40*(7): e487–e488.

Hamilton, R.H., E.G. Chrysikou and B. Coslett (2011). "Mechanisms of aphasia recovery after stroke and the role of noninvasive brain stimulation." *Brain and Language 118*(1–2): 40–50.

Harris, R.P., M. Helfand, S.H. Woolf, K.N. Lohr, C.D. Mulrow, S.M. Teutsch and D. Atkins (2001). "Current methods of the U.S. Preventive Services Task Force: A review of the process." *American Journal of Preventive Medicine 20*(3, Supplement 1): 21–35.

Heiss, W.-D., H. Karbe, G. Weber-Luxemburger, K. Herholz, J. Kessler, U. Pietrzyk and G. Pawlik (1997). "Speech-induced cerebral metabolic activation reflects recovery from aphasia." *Journal of the Neurological Sciences 145*(2): 213–217.

Hermann, D.M. and M. Chopp (2012). "Promoting brain remodelling and plasticity for stroke recovery: therapeutic promise and potential pitfalls of clinical translation." *The Lancet Neurology 11*(4): 369–380.

Hilari, K. and S. Byng (2009). "Health-related quality of life in people with severe aphasia." *International Journal of Language & Communication Disorders 44*(2): 193–205.

Hiramoto, T., Y. Ihara and Y. Watanabe (2006). "[alpha]-1 Adrenergic receptors stimulation induces the proliferation of neural progenitor cells in vitro." *Neuroscience Letters 408*(1): 25–28.

Hong, J.M., D.H. Shin, T.S. Lim, J.S. Lee and K. Huh (2012). "Galantamine administration in chronic post-stroke aphasia." *Journal of Neurology, Neurosurgery & Psychiatry 83*(7): 675–680.

Huber, W. (1999). "The role of piracetam in the treatment of acute and chronic aphasia." *Pharmacopsychiatry 32*(Suppl 1): 38–43.

Huber, W., K. Willmes, K. Poeck, B. Van Vleymen and W. Deberdt (1997). "Piracetam as an adjuvant to language therapy for aphasia: A randomized double-blind placebo-controlled pilot study." *Archives of Physical Medicine and Rehabilitation 78*(3): 245–250.

Hughes, J.D., D.H. Jacobs and K.M. Heilman (2000). "Neuropharmacology and linguistic neuroplasticity." *Brain and Language 71*(1): 96–101.

Iacoboni, M., A. Padovani, V. Di Piero and G. Lenzi (1995). "Post-stroke depression: Relationships with morphological damage and cognition over time." *The Italian Journal of Neurological Sciences 16*(3): 209–216.

Jaenisch, N., O.W. Witte and C. Frahm (2010). "Downregulation of potassium chloride cotransporter KCC2 after transient focal cerebral ischemia." *Stroke 41*(3): e151–e159.

Jambaqué, I., C. Chiron, A. Kaminska, P. Plouin and O. Dulac (1998). "Transient motor aphasia and recurrent partial seizures in a child: language recovery upon seizure control." *Journal of Child Neurology 13*(6): 296–300.

Jenkins, W.M. and M.M. Merzenich (1987). "Reorganization of neocortical representations after brain injury: A neurophysiological model of the bases of recovery from stroke." *Progress in Brain Research 71*: 249–266.

Jitsuki, S., K. Takemoto, T. Kawasaki, H. Tada, A. Takahashi, C. Becamel, A. Sano, M. Yuzaki, R.S. Zukin and E.B. Ziff (2011). "Serotonin mediates cross-modal reorganization of cortical circuits." *Neuron 69*(4): 780–792.

Johnson, J.W. and S.E. Kotermanski (2006). "Mechanism of action of memantine." *Current Opinion in Pharmacology 6*(1): 61–67.

Jordaan, B., D. Oliver, I. Dormehl and N. Hugo (1996). "Cerebral blood flow effects of piracetam, pentifylline, and nicotinic acid in the baboon model compared with the known effect of acetazolamide." *Arzneimittel-Forschung 46*(9): 844–847.

Jorge, R.E., L. Acion, D. Moser, H.P. Adams Jr. and R.G. Robinson (2010). "Escitalopram and enhancement of cognitive recovery following stroke." *Archives of General Psychiatry 67*(2): 187.

Kahle, M.P. and G.J. Bix (2013). "Neuronal restoration following ischemic stroke influences, barriers, and therapeutic potential." *Neurorehabilitation and Neural Repair 27*(5): 469–478.

Kang, E.K., Y.K. Kim, H.M. Sohn, L.G. Cohen and N.-J. Paik (2011). "Improved picture naming in aphasia patients treated with cathodal tDCS to inhibit the right Broca's homologue area." *Restorative Neurology and Neuroscience 29*(3): 141–152.

Karbe, H., A. Thiel, G. Weber-Luxemburger, K. Herholz, J. Kessler and W.-D. Heiss (1998). "Brain plasticity in poststroke aphasia: What is the contribution of the right hemisphere?" *Brain and Language 64*(2): 215–230.

Kessler, J., A. Thiel, H. Karbe and W. Heiss (2000). "Piracetam improves activated blood flow and facilitates rehabilitation of poststroke aphasic patients." *Stroke 31*(9): 2112–2116.

Kilgard, M.P. and M.M. Merzenich (1998). "Cortical map reorganization enabled by nucleus basalis activity." *Science 279*(5357): 1714–1718.

Kimura, M., R.G. Robinson and J.T. Kosier (2000). "Treatment of cognitive impairment after poststroke depression: A double-blind treatment trial." *Stroke 31*(7): 1482–1486.

Korchounov, A. and U. Ziemann (2011). "Neuromodulatory neurotransmitters influence LTP-like plasticity in human cortex: A pharmaco-TMS study." *Neuropsychopharmacology 36*(9): 1894–1902.

Larson, E.B. and F.S. Zollman (2010). "The effect of sleep medications on cognitive recovery from traumatic brain injury." *Journal of Head Trauma Rehabilitation 25*(1): 61–67.

Laska, A.C., B. Mårtensson, T. Kahan, M. von Arbin and V. Murray (2007). "Recognition of depression in aphasic stroke patients." *Cerebrovascular Diseases 24*(1): 74–79.

Laska, A.C., M. Von Arbin, T. Kahan, A. Hellblom and V. Murray (2005). "Long-term antidepressant treatment with moclobemide for aphasia in acute stroke patients: A randomised, double-blind, placebo-controlled study." *Cerebrovascular Diseases 19*(2): 125–132.

Leemann, B., M. Laganaro, D. Chetelat-Mabillard and A. Schnider (2011). "Crossover trial of subacute computerized aphasia therapy for anomia with the addition of either levodopa or placebo." *Neurorehabilitation and Neural Repair 25*(1): 43–47.

Lees, J.S., E.S. Sena, K.J. Egan, A. Antonic, S.A. Koblar, D.W. Howells and M.R. Macleod (2012). "Stem cell-based therapy for experimental stroke: A systematic review and meta-analysis." *International Journal of Stroke 7*(7): 582–588.

Li, W.L., H.H. Cai, B. Wang, L. Chen, Q.G. Zhou, C.X. Luo, N. Liu, X.S. Ding and D.Y. Zhu (2009). "Chronic fluoxetine treatment improves ischemia-induced spatial cognitive deficits through increasing hippocampal neurogenesis after stroke." *Journal of Neuroscience Research 87*(1): 112–122.

Lichtenwalner, R.J. and J.M. Parent (2005). "Adult neurogenesis and the ischemic forebrain." *Journal of Cerebral Blood Flow & Metabolism 26*(1): 1–20.

Linn, L. (1947). "Sodium amytal in treatment of aphasia." *Archives of Neurology and Psychiatry 58*(3): 357.

Lipton, S.A. (2006). "Paradigm shift in neuroprotection by NMDA receptor blockade: Memantine and beyond." *Nature Reviews. Drug Discovery. 5*(2): 160–170.

Lloyd, S.A., Z.R. Balest, F.S. Corotto and R.J. Smeyne (2010). "Cocaine selectively increases proliferation in the adult murine hippocampus." *Neuroscience Letters 485*(2): 112–116.

Lossius, M., O. Rønning, P. Mowinckel and L. Gjerstad (2002). "Incidence and predictors for post-stroke epilepsy. A prospective controlled trial. The Akershus stroke study." *European Journal of Neurology 9*(4): 365–368.

Malykh, A.G. and M.R. Sadaie (2010). "Piracetam and piracetam-like drugs." *Drugs 70*(3): 287–312.

Martinowich, K. and B. Lu (2007). "Interaction between BDNF and serotonin: Role in mood disorders." *Neuropsychopharmacology 33*(1): 73–83.

McNeil, M., P. Doyle, K. Spencer, A.J. Goda, D. Flores and S. Small (1997). "A double-blind, placebo-controlled study of pharmacological and behavioural treatment of lexical-semantic deficits in aphasia." *Aphasiology 11*(4–5): 385–400.

Mikami, K., R.E. Jorge, D.J. Moser, S. Arndt, M. Jang, A. Solodkin, S.L. Small, P. Fonzetti, M.T. Hegel and R.G. Robinson (2011). "Increased frequency of first-episode poststroke depression after discontinuation of escitalopram." *Stroke 42*(11): 3281–3283.

Mikami, K., R.E. Jorge, D.J. Moser, S. Arndt, M. Jang, A. Solodkin, S.L. Small, P. Fonzetti, M.T. Hegel and R.G. Robinson (2013). "Prevention of poststroke apathy using escitalopram or problem-solving therapy." *American Journal of Geriatric Psychiatry 21*(9): 855–862.

Monti, A., R. Ferrucci, M. Fumagalli, F. Mameli, F. Cogiamanian, G. Ardolino and A. Priori (2012). "Transcranial direct current stimulation (tDCS) and language." *Journal of Neurology, Neurosurgery & Psychiatry 84*(8): 832–842.

Morris, P., B. Raphael and R.G. Robinson (1992). "Clinical depression is associated with impaired recovery from stroke." *Medical Journal of Australia 157*(4): 239–242.

Morris, P.L., R.G. Robinson, M. De Carvalho, P. Albert, J.C. Wells, J.F. Samuels, D. Eden-Fetzer and T.R. Price (1996). "Lesion characteristics and depressed mood in the stroke data bank study." *Journal of Neuropsychiatry and Clinical Neurosciences 8*(2): 153–159.

Mula, M., M.R. Trimble, P. Thompson and J.W. Sander (2003). "Topiramate and word-finding difficulties in patients with epilepsy." *Neurology 60*(7): 1104–1107.

Müller, W., G. Eckert and A. Eckert (1999). "Piracetam: Novelty in a unique mode of action." *Pharmacopsychiatry 32*(Suppl 1): 2–9.

Murphy, T.H. and D. Corbett (2009). "Plasticity during stroke recovery: From synapse to behaviour." *Nature Reviews Neuroscience 10*(12): 861–872.

Narushima, K., K.-L. Chan, J.T. Kosier and R.G. Robinson (2003). "Does cognitive recovery after treatment of poststroke depression last? A 2-year follow-up of cognitive function associated with poststroke depression." *American Journal of Psychiatry 160*(6): 1157–1162.

Nudo, R. and K. Friel (1998). "Cortical plasticity after stroke: implications for rehabilitation." *Revue Neurologique 155*(9): 713–717.

Nudo, R.J., B.M. Wise, F. SiFuentes and G.W. Milliken (1996). "Neural substrates for the effects of rehabilitative training on motor recovery after ischemic infarct." *Science 272*(5269): 1791–1794.

Olsen, T.S. (2001). "Post-stroke epilepsy." *Current Atherosclerosis Reports 3*: 340–344.

Orgogozo, J.-M. (1999). "Piracetam in the treatment of acute stroke." *Pharmacopsychiatry 32*(Suppl 1): 25–32.

Overman, J.J., A.N. Clarkson, I.B. Wanner, W.T. Overman, I. Eckstein, J.L. Maguire, I.D. Dinov, A.W. Toga and S.T. Carmichael (2012). "A role for ephrin-A5 in axonal sprouting, recovery, and activity-dependent plasticity after stroke." *Proceedings of the National Academy of Sciences 109*(33): E2230–E2239.

Papadopoulos, C.M., S.-Y. Tsai, V. Guillen, J. Ortega, G.L. Kartje and W.A. Wolf (2009). "Motor recovery and axonal plasticity with short-term amphetamine after stroke." *Stroke 40*(1): 294–302.

Pashek, G.V. and D.L. Bachman (2003). "Cognitive, linguistic and motor speech effects of donepezil hydrochloride in a patient with stroke-related aphasia and apraxia of speech." *Brain and Language 87*(1): 179–180.

Pedersen, P.M., H. Stig Jørgensen, H. Nakayama, H.O. Raaschou and T.S. Olsen (1995). "Aphasia in acute stroke: Incidence, determinants, and recovery." *Annals of Neurology 38*(4): 659–666.

Platz, T., I. Kim, U. Engel, C. Pinkowski, C. Eickhof and M. Kutzner (2005). "Amphetamine fails to facilitate motor performance and to enhance motor recovery among stroke patients with mild arm paresis: interim analysis and termination of a double blind, randomised, placebo-controlled trial." *Restorative Neurology and Neuroscience 23*: 271–280.

Ploughman, M., V. Windle, C.L. MacLellan, N. White, J.J. Doré and D. Corbett (2009). "Brain-derived neurotrophic factor contributes to recovery of skilled reaching after focal ischemia in rats." *Stroke 40*(4): 1490–1495.

Plow, E.B., J.R. Carey, R.J. Nudo and A. Pascual-Leone (2009). "Invasive cortical stimulation to promote recovery of function after stroke: A critical appraisal." *Stroke 40*(5): 1926–1931.

Pomara, N., B.R. Ott, E. Peskind and E.M. Resnick (2007). "Memantine treatment of cognitive symptoms in mild to moderate Alzheimer disease: Secondary analyses from a placebo-controlled randomized trial." *Alzheimer Disease and Associated Disorders 21*(1): 60–64.

Porch, B.E. and D.M. Feeney (1986). *Effects of antihypertensive drugs on recovery from aphasia.* Minneapolis, MN: BRK Publishers.

Rajashekaran, P., K. Pai, R. Thunga and B. Unnikrishnan (2013). "Post-stroke depression and lesion location: A hospital based cross-sectional study." *Indian Journal of Psychiatry 55*(4): 343.

Ramic, M., A.J. Emerick, M.R. Bollnow, T.E. O'Brien, S.-Y. Tsai and G.L. Kartje (2006). "Axonal plasticity is associated with motor recovery following amphetamine treatment combined with rehabilitation after brain injury in the adult rat." *Brain Research 1111*(1): 176–186.

Rasmussen, R., K. Overgaard, E. Hildebrandt-Eriksen and G. Boysen (2006). "d-Amphetamine improves cognitive deficits and physical therapy promotes fine motor rehabilitation in a rat embolic stroke model." *Acta Neurologica Scandinavica 113*(3): 189–198.

Rasmusson, D. (2000). "The role of acetylcholine in cortical synaptic plasticity." *Behavioural Brain Research 115*(2): 205–218.

Robinson, R.G. (1998). *The clinical neuropsychiatry of stroke: Cognitive, behavioral and emotional disorders following vascular brain injury.* Cambridge, England, Cambridge University Press.

Robinson, R.G., R.E. Jorge, D.J. Moser, L. Acion, A. Solodkin, S.L. Small, P. Fonzetti, M. Hegel and S. Arndt (2008). "Escitalopram and problem-solving therapy for prevention of poststroke depression." *Journal of the American Medical Association 299*(20): 2391–2400.

Robinson, R.G., W.J. Shoemaker and M. Schlumpf (1980). "Time course of changes in catecholamines following right hemispheric cerebral infarction in the rat." *Brain Research 181*(1): 202–208.

Robinson, R.G., W.J. Shoemaker, M. Schlumpf, T. Valk and F.E. Bloom (1975). "Effect of experimental cerebral infarction in rat brain on catecholamines and behaviour." *Nature 255*(5506): 332–334.

Rogers, S., M. Farlow, R. Doody, R. Mohs and L. Friedhoff (1998). "A 24-week, double-blind, placebo-controlled trial of donepezil in patients with Alzheimer's disease." *Neurology 50*(1): 136–145.

Rösser, N., P. Heuschmann, H. Wersching, C. Breitenstein, S. Knecht and A. Flöel (2008). "Levodopa improves procedural motor learning in chronic stroke patients." *Archives of Physical Medicine and Rehabilitation 89*(9): 1633–1641.

Sabe, L., F. Salvarezza, A.G. Cuerva, R. Leiguarda and S. Starkstein (1995). "A randomized, double-blind, placebocontrolled study of bromocriptine in nonfluent aphasia." *Neurology 45*(12): 2272–2274.

Saxton, J., R.K. Hofbauer, M. Woodward, N.L. Gilchrist, F. Potocnik, H.-A. Hsu, M.L. Miller, V. Pejović, S.M. Graham and J.L. Perhach (2012). "Memantine and functional communication in Alzheimer's disease: Results of a 12-week, international, randomized clinical trial." *Journal of Alzheimer's Disease 28*(1): 109–118.

Schäbitz, W.-R., T. Steigleder, C.M. Cooper-Kuhn, S. Schwab, C. Sommer, A. Schneider and H.G. Kuhn (2007). "Intravenous brain-derived neurotrophic factor enhances poststroke sensorimotor recovery and stimulates neurogenesis." *Stroke 38*(7): 2165–2172.

Scheidtmann, K., W. Fries, F. Müller and E. Koenig (2001). "Effect of levodopa in combination with physiotherapy on functional motor recovery after stroke: a prospective, randomised, double-blind study." *The Lancet 358*(9284): 787–790.

Schiff, N.D. (2010). "Recovery of consciousness after brain injury: a mesocircuit hypothesis." *Trends in Neurosciences 33*(1): 1–9.

Schultz, W. (2002). "Getting formal with dopamine and reward." *Neuron 36*(2): 241–263.

Seniów, J., M. Litwin, T. Litwin, M. Leśniak and A. Członkowska (2009). "New approach to the rehabilitation of post-stroke focal cognitive syndrome: Effect of levodopa combined with speech and language therapy on functional recovery from aphasia." *Journal of the Neurological Sciences 283*(1–2): 214–218.

Skidmore, E.R., E.M. Whyte, M.B. Holm, J.T. Becker, M.A. Butters, M.A. Dew, M.C. Munin and E.J. Lenze (2010). "Cognitive and affective predictors of rehabilitation participation after stroke." *Archives of Physical Medicine and Rehabilitation 91*(2): 203–207.

Small, S.L. (1994). "Pharmacotherapy of aphasia. A critical review." *Stroke 25*(6): 1282–1289.

Smith, H.K. and F.N. Gavins (2012). "The potential of stem cell therapy for stroke: Is PISCES the sign?" *The FASEB Journal 26*(6): 2239–2252.

So, E., J. Annegers, W. Hauser, P. O'Brien and J. Whisnant (1996). "Population-based study of seizure disorders after cerebral infarction." *Neurology 46*(2): 350–355.

Sonde, L. and J. Lökk (2007). "Effects of amphetamine and/or l-dopa and physiotherapy after stroke; a blinded randomized study." *Acta Neurologica Scandinavica 115*(1): 55–59.

Spiegel, A., S. Shivtiel, A. Kalinkovich, A. Ludin, N. Netzer, P. Goichberg, Y. Azaria, I. Resnick, I. Hardan, H. Ben-Hur, A. Nagler, M. Rubinstein and T. Lapidot (2007). "Catecholaminergic neurotransmitters regulate migration and repopulation of immature human CD34+ cells through Wnt signaling." *Nature Immunology 8*(10): 1123–1131.

Sprigg, N., M.R. Willmot, L.J. Gray, A. Sunderland, V. Pomeroy, M. Walker and P.M.W. Bath (2007). "Amphetamine increases blood pressure and heart rate but has no effect on motor recovery or cerebral haemodynamics in ischaemic stroke: A randomized controlled trial (ISRCTN 36285333)." *Jounral of Human Hypertension 21*(8): 616–624.

Starkstein, S.E., J.B. Bryer, M.L. Berthier, B. Cohen, T.R. Price and R.G. Robinson (1991). "Depression after stroke: The importance of cerebral hemisphere asymmetries." *Journal of Neuropsychiatry and Clinical Neuroscience 3*(3): 276–285.

Starkstein, S.E. and R.G. Robinson (1989). "Affective disorders and cerebral vascular disease." *British Journal of Psychiatry 154*: 170–182.

Szaflarski, J.P., J.B. Allendorfer, C. Banks, J. Vannest and S.K. Holland (2013). "Recovered vs. not-recovered from post-stroke aphasia: The contributions from the dominant and non-dominant hemispheres." *Restorative Neurology and Neuroscience 31*(4): 347–360.

Tanaka, Y., M. Albert, S. Aketa, K. Hujita, E. Noda, M. Takashima, C. Nonaka, E. Yokoyama and M. Tanaka (2004). *Serotonergic therapy for fluent aphasia.* Philadelphia: Lippencott Williams and Wilkins.

Tanaka, Y., M. Miyazaki and M.L. Albert (1997). "Effects of increased cholinergic activity on naming in aphasia." *The Lancet 350*(9071): 116–117.

Tariot, P.N., M.R. Farlow, G.T. Grossberg, S.M. Graham, S. McDonald, I. Gergel and Metamine Study Group (2004). "Memantine treatment in patients with moderate to severe Alzheimer disease already receiving donepezil: A randomized controlled trial." *Jounral of the American Medical Association 291*(3): 317–324.

Thiel, A., B. Schumacher, K. Wienhard, S. Gairing, L.W. Kracht, R. Wagner, W.F. Haupt and W.-D. Heiss (2006). "Direct demonstration of transcallosal disinhibition in language networks." *Jounral of Cerebral Blood Flow and Metabolism 26*(9): 1122–1127.

Thomas, P., C. Rascle, B. Mastain, M. Maron and G. Vaiva (1997). "Test for catatonia with zolpidem." *The Lancet 349*(9053): 702.

Tsai, S.-Y., T.M. Markus, E.M. Andrews, J.L. Cheatwood, A.J. Emerick, A.K. Mir, M.E. Schwab and G.L. Kartje (2007). "Intrathecal treatment with anti-Nogo-A antibody improves functional recovery in adult rats after stroke." *Experimental Brain Research 182*(2): 261–266.

Tsai, S.-Y., C.M. Papadopoulos, M.E. Schwab and G.L. Kartje (2011). "Delayed anti-Nogo-A therapy improves function after chronic stroke in adult rats." *Stroke 42*(1): 186–190.

Tsikunov, S.G. and S.G. Belokoskova (2007). "Psychophysiological analysis of the influence of vasopressin on speech in patients with post-stroke aphasias." *Spanish Journal of Psychology 10*(1): 178–188.

Tsz-Ming, C. and D. Kaufer (2001). "Effects of donepezil on aphasia, agnosia, and apraxia in patients with cerebrovascular lesions." *Jounral of Neuropsychiatry and Clinical Neurosciences 13*: 140.

Ueno, Y., M. Chopp, L. Zhang, B. Buller, Z. Liu, N.L. Lehman, X.S. Liu, Y. Zhang, C. Roberts and Z.G. Zhang (2012). "Axonal outgrowth and dendritic plasticity in the cortical peri-infarct area after experimental stroke." *Stroke 43*(8): 2221–2228.

van de Weg, F.B., D.J. Kuik and G.J. Lankhorst (1999). "Post-stroke depression and functional outcome: A cohort study investigating the influence of depression on functional recovery from stroke." *Clinical Rehabilitation 13*(3): 268–272.

Vernon, M.W. and E.M. Sorkin (1991). "Piracetam." *Drugs and Aging 1*(1): 17–35.

Vetencourt, J.F.M., E. Tiraboschi, M. Spolidoro, E. Castrén and L. Maffei (2011). "Serotonin triggers a transient epigenetic mechanism that reinstates adult visual cortex plasticity in rats." *European Journal of Neuroscience 33*(1): 49–57.

Volbracht, C., J. Van Beek, C. Zhu, K. Blomgren and M. Leist (2006). "Neuroprotective properties of memantine in different in vitro and in vivo models of excitotoxicity." *European Journal of Neuroscience 23*(10): 2611–2622.

Wade, D.T., R.L. Hewer, R.M. David and P. M. Enderby (1986). "Aphasia after stroke: Natural history and associated deficits." *Journal of Neurology, Neurosurgery & Psychiatry 49*(1): 11–16.

Waldowski, K., J. Seniów, M. Leśniak, S. Iwański and A. Członkowska (2012). "Effect of low-frequency repetitive transcranial magnetic stimulation on naming abilities in early-stroke aphasic patients: A prospective, randomized, double-blind sham-controlled study." *The Scientific World Journal 2012*.

Walker-Batson, D., S. Curtis, R. Natarajan, J. Ford, N. Dronkers, E. Salmeron, J. Lai and D.H. Unwin (2001). "A double-blind, placebo-controlled study of the use of amphetamine in the treatment of aphasia." *Stroke 32*(9): 2093–2098.

Whiting, E., H.J. Chenery, J. Chalk, D.A. Copland, B. Angrist, J. Corwin, B. Bartlik, T. Cooper, S. Asghar and V. Tanay (2007). "Dexamphetamine boosts naming treatment effects in chronic aphasia." *Journal of the International Neuropsychological Society 13*(6): 972.

Wolf, M., S. Mangiavacchi and X. Sun (2003). "Mechanisms by which dopamine receptors may influence synaptic plasticity." *Annals of the New York Academy of Sciences 1003*: 241–249.

Wong, I.C. and S.D. Lhatoo (2000). "Adverse reactions to new anticonvulsant drugs." *Drug Safety 23*(1): 35–56.

Xerri, C., M.M. Merzenich, B.E. Peterson and W. Jenkins (1998). "Plasticity of primary somatosensory cortex paralleling sensorimotor skill recovery from stroke in adult monkeys." *Journal of Neurophysiology 79*(4): 2119–2148.

Yao, C., A. Williams, J. Hartings, X. Lu, F. Tortella and J. Dave (2005). "Down-regulation of the sodium channel Na(v)1.1 alpha-subunit following focal ischemic brain injury in rats: In situ hybridization and immuno-histochemical analysis." *Life Sciences 77*(10): 1116–1129.

You, D.S., D.-Y. Kim, M.H. Chun, S.E. Jung and S.J. Park (2011). "Cathodal transcranial direct current stimulation of the right Wernicke's area improves comprehension in subacute stroke patients." *Brain and Language 119*(1): 1–5.

22

TRANSCRANIAL DIRECT CURRENT STIMULATION AND APHASIA THERAPY POST STROKE

Jenny Crinion

Introduction

Being able to communicate is something most of us take for granted. But when a person has aphasia (speech and language disorder), most commonly caused by stroke, this becomes a source of profound frustration and anxiety for them and their families. While some people do recover, many do not. Centralized stroke centers that specialize in stroke diagnosis and care along with rapidly rendering appropriate treatment have significantly improved mortality and morbidity of stroke. For example, mortality from stroke in the UK has decreased from 21% in 1999 to 12% in 2008, and in the USA from 2000 to 2010 the relative rate of stroke death fell by 35.8% and the actual number of stroke deaths declined by 22.8% (Go et al., 2014). However, while the rates of death attributable to stroke have declined, the burden of the disease remains high. Stroke prevalence has been increasing, meaning that more people are surviving with long-standing disability. Speech and language disorders (aphasia) are the most feared outcome by patients at risk of stroke (Samsa et al., 1998). Aphasia is an unpleasant disorder, with a high social cost (Lam and Wodchis, 2010). Patients with impoverished speech are more likely to withdraw socially and suffer from depression (Northcott and Hilari, 2011). Indeed, aphasia is the second most common major impairment after stroke, with a prevalence of ~250,000 in the UK and 1 million in the USA.

As the prevalence of post-stroke aphasia is increasing, so will the demand for already limited speech and language therapy (SALT). SALT is effective at treating aphasia. The recent Cochrane review (Brady et al., 2012) concluded, "Significant differences [SALT vs. no SALT] were evident in measures of spoken language." Treatment of aphasia can also improve depression (Ayerbe et al., 2011). Importantly, therapy-driven gains can be made at any point after stroke, not just in the early phase (Moss and Nicholas, 2006). As such, SALT works (Brady et al., 2012), but the big issue is making sure aphasic patients with speech impairments have access to the correct therapies. Indeed aphasia may respond to therapy many months and years after the stroke occurs, but a very large dose is required to improve. Meta-analyses show that aphasic patients need to complete around 100 hours of behavioral therapy to significantly improve their real-world communicative outcomes (Bhogal et al., 2003).

Unfortunately, provision of specialist therapy (SALT) is far below that needed to provide optimal rehabilitation (Code and Heron, 2003), and the majority of patients do not get the correct dose (Code, 2003; Code and Heron, 2003). Depressingly, most patients in the UK get around 10 hours total therapy input from the National Health Service (Code, 2003). This is very disabling and frustrating for patients and their families and can impair patient's participation and compliance with rehabilitation programs for associated disabilities (Hilari, 2011; Hilari et al., 2012; Jette et al., 2005). This is unacceptable and healthcare commissioners need to address this growing unmet need urgently. However, it is not economically feasible to solve this unmet need by massively increasing the amount of SALT face-to-face time.

To address how the treatment of aphasia might be made more effective, researchers are now investigating using an emerging, safe brain stimulation method called transcranial direct current stimulation (tDCS). The aim is to test whether tDCS paired with SALT is an effective and acceptable method to boost patients' recovery after aphasic stroke. Research to date has primarily assessed whether aphasic patients can improve their spoken language function with targeted and sustained computer-delivered practice (Palmer et al., 2012) in combination with tDCS brain stimulation technology. In this chapter I will outline some of the key concepts that I think readers may want to keep in mind when following this area of fast developing research and its potential application to aphasia treatment. Firstly I will highlight (1) current understanding of mechanisms of tDCS and (2) how it can be applied/used in patient populations. Then I will review (3) tDCS as a novel method for enhancing aphasia (post-stroke) treatment effects. Here I will focus on the latest group studies (minimum six patients) that have used tDCS as an adjunct to SALT in aphasic stroke patients. I divide this section into studies of (i) chronic aphasia—(a) stimulating the perilesional left hemisphere and (b) stimulating the right hemisphere—and (ii) sub-acute aphasia. I then finish with (4) future considerations for brain stimulation as a novel home-therapeutic intervention in aphasia treatment.

1   TDCS: The Mechanisms

To use tDCS in aphasia, it is important to understand not only how tDCS functions but also the brain mechanisms being studied and the features of the language function of interest. tDCS is the most used and best-known method of transcranial electrical stimulation (tES). tDCS involves the non-invasive application of continuous (~10 to 20 minutes) weak (1–2 mA) electrical currents directly to the scalp through a pair of electrodes (anodal or cathodal) to target brain regions (Nitsche and Paulus, 2000; Priori et al., 1998). As a result, tDCS induces a subthreshold polarization of cortical neurons in the target brain regions (e.g., language network) that is too weak to generate an action potential but instead modulates the neuronal response threshold so that it can be defined as subthreshold stimulation. However, by changing the intrinsic neuronal excitability, tDCS can induce changes in the resting membrane potential and the postsynaptic activity of cortical neurons. This, in turn, can alter the spontaneous firing rate of neurons and modulate their response to afferent signals (Bindman et al., 1962; Bindman et al., 1964; Bindman et al., 1979; Creutzfeldt et al., 1962), leading to changes in synaptic efficacy, which, in turn, influences the response of the brain network engaged during the task and correlates with a change in behavior (i.e., task performance). In this sense, it is interpreted that tDCS primes the behavioral system by increasing/decreasing cortical excitability, promoting mechanisms of long-term potentiation and long-term depression (LTP/LTD) and producing corresponding effects in the task-engaged brain networks. If we are to induce long-term consolidation or the re-learning of information (a goal of aphasia therapy; Liebetanz et al., 2002), a neuromodulatory method that has features of LTP-like processes is attractive.

The hypotheses concerning the application of tDCS in language functioning are that, depending on the polarity of the stimulation, tDCS can increase or decrease cortical excitability in the stimulated and task-engaged brain regions and facilitate or inhibit language function/behavior accordingly, thereby enabling the investigation of the causal relationships between brain activity and behavior by means of neural modulation. In the motor system it has been shown that anodal tDCS induces membrane depolarization during task execution that, in turn, facilitates motor function both for the duration of the stimulation (e.g., 20 minutes) with the gains persisting for at least the same amount of time afterwards, while cathodal tDCS induces membrane hyperpolarization and inhibition of task performance (Liebetanz et al., 2002; Nitsche et al., 2003a; Nitsche et al., 2003b; Nitsche et al., 2005). However, in many cognitive neuroscience experiments, the stimulation of non-motor areas, including language cortices, has led to the observation that behavioral effects are often not unequivocal, with anodal stimulation usually inducing facilitation and cathodal stimulation inducing a range of (if any) effects (see Jacobson et al., 2012, for a comprehensive review). Because tDCS as a neuromodulator does not induce neuronal firing directly, unlike TMS, it will only induce the firing of neurons that are near threshold. That is, neurons that are not influenced by the task subjects are engaged in during tDCS are less likely to discharge. Therefore, while the spatial and temporal resolution of the tDCS effects are reduced compared with those of TMS, it may be overcome by considering the state of the active task-engaged brain network in the vicinity of the stimulating tDCS electrodes. See Miniussi (Miniussi and Ruzzoli, 2013) for an excellent review of the mutual interactions between non-invasive brain stimulation methods (NIBS), including tDCS, and brain activity and an updated and precise perspective on the theoretical frameworks of NIBS and their impact on cognitive neuroscience. Miniussi proposes that given NIBS necessarily involves the relatively indiscriminate activation of large numbers of neurons one can interpret its impact on a neural system as modulation of neural activity that changes the relation between noise and signal.

From a language standpoint, what this means is that tDCS-induced effects are more likely to be sensitive to the state of the brain-language network (language signal within a region) in the vicinity of the stimulating electrode that is active at that moment during stimulation. Thus, the polarization of neurons in combination with ongoing synaptic input can be contextualized in a framework of synaptic co-activation akin to Hebbian-like plasticity mechanisms. In this sense, tDCS neuromodulation will interact with the level of excitation of the brain system, driven by the behavioral task to shape the final result. The combination of anodal tDCS with a language task execution is like the co-activation of a specific language network. My own previous functional magnetic resonance neuroimaging (fMRI) research has shown that left frontal anodal tDCS in healthy older subjects delivered during a phonemically cued naming task, results in on-line faster naming reaction times (RT) and focal neural priming in Broca's area (Holland et al., 2011). Furthermore, faster naming responses correlated with decreased BOLD signal in Broca's area. Likewise, anodal tDCS by depolarizing neurons nearer to threshold can reduce the amount of excitatory input required to produce a naming response. Thus, we have a situation in which there is increased excitability (manifest as a faster naming response time) accompanied by reduced BOLD (less synaptic input for a given output; i.e., naming). The reduction of BOLD signal in Broca's area may be analogous to the neural priming effects seen in behavioral priming experiments. This suggests that anodal tDCS concurrent with naming may facilitate responses through a regionally specific neuronal adaptation mechanism in Broca's area. Similar results have been observed by Antal and colleagues (Antal et al., 2011) where anodal stimulation of motor cortex reduced supplementary motor area (SMA) activation during a finger-thumb motor skill task.

In our fMRI study not all regions in the vicinity of the stimulating electrode were affected by tDCS-only activation in left Broca's area (i.e., the region that was significantly engaged by the phonemically cued naming task). Anodal tDCS had no detectable impact on neural response in left precentral gyrus and left anterior insula, regions also directly beneath the anode electrode. This indicated that tDCS can have a regionally specific rather than global cortical facilitation effect and that anodal tDCS effects were maximal in regions directly associated with the task manipulation. In this study, anodal tDCS delivered to left frontal regions during a cued-naming task facilitated activation of Broca's area and sped up subjects' word retrieval performance, but had no effect on other brain regions that were also in the vicinity of the stimulating electrode, as the task chosen did not selectively engage these nearby regions. This finding is consistent with Miniussi's signal-to-noise ratio interpretation of tDCS effects—where anodal tDCS boosted task-relevant neural signal in Broca's area, relative to unrelated neural noise within the brain network.

The presentation of a concurrent task during anodal tDCS, as reported here, may be critical to maximally facilitate task-relevant depolarization of membranes so that less synaptic activity is needed to reach a threshold, thereby aiding synaptic modification and resulting in a decreased BOLD response. While the sole increase in excitability induced by anodal tDCS (e.g., increased neuronal firing rates, which is likely chaotic; Bindman et al., 1964) may not be sufficient to induce long-term changes, an additional synaptic activation (by co-stimulation or language training) may lead to synapse specificity as a source for long-term plasticity. For example, synapses within the motor cortex are functionally potentiated and structurally stabilized during motor training (Rioult-Pedotti et al., 1998; Rioult-Pedotti et al., 2000; Xu et al., 2009), a process that may be catalyzed when anodal tDCS is applied to a cortical region involved in this process. From an aphasia treatment point of view this means that anodal tDCS–induced facilitatory effects are more likely when stimulation is delivered during aphasia treatment and the stimulating electrode is positioned over the patient's residual cortex actively engaged by the treatment task. This approach should induce immediate on-line improvement in the patient's language performance (e.g., if delivered during anomia treatment the patients' naming accuracy and reaction time will improve). Then, when tDCS is paired with aphasia treatment on multiple occasions, this will lead to a longer-term boost (i.e., consolidation in rehabilitation gains). Our fMRI data supports the importance of Broca's area in naming and as a candidate site for tDCS in neurorehabilitation of anomic brain-damaged patients.

2 TDCS: Application/Usability

tDCS technology is easy to use, relatively inexpensive and well suited to on-line application (i.e., brain stimulation concurrent with behavioral intervention). As highlighted earlier (Holland et al., 2011), inferior frontal cortex (Broca's area) can be easily and comfortably targeted with tDCS during speech production. At the start of stimulation, most subjects will perceive a slight itching sensation under the electrodes as the current is ramped up (slower ramping, e.g., 15 seconds to reach 2 mA, produces less pronounced sensations), which then quickly fades in most cases. In contrast, transcranial magnetic stimulation (TMS) and in particular repetitive TMS of the same region, can inadvertently stimulate the facial nerve, causing facial twitches, or even the trigeminal nerve, resulting in painful sensations making certain on-line tasks, such as spoken picture naming, very difficult. Therefore, for a treatment study that requires multiple sessions, tDCS may be a more suitable option. Figure 22.1 illustrates the neuroimaging data (structural and functional) supporting the setup for anodal tDCS delivered to left inferior frontal gyrus (Broca's area) of an aphasic patient during anomia treatment delivered in my lab. The patient whose stroke anatomically spared Broca's area had 20 minutes of anodal tDCS delivered concurrently with anomia treatment three times a week for 6 weeks.

For research purposes it is also easier to conduct placebo (sham) stimulation-controlled studies with tDCS than TMS, because, with the exception of a slight itching sensation, when the current is ramped up subjects rarely experience sensations related to the treatment (Gandiga et al., 2006). In an active sham tDCS condition the current is ramped up slowly in the same manner as the 'real' tDCS condition to mirror the initial sensations but when the target stimulation intensity is reached (e.g., 2 mA) the current is turned off. In addition, a small current pulse can be set to occur every 550 ms instead of the stimulation current. This has no therapeutic effect but is to keep the electrodes warm throughout the experiment, mirroring the local electrode heating found with

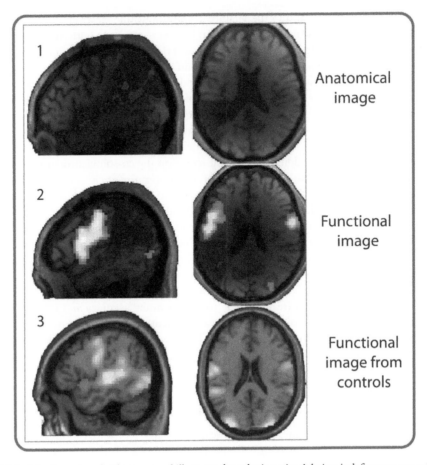

Figure 22.1 Naming network. The top panel illustrates the aphasic patient's lesion in left temporo-parietal cortices. The middle panel illustrates the left perilesional network that the same patient activated during an fMRI study of confrontation naming. The contrast was naming nouns > rest, $p = 0.001$ uncorrected. The last panel illustrates the language network activated by a group of age-matched healthy older controls (n = 24) completing the same task, $p = 0.05$ corrected. Anodal tDCS was delivered to the patient's structurally intact left inferior frontal gyrus, which was activated by the naming task to boost anomia treatment outcomes.

'real' tDCS. Therefore, reliable effects of stimulation in the absence of any confounding "placebo effects" (i.e., the influence of participants' expectation of an effect on the observed results) may be achieved using tDCS.

Patient Recruitment and Inclusion/Exclusion Criteria

There are no known serious risks of tDCS. No side effects have been observed in previous studies using these treatments/techniques in the limited number of studies of chronic aphasic stroke patients to date (see Tables 22.1 and 22.2). Large-scale cohort testing from different research centers have reported that the most common adverse sensation is a slight itching sensation under the electrode and seldom-occurring headache, fatigue, and nausea (see Nitsche et al., 2008, Table 1; Poreisz et al., 2007). Although reports of skin burns associated with tDCS have been reported (Frank et al., 2011; Lagopoulos and Degabriele, 2008; Palm et al., 2008), these occurred in the context of extending stimulation periods (30 minutes), drying of electro-conductive gel, abraded skin surface and the use of tap water to soak the sponge sheaths, respectively. When conventional tDCS protocols were employed (i.e., 1–2 mA stimulation for up to 20 minutes), using optimized safety protocols, significant adverse effects, such as burning of the skin (Dundas et al., 2007; Loo et al., 2011; Minhas et al., 2010) or heating of the electrodes and scalp surface (Datta et al., 2009; Nitsche and Paulus, 2000; Nitsche and Paulus, 2001) was avoided. Under these protocol guidelines, tDCS may be considered safe (Nitsche et al., 2003b). However, tDCS must not be used on patients with a pacemaker or brain stimulator as it can interfere or damage these devices. Similarly it must not be used on patients with implanted intracranial metals such as clippings, coilings, ventriculo-peritoneal shunts, endoprosthesis, etc.

To date, studies combing tDCS and aphasia treatment have tended to focus on patients more than 12 months post-ischemic stroke with no history of epilepsy or post-stroke seizures (while considered safe, there are theoretical risks of tDCS inducing seizures in stroke patients). tDCS has not been reported to provoke seizures in non-acute neurological deficits (i.e., intervention protocols are well below the threshold of tissue damage; Liebetanz et al., 2009; Nitsche et al., 2003b). Therefore, compared with TMS, tDCS may be a viable option for stimulation of perilesional cortex where the threshold to induce seizures is lower. In a clinical context, this makes tDCS an appealing form of neurostimulation in chronic stroke populations (Priori et al., 2009). However, further investigation of tDCS hazards is certainly warranted in acute and non-acute patients, both for existing protocols and those under development (Bikson et al., 2009), in particular, the interaction of stimulation with different disease etiologies and potential risk factors of seizure, such as lack of sleep (Nitsche et al., 2008). Therefore, appropriate safety criteria are unknown, especially in the context of repeated protocols that may be required for rehabilitation.

3 Investigating tDCS as a Novel Method for Enhancing Aphasia (Post-Stroke) Treatment Effects.

i. *Chronic Aphasia: Speech Production*

A recent study found that in chronic aphasic patients tDCS applied off-line (i.e., in isolation or not concurrently with SALT) had no effect on language function (Volpato et al., 2013). In direct contrast, there is a precedent for combining on-line tDCS with anomia (word-finding problems) treatment with positive results. Interestingly all the treatment studies to date using on-line tDCS in chronic aphasic patients have focused on speech production (see Table 22.1). This combinatorial approach is important because intensive therapy is required for best aphasia recovery (Bhogal et al., 2003), and tDCS may help consolidate practice rather than simply affect performance alone (Reis et al., 2009). By pairing tDCS (delivered to the patient's structurally intact, residual language cortices) with intensive aphasia rehabilitation the aim is to enhance long-term treatment outcomes. The hypothesis underlying these studies is that the short-lasting gain observed from a single session of tDCS will accumulate with repeated sessions and eventually lead to a permanent improvement in function; that is, tDCS requires Hebbian pairing with training to facilitate learning processes (Reis et al., 2009). This approach has been influenced, at least in part, by (1) the facilitatory effects observed in multiple-exposure studies of healthy participants and (2) the idea that the favorable effects of mass-practice seen in behavior-only anomia treatments may also be valid in combined tDCS and behavioral training approaches.

In healthy participants, multiple sessions of left-sided anodal stimulation can improve overall performance when learning new information and associations relative to sham (e.g., de Vries et al., 2010; Fiori et al., 2010; Floël et al., 2008). For language learning, a recent study applied anodal stimulation to left Broca's area on-line during the acquisition phase of an artificial grammar and demonstrated enhanced performance at detecting syntactic violations along with an increased use

Table 22.1 Group Studies of tDCS Delivered Concurrently with Aphasia Therapy in Chronic Aphasic Stroke Patients (minimum of six patients)

No. Authors	n	Lesion location	Time PSMean (range)	Design	tDCS	tDCS parameters	Exposure	Task	Results	tDCS effect	Bx effect	Duration of effect
1 Baker et al. (2010)	10	3 – L frontal 4 – L TP 1 – L FP 1 – L FTP 1 – L temporal	Chronic 64.6 months (10–242)	Crossover Randomized Sham controlled 1 wk between interventions	A, S	1 mA 20 min. L frontal-precentral	5 days	Spoken WPM	Naming accuracy improved for treated items, A (14%) > S (6%)	8%	6%	1 week post-treatment
2 Fridriksson et al. (2011)	8	All had posterior cortical or subcortical lesions	Chronic 58.4 months (10–150)	Crossover Randomized Sham controlled 3 wks between interventions	A, S	1 mA 20 min. L posterior cortex	5 days	Spoken WPM	Naming reaction time was faster A (−456 ms) > S (−281 ms)	174 ms faster	281 ms faster	3 weeks post-treatment
3 Kang et al. (2011)	10	1 – L frontal 1 – L TP 3 – L FT 2 – L FTP 3 – L subcortical	Chronic 52.4 months (6.0–180.6)	Crossover Randomized Sham controlled 1 wk between interventions	C, S	2 mA 20 min. R Broca's	5 days	Word retrieval training	Naming accuracy improved in C (4%) > S (2%) 1 hour following the last (5th) ctDCS treatment session	2%	2%	Not assessed
4 Vines et al. (2011)	6	All had left frontal damage	Chronic 4.6 years (1.3–10)	Crossover Randomized Sham controlled 1 wk between interventions	A, S	1.2 mA 20 min. R posterior inferior frontal gyrus (F8)	3 days	Melodic intonation therapy	Speech rate of fluency improved A (−10.9%) > S (+2.5%) Cohen d −1.98	10.9% faster	2.5% slower	Not assessed

	Study	N	Lesion location	Chronicity	Design	Stimulation	Treatment	Increased naming accuracy	%	%	
5	Floël et al. (2011)	12	1 – L frontal 5 – L TP 1 – L FT 5 – L FTP	Chronic 84.2 months (14–260)	Crossover Randomized Sham controlled 1 wk between interventions	A, C, S 1 mA 20 min. Twice per day R TP	Naming therapy	Increased naming accuracy A (89%) > S (83%) = C (84%)	6%	83%★	2 weeks post-treatment
6	Fiori et al. (2013)	7	2 – L FT 2 – L FTP 1 – L temporal – insula 1 – L temporal 1 – L TP	Chronic 32.8 months (7–84)	Crossover Randomized Sham controlled 6 days between interventions	A, S 1 mA 20 min. Wernicke's area (CP5) Broca's area (F5)	Naming therapy: Nouns and verbs	Naming accuracy improved Nouns: W (31%) > B (12) > S (10) Verbs: B (42%) > W (15) > S (13)	Nouns: W (21%) Verbs: B (29%)	Nouns: 10% Verbs: 13%	4 weeks post-treatment
7	Marangolao et al. (2014)	8	4 – L-temporal 4 – L FT	Chronic 41.1 months (14–84)	Crossover Sham controlled 14 days between interventions	A, S 1 mA 20 min. Broca's Wernicke's	Conversation therapy with SALT	Increased speech coherence B (64%) > W (30%) = S (25%)	39%	25%	Not assessed

PS-post stroke. Bx effect-behavioral effect. L-left. R-right. TP-temporoparietal. FTP-fronto-temporoparietal. FT-frontotemporal. A-anodal stimulation; C-cathodal stimulation; S-sham stimulation. WPM-word-to-picture matching. SALT-speech and language therapy. K-WAB-Korean version of Western Aphasia Battery.

★ This figure is surprisingly large due to the fact that patients started off at a baseline level of 0% naming success on items subsequently treated until they reached a naming accuracy of at least 80%.

Table 22.2 Group Studies of tDCS Delivered Concurrently with Aphasia Therapy in Subacute Aphasic Stroke Patients (minimum of six patients)

No.	Authors	n	Lesion location	Time PSMean (range)	Design	tDCS	TDCS parameters	Exposure	Task	Results	tDCS effect	Bx effect	Duration of effect
1	You et al. (2011)	21	Cathodal: 5 – L frontal 1 – L temporal 1 – L subcortical Anodal: 4 – L temporal 3 – L frontal Sham: 6 – L frontal 1 – L parietal	Subacute (16–38 days)	Three-group comparison	C, A, S	2mA30 min. C- RSTG-CP6 A-LSTG-CP5 S-LSTG-CP5	10 days 5 days × 2 weeks	Conventional SALT	Auditory comprehension improved in all groups but C (17%) > A (10) = S (10)	7%	10%	Not assessed
2	Jung et al. (2011)	37	Range of LMCAInfarct/hemorrhage	Subacute 220.9 days (13 < 30; 10 > 90)	Within group-all had C-tDCS	C	1 mA20 min. Brodmann area 45	10 days	Conventional SALT	AQ K-WAB % improved from pre- to post-therapy (14.94 ± 6.73%) Lower initial severity = better AQ% change.	Not assessed	Not assessed	Not assessed

PS-post stroke. Bx effect-behavioral effect. L-left. R-right. A-anodal stimulation; C- cathodal stimulation; S-sham stimulation. SALT-speech and language therapy. K-WAB-Korean version of Western Aphasia Battery. AQ-aphasia quotient.

of rule-based decision making (de Vries et al., 2010). Similarly, anodal stimulation applied to left Wernicke's area during acquisition of an artificial lexicon increased the rate and overall success of language learning compared to sham stimulation after a single exposure to tDCS (Floël et al., 2008). In other words, the hypothesis is that brain stimulation itself would not produce any lasting changes in language function; instead, it would temporarily create a state that optimizes learning or, in the case of aphasic patients, re-learning and rehabilitation. By boosting this natural process in aphasic patients tDCS could lead to additional improvements in language function, on top of the main effect of SALT, and lead to further improvement in language function.

(a)   Stimulating the Perilesional Left Hemisphere

In relatively well-recovered aphasic patients, as in normal individuals, successful speech production has been correlated with brain activity in the left hemisphere (Fridriksson et al., 2010). In this context, one may predict that facilitating the remaining left perilesional cortex with excitatory stimulation could improve speech recovery. Preliminary results suggest that anodal tDCS applied to the remaining structurally intact cortex in the lesioned left hemisphere can facilitate naming performance post-treatment. Four tDCS group studies (see Table 22.1, study numbers 1, 2, 6, and 7) adopted this approach using a repeated intervention protocol in chronic aphasic patients that spanned several days with anodal tDCS delivered during a given speech production task. The latter two studies are the latest papers by two groups who have published additional papers using similar protocols/data, so I will not refer to those other papers here.

In the first treatment study, (Table 22.1, study 1), 10 aphasic speakers were trained for 5 consecutive days using a spoken word-to-picture match task during which they received 20 minutes of anodal (1 mA) or sham stimulation of left frontal and precentral cortex (Baker et al., 2010). The patients' naming accuracy improved on average by 14% after anodal stimulation compared to sham (6%); that is, tDCS had an additive effect of 8% on top of the behavioral training effect, which was 6% improvement in naming. These improvements in naming were retained for at least 1 week for items that had been treated. Consistent with the behavioral rehabilitation literature, the observed facilitatory effects did not generalize to untreated items matched for psycholinguistic complexity. In a second study by this group (Table 22.1, study 2), the same treatment paradigm was used in eight mild-fluent aphasic patients with lesions restricted to left posterior cortical and subcortical regions. Anodal stimulation was applied to left posterior perilesional cortex (Fridriksson et al., 2011), and as accuracy for naming was high at baseline in these patients, the outcome measure was reaction time. Anodal stimulation resulted in faster naming responses compared to sham stimulation. This naming improvement persisted for at least 3 weeks. Again, the facilitatory effect of anodal stimulation was restricted to the treated items only.

In the third naming study (Table 22.1, study 6), Fiori and colleagues (2013) trained seven non-fluent aphasic patients to name 102 nouns and 102 verbs they could comprehend but not accurately produce. Naming practice was paired with 1 mA of anodal tDCS applied to left Wernicke's area, left Broca's area and with sham stimulation of the same region. Overall, as a group, patients showed improved naming accuracy in response to the behavioral training (12% sham) after 5 days of intervention. The authors further discuss how patients were much more accurate in noun naming after anodal left temporal stimulation (Wernicke's, 31%; Broca's, 12%; sham, 10%) and in verb naming after anodal left frontal stimulation (Wernicke's, 15%; Broca's, 42%; sham, 13%). Importantly, these gains were maintained 4 weeks after tDCS. However, considering that it was a small study and that all of their patients had left hemisphere damage involving the temporal lobe to some degree, it is not clear that the better recovery observed after the left temporal and frontal stimulation, respectively, for nouns and verbs, was directly related to activation of these areas per se. That is, it is not clear how many patients actually had structurally intact cortex underneath the anode electrode for each intervention and how the current flow would have been affected by their different lesions in the vicinity of the stimulating electrodes. The same criticism could be applied to Marangolo's study (Marangolo et al., 2014) (Table 22.1, study 6). Here the authors extend the speech training approach to look at effects of frontal versus temporal tDCS on conversational therapy outcomes. All eight chronic aphasic individuals had temporal lobe damage and four also had frontal damage. Nevertheless, frontal anodal tDCS did have an additive effect and significantly improved the patients' speech coherence directly after treatment compared to behavioral training alone. This confirms the findings from the earlier studies that highlight the importance of coupling tDCS with the treatment for both immediate and longer-term gains and suggests that using anodal tDCS stimulation in the vicinity of perilesional tissue is possible, well-tolerated and can enhance chronic patients' response to SALT.

(b) Stimulating the Right Hemisphere

An alternative possibility for aphasia recovery relies on recruitment of the right hemisphere to facilitate language improvement. Previous neuroimaging and behavioral studies found that right hemisphere homologues of "classical" language regions are activated by language tasks in aphasic stroke patients (Blank et al., 2003; Crinion and Price, 2005; Leff et al., 2002; Saur et al., 2006). What is not always clear is whether increased right hemisphere activation might be the consequence of a loss of active inter-hemispheric inhibition from homologous regions in the lesioned hemisphere or a compensatory neural response, contributing to functional recovery (for a useful review, see Geranmayeh et al., 2014; Saur and Hartwigsen, 2012). What is clear is that there is little evidence for takeover of function in areas previously unrelated to language processing (i.e., it appears to be a preexisting bilateral language network). For aphasic patients with extensive left hemisphere lesions, upregulation of right hemispheric language homologues might be crucial; indeed, their only option for recovery (Schlaug et al., 2009; Winhuisen et al., 2005). This is the approach that Vines and colleagues used (Vines et al., 2011) (Table 22.1, study 4). They paired anodal tDCS with melodic intonation therapy in severely aphasic patients with extensive left IFG lesions and found it significantly improved patients' speech fluency. This suggests that, in these patients at least, the right IFG was contributing to their speech recovery.

By contrast, in aphasic patients whose lesions only partially damage left hemisphere cortices, the role of right IFG Broca's homologue in speech recovery is not always deemed facilitatory. An open-protocol TMS study showed that 10 sessions of inhibitory 1 Hz rTMS over the posterior inferior portion of the right pars triangularis significantly improved picture naming in four chronic aphasic patients. This effect was maintained 2 months later (Naeser et al., 2005). The hypothesis behind this paradoxical effect is that language improvement was due to suppression of activity in the 'overactive' right hemisphere. That is, rTMS downregulated inhibitory activity in the right healthy Broca's homologue area, which, in turn, reduced the abnormally increased inter-hemispheric inhibition from the contralesional to the ipsilesional hemisphere. This theory borrows directly from the motor recovery literature where recovery after stroke is seen a dynamic process that may involve a variety of plastic changes in both hemispheres to achieve inter-hemisphere balance (Fregni and Pascual-Leone, 2006; Mansur et al., 2005; Oliveri et al., 2001; Ward and Cohen, 2004). In the case of tDCS application of inhibitory cathodal tDCS (ctDCS) to the primary motor cortex can decrease motor cortical excitability at this site (Nitsche and Paulus, 2000; Nitsche et al., 2003a; Purpura and McMurtry, 1965; Wassermann and Grafman, 2005). Furthermore, ipsilesional facilitatory anodal tDCS or contralesional ctDCS elicited motor improvements in chronic stroke patients (Boggio et al., 2007; Hummel et al., 2005). This led Kang and colleagues (Kang et al., 2011) (Table 22.1, study 3) to test the hypothesis that ctDCS applied to the right healthy Broca's homologue area simultaneously with word-retrieval training might improve picture naming task performance in patients with chronic post-stroke aphasia.

Ten right-handed patients with post-stroke aphasia were enrolled in this double-blind, counterbalanced, sham-controlled, crossover study. Each patient received an intervention of ctDCS (2 mA for 20 minutes) and of sham tDCS (2 mA for 1 minute) daily for 5 consecutive days in a randomized crossover manner with a minimum interval of 1 week between interventions, over a healthy right Broca's homologue area using a left supraorbital anode and simultaneous daily sessions of conventional word-retrieval training. ctDCS was found to have a small (4%) but significant improvement in picture naming ($p = 0.02$) 1 hour following the last (fifth) ctDCS treatment session, but no statistically significant changes were observed after sham tDCS (2%). It was not assessed whether these effects persisted. However, it is interesting to directly contrast the size of these effects with the Baker (Baker et al., 2010) study (Table 22.1, study 1). Baker and colleagues also combined tDCS with anomia treatment for 5 days but used anodal tDCS delivered to left Broca's area. They found tDCS resulted in large effects (14% improvement in naming, compared to sham, 6%) that persisted for at least 1 week after intervention. It is tempting to think that this might suggest that anodal tDCS to the left perilesional cortex is more effective than cathodal to the right. However, the question of whether left perilesional areas, or homologous areas of the right hemisphere, are more crucial for speech recovery can only be addressed in a study that directly compares tDCS effects when delivered to both these areas (i.e., a within-group crossover design). Irrespective, it does highlight that choosing the 'right' behavioral treatment is key (Baker's sham = 6% > Kang's tDCS = 4%; sham = 2%), both for observing statistically significant and clinically meaningful treatment and adjuvant tDCS effects that enhance aphasic individuals' language recovery immediately post treatment and longer term.

In a complementary approach, Floël and colleagues (Table 22.1, study 5) delivered anodal, cathodal and sham tDCS to right temporo-parietal regions during anomia treatment. Patients practiced a small number of items over 3 days that they consistently at baseline could not name (0%) until they reached 80% accuracy. The sham effect (behavioral treatment alone) in their study was therefore 83%. This meant the tDCS effect could maximally be 27% (i.e., if the patients' naming improved to a perhaps unrealistic 100%). A more sensitive design would have included a larger pool of items, with treated and untreated lists of items being balanced for naming accuracy, avoiding the problem of regression to a mean of 0% and overinflating the main effect of the sham (e.g., naming baseline accuracy 40%, allowing 60% room for improvement). Having said that, the patients' naming did statistically improve further to 89% with anodal tDCS. This effect persisted for 2 weeks post treatment. Interestingly, cathodal tDCS had no effect in these patients. Taken together with Kang's study, it suggests that, in the context of a strong behavioral treatment effect, cathodal tDCS may offer little advantage but anodal tDCS can still boost recovery. See Miniussi (Miniussi and Ruzzoli, 2013) for a discussion of the potential physiological mechanisms underlying why this may be the case. Alternatively, it may be that right temporal and frontal regions respond differently to anodal and cathodal tDCS, respectively when paired with anomia treatment. Further studies are clearly needed to explore this.

ii.   *Subacute Aphasia*

Consistent with the chronic aphasia studies (Polanowska et al., 2013) found that in subacute aphasic patients tDCS applied off-line (i.e., in isolation or not concurrently with SALT) had no effect on language treatment outcomes. Only two tDCS group studies have been conducted to date in subacute aphasic stroke patients (see Table 22.2). Both investigated tDCS as an adjunct to conventional SALT and its impact on standardized aphasia outcomes. Jung and colleagues (Jung et al., 2011) (Table 22.2, study 2) applied 1 mA cathodal tDCS to Broca's area in all 37 patients. There was no sham, so interpretation of tDCS effects on behavioral outcomes is not possible. Lesion distribution was not controlled, so it is not clear how many patients had structurally intact tissue in the vicinity of the stimulating electrode. Hemorrhagic stroke patients, in whom the risk of post-stroke epilepsy is higher, were included. Nevertheless, tDCS was well tolerated by all, and no adverse events were reported. Behaviorally, the least aphasic patients made the best language improvements (i.e., recovered quickly), while more severely aphasic patients changed little following 10 days of SALT paired with tDCS.

You and colleagues (You et al., 2011) (Table 22.2, study 1) conducted a between-group study of 2 mA tDCS (cathodal right STG, anodal left STG, sham) paired with SALT in 21 aphasic individuals. The cathodal tDCS group recovered significantly more auditory comprehension (17%) than the sham group (10%) and the anodal tDCS group (10%). The authors interpret this result as evidence that suppression of activity in the 'overactive' right hemisphere after left hemisphere stroke may promote recovery. Interestingly, the cathodal group were behaviorally the least impaired on auditory comprehension testing at baseline. This is consistent with Jung's study showing that aphasia severity is a reliable predictor of outcome in the subacute stage post stroke. However, this difference in baseline does make it difficult to interpret the between-groups comparisons and to sort out the effects of tDCS. In addition, if baseline performance is not stable or equivalent between groups, it is more difficult to detect a difference between groups, especially if the effects of the treatment are small or variable (such as in this study, where sham was equivalent to anodal). Contributing to this variability, lesion distribution was not equivalent in the three groups. Of particular note is that four of the seven patients in the anodal tDCS group had lesions to the left temporal lobe, and it is not clear whether they had structurally intact cortex underneath the left STG stimulating electrode. In conclusion, it is impossible to judge at this stage whether tDCS offers any benefit to aphasia treatment in the subacute stage post stroke. Importantly, however, these two studies have shown in a relatively large number of patients (n = 58) that 2 mA and 1 mA tDCS was well tolerated and safe when delivered for 10 days in combination with SALT. This is encouraging, and tDCS plus aphasia treatment studies in this early stage post stroke are feasible.

Summary

By linking data and theoretical models from these complementary studies I hoped to deliver an integrated picture of current aphasia rehabilitation targeting subgroups of aphasic patients using tDCS. These are early days in this field, but the most compelling evidence to date suggests that in chronic aphasia post stroke anodal tDCS delivered to the patient's residual spoken language network (left hemisphere if preserved post stroke or when more extensively damaged right hemisphere homologue) when paried with rehabilitation training has a potential role in boosting consolidation of anomia rehabilitation practice rather than a simple effect on language performance. The effects of anodal tDCS are, in the majority of studies, greater than or at least equivalent to the size of the behavioral treatment effects alone (see Table 22.1). tDCS paired with SALT is feasible in the early days post stroke, but little work has been done to assess its efficacy. We are far from tailoring treatment to individual patients. Future studies in larger groups of patients that control for lesion distribution and aphasia severity may provide us with a means of identifying those who are likely to respond to specific tDCS and behavioral therapies. This would provide an empirical basis from which to investigate specific aphasia interventions in future multi-center clinical trials and could greatly improve the quality of aphasia treatment for stroke patients.

4   Future Directions

Brain Stimulation as a Novel Home Therapeutic Intervention?

tDCS use is currently largely restricted to lab-based experiments, limiting its translational impact. Most chronic stroke patients living in the community often have mobility issues, limiting how many can take part in intensive clinical studies and increasing the associated labor and travel costs.

Giving patients a home tool to improve their aphasia rehabilitation may be empowering and give them a sense that they are able to affect their own recovery (Palmer et al., 2013). Economic analyses of SALTs and computer-based aphasia treatment have demonstrated that they provide good value for the money regarding their benefit to society (Marsh, 2010; Latimer et al., 2013). There is evidence to suggest that when patients with aphasia are successfully treated they interact more efficiently with other therapists (e.g., physiotherapists, occupational therapists) and thus make greater gains in other, non-language domains (Hilari et al., 2012; Jette et al., 2005).

Home-tDCS kits are now currently being designed to combine the benefits of tDCS—namely low-intensity, safe, neuromodulation with home behavioral practice—while minimizing costs. Combined with the ability to robustly sham home-tDCS, this provides clinical researchers with a compelling platform and much promise as an adjunct to neurorehabilitation. A few home-tDCS kits have been developed, but none have been designed for use with stroke patient populations with cognitive impairments. An American product, the Soterix-Stimulator, is available, but only to approved American physicians and institutions. It currently does not have a CE marking, which is mandatory for use in Europe. It is also not optimally designed for home use in patients with cognitive impairments, which may limit its usability with aphasic patients. Nevertheless, this exciting area of development is of significant interest to academia, industry and clinical practice, with many global manufacturers interested in developing an effective and acceptable home-tDCS kit for use in clinical rehabilitation.

If tDCS proves to be an effective adjunct to aphasia treatment, then a home-tDCS kit suitable for use in this patient population would ensure translation and successful implementation of aphasia treatment research findings into novel and timely clinical treatment practice. Successful home-tDCS could increase the amount of aphasia recovery individual patients make, as well as free up more SALT time. In my opinion, a practical home-tDCS treatment product is therefore, necessary to address existing clinical research needs and, if successful, emerging healthcare needs for low-cost home-based solutions.

References

Antal, A., Polania, R., Schmidt-Samoa, C., Dechent, P., Paulus, W., 2011. Transcranial direct current stimulation over the primary motor cortex during fMRI. Neuroimage. 55, 590–6.

Ayerbe, L., Ayis, S., Rudd, A.G., Heuschmann, P.U., Wolfe, C.D., 2011. Natural history, predictors, and associations of depression 5 years after stroke: the South London Stroke Register. Stroke: a journal of cerebral circulation. 42, 1907–11.

Baker, J.M., Rorden, C., Fridriksson, J., 2010. Using transcranial direct-current stimulation to treat stroke patients with aphasia. Stroke: a journal of cerebral circulation. 41, 1229–36.

Bhogal, S.K., Teasell, R., Speechley, M., 2003. Intensity of aphasia therapy, impact on recovery. Stroke: a journal of cerebral circulation. 34, 987–93.

Bikson, M., Datta, A., Elwassif, M., 2009. Establishing safety limits for transcranial direct current stimulation. Clinical neurophysiology. 120, 1033–4.

Bindman, L.J., Lippold, O.C., Milne, A.R., 1979. Prolonged changes in excitability of pyramidal tract neurones in the cat: a post-synaptic mechanism. Journal of physiology. 286, 457–77.

Bindman, L.J., Lippold, O.C., Redfearn, J.W., 1962. Long-lasting changes in the level of the electrical activity of the cerebral cortex produced bypolarizing currents. Nature. 196, 584–5.

Bindman, L.J., Lippold, O.C., Redfearn, J.W., 1964. The action of brief polarizing currents on the cerebral cortex of the rat (1) during current flow and (2) in the production of long-lasting after-effects. Journal of physiology. 172, 369–82.

Blank, S.C., Bird, H., Turkheimer, F., Wise, R.J., 2003. Speech production after stroke: the role of the right pars opercularis. Annals of neurology. 54, 310–20.

Boggio, P.S., Nunes, A., Rigonatti, S.P., Nitsche, M.A., Pascual-Leone, A., Fregni, F., 2007. Repeated sessions of noninvasive brain DC stimulation is associated with motor function improvement in stroke patients. Restorative neurology and neuroscience. 25, 123–9.

Brady, M.C., Kelly, H., Godwin, J., Enderby, P., 2012. Speech and language therapy for aphasia following stroke. The Cochrane database of systematic reviews. 5, CD000425.

Code, C., 2003. The quantity of life for people with chronic aphasia. Neuropsychological rehabilitation. 13, 379–90.

Code, C., Heron, C., 2003. Services for aphasia, other acquired adult neurogenic communication and swallowing disorders in the United Kingdom, 2000. Disability and rehabilitation. 25, 1231–7.

Creutzfeldt, O.D., Fromm, G.H., Kapp, H., 1962. Influence of transcortical d-c currents on cortical neuronal activity. Experimental neurology. 5, 436–52.

Crinion, J., Price, C.J., 2005. Right anterior superior temporal activation predicts auditory sentence comprehension following aphasic stroke. Brain. 128, 2858–71.

Datta, A., Elwassif, M., Bikson, M., 2009. Bio-heat transfer model of transcranial DC stimulation: comparison of conventional pad versus ring electrode. *Conference proceedings: Annual International Conference of the IEEE Engineering in Medicine and Biology Society.* 2009, 670–3.

de Vries, M.H., Barth, A.C.R., Maiworm, S., Knecht, S., Zwitserlood, P., Flöel, A., 2010. Electrical stimulation of Broca's area enhances implicit learning of an artificial grammar. Journal of cognitive neuroscience. 22, 2427–36.

Dundas, J.E., Thickbroom, G.W., Mastaglia, F.L., 2007. Perception of comfort during transcranial DC stimulation: effect of NaCl solution concentration applied to sponge electrodes. Clinical neurophysiology. 118, 1166–70.

Fiori, V., Cipollari, S., Di Paola, M., Razzano, C., Caltagirone, C., Marangolo, P., 2013. tDCS stimulation segregates words in the brain: evidence from aphasia. Frontiers in Human Neuroscience. 14, 269.

Fiori, V., Coccia, M., Marinelli, C.V., Vecchi, V., Bonifazi, S., Ceravolo, M.G., Provinciali, L., Tomaiuolo, F., Marangolo, P., 2010. Transcranial direct current stimulation improves word retrieval in healthy and non-fluent aphasic subjects. Journal of cognitive neuroscience. 23, 2309–23.

Flöel, A., Meinzer, M., Kirstein, R., Nijhof, S., Deppe, M., Knecht, S., Breitenstein, C., 2011. Short-term anomia training and electrical brain stimulation. Stroke. 42, 2065–7.

Flöel, A., Rosser, N., Miichka, O., Knecht, S., Breitenstein, C., 2008. Noninvasive brain stimulation improves language learning. Journal of cognitive neuroscience. 20, 1415–22.

Frank, E., Eichhammer, P., Burger, J., Zowe, M., Landgrebe, M., Hajak, G., Langguth, B., 2011. Transcranial magnetic stimulation for the treatment of depression: feasibility and results under naturalistic conditions: a retrospective analysis. European archives of psychiatry and clinical neuroscience. 261, 261–6.

Fregni, F., Pascual-Leone, A., 2006. Hand motor recovery after stroke: tuning the orchestra to improve hand motor function. Cognitive and behavioral neurology: official journal of the Society for Behavioral and Cognitive Neurology. 19, 21–33.

Fridriksson, J., Bonilha, L., Baker, J.M., Moser, D., Rorden, C., 2010. Activity in preserved left hemisphere regions predicts anomia severity in aphasia. Cerebral cortex. 20, 1013–9.

Fridriksson, J., Richardson, J.D., Baker, J.M., Rorden, C., 2011. Transcranial direct current stimulation improves naming reaction time in fluent aphasia: a double-blind, sham-controlled study. Stroke. 42, 819–21.

Gandiga, P.C., Hummel, F.C., Cohen, L.G., 2006. Transcranial DC stimulation (tDCS): a tool for double-blind sham-controlled clinical studies in brain stimulation. Clinical Neurophysiology. 117, 845–50.

Geranmayeh, F., Brownsett, S.L., Wise, R.J., 2014. Task-induced brain activity in aphasic stroke patients: what is driving recovery? Brain: a journal of neurology. **137**, 2632–48.

Go, A.S., Mozaffarian, D., Roger, V. L., Benjamin, E. J., Berry, J. D., Blaha, M. J., Dai, S., Ford, E. S., Fox, C. S., Franco, S., Fullerton, H. J., Gillespie, C., Hailpern, S. M., Heit, J.A., Howard, V. J., Huffman, M. D., Judd, S. E., Kissela, B. M., Kittner, S. J., Lackland, D. T., Lichtman, J. H., Lisabeth, L. D., Mackey, R.H., Magid, D.J., Marcus, G.M., Marelli, A., Matchar, D. B., McGuire, D. K., Mohler, E. R., 3rd, Moy, C. S., Mussolino, M. E., Neumar, R.W., Nichol, G., Pandey, D. K., Paynter, N. P., Reeves, M. J., Sorlie, P. D., Stein, J., Towfighi, A., Turan, T. N., Virani, S. S., Wong, N. D., Woo, D., Turner, M. B., 2014. Heart disease and stroke statistics—2014 update: a report from the American Heart Association. Circulation. 129, e28–e292.

Gupta, S. R., Naheedy, M. H., Elias, D., Rubino, F.A., 1988. Postinfarction seizures. a clinical study. Stroke: a journal of cerebral circulation. 19, 1477–81.

Hilari, K., 2011. The impact of stroke: are people with aphasia different to those without? Disability and rehabilitation. 33, 211–8.

Hilari, K., Needle, J. J., Harrison, K. L., 2012. What are the important factors in health-related quality of life for people with aphasia? A systematic review. Archives of physical medicine and rehabilitation. 93, S86–95.

Holland, R., Leff, A. P., Josephs, O., Galea, J. M., Desikan, M., Price, C. J., Rothwell, J. C., Crinion, J., 2011. Speech facilitation by left inferior frontal cortex stimulation. Current biology. 21, 1403–7.

Hummel, F., Celnik, P., Giraux, P., Floel, A., Wu, W. H., Gerloff, C., Cohen, L. G., 2005. Effects of non-invasive cortical stimulation on skilled motor function in chronic stroke. Brain: a journal of neurology. 128, 490–9.

Jacobson, L., Koslowsky, M., Lavidor, M., 2012. tDCS polarity effects in motor and cognitive domains: a meta-analytical review. Experimental brain research. 216, 1–10.

Jette, D. U., Warren, R. L., Wirtalla, C., 2005. The relation between therapy intensity and outcomes of rehabilitation in skilled nursing facilities. Archives of physical medicine and rehabilitation. 86, 373–9.

Jung, I. Y., Lim, J. Y., Kang, E. K., Sohn, H. M., Paik, N. J., 2011. The factors associated with good responses to speech therapy combined with transcranial direct current stimulation in post-stroke aphasic patients. Annals of rehabilitation medicine. 35, 460–9.

Kang, E. K., Kim, Y. K., Sohn, H. M., Cohen, L. G., Paik, N. J., 2011. Improved picture naming in aphasia patients treated with cathodal tDCS to inhibit the right Broca's homologue area. Restorative neurology and neuroscience. 29, 141–52.

Lagopoulos, J., Degabriele, R., 2008. Feeling the heat: the electrode-skin interface during DCS. Acta Neuropsychiatry. 20, 98–100.

Lam, J. M., Wodchis, W. P., 2010. The relationship of 60 disease diagnoses and 15 conditions to preference-based health-related quality of life in Ontario hospital-based long-term care residents. Medical care. 48, 380–7.

Latimer, N. R., Dixon, S., Palmer, R., 2013. Cost-utility of self-managed computer therapy for people with aphasia. International journal of technology assessment in health care. 29, 402–9.

Leff, A., Crinion, J., Scott, S., Turkheimer, F., Howard, D., Wise, R., 2002. A physiological change in the homotopic cortex following left posterior temporal lobe infarction. Annals of neurology. 51, 553–8.

Liebetanz, D., Koch, R., Mayenfels, S., Konig, F., Paulus, W., Nitsche, M. A., 2009. Safety limits of cathodal transcranial direct current stimulation in rats. Clinical neurophysiology. 120, 1161–7.

Liebetanz, D., Nitsche, M. A., Tergau, F., Paulus, W., 2002. Pharmacological approach to the mechanisms of transcranial DC-stimulation-induced after-effects of human motor cortex excitability. Brain: a journal of neurology. 125, 2238–47.

Loo, C. K., Martin, D. M., Alonzo, A., Gandevia, S., Mitchell, P. B., Sachdev, P., 2011. Avoiding skin burns with transcranial direct current stimulation: preliminary considerations. International journal of neuropsychopharmacology. 14, 425–6.

Mansur, C. G., Fregni, F., Boggio, P. S., Riberto, M., Gallucci-Neto, J., Santos, C. M., Wagner, T., Rigonatti, S. P., Marcolin, M. A., Pascual-Leone, A., 2005. A sham stimulation-controlled trial of rTMS of the unaffected hemisphere in stroke patients. Neurology. 64, 1802–4.

Marangolo, P., Fiori, V., Campana, S., Calpagnano, M. A., Razzano, C., Caltagirone, C., Marini, A., 2014. Something to talk about: enhancement of linguistic cohesion through tdCS in chronic non fluent aphasia. Neuropsychologia. 53, 246–56.

Marsh K., Bertranou, E., Suominen H, Venkatachalam M., 2010. *An economic evaluation of speech and language therapy*. London: Matrix Evidence.

Minhas, P., Bansal, V., Patel, J., Ho, J. S., Diaz, J., Datta, A., Bikson, M., 2010. Electrodes for high-definition transcutaneous DC stimulation for applications in drug delivery and electrotherapy, including tDCS. Journal of neuroscience methods. 190, 188–97.

Miniussi, C., Ruzzoli, M., 2013. Transcranial stimulation and cognition. Handbook of clinical neurology. 116, 739–50.

Moss, A., Nicholas, M., 2006. Language rehabilitation in chronic aphasia and time postonset: a review of single-subject data. Stroke: a journal of cerebral circulation. 37, 3043–51.

Naeser, M.A., Martin, P.I., Nicholas, M., Baker, E.H., Seekins, H., Kobayashi, M., Theoret, H., Fregni, F., Maria-Tormos, J., Kurland, J., Doron, K.W., Pascual-Leone, A., 2005. Improved picture naming in chronic aphasia after TMS to part of right Broca's area: an open-protocol study. Brain and language. 93, 95–105.

Nitsche, M.A., Cohen, L.G., Wassermann, E.M., Priori, A., Lang, N., Antal, A., Paulus, W., Hummel, F., Boggio, P.S., Fregni, F., Pascual-Leone, A., 2008. Transcranial direct current stimulation: State of the art 2008. Brain stimulation. 1, 206–223.

Nitsche, M.A., Nitsche, M.S., Klein, C.C., Tergau, F., Rothwell, J.C., Paulus, W., 2003a. Level of action of cathodal DC polarisation induced inhibition of the human motor cortex. Clinical neurophysiology. 114, 600–4.

Nitsche, M.A., Paulus, W., 2000. Excitability changes induced in the human motor cortex by weak transcranial direct current stimulation. Journal of physiology. 527 Pt 3, 633–9.

Nitsche, M.A., Paulus, W., 2001. Sustained excitability elevations induced by transcranial DC motor cortex stimulation in humans. Neurology. 57, 1899–901.

Nitsche, M.A., Schauenburg, A., Lang, N., Liebetanz, D., Exner, C., Paulus, W., Tergau, F., 2003b. Facilitation of implicit motor learning by weak transcranial direct current stimulation of the primary motor cortex in the human. Journal of Cognitive Neuroscience. 15, 619–26.

Nitsche, M.A., Seeber, A., Frommann, K., Klein, C.C., Rochford, C., Nitsche, M.S., Fricke, K., Liebetanz, D., Lang, N., Antal, A., Paulus, W., Tergau, F., 2005. Modulating parameters of excitability during and after transcranial direct current stimulation of the human motor cortex. Journal of physiology. 568, 291–303.

Northcott, S., Hilari, K., 2011. Why do people lose their friends after a stroke? International journal of language and communication disorders/Royal College of Speech & Language Therapists. 46, 524–34.

Oliveri, M., Bisiach, E., Brighina, F., Piazza, A., La Bua, V., Buffa, D., Fierro, B., 2001. rTMS of the unaffected hemisphere transiently reduces contralesional visuospatial hemineglect. Neurology. 57, 1338–40.

Palm, U., Keeser, D., Schiller, C., Fintescu, Z., Nitsche, M., Reisinger, E., Padberg, F., 2008. Skin lesions after treatment with transcranial direct current stimulation (tDCS). Brain Stimulation. 1, 386–7.

Palmer, R., Enderby, P., Cooper, C., Latimer, N., Julious, S., Paterson, G., Dimairo, M., Dixon, S., Mortley, J., Hilton, R., Delaney, A., Hughes, H., 2012. Computer therapy compared with usual care for people with long-standing aphasia poststroke: a pilot randomized controlled trial. Stroke: a journal of cerebral circulation. 43, 1904–11.

Palmer, R., Enderby, P., Paterson, G., 2013. Using computers to enable self-management of aphasia therapy exercises for word finding: the patient and carer perspective. International journal of language and communication disorders/Royal College of Speech & Language Therapists. 48, 508–21.

Polanowska, K. E., Lesniak, M., Seniow, J. B., Czlonkowska, A., 2013. No effects of anodal transcranial direct stimulation on language abilities in early rehabilitation of post-stroke aphasic patients. Neurologia i neurochirurgia polska. 47, 414–22.

Poreisz, C., Boros, K., Antal, A., Paulus, W., 2007. Safety aspects of transcranial direct current stimulation concerning healthy subjects and patients. Brain research bulletin. 72, 208–14.

Priori, A., Berardelli, A., Rona, S., Accornero, N., Manfredi, M., 1998. Polarization of the human motor cortex through the scalp. Neuroreport. 9, 2257–60.

Priori, A., Hallett, M., Rothwell, J. C., 2009. Repetitive transcranial magnetic stimulation or transcranial direct current stimulation? Brain stimulation. 2, 241–5.

Purpura, D. P., McMurtry, J. G., 1965. Intracellular activities and evoked potential changes during polarization of motor cortex. Journal of neurophysiology. 28, 166–85.

Reis, J., Schambra, H. M., Cohen, L. G., Buch, E. R., Fritsch, B., Zarahn, E., Celnik, P. A., Krakauer, J. W., 2009. Noninvasive cortical stimulation enhances motor skill acquisition over multiple days through an effect on consolidation. Proceedings of the National Academy of Sciences of the United States of America. 106, 1590–5.

Rioult-Pedotti, M. S., Friedman, D., Donoghue, J. P., 2000. Learning-induced LTP in neocortex. Science. 290, 533–6.

Rioult-Pedotti, M. S., Friedman, D., Hess, G., Donoghue, J. P., 1998. Strengthening of horizontal cortical connections following skill learning. Nature neuroscience. 1, 230–4.

Samsa, G. P., Matchar, D. B., Goldstein, L., Bonito, A., Duncan, P. W., Lipscomb, J., Enarson, C., Witter, D., Venus, P., Paul, J. E., Weinberger, M., 1998. Utilities for major stroke: results from a survey of preferences among persons at increased risk for stroke. American heart journal. 136, 703–13.

Saur, D., Hartwigsen, G., 2012. Neurobiology of language recovery after stroke: lessons from neuroimaging studies. Archives of physical medicine and rehabilitation. 93, S15–25.

Saur, D., Lange, R., Baumgaertner, A., Schraknepper, V., Willmes, K., Rijntjes, M., Weiller, C., 2006. Dynamics of language reorganization after stroke. Brain. 129, 1371–84.

Schlaug, G., Marchina, S., Norton, A., 2009. Evidence for plasticity in white-matter tracts of patients with chronic Broca's aphasia undergoing intense intonation-based speech therapy. Annals of the New York Academy of Sciences. 1169, 385–94.

Vines, B. W., Norton, A. C., Schlaug, G., 2011. Non-invasive brain stimulation enhances the effects of melodic intonation therapy. Frontiers in psychology. 2, 230.

Volpato, C., Cavinato, M., Piccione, F., Garzon, M., Meneghello, F., Birbaumer, N., 2013. Transcranial direct current stimulation (tDCS) of Broca's area in chronic aphasia: a controlled outcome study. Behavioural brain research. 247, 211–6.

Ward, N. S., Cohen, L. G., 2004. Mechanisms underlying recovery of motor function after stroke. Archives of neurology. 61, 1844–8.

Wassermann, E. M., Grafman, J., 2005. Recharging cognition with DC brain polarization. Trends in cognitive sciences. 9, 503–5.

Winhuisen, L., Thiel, A., Schumacher, B., Kessler, J., Rudolf, J., Haupt, W. F., Heiss, W. D., 2005. Role of the contralateral inferior frontal gyrus in recovery of language function in poststroke aphasia: a combined repetitive transcranial magnetic stimulation and positron emission tomography study. Stroke: a journal of cerebral circulation. 36, 1759–63.

Xu, T., Yu, X., Perlik, A.J., Tobin, W.F., Zweig, J.A., Tennant, K., Jones, T., Zuo, Y., 2009. Rapid formation and selective stabilization of synapses for enduring motor memories. Nature. 462, 915–9.

You, D.S., Kim, D.Y., Chun, M. H., Jung, S.E., Park, S.J., 2011. Cathodal transcranial direct current stimulation of the right Wernicke's area improves comprehension in subacute stroke patients. Brain and language. 119, 1–5.

23

A FOCUS ON LIFE PARTICIPATION

Jacqueline J. Hinckley and Audrey L. Holland

Introduction

The Life Participation Approach to Aphasia (LPAA; LPAA Project Group, 2001) is a statement of values and priorities that emphasize the consumer's viewpoint, attainment of meaningful life changes and outcomes, and participation in desired social roles and activities. Its development was influenced over a decade ago by the prescient need to address real changes in an efficient and effective way and to acknowledge the unmet needs of consumers with aphasia and their families. Since its first formal articulation, incorporating consumer values and targeting those supports that can lead to return to participation in life has grown. Assessments and intervention approaches that are consistent with this statement of values have been investigated and disseminated.

Core Values of LPAA

The goal of the LPAA is to help individuals return as fully to life as possible after stroke or other injury. Thus, a practice that is consistent with this set of values would "begin at the end" (Kagan & Simmons-Mackie, 2007) by thinking ahead to the specific activities that an individual may want to engage in and prioritizing clinical work that supports those activities. For example, Susan has a reading impairment as a result of her aphasia, and when questioned about what sort of reading was most important to her, she noted that reading recipes and cooking magazines were what she missed the most. These activities became the focus of her reading therapy, rather than a broad-based approach to the skill of reading.

The LPAA also broadens our clinical attention to individuals such as family members, close friends, caregivers, or others who are routinely in close proximity to the person with aphasia. Thus, life participation approaches focus not only on the persons who have impairment, but also on those around them and how together they construct reality (Armstrong & Ferguson, 2010). Clinical activities therefore are likely to target important others, including their skills, strategies, and abilities to communicate with and support the communication of individuals with aphasia. When important others are ineffective at the use of communication supports, then *their* skills are one focus of rehabilitation.

The consequences of aphasia often endure for the rest of one's life. LPAA principles include the notion that lifelong supports should be made available to them. This may be done in a variety of ways, but the proliferation of aphasia centers around the United States that provide ongoing support is one clear example.

Finally, the success of LPAA approaches is realized by changes in perceived quality of life, social interaction, well-being, social participation, life satisfaction, and related parameters. Such changes may not be associated with specific linguistic performances on decontextualized measures, but are regarded as equally valid foci for aphasia treatment. Indeed, any change that does not impact the person's ultimate lifestyle or wellness can be questioned for its usefulness. For example, confidence, manifested both by being able to return to previous activities, such as John re-joining his church choir, and manifesting higher scores on a measure of communication confidence are both suggestive of positive change, despite minimal linguistic improvements.

The core values of LPAA are similar to the defining characteristics of patient-centered care. For example, an evidence-based, stroke-specific definition of patient-centered care (Lawrence & Kinn, 2011) elevates the importance of the individual, identifies outcomes that reflect life participation and are prioritized and valued by the individual, monitors and measures outcomes that are valued by the individual, and applies all of this to the clinical process. Thus, the LPAA can be thought of as a forerunner of sorts for the current discussion of patient-centered care. Of course, the LPAA is specifically translated for the needs and priorities of individuals with aphasia.

Research and Clinical Examples

As the forgoing suggests, focus on life participation has led researchers and clinicians to consider different research questions, measures, and practices, expanding their view of the consequences of life with aphasia. Although consideration of long-term consequences is not new to either research or clinical practice, tools and techniques to incorporate life participation have proliferated since the articulation of the LPAA.

Prior to 2001, much of aphasia research concerned understanding the nature of an individual's linguistic impairments and developing interventions that followed conceptually or theoretically from those impairments. Researchers now also focus on the experience of people living with aphasia and what people with aphasia think. For example, research has focused on whether people with aphasia want health information in the hospital, whether they perceive that they receive sufficient health information, whether written materials are suitable, what people with aphasia think about the therapeutic process and discharge, and what people with aphasia think about the availability of aphasia information and resources (e.g., Dalemans, de Witte, Wade, & van den Heuven, 2010; Hinckley, Hasselkus, & Ganzfried, 2013; Worrall et al., 2011).

An extension of the life participation approach is the incorporation of people with aphasia into the research process itself. People with aphasia have participated in research as collaborators, providing viewpoints on barriers or facilitators for returning to work (Garcia, Barrette, & Laroche, 2000) or on the quality of stroke-related websites (Moss, Parr, & Petheram, 2004). People with aphasia can serve as advisors to ongoing research projects, making contributions to participant recruitment, refining training protocols and instructions, and reviewing easy-to-read summaries of a research project's results (Palmer & Patterson, 2013). This level of participation is achieved by providing a number of different communication supports that allow the people with aphasia to follow the advisory group meetings and express their opinions through pictorial, written, and other graphic means (Dalemans, Wade, van den Heuvel, & de Witte, 2009). Finally, people with aphasia can express their views about aphasia research priorities in commonly accepted techniques such as nominal group technique (Hinckley, Boyle, Lombard, & Bartels-Tobin, 2013).

Research targeting treatment effects that were primarily limited to analyzing performance on standardized, decontextualized measures now include measures that assess aspects of life participation such as quality of life, community integration, or wellness. Evaluating multiple levels of potential outcomes for any given intervention allows us to consider the possibility that, regardless of the intention of the intervention, outcomes may be far-reaching or unexpected (Hinckley & Carr, 2001).

Clinical practice has also been substantially affected by a life participation approach. The assessment process, according to a life participation view, actively includes the perceptions of the person with aphasia and significant others about activity and life priorities. Tools designed to collect information about life participation such as community integration, perceived quality of life, or wellness are included in pre- and post-treatment evaluations.

The nature of intervention itself has been affected by the LPAA. Consistent with LPAA's core values, intervention is now more likely to target important others, communication partners, the community, and the social environment as ways to improve the communication abilities and life of an individual with aphasia. These interventions may be focused on communication behaviors, knowledge and use of communication supports, or counseling. The use of personally relevant contexts and activities, such as conversation or a particular hobby, can be effectively used as a way to address communication. Specialized aphasia centers and programs connect people with aphasia to others living with the condition, community volunteers and activities, and a new way of living.

The value of the LPAA approach is acknowledged by all those who actively work to create these kinds of supports and environments. As we learn more about interventions, long-term effects on health and wellness, and the individual differences of the functioning of the human brain, we also begin to understand why this approach has taken such a foothold in the aphasia community.

Life Participation as a Framework for Intervention

Participating in life is the ultimate goal of any course of intervention. In order for individuals with aphasia to participate in life, communication has to be supported in a variety of ways to enable access to typical life activities.

Intervention with an exclusive emphasis on language skills and impairments may delay participation in activities such as conversation, participation in health care decisions, and comprehension of health information. In some cases, a focus on language skills or components may fail to enable the individual to achieve participation.

Take, for example, a client who would like to order independently at a favorite restaurant. Exercising independence and personal choice about the food one eats during the day is a simple and basic element of dignity. It is also a common complaint among individuals with aphasia who end up having their food selected and/or ordered for them.

In a strictly impairment-focused approach, the language skills and components that present the biggest barrier for ordering in a restaurant would be targeted. Lexical retrieval skills, oral reading, or other word production skills might be targeted via specific semantic or phonological interventions. These interventions might incorporate restaurant-relevant vocabulary, but not necessarily. The notion would be to improve the underlying skills that are necessary for restaurant ordering, so that the individual could order any item in any restaurant (Hinckley & Carr, 2001, 2005).

If life participation is the focus from the initiation of treatment, then the specific, personally relevant items that the individual is most likely to want to order in a particular restaurant will be the focus of intervention. Importantly, the supports that will be most successful for the individual for ordering those menu items in those restaurants will be identified, developed, and established. These supports could include a variety of techniques that the individual with aphasia might use, such as pointing or gesturing, using written cues, or selecting from pictured items in a communication notebook. Other supports could focus on the communication partner and ways in which the partner can support menu-ordering without compromising the individual's independence. Selecting the communication supports used by either the person with aphasia or a primary communication partner would depend not only on the person's linguistic abilities, but also on personality and personal preferences. Finally, employees at the restaurants where the person with aphasia commonly goes can be trained in supportive communication techniques. Any or all of these routes would achieve the life participation goal of allowing the individual with aphasia to order in a restaurant.

The interaction and overlap of the components that contribute to living successfully with aphasia are depicted by a framework based on the World Health Organization's (WHO) *International Classification of Functioning, Disability, and Health* (ICF). The Aphasia Framework for Outcome Measurement (A-FROM; Kagan et al, 2008) depicts four different domain areas that contribute to life with aphasia and are illustrated in the menu-ordering example above. The *Language and Related Processing* domain comprises all aspects of comprehension, reading, writing, and spoken language.

The *Participation* domain consists of the roles, relationships, and activities in which individuals with aphasia might typically take part. In the example above, going to the restaurant with a partner is the activity. However, this activity encompasses more than just ordering food, because inherent in this activity is sharing the experience and conversation with other people.

The *Environment* domain focuses on other people in the environment, their knowledge and attitudes, including their ability to support communication. For a restaurant outing, a primary communication partner might play an important role in providing the right communication supports for that activity. Alternatively, restaurant staff could also be trained to seat the individual with aphasia in a quiet section of the restaurant, allow sufficient time, and provide choices with written or gestural supports.

The fourth domain is the *Personal Factors and Identity* domain, and this includes personal attributes, such as age and gender, along with qualities like confidence, extroversion, and optimism. These personal factors will determine which supports are acceptable to the individual with aphasia and which ones will be most successful.

Each of these four domains is associated with outcome measures and also intervention types and targets. One of the purposes of the A-FROM is to help clinicians and researchers consider all aspects of living with aphasia and identify areas of participation, the environment, and personal factors that should be part of providing comprehensive communication support and intervention.

The preceding chapters in this volume have focused on the science and processes of interventions that primarily focus on the domain *Language and Related Processing*. In the remainder of this chapter, we will describe examples of interventions and outcomes associated with the other three domains: *Participation, Environment*, and *Personal Factors and Identity*.

Examples of Life Participation Approaches

Participation Domain Interventions and Outcomes

The *Participation* domain of the A-FROM encompasses the roles, relationships, and activities that are typical for that individual. Interventions that affect this domain should be those that enable and empower persons with aphasia to participate more comfortably in those aspects of society that appeal to them. These interventions are characterized by providing communication supports and communication access, in whatever way is needed, to promote engagement in the normal commerce of social interaction.

Participation in Health Care

The first thing that most people with aphasia want to be a part of is their own health care. To carry out this role in the hospital environment requires moderate understanding of what has happened, what treatments or medications are being provided, and the ability to express choices or preferences about the care that is being provided. Perhaps as many as 88% of individuals admitted into a stroke inpatient ward have some form of disability that affects their ability to comprehend or express health information while in the hospital (O'Halloran, Worrall, & Hickson, 2009).

Unfortunately, individuals experiencing stroke often report that they do not receive the information they would like (Haffensteindottir, Vergunst, Lindeman, & Schuurmans, 2011), and the presence of aphasia due to stroke exacerbates this problem (Cruice, 2007; Holland & Fridriksson, 2001; Parr, Byng, Gilpin, & Ireland, 1997; Worrall, Rose, Howe, McKenna, & Hickson, 2007). It is unfortunately true that both people with aphasia and their significant others are less likely to receive information about stroke than those without aphasia (Avent et al., 2005; Eames, McKenna, Worrall, & Read, 2003; Howe et al., 2008; Knight, Worrall, & Rose, 2006; Worrall et al., 2011).

Speech-language pathologists should play a central role in ensuring that people with aphasia are provided with the supports necessary for them to participate as much as possible in their own health care. Being able to participate in the exchange of health information bears on the overall health of the patient and fits well within the scope of practice for speech-language pathology (ASHA, 2007). Education, counseling, and maximizing communication through compensatory efforts are the primary goals of speech pathology intervention in acute care (Duffy, Fossett, & Thomas, 2011). In order to fully assist patients with communication impairments in the acute care setting, speech-language pathologists must identify potential communication challenges, and also serve as a conduit and educator for ensuring that patients and their families are provided information in an accessible way.

Written information in conjunction with verbal explanation is preferred in the acute care setting, and this information will be most effective if patients and families have repeated opportunities to discuss the information and ask questions (Eames, McKenna, Worrall, & Read, 2003; Rose, Worrall, Hickson, & Hoffmann, 2010; Rose, Worrall, Hickson, & Hoffmann, 2011). Recommendations for aphasia-friendly written materials are shown in Table 23.1. Repeated education opportunities while in the hospital are associated with much better overall rehabilitation outcomes than information that is provided on a single occasion (Forster et al., 2012). Holland and Nelson (2014) provide information concerning the importance of counseling at this stage of the recovery/rehabilitation as well.

Participation in rehabilitation means that individuals with aphasia and their families are putatively ready to communicate preferences about treatment and to identify personally relevant goals and personally meaningful outcomes. In a person-focused approach to assessment and goal setting, this process begins with therapists defining goal setting and aphasic persons and families identifying rehabilitation goals. After that, clinicians typically conduct a formal assessment. The results of this evaluation are discussed together with families and persons with aphasia in relationship to their personally relevant goals in a fully collaborative goal-setting session (Leach et al., 2010).

Table 23.1 Recommendations for aphasia-friendly written materials (based on Aleligay, Worrall, & Rose, 2008; Brennan, Worrall, & McKenna, 2005; Rose, Worrall, & McKenna, 2003).

Use simple sentences.
Shorten all long and complex sentences.
Make passive sentences active.
Clarify the referents of pronouns.
Substitute more frequent words for infrequent words.
Use large print.
Increase white space (vertical spacing).
Flesch-Kincaid Reading Grade level approximately 5–6.

Goal attainment scaling is a collaborative process for clinician and family evaluation of goals that has the strongest empirical support for its validity and effects (Hurn, Kneebone, & Cropley, 2006) and is a useful tool for goal setting and outcome measurement. There are six steps in the process of using goal attainment scaling (Malec, 1999). Goals that are relevant and meaningful are identified and prioritized. For example, the person with aphasia might want to be able to answer the telephone. A timeline is established for each goal, during which a pre-assessment and final assessment will be conducted for progress on that particular goal. Next, persons with aphasia, their significant others, and their clinician collaboratively establish the expected level of outcome and other possible outcomes of the goal. These outcomes should be articulated in clear behavioral terms.

Applying a collaborative framework and using appropriate clinical tools for the rehabilitation setting, the clinician can engage the person with aphasia in active participation in the rehabilitation process. Demonstrating that continued improvement and life participation is dependent on their actions will increase the likelihood that persons with aphasia will embrace opportunities for life participation after rehabilitation and may reduce the distress and disappointment that is often associated with discharge from rehabilitation services (Cott, Wiles, & Devitt, 2007).

It should be noted here that in many cases individuals with aphasia and their families frequently still have an ill-defined and murky notion of the rehabilitation process itself, which may only be minimally modulated by the quality of information and counseling provided. This requires not only highly focused activities such as goal attainment scaling, but good counseling as well. One such approach for this early phase of recovery is provided by Holland and Nelson (2014).

Participation in Personally Meaningful Activities

As rehabilitation progresses and the person with aphasia moves toward discharge, there should be significant emphasis on participation in other activities in addition to participation in the health care process. This can be accomplished by focusing on activities that are preferred by the person with aphasia.[1]

An individual's preferred activities can be successfully identified by using available tools and providing communication supports. For example, Appendix 2 of the WHO's ICF Checklist (2003) provides an interview that helps the clinician gather information about which activities are most important to the client. Examples of the interview probes are shown in Table 23.2.

One tool that was specifically created for aphasia is the Life Interests and Values (LIV) card sort (www.livcards.org). In this tool, four categories of life activities are depicted in a set of 95 pictures that represent activities in each of four categories. Examples of categories and activities included in

Table 23.2 Probes and examples from the WHO ICF Checklist for gathering perceptions about specific activities and participation.

Probes from the WHO ICF Checklist, Appendix 2	*Examples of Communication and Interaction Activity and Participation Domains*
How much difficulty do you have NOW doing [specific activity]?	Receiving spoken and non-verbal messages
How does this compare (more or less difficult) to before your aphasia?	Speaking
How much problem do you actually have [doing specific activity]?	Producing non-verbal messages
Is this problem [doing specific activity] made better or worse by anything or anyone?	Conversation
Is your ability to [do the specific activity] without assistance more or less than what you actually do?	Making friends

Table 23.3 The four categories included in the LIV with examples of activities in each category.

Category	Examples of Activities
Home & Community Activities	Cleaning the house, doing laundry, grocery shopping, going to the doctor, voting
Creative & Relaxing Activities	Using a computer, bird watching, drawing/painting, listening to music, going to the movies
Physical Activities	Golfing, yoga, walking, swimming, fishing
Social Activities	Family gatherings, eating out, picnic, storytelling, using the phone

the inventory are shown in Table 23.3. As each pictured activity is presented, the interviewer asks, "Do you do this now?" If the person with aphasia responds "no," the follow-up question is, "Do you want to start doing this?" If the client is already doing the activity, the follow-up question is, "Do you want to do this more?" (Haley et al., 2012). Note that this activity can be modified as a card-sorting task, with help provided in understanding the cards and the task of individuals with aphasia being to sort the cards into the above categories. We believe using LIV in this manner permits more autonomous decision making.

Once the person with aphasia has chosen the most highly valued activities in which to participate, a number of specific approaches can be selected to facilitate participation. Participating in reading for enjoyment, for example, can be facilitated through communication supports like those found in Aphasia Book Clubs (Bernstein-Ellis & Elman, 1998; Elman & Bernstein-Ellis, 2003). In Aphasia Book Clubs, a group of individuals with aphasia read a selected book together making use of character sketches, outlines, lists of key events, and other techniques that support comprehension of the text and narrative. The Aphasia Book Club approach enables an individual with aphasia to return to pleasurable reading that is enjoyed in a social context. A similar approach can be applied for a group of film lovers with aphasia. A useful technique in this regard is the Aphasia Film Forum (www.speakingofaphasia.com).

The communication partner approach foregrounds participation in any activity in which the person with aphasia is interested, like gardening, bowling, or sailing (Lyon et al, 1997). In this approach, a person with aphasia is matched with a community member who shares an interest in one of the client's preferred activities. The partner may be supplied with strategies to support communication, but the primary goal is for the person with aphasia to engage in the activity, focusing on enjoyment of the activity without a focus on communication difficulties. A very successful recent adaptation has been developed by Silverman (2011).

Return to participating in other community activities can also be supported through reciprocal scaffolding (Avent & Austermann, 2003; Avent, Patterson, Liu, & Small, 2009). For example, a science teacher with aphasia might work on short science lessons that can be used as part of a volunteer job at the local school. If the person with aphasia has difficulties with vocabulary or particular aspects of the lesson, the interaction with the students provides cues, scaffolds, and supports in order for the client with aphasia to be successful.

Participation in Conversation and Relationships

Participation in conversation and relationships can occur with the use of a variety of communication supports. Email, texting, and video calls provide methods for interaction that can be targeted in addition to face-to-face conversation. The clinician can help with determining appropriate methods and training the individual with aphasia to use these communication methods regularly to maintain important social connections. One of the very interesting approaches used among and across aphasia centers in North America has been building relationships among center members through the use of Skype and similar programs. Some programs also encourage communication with other persons with aphasia or in some cases college and graduate students who are interested in learning more about aphasia in this manner. Here the usual form of media used is *FaceTime* (by Apple).

New friendships with others who are facing similar circumstances are an important aspect of participation in relationships and can offer multiple potential benefits. One effective way to support this type of participation is through aphasia groups. Aphasia groups have an important effect on number of friendships and social networks (Lanyon, Rose, & Worrall, 2013; Vickers, 2010), as well as on the improvement of linguistic functions.

Improvement in conversation is partially dependent on the skills of a conversational partner. Partner training is at least equally important in facilitating participation in conversation as improved communication abilities on the part of the person with aphasia. Partner training approaches will be described in the next section.

Environment Domain Interventions and Outcomes

A focus on the environment to support life participation includes modifying the physical environment, the communication environment, and training others in the environment to support communication access.

Characteristics of the physical environment can significantly affect the communication success of an individual with aphasia. Analysis of 25 in-depth interviews of people with aphasia suggested several physical barriers that hindered life participation (Howe, Worrall, & Hickson, 2008). Characteristics of objects, such as highly varied presentation or unclear pictures or signs, are a physical barrier that can be improved on by professionals in controlled environments, such as clinics and hospitals. Noise, visual distractions, and spatial location of key objects or people were also reported as physical barriers to activity participation. Reducing noise, using visual supports such as color coding, and having easy-to-read written information as a supplement are examples of facilitators identified by people with aphasia. Attempting conversation in noisy, crowded, or unfamiliar locations is also perceived as physical barriers to conversation participation (Johansson, Carlsson, & Sonnander, 2012). Speech-language pathologists play a key role in educating other professionals, caregivers, and communication partners about the importance of managing the physical environment in ways that support successful communication.

Communication supports are defined as communication strategies, contextual resources, and environmental adaptations that provide access to communication, events, and activities (King, 2013). Speech-language pathologists play a key role in identifying the effective communication supports for the patient. In acute care, clinicians can determine the best way to ask the patient about pain level, to train the patient to use the call button, to explain the purpose of medications, or to ask for consent for a specific medical procedure. A number of apps are available for use in these circumstances.

The presence of communication supports such as communication notebooks, pictures, objects, and paper and pen for writing and drawing can improve the effectiveness and efficiency of an interaction. Interventions that enhance the use of various communication modalities are generally effective in improving communication (Rose, 2013). For example, the presence of low-tech visual scene displays that incorporate a personally relevant photo and key phrases can increase conversational turns and information transfer (Hux, Buechter, Wallace, & Wilson, 2010). Partner training may contribute most to modifying the environment for successful communication. Partner training has been investigated in several studies and has been the subject of a systematic review (Simmons-Mackie et al., 2010). Communication partner training improves communication activity level and participation for individuals with chronic aphasia. "A skilled communication partner is able to facilitate and support the communication of people with aphasia and should be considered a method of providing environmental support and access" (Simmons-Mackie et al., 2010, p. 1836). The known outcomes of communication partner training of any kind are improved participation in conversation, activities, and social interaction (Simmons-Mackie et al., 2010). The most comprehensive view of the spectrum of supported communication techniques in aphasia is the recent text by Simmons-Mackie, King, and Beukelman (2013).

There are several key principles and techniques that result in effective partner training. Supported Conversation for Aphasia (SCA™) is a method for training communication partners to better facilitate communication with a person with aphasia. The principles and training techniques of SCA can be used to effectively train family members, community volunteers, and health care workers (Kagan et al., 2001; Legg, Young, & Bryer, 2005; Rayner & Marshall, 2003; Simmons-Mackie et al., 2007). The two basic principles for the communication partner are to learn how to (1) acknowledge the competence of the person with aphasia and (2) reveal the competence of the person with aphasia by using a number of different communication tools and strategies that support both comprehension and expression.

Conversational Coaching (Hopper, Holland, & Rewega, 2002) is intended to target the person with aphasia along with the primary communication partner, such as a spouse, who will be able to continue to use the targeted strategies over time. In Conversational Coaching, an intervention designed for targeting a primary communication relationship, strategies are selected by considering (1) the ability of the person to use the strategy (in other words, circumlocution might be an ineffective strategy for a person with a severe expressive deficit), (2) desire of the person to use the strategy (if a person is adamantly refusing a strategy, it won't get used anyway), and (3) potential of the strategy to improve the quality of the communication (perhaps because the strategy was already observed to be effective on certain occasions or appeared to have potential) (Hopper, Holland, & Rewega, 2002).

Targets for communication training extend beyond the most immediate communication partners to those in the community. One of the most ingenious of such projects occurs at the Snyder Center for Aphasic Life Enhancement (SCALE). This ongoing community project targets local businesses located near SCALE in Baltimore, Maryland. Persons with aphasia check out the "aphasia friendliness" of restaurants in the area and then rate them on the quality of their communication environment. Those that "pass" are rewarded with a window sticker saying that they are indeed aphasia-friendly. Those that do not are offered an opportunity to be educated as to how to achieve this.[2]

A program for training emergency responders such as law enforcement officers and emergency medical personnel has been developed and disseminated (Ganzfried & Symbolik, 2011). Other medical personnel, such as nurses, nursing assistants, social workers, medical students, and doctors have also been the targets of organized communication training (Legg, Young, & Bryer, 2005; Rowland & McDonald, 2009; Welsh & Szabo, 2011). Like the widespread compliance with physical and building accessibility issues, training 201 community members offers access to important services through communication supports.

Personal Factors and Identity Domain Interventions and Outcomes

Communication support can enhance social engagement and belongingness. The belongingness hypothesis suggests that people need frequent, positive interactions with the same individuals, occurring in a framework of stable caring (Baumeister & Leary, 1995). Deficits in belongingness can result in detriments to physical and mental health, and this oft-supported observation implies that interpersonal relationships are a need, not just a want (Baumeister & Leary, 1995). Speech-language interventions that address social interactions and communication confidence, for example, can have direct and indirect effects on depression, well-being, and physical health.

One outgrowth of incorporating personal identity into a person-centered, life participation approach to intervention is to support self-advocacy activities. To do this, the clinician must help people with aphasia develop the tools they need to request communication supports themselves, and to express their choices. A key characteristic of self-advocacy is the option to engage in or opt out of any particular choice or activity (Threats, 2007). Choices made by people with aphasia will be outgrowths of their lifestyle, habits, coping style, education, and past experiences. The trick is to remember that choice is neither the obligation nor the right of one's clinician.

Self-advocacy can include learning a script to request certain communication supports or environmental manipulations or the use of a written card that provides information about the person's communication needs. Indeed, telling the story of the stroke and the effects of living with its consequences is the most frequently chosen topic for script development (Holland, Halper, & Cherney, 2010). It is critical that any person with a disability be able to request needed accommodations in order to ensure the ability to participate in chosen activities.

There is no doubt that aphasia substantially affects one's self-concept and requires a process of adaptation (Shadden, 2005; Shadden & Agan, 2004). A strong argument can be made for a positive psychology approach in aphasia in which the study of strength, resilience, and happiness can be applied to issues of concern in health care, such as depression, illness, and well-being (Holland & Nelson, 2014; Worrall et al., 2010). Individuals with aphasia can re-negotiate their identity with aphasia through effectively led conversation groups and support groups (Shadden & Koski, 2007; Simmons-Mackie & Elman, 2011).

Counseling techniques within the scope of practice of the speech-language pathologist are also relevant to the Personal Factors and Identity domain. Holland and Nelson (2014) focus their recent counseling text in accordance with Seligman's positive psychology approach (see, most recently, Seligman's book *Flourish*, 2011). In effect, Holland and Nelson (2014) argue that Seligman's model of well-being is more appropriate with people and families who were mostly living productive lives before the intrusion of a communication disorder in their lives than are models built on conceptions of psychopathology. There are a number of ways to increase living the full and engaged life following stroke and aphasia, such as recognizing what is good in one's everyday life, learning to become more resilient, and learning how self-efficacy is done successfully. Holland and Nelson (2014) provide practicing clinicians with exercises, and experiential learning approaches adapted to language-impaired clients and their families.

Life with Aphasia: Integrating the Domains

Aphasia Centers

Aphasia centers have developed as places where people with aphasia can access supports that address the Participation, Environment, and Personal Factors and Identity domains. Aphasia centers are places where a holistic approach to living with aphasia is fostered in a community atmosphere through a variety of non-traditional services (Simmons-Mackie & Holland, 2011). Aphasia centers create a model for life participation through various programs. Aphasia center programs are typically oriented around participant choice of activities that relate to successful return to life. Engaging in these activities in a supported, group environment enhances coping and self-efficacy, which leads to more life participation. Participation in activities is done in a supported, adapted environment so that each individual can re-negotiate identity with aphasia through successful social interaction.

The first independent community-based aphasia center was started in 1979 by Pat Arato in Toronto, Canada, and exists today as the Aphasia Institute, providing programs, training, and products that support life participation. The first independent community-based aphasia center in the United States was the Aphasia Center of California, started by Roberta Elman in 1996. Today, there are more than 33 aphasia centers across the United States and Canada. Centers in the original survey varied in both size and intensity of programming, but all met at least once a week for an hour of programming with the majority offering 4–6 hours of weekly programming.

Case Example: Integrating the Domains

The following case example will illustrate how the four domains of the A-FROM (Kagan et al., 2008)—Language Processing, Participation, Environment, and Personal Factors and Identity—contribute to a particular activity goal. Bob is a 48-year-old gentleman who was working as an aerospace technician prior to a single left hemisphere stroke that left him with a moderate non-fluent aphasia. He lives with his wife, who works full time as a paralegal. Bob does not feel confident about returning to driving, but wants to be able to get around town independently. He would like to be able to use the public bus service successfully. Using public transportation is important to independence and depends on successful communication abilities (Ashton et al., 2008).

Going with Bob on a bus trip to a nearby location offers an opportunity to directly observe potential communication challenges and successes, as well as the barriers and facilitators that affect his use of public transportation. Key communication stages of using public transport are (1) planning the route, (2) identifying and finding the correct departure point and vehicle, (3) paying the fare, and (4) communicating the destination (Ashton et al., 2008).

The four A-FROM domains each contribute to successful participation in the use of public transportation. The Language Processing domain encompasses training the vocabulary needed for using public transportation, practicing scripts needed to get information or get to the appropriate destination, or understanding questions or directions that might be offered in the transportation context. In addition, Bob will need to be able to read and identify correct route or destination names, route numbers, and similar information. Treatment strategies in this volume can be matched successfully to Bob's need to improve language processes for using public transportation.

The Environment domain can be targeted by contacting the transportation system and providing training to bus drivers and information desk personnel about how to support communication. In addition, Bob and other people with aphasia can be encouraged and supported to attend public meetings about improvements to the public transportation system that would better support their use of the system. The technology and other supports that Bob can use should also be investigated and practiced to make his trips more successful.

The Participation domain is foregrounded here because the focus is on a specific activity that Bob wants to do (ride the bus). One way to facilitate this further is to find a "buddy" for Bob who will accompany him on the first few trips or to find someone else who is taking the same route at the same time.

We can address Personal Factors and Identity by pinpointing and discussing Bob's anxieties about what might go wrong during one of his trips. Counseling approaches can be used to identify solutions to potential problems. Bob's lack of confidence for being able to independently use the bus can be addressed by capitalizing on the sources of self-efficacy (Berry & West, 1993). The sources of self-efficacy are vicarious observation (knowing others with aphasia who successfully ride the bus), verbal encouragement, counseling and reduction of anxiety and stress, and mastery experiences.

The example of Bob riding public transportation illustrates the holistic nature of the life participation approach. Attending solely to Language Processing might mean that Bob can understand

and produce transportation-related words, produce transportation-related scripts in the clinic, or successfully read a bus schedule in a treatment room. A full-on, life participation approach to aphasia takes into account the Environment in which Bob actually has to ride the bus and his personal characteristics, including his personality, past experiences, and attitudes that will further affect his ability to successfully participate in public transportation. The issues of Environment and Personal Factors may weigh as heavily in Bob's ultimate success as aspects of his Language Processing.

Conclusions

A life participation approach simply refers to helping the individual return to meaningful appropriate and personally fulfilling activities. While this ultimate goal can be achieved with different routes (e.g., training a "skill" like "improving generalized naming"), when these skills are the sole focus of treatment, they are unlikely to result in a meaningful change in the person's life participation (Ross & Wertz, 1999, 2002). An active, explicit focus on what the person is going to do with the rest of his or her life is necessary to achieve this goal.

Notes

1 We have carefully avoided the use of the term "patient" in this section. This is because the "patient" label rightfully should be cast aside once the immediate, acute phase is over and the person moves into rehabilitation. Certainly, once released from rehab, then personhood should be the focus. We understand the political correctness in the terms "persons with aphasia" and "individuals with aphasia," but reject the distancing use of the acronyms PWA and IWA.
2 Personal communication, Denise McCall, MS. Program Director—SCALE.

References

Aleligay, A., Worrall, L.E., & Rose, T.A. (2008). Readability of written health information provided to people with aphasia. *Aphasiology, 22*, 383–407.

American Speech-Language-Hearing Association (ASHA). (2007). *Scope of Practice in Speech-Language Pathology* [Scope of Practice]. Available from www.asha.org/policy.

Armstrong, E., & Ferguson, A. (2010). Language, meaning, context, and functional communication. *Aphasiology, 24*, 480–496.

Ashton, C., Aziz, N.A., Barwood, C., French, R., Savina, E., & Worrall, L. (2008). Communicatively accessible public transport for people with aphasia: A pilot study. *Aphasiology, 22*, 305–320.

Avent, J.R., & Austermann, S. (2003). Reciprocal scaffolding: A context for communication treatment in aphasia. *Aphasiology, 17*, 397–404.

Avent, J., Glista, S., Wallace, S., Jackson, J., Nishioka, J., & Yip. W. (2005). Family information needs about aphasia. *Aphasiology, 19*, 365–375.

Avent, J., Patterson, J., Lu, A., & Small, K. (2009). Reciprocal scaffolding treatment: A person with aphasia as clinical teacher. *Aphasiology, 23*, 110–119.

Baumeister, R.F., & Leary, M.R. (1995). The need to belong: Desire for interpersonal attachments as a fundamental human motivation. *Psychological Bulletin, 117*, 497–529.

Bernstein-Ellis, E., & Elman, R.J. (1998). Aphasia group communication treatment: The Aphasia Center of California approach. In R.J. Elman (Ed.), *Group treatment of neurogenic communication disorders: The expert clinician's approach*. New York: Butterworth-Heinemann.

Berry, J.M., & West, R.L. (1993). Cognitive self-efficacy in relation to personal mastery and goal setting across the life span. *International Journal of Behavioral Development, 16*, 351–379.

Brennan, A., Worrall, L., & McKenna, K. (2005). The relationship between specific features of aphasia-friendly written material and comprehension of written material for people with aphasia: An exploratory study. *Aphasiology, 19*, 693–711.

Cott, C.A., Wiles, R., & Devitt, R. (2007). Continuity, transition, and participation: Preparing clients for life in the community post-stroke. *Disability and Rehabilitation, 29*, 1566–1574.

Cruice, M. (2007). Issues of access and inclusion in aphasia. *Aphasiology, 21*, 3–8.

Dalemans, R.J.P., de Witte, L., Wade, D., & van den Heuvel, W. (2010). Social participation through the eyes of people with aphasia. *International Journal of Language and Communication Disorders, 45*, 537–550.

Dalemans, R., Wade, D.T., van den Heuvel, W.J.A., & de Witte, L.P. (2009). Facilitating the participation of people with aphasia in research: A description of strategies. *Clinical Rehabilitation, 23*, 948–959.

Duffy, J.R., Fossett, T.R.D., & Thomas, J.E. (2011). Clinical practice in acute care hospital settings. In L.L. LaPointe (Ed.), *Aphasia and related neurogenic communication disorders* (pp. 48–58). New York: Thieme.

Eames, S., McKenna, K., Worrall, L., & Read, S. (2003). The suitability of written education material for stroke survivors and their carers. *Topics in Stroke Rehabilitation, 10*, 70–83.

Elman, R.J., & Bernstein-Ellis, E. (2003). Promoting literature for individuals with aphasia: "Reading for Life: A book club for individuals with aphasia." *ASHA Leader, 8*, 38.

Forster, A., Brown, L., Smith, J., House, A., Knapp, P., Wright, J.J., & Young, J. (2012). Information provision for stroke patients and their caregivers. *The Cochrane Library, 11*, 1–131.

Ganzfried, E.S., & Symbolik, S.N. (2011). Aphasia awareness training for emergency responders: Train the trainers. Presented at the Clinical Aphasiology Conference, Fort Lauderdale, FL, May 31 through June 4.

Garcia, L.J., Barrette, J., & Laroche, C. (2000). Perceptions of the obstacles to work reintegration for persons with aphasia. *Aphasiology, 14*, 269–290.

Haffensteindottir, T.B., Vergunst, N., Lindeman, E., & Schuurmans, M. (2011). Educational needs of patients with a stroke and their caregivers: A systematic review of the literature. *Patient Education and Counseling, 85*, 14–25.

Haley, K.L., Womack, J., Helm-Estabrooks, N., Lovette, B., & Goff, R. (2012). Supporting autonomy for people with aphasia: Use of the Life Interests and Values (LIV) cards. *Topics in Stroke Rehabilitation, 20*(1), 22–35.

Hinckley, J.J., Boyle, E., Lombard, D., & Bartels-Tobin, L. (2013). Towards a public research agenda in aphasia: Preliminary work. *Disability and Rehabilitation*.

Hinckley, J.J., & Carr, T.H. (2001). Differential contributions of cognitive abilities to success in skill-based versus context-based aphasia treatment. *Brain and Language, 79*, 3–6.

Hinckley, J.J., & Carr, T.H. (2005). Comparing the outcomes of intensive and nonintensive aphasia treatment. *Aphasiology, 19*, 965–974.

Hinckley, J.J., Hasselkus, A., & Ganzfried, E. (2013). What people with aphasia think about availability of aphasia resources. *American Journal of Speech-Language Pathology, 22*, S310–S317.

Holland, A.L., & Fridriksson, J. (2001). Management for aphasia in the acute phases post stroke. *American Journal of Speech-Language Pathology, 10*, 19–28.

Holland, A.L., Halper, A.S., & Cherney, L.R. (2010). Tell me your story: Analysis of script topics selected by persons with aphasia. *American Journal of Speech-Language Pathology, 19*, 198–203.

Holland, A.L., & Nelson, R.L. (2014). *Counseling in communication disorders: A wellness perspective* (2nd ed.). San Diego: Plural Publishing.

Hopper, T., Holland, A., & Rewega, M. (2002). Conversational coaching: Treatment outcomes and future directions. *Aphasiology, 16*, 745–761.

Howe, T.J., Worrall, L.E., & Hickson, L.M.H. (2008). Interviews with people with aphasia: Environmental factors that influence their community participation. *Aphasiology, 22*, 1092–1100.

Hurn, J., Kneebone, I., & Cropley, M. (2006). Goal setting as an outcome measure: A systematic review. *Clinical Rehabilitation, 20*, 756–772.

Hux, K., Buechter, M., Wallace, S., & Weissling, K. (2010). Using visual scene displays to create a shared communication space for a person with aphasia. *Aphasiology, 24*, 643–660.

Johansson, M.B., Carlsson, M., & Sonnander, K. (2012). Communication difficulties and the use of communication strategies: from the perspective of individuals with aphasia. *International Journal of Language & Communication Disorders, 47*, 144–155.

Kagan, A., Black, S.E., Duchan, J.F., Simmons-Mackie, N., & Square, P. (2001). Training volunteers as conversation partners using "supported conversation for adults with aphasia" (SCA): A controlled trial. *Journal of Speech, Language and Hearing Research, 44*(3), 624–638.

Kagan, A., & Simmons-Mackie, N. (2007). Beginning with the end: Outcome-driven assessment and intervention with life participation in mind. *Topics in Stroke Rehabilitation, 27*, 309–317.

Kagan, A., Simmons-Mackie, N., Rowand, A., Huijbregts, M., Shumway, E., McEwen, S., Threats, T., & Sharp, S. (2008). Counting what counts: A framework for capturing real-life outcomes in aphasia intervention. *Aphasiology, 22*, 258–280.

King, J.M. (2013). Communication supports. In N. Simmons-Mackie, J.M. King, & D. Beukelman (Eds.), *Supporting communication for adults with acute and chronic aphasia*. Baltimore: Brookes Publishing.

Knight, K., Worrall, L., & Rose, T. (2006). The provision of stroke information to stroke patients within an acute hospital setting: What actually happens and how do patients feel about it? *Topics in Stroke Rehabilitation, 13*, 78–97.

Lanyon, L.E., Rose, M.L., & Worrall, L.E. (2013). The efficacy of outpatient and community-based aphasia interventions: A systematic review. *International Journal of Speech-Language Pathology, 15*, 359–374

Lawrence, M., & Kinn, S. (2011). Defining and measuring patient-centered care: An example from mixed-methods systematic review of the stroke literature. *Health Expectations, 15*, 295–326.

Leach, E., Cornwell, P., Fleming, J., & Haines, T. (2010). Patient-centered goal setting in a subacute rehabilitation setting. *Disability and Rehabilitation, 32*, 159–172.

Legg, C., Young, L., & Bryer, A. (2005). Training sixth-year medical students in obtaining case-history information from adults with aphasia. *Aphasiology, 19*(6), 559–575.

LPAA Project Group (in alphabetical order: Chapey, R., Duchan, J., Elman, R., Garcia, L., Kagan, A., Lyon, J., & Simmons-Mackie, N). (2001). Life participation approach to aphasia: A statement of values for the future. In R. Chapey (Ed.), Language intervention strategies in aphasia and related neurogenic communication disorders (4th ed.) (pp. 235–248). Philadelphia, PA: Lippincott Williams & Wilkins.

Lyon, J., Cariski, D., Keisler, L., Rosenbek, J., Levine, R., Kumpula, J., Ryff, C., Coyne, S., & Blanc, M. (1997). Communication Partners: Enhancing participation in life and communication for adults with aphasia in natural settings. *Aphasiology, 11*, 693–708.

Malec, J.F. (1999). Goal attainment scaling in rehabilitation. *Neuropsychological Rehabilitation, 9*, 253–275.

Moss, B., Parr, S., & Petheram, B. (2004). "Pick me up and not a down, up": How are the identities of people with aphasia represented in aphasia, stroke and disability websites? *Disability and Society, 19*, 759–768.

O'Halloran, R., Worrall, L.E., & Hickson, L. (2009). The number of patients with communication related impairments in acute hospital stroke units. *International Journal of Speech-Language Pathology, 11*, 438–449.

Palmer, R., & Paterson, G. (2013). To what extent can people with communication difficulties contribute to health research? *Nurse Researcher, 20*, 12–16.

Parr, S., Byng, S., Gilpin, S., & Ireland, C. (1997). *Talking about aphasia: Living with loss of language after stroke.* Buckingham: Open University Press.

Rayner, H., & Marshall, J. (2003). Training volunteers as conversation partners for people with aphasia. *International Journal of Language and Communication Disorders, 38*(2), 149–164.

Rose, M.L. (2013). Releasing the constraints on aphasia therapy: The positive impact of gesture and multi-modality treatments. *American Journal of Speech-Language Pathology, 22*, S227–S239.

Rose, T., Worrall, L., Hickson, L., & Hoffmann, T. (2010). Do people with aphasia want written stroke and aphasia information? A verbal survey exploring preferences for when and how to provide stroke and aphasia information. *Topics in Stroke Rehabilitation, 17*, 79–98.

Rose, T., Worrall, L., Hickson, L., & Hoffmann, T. (2011). Aphasia friendly written health information: Content and design characteristics. *International Journal of Speech-Language Pathology, 13*, 355–347.

Rose, T., Worrall, L., & McKenna, K. (2003). The effectiveness of aphasia-friendly principles for printed health education materials for people with aphasia following stroke. *Aphasiology, 17*, 947–963.

Ross, K.B., & Wertz, R.T. (1999). Comparison of impairment and disability measures for assessing severity of, and improvement in, aphasia. *Aphasiology, 13*, 113–124.

Ross, K., & Wertz, R.W. (2002). Relationships between language-based disability and quality of life in chronically aphasic adults. *Aphasiology, 16*, 791–800.

Rowland, A., & McDonald, L. (2009). Evaluation of social work communication skills to allow people with aphasia to be part of the decision making process in health care. *Social Work Education, 28*, 128–144.

Seligman, M.E.P. (2011). *Flourish.* New York: Free Press.

Shadden, B.B. (2005). Aphasia as identify theft: Theory and practice. *Aphasiology, 19*, 211–223.

Shadden, B.B., & Agan, J.P. (2004). Renegotiation of identity: The social context of support groups. *Topics in Language Disorders, 24*, 174–186.

Shadden, B.B., & Koski, P.R. (2007). Social construction of self for persons with aphasia: When language as a cultural tool is impaired. *Journal of Medical Speech-Language Pathology, 15*, 99–105.

Silverman, M. (2011). Community: The key to building and extending engagement for individuals with aphasia. *Seminars in Speech and Language, 23*, 256–267.

Simmons-Mackie, N., & Elman, R. (2011). Negotiation of identity in group therapy for aphasia: the Aphasia Café. *International Journal of Language & Communication Disorders, 46*, 312–323.

Simmons-Mackie, N., & Holland, A.L. (2011). Aphasia centers in North America: A survey. *Seminars in Speech & Language, 32*, 203–215.

Simmons-Mackie, N., Kagan, A., Christie, C., Huijbregts, M., McEwen, S., & Willems J. (2007). Communicative access and decision making for people with aphasia: Implementing sustainable healthcare systems change. *Aphasiology, 21*, 39–66.

Simmons-Mackie, N., King, J., & Beukelman, D. (2013). *Supporting communication for adults with acute and chronic aphasia*. Baltimore MD: Brookes.

Simmons-Mackie, N., Raymer, A., Armstrong, E., Holland, A., & Cherney, L.R. (2010). Communication partner training in aphasia: A systematic review. *Archives of Physical Medicine Rehabilitation, 91*, 1814–1837.

Threats, T. (2007). Access for persons with neurogenic communication disorders: Influences of Personal and Environmental Factors of the ICF. *Aphasiology, 21*, 67–80.

Vickers, C. (2010). Social networks after the onset of aphasia: The impact of aphasia group attendance. *Aphasiology, 24*, 902–910.

Welsh, J.D., & Szabo, G.B. (2011). Teaching nursing assistant students about aphasia and communication. *Seminars in Speech and Language, 32*, 243–255.

Worrall, L., Brown, K., Cruice, M., Davidson, B., Hersh, D., Howe, T., & Sherratt, S. (2010). The evidence for a life-coaching approach to aphasia. *Aphasiology, 24*, 497–514.

Worrall, L., Rose, M., Howe, T., McKenna, K., & Hickson, L. (2007). Developing an evidence base for accessibility for people with aphasia. *Aphasiology, 21*, 124–136.

Worrall, L., Sherratt, S., Rogers, P., Howe, T., Hersh, D., Ferguson, A., & Davidson, B. (2011). What people with aphasia want: Their goals according to the ICF. *Aphasiology, 25*, 309–322.

World Health Organization. (2003). *ICF Checklist*. Geneva: World Health Organization.

24

THE NATURE AND IMPLICATIONS OF RIGHT HEMISPHERE LANGUAGE DISORDERS

Connie A. Tompkins, Chia-Ming Lei, and Alexandra Zezinka

Historically, the study of neurologically-based language disorders has focused on aphasia, which most often is a consequence of damage to the language-dominant left cerebral hemisphere (LH). Over the past 30 years, nonaphasic language impairments associated with right hemisphere damage (RHD) have received increasing attention. About 50% of unselected patients with RHD have such deficits (Benton & Bryan, 1996), and in a rehabilitation setting the estimates exceed 80% (Blake, Duffy, Myers, & Tompkins, 2002; Côté, Payer, Giroux, & Joanette, 2007). Communication disorders in RHD clearly can affect daily function, social interaction, and quality of life. Thus, one important goal of the quest to understand RHD language disorders is to derive implications for diagnosis, prognosis, and clinical intervention. From a theoretical perspective, language impairments in adults with RHD have been studied not only in their own right, but also as a window on the nature of language representation and processing in the so-called minor hemisphere. The research on RHD converges with other investigations, including those of individuals with intact (e.g., Beeman & Chiarello, 1998; Vigneau, Beaucousin, Hervé et al., 2011) and surgically disconnected right hemispheres (e.g., Baynes & Eliassen, 1998; Zaidel, 1998) and of people who are recovering from aphasia (e.g., Turkeltaub, Messing, Norise, & Hamilton, 2011) to indicate that the right hemisphere (RH) potential for language processing is far from minor.

This chapter focuses on the most definitive evidence about RHD language functioning, which comes from right-handed adults with acquired neuropathology confined to the right cerebral hemisphere. Such damage typically results from a cerebrovascular accident rather than etiologies with more diffuse consequences like traumatic brain injury or Alzheimer's disease.

The chapter is organized into four parts. The first outlines some conceptual and methodological issues that influence the conduct and interpretation of RHD language research. Next we provide an overview of evidence about RHD language disorders in lexical-semantic and pragmatic-discourse function, discuss current attributions about the nature of these difficulties, and identify considerations for future research. We focus on these domains because of the wealth of evidence for their potential disruption after RHD, in contrast to phonological and syntactic functions that RHD leaves essentially unimpaired. Language processing in the intact RH and hemispheric cooperation in language functioning also are addressed in this section as frameworks to guide and interpret the investigation of RHD disorders. While deficits in prosodic (e.g., Baum & Pell, 1999; Ross & Monnot, 2011) and emotional processing (e.g., Heilman, 2009) also may be hallmarks of RHD and contribute crucially to social communication, these are discussed by Tippett and Elliott in chapter 25, this volume. The third section considers how evidence and perspectives on RHD language disorders and intact RH language function inform one another. Finally, we address briefly some issues in clinical management of RHD language disorders.

Designing and Reading the Research: Conceptual and Methodological Considerations

Planning and interpreting studies of RHD presents a number of challenges. Chief among these are a dearth of explicit, testable models of the cognitive and linguistic domains or systems that support social exchange and philosophical and empirical issues related to the validity of predicting from normal to disordered function (or vice versa). These issues are discussed in the third section of the chapter.

Theory building is further complicated by limited information on whether there is more than one variant of RHD language disorders, or whether there are predictable sets of co-occurring symptoms. Some progress is beginning on this front: potential subgroups have been identified based on performance on a relatively new standardized test of verbal communication (e.g., Côté et al. 2007; Ferré, Fonseca, Ska, & Joanette, 2012).[1] Another major problem is that there is little consensus on how to define or even what to call RHD language deficits, in totality or as individual components of an aggregate "syndrome." Conceptual and terminological imprecision and overlap are common in referring to targets of inquiry like nonliteral language processing, inferencing, integration, and reasoning from a theory of mind (Stemmer & Joanette, 1998; Tompkins, 1995). This definitional difficulty both derives from and contributes to most of the other challenges described below (for further discussion, see, e.g., Joanette & Ansaldo, 1999; Myers, 1999; Stemmer & Joanette, 1998).

Other notable considerations in the investigation of RHD include those related to the following.

Accounting for Variability

Adults with RHD are heterogeneous, varying widely in lesion characteristics, presence and severity of impairments, and reactions to and eventual outcomes of their condition (Tompkins, Lehman, Wyatt, & Schulz, 1998). Attributes unrelated to the neurological event, such as age-related sensory changes, educational attainment, and premorbid knowledge, skills, and cognitive capacities, add to these sources of heterogeneity. Characteristics like handedness (Shapleske, Rossell, Woodruff, & David, 1999), sex (Shapleske et al., 1999; Ingalhalikar, Smith, Parker et al., 2014), or age (Federmeier, 2007; Guzzetti & Daini, 2014) also may interact with hemispheric contributions to language functioning. Intrasubject performance variability also is evident in adults with RHD. Some of this undoubtedly reflects physiological and psychological adaptation and compensation to the consequences of the neurological insult, though little is known yet about this kind of change over time. Some also can be task induced, for example, by purposeful manipulation of attentional processing requirements (e.g., Tompkins & Lehman, 1998). Among the hurdles this pervasive variability poses for RHD language research, it is essentially impossible for studies to account for a full range of potential components of and contributors to communication performance. It is also extremely difficult to match subsets of participants for between-subjects comparisons. Additionally, particularly in combination with frequently limited participant descriptions, it can be quite challenging to generalize results.

Selecting Participant Samples

In the RHD language disorders literature, sample sizes generally are quite small and sampling biases are common, such as selecting participants solely from those in rehabilitation. Another sampling issue concerns the question of which RHD participants to study. Some suggest that to understand RHD language disorders, one should investigate only individuals who have them (Myers, 1999). On the other hand, a sample that is not selected for language disorders confers advantages for discovering subgroups of the RHD population, developing prognostic profiles, and/or inferring potential mechanisms of deficit by assessing factors associated with spared and impaired performances. Of course, an unselected sample will include an unknown mix of individuals with and without language disorders, or with and without particular processing deficits. Either way, results that reflect only the group mean performance may be entirely uninformative.

Designating Disordered Performances

Beyond the general difficulty of determining who has a language disorder is a more specific challenge. For many variables of interest, especially in the realm of pragmatics and interpersonal communication, normative information is not available, and individual differences and sociocultural variations are not well understood. Control groups are a start, but due to their typically small sizes in the RHD literature, the variety of attributes that may influence performance, and the potentially vast range of "normal," it often remains quite difficult to decide what constitutes a "deficit."

Establishing Control Groups

When the research goal is to determine whether RHD is responsible for performances of interest, it becomes especially problematic to select an appropriate control group. Adults with left hemisphere damage (LHD) and aphasia often cannot be used because their linguistic processing difficulties may invalidate their performance with complex stimuli and task instructions typical of RHD language studies. When participants with LHD are included, issues arise of equating the groups for severity (Duffy & Myers, 1991). Adults with LHD who are sufficiently accurate on an experimental task may be less neurologically involved than the RHD group, particularly if the RHD sample is relatively severe (e.g., includes only people who receive cognitive-language rehabilitation). It is important in such circumstances that conditions be included to probe for compelling double dissociations in performance or for paradoxical functional facilitation effects (Kapur, 1996). It also helps to evaluate potentially different reasons for quantitatively similar performances of participants with RHD and LHD (Kasher, Batori, Soroker, Graves, & Zaidel, 1999; Tompkins, 1990). However, such a rarefied sample of adults with LHD raises questions about its representativeness (Joanette & Goulet, 1994). It is less difficult to constitute a control group when the research question asks only whether certain kinds of deficits can occur in adults with RHD. In such cases, nonspecific performance differences can be reduced by using control groups of patients with peripheral nervous system involvement (Lojek-Osiejuk, 1996) or of neurologically normal adults who have experienced the "patient" role (e.g., people with orthopedic injuries; Blonder, Burns, Bowers, Moore, & Heilman, 1993).

Inferring Lesion-Behavior Correspondences

Few studies of adults with RHD have attempted to discover relationships between cognitive and communicative performances and lesion site, despite the potential diagnostic, prognostic, and explanatory value of doing so. Recent work has begun to tackle this important issue (e.g., Griffin, Friedman, Ween, Winner, Happé, & Brownell, 2006; Prabhakaran, Raman, Grunwald et al., 2007; Marini, 2012; Schmidt, Cardillo, Kranjec, Lehet, Widick, & Chatterjee, 2012; Tompkins, Fassbinder, Scharp, & Meigh, 2008; Yang, Tompkins, Meigh, & Prat, submitted). The typically small sample sizes and inherent heterogeneity in RHD language studies complicate efforts to align lesion and

language characteristics. Another obstacle is the various "unknowns" about the specific physiological consequences of neurological injury, discussed later in this chapter.

Other Methodological Issues

It can be difficult to apply many of the psycholinguistic or cognitive-neuropsychological research
paradigms that allow fine-grained analysis of component strengths and weaknesses in adults with
RHD. Performance on tasks that involve precisely timed stimulus presentation methods may be
confounded by concomitant deficits, such as hemispatial neglect or visuoperceptual difficulties,
or by general and/or specific slowing (Howes & Boller, 1975). Such considerations contribute to
the fact that the overwhelming majority of research has used offline methods and explicit/meta-
linguistic tasks to evaluate language processing in adults with RHD. This fact also has skewed the
accumulated observations, because such methods introduce multiple demands that are not part of
natural language processing and that may confound or obscure the processes of interest. In comparison, less cognitively demanding implicit or online measures have revealed strengths that are not
evident from offline, metalinguistic tasks; thus such methods may help to sort out potential reasons for impaired end-product performance (see Tompkins & Baumgaertner, 1998; Tompkins &
Lehman, 1998). Of course, some online measurements have their own sets of problems, such as
determining how and where to probe to evaluate a process as it is happening. Well-elaborated
theoretical models of the mechanisms in question are needed to help address such issues. A final
methodological point is that it also challenging to validate stimulus materials. Norms do not exist
for many stimulus parameters of interest. Those that are available, such as category norms, usually
are based on young adults' metalinguistic judgments, raising questions about the validity of applying them with older adults or in more implicit tasks.

Evidence and Attributions about RHD Language Disorders

Lexical-Semantic Processing

Individuals with RHD may have difficulties on measures that require lexical processing, like
word-picture matching, picture naming, semantic judgment, and verbal fluency tasks. Results from
studies using the same tasks often are contradictory, but these investigations may have enrolled
different patient samples, as discussed above.

One major problem in evaluating studies of RHD lexical-semantic disorders is that many
have not specified a model of lexical semantics or an account of how lexical-semantic representations or computations are hypothesized to be impaired. Broadly speaking, such impairments can
reflect degradation of stored representations or disorders of processes that map phonological or
orthographic lexical information onto meaning (or vice versa). For activation of related meanings, as evaluated in priming studies, effects could derive from associations between phonological or orthographic information, associations of word meanings based on semantic similarity or
co-occurrence probability, or an interaction. Because many studies reviewed here do not allow
a clear differentiation of such factors, the term *lexical-semantic* as used herein subsumes all such
aspects of the lexical-semantic system.

One early line of research investigated whether RHD can cause subtle, general deficits in
the lexical-semantic system. Results from word-picture matching and picture naming studies
are inconclusive. Although various studies show that individuals with RHD can be impaired on
such tasks (Gainotti, Caltagirone, Miceli, & Masullo, 1983; Lesser, 1974), the participants' errors
could be due to visual perceptual impairment (Chieffi, Carlomagno, Silveri, & Gainotti, 1989;
Gainotti et al., 1983). The common finding that adults with RHD make more visual-semantic

errors than pure visual errors could reflect either an interaction of visual-perceptual and semantic deficits or the products of impaired visual-perceptual recognition as filtered through an intact lexical-semantic system.

Results of early priming studies also provide little evidence of lexical-semantic disorders, in that individuals with RHD have no deficit in associative lexical priming at short and long stimulus onset asynchronies (Gagnon, Goulet, & Joanette, 1989; Henik, Dronkers, Knight, & Osimani, 1993; Tompkins, 1990). Such findings suggest that lexical-semantic activation processes are preserved to some degree in RHD, but they do not rule out the possibility that these processes are in some way less efficient. For instance, in a study of lexical metaphor processing, reaction times of participants with RHD were slower even after being adjusted for basic response speed (Tompkins, 1990), a finding that could reflect slowed activation.

A recent systematic review of 11 studies of semantic priming in adults with RHD catalogues difficulties in 5 of the 11 and concludes that impairments are more evident for polysemic (words with multiple meanings or senses) than for monosemic words (de Lima Müller & de Salles, 2013). However, the selection criteria for the review were somewhat idiosyncratic. Despite the inclusion of an unpublished master's thesis and a chapter, several peer-reviewed publications are omitted (e.g., Fassbinder & Tompkins, 2001; Lincoln, Long, Swick, Larsen, & Baynes, 2008; Tompkins, 1990). The conclusions of the review also are not tempered for interindividual differences emphasized in some of the original studies.

Other data are consistent with a possible subtle lexical-semantic deficit, but perhaps only when processing is relatively demanding of cognitive effort. In several studies using metalinguistic tasks, individuals with RHD had difficulty in conditions requiring retrieval of semantic information, as compared to phonological or orthographic aspects of words (Chiarello & Church, 1986; Joanette & Goulet, 1989; Lesser, 1974). From these results, the authors infer an impairment of lexical-semantic processing in RHD. However, this inference is valid only if stimuli in contrasting conditions have the same cognitive resource demands. That this is a questionable assumption has been shown for verbal fluency tasks. When semantic and orthographic conditions are equated for the average number of words that control subjects produce to criterion, individuals with RHD are impaired in both conditions (Goulet, Joanette, Sabourin, & Giroux, 1997). This suggests a general search inefficiency in retrieving items for this task, more than a problem of lexical-semantics. Overall, this evidence does not definitively indicate whether a lexical-semantic deficit is a direct consequence of RHD, or whether the accumulated results reflect more generalized difficulties with attentional or working memory processes.

Another line of research has investigated whether RHD impairs the processing of specific meaning domains, such as those carried by nonliteral or emotional words. Although one study found that adults with RHD did not prime for metaphoric word meanings, neither did the control group (Klepousniotou & Baum, 2005a). In an earlier investigation, adults with RHD did prime for such meanings, similarly to control subjects (Tompkins, 1990). Evidence for a specific deficit for nonliteral meanings again may be linked to demands for effortful processing. Individuals with RHD do more poorly on semantic judgment tasks involving metaphoric or emotional meanings than do control subjects with LHD and without brain damage, but RHD participants perform equally to LHD subjects in judging literal or affectively neutral meanings (Borod, Andelman, Olber, Tweedy, & Welkowitz, 1992; Brownell, Simpson, Bihrle, Potter, & Gardner, 1990). Adults with RHD also are less likely to group word triplets based on metaphoric relations (Brownell, Potter, Michelow, & Gardner, 1984). Extending this word-triplet study to include nonmetaphoric ambiguous nouns, Brownell and colleagues (1990) reinterpreted the results to indicate that adults with RHD are generally insensitive to alternative meanings.[2] In any case, to infer a specific impairment in the effortful processing of "metaphoric" or "emotional" semantic meanings, it is necessary to demonstrate that such differences do not derive from an interaction of general processing limitations and differences in processing difficulty between domains. On the whole, these findings do not rule out domain-specific lexical-semantic deficits, but neither do they provide compelling evidence.

Much recent work has been driven by or interpreted in light of models of RH lexical-semantic processing derived from studies of people with healthy brains. The underlying assumption in relating these models to RHD disorders has most often been one of direct mapping. That is, RHD is presumed to cause a loss (or diminution) of function that has been attributed to the intact RH and a corresponding over-reliance on LH processes. The direct mapping assumption is problematic, as elaborated later in this chapter. However, two prominent applications of normal processing models are considered next.

One relatively long-standing hypothesis is that RHD will disrupt the activation of, for example, metaphoric meanings or subordinate interpretations of lexical ambiguities (the "intelligence-related" interpretation of the adjective *sharp* or the "sides-of-a-river" interpretation of the noun *bank*). This prediction is based on evidence suggesting that the intact RH serves the purpose of "coarsely coding" semantic input, activating or maintaining weak associates of lexical items or distant semantic relations (for reviews, see Beeman, 1998; Jung-Beeman, 2005). A second hypothesis, linked to the previous one, is that the LH quickly selects dominant or contextually appropriate meanings, while the RH hemisphere maintains activation of subordinate meanings and remote associates (for reviews, see Beeman, 1998; Chiarello, 1998; Jung-Beeman, 2005). Assuming the direct mapping between normal and disordered RH functions, this hypothesis predicts that individuals with RHD should not have access to nondominant or alternative interpretations. Assuming that LH processes predominate, adults with RHD should show inhibition effects for subordinate meanings of ambiguous words or remotely associated words. Such effects have been reported for right visual field/LH presentations in priming studies with non-brain-damaged individuals (Burgess & Simpson, 1988; Nakagawa, 1991), though not always (Anaki, Faust, & Kravetz, 1998). Priming of (subordinate) metaphoric interpretations of lexical ambiguities at both short and long interstimulus intervals (Tompkins, 1990) is at odds with the notion that such meanings are unavailable to adults with RHD, either early or over extended periods of time.

Priming studies of lexical ambiguity resolution, investigating when and how adults with RHD activate multiple word meanings and select those that are contextually appropriate, also paint a different picture from this direct mapping assumption. Integrating the broader literature on language processing and language disorders in RHD, Tompkins, Baumgaertner, Lehman, and Fassbinder (2000; see also Tompkins, 2008) proposed a suppression deficit hypothesis. The first premise of this hypothesis is that adults with RHD, rather than failing to activate nondominant or alternative interpretations, routinely activate multiple interpretations but hold on too long to those that become contextually inappropriate. The second premise is that interindividual differences in the suppression of contextually incompatible meanings will predict narrative comprehension in adults with RHD and, potentially, performance in many other problem domains.

The authors first evaluated this hypothesis by placing balanced lexical ambiguities—words with two relatively equally probable meanings (e.g., *spade*)—at the end of short sentences that biased one interpretation and ruled out the other. Results of a relatedness judgment task demonstrated that shortly after hearing an ambiguity, average response times of both RHD and control groups were influenced by both its meanings. At a later time interval, though, the control group had suppressed the contextually incompatible meaning—their response time was no longer influenced by that meaning—while the RHD group had not. Because the RHD group was accurate in their relatedness judgments, their suppression mechanism must have worked, but in a delayed or inefficient manner. Intragroup variability in suppression function was clear, in that interindividual differences in suppression effectiveness predicted general narrative comprehension for the RHD group.

Fassbinder and Tompkins (2001) report a lexical-level suppression deficit for adults with RHD, as well. Klepousnioutou and Baum's (2005b) results also are mostly consistent with the suppression deficit hypothesis: no RHD deficit for early priming of subordinate meanings of homonyms or weak associates of metonyms, but abnormally prolonged priming for contextually incompatible meanings or associates.[3] Also, the absence of early priming for metaphoric senses of words was taken as evidence of a potential metaphor-specific processing deficit in adults with RHD; alternative interpretations are offered below.

Grindrod and Baum evaluated lexical ambiguity resolution in single sentence (2003) and two-sentence discourse contexts (2005) using balanced ambiguities. The pattern of results is complicated and not entirely consistent. In the sentence study, in unbiased contexts, the RHD group primed only for the slightly more frequent, first-meaning of the ambiguity, both immediately after its offset and at a later test point. In biased contexts, at the immediate test point, they primed for only the slightly less frequent, second-meaning regardless of its contextual congruity. In the discourse study there was no significant priming, but the "majority" of the RHD group reportedly primed for second-meanings regardless of context immediately after the ambiguity, and for first meanings regardless of context at the later test point. The authors conclude that the RHD group was impaired in using context to process and resolve lexical ambiguity.

One particularly commendable aspect of this work is the examination of intragroup consistency. The authors note that even for the statistically significant effects, only 44% of RHD participants' results fit the group pattern. This figure again highlights the need for caution in interpreting group average findings and the importance of accounting for individual differences. Methodological discrepancies between these studies and those reviewed previously include differences in stimulus presentation (visual context + auditory target for Grindrod & Baum; all auditory for the others) and in early test intervals (0 ms ISI between ambiguity offset and target onset for Grindrod & Baum; 100 or 175 ms ISI for others). The need to switch so rapidly between presentation modalities may have disrupted contextual processing for Grindrod and Baum's RHD group, relative to their control subjects.

Returning to the hypothesis that the intact RH "coarsely codes" language input, some adults with RHD may have a coarse semantic coding deficit; that is, that they may have difficulty activating and/or sustaining broad-based meaning representations that include particularly distant features and remote associates of words. In a priming study of the early activation and later maintenance of more and less remote subordinate features of unambiguous words (e.g., "rotten" vs. "crunchy" as features of an *apple*), a group with RHD was less accurate than a healthy control group only for the more distant (or less frequent) subordinate semantic features (Tompkins, Fassbinder et al., 2008). Hagoort, Brown, and Swaab (1996) also report a trend for adults with RHD to be impaired in processing distantly related word pairs (members of the same category that were unassociated) but not closely related pairs (associated words).

Because their group with RHD primed for subordinate meanings of homonyms and weak associates of metonyms, Klepousnioutou and Baum (2005a, 2005b) rule out a coarse coding deficit and favor a metaphor-specific processing deficit to account for their results. However, a coarse coding deficit may only be evident for the most remote relationships among word meanings or features (Tompkins, Fassbinder et al., 2008; Tompkins, Scharp, Meigh, & Fassbinder, 2008). If so, Klepousniotou and Baum's metaphor results may reflect a coarse coding deficit, in that their metaphorically related primes and targets appear to be quite loosely connected. An alternative account derives from Lincoln and colleagues (2008), who report that RHD disrupted the use of visual perceptual information about words. Control subjects, and LHD subjects with comprehension level and lesion size controlled, recognized pictures that matched the implied state or shape of an object (e.g., an apple in a bag versus in a salad) better than the unmatched pictures. The RHD group did not show the match effect.[4] The vast majority of Tompkins and colleagues' features are perceptual, though they encompass taste, audition, olfaction, and combinations as much as visual features. A good proportion of Klepousniotou and Baum's metaphoric target words also reflect visual perceptual features of their primes.

Although the suppression deficit and coarse coding deficit hypotheses have often been cast as competitors, they are not mutually incompatible. A suppression deficit can yield prolonged activation of contextually incompatible word meanings or features most anywhere along a semantic distance continuum, while a coarse coding deficit may affect only the most remote aspects of meaning. The two deficits result from different lesion complexes (Tompkins, 2012; Yang, et al., submitted) and co-occur in a sizeable proportion of adults with RHD (Blake, Tompkins, Scharp, Meigh, & Wambaugh, 2015). In addition, reports of suppression deficit in some adults with RHD fit easily into a recent revision of the coarse coding hypothesis, the bilateral activation, inhibition, and selection (BAIS) model, which proposes bilateral hemispheric roles for semantic integration and selection as well as for early meaning activation and maintenance (Jung-Beeman, 2005).

In summary, evidence remains sparse as to whether or how RHD affects the lexical-semantic system. To address this issue, studies are needed that are based on models of lexical-semantic processing, and from which directly testable predictions can be derived. To differentiate lexical-semantic deficits from generalized processing difficulties, various attentional, retrieval, and/ or timing demands of the experimental tasks need to be directly manipulated. Evidence about lesion-performance associations will be critical to advance knowledge in this area, as well.

Updated models of hemispheric contributions to lexical-semantic processing also should be considered. It is now well documented that bilaterally distributed brain networks contribute to lexical-semantic processing (e.g., Donnelly, Allendorfer, & Szaflarski, 2011; Gow, 2012; Jung-Beeman, 2005; Vigneau et al., 2011). Some of this evidence comes from methods that allow more causal attributions than others, including repetitive transcranial magnetic stimulation (rTMS; Harpaz, Levkovitz, & Lavidor, 2009) and transcranial direct current stimulation (Peretz & Lavidor, 2013; Weltman & Lavidor, 2013). The nature of hemispheric contributions and interactions, however, remains under substantial debate.

Many studies continue to report evidence consistent with the coarse semantic coding hypothesis or its update, the BAIS model (e.g., Forgács et al., 2012; Lovseth & Atchley, 2010; Meyer & Federmeier, 2007, 2008; Sass, Krach, Sachs, & Kircher, 2009), extending it to less frequent verbs (Chiarello, Kacinik, Shears, Arambel, Halderman, & Robinson, 2006) and "punch words" that reflect the endings of jokes (Coulson & Williams, 2005). However, inconsistent results also are mounting (e.g., Coney, 2002; Frishkoff, 2007; Gouldthorp & Coney, 2011; Kandhadai & Federmeier, 2008; Meyer and Federmeier, 2007, 2008). Coulson and Wu's (2005) findings, for instance, suggest that the RH is involved in coding thematically related information rather than semantic distance. Other results indicate that coarse coding alone does not account for some comprehension phenomena it has been suggested to undergird (e.g., metaphor processing; Forgács et al., 2012).

Debate also remains ongoing about hemispheric differences in time course of meaning activation. Some divided visual field studies suggest earlier LH activation of subordinate meanings (e.g., Burgess & Simpson, 1988) and categorical relationships (e.g., Koivisto & Laine, 2000). Other work, using more sensitive magnetoencephalographic (MEG) methods, finds that while hemispheric time courses are highly correlated, RH activation precedes that of the LH (Assaf, Jagannathan, Calhoun, et al., 2009).[5]

Whether or how the RH preferentially maintains features or meanings of words remains controversial, as well. Some work suggests that rather than maintaining weakly related, categorical, connections between words, the RH maintains activation only for targets that are both categorically and associatively related (Bouaffre & Faita-Ainseba, 2007). Harpaz, Lavidor, and Goldstein (2013) also report no evidence of RH contribution to maintaining subordinate meanings. Their MEG results indicate that the RH perisylvian network that is preferentially involved in processing subordinate meanings in a 153–235 ms time range is no longer engaged in the 235–390 ms processing range. Meyer and Federmeier's (2008) ERP results, obtained in an eye-tracking study, suggest that the RH actually may dampen (or let decay) subordinate meanings, and then reactivate them more quickly than the LH in contextually incompatible contexts. If experimental methods miss this inhibition/decay interval, this dynamic pattern could be mistaken for maintenance of context-inconsistent meanings. Various other results also implicate flexible RH participation in lexical-semantic processing, potentially to incorporate unanticipated or surprising aspects of meaning into prior context (Coulson & Williams, 2005; Federmeier, 2007; Meyer & Federmeier, 2007, 2008).

The dynamics of hemispheric cooperation and competition have received additional attention of late. For example, Evans and Federmeier (2009) report different hemispheric asymmetries at different processing stages (i.e., encoding vs. retrieval). Rutherford and Lutz (2004) found better nonword and pseudoword processing when one visual field was distracted, suggesting that the hemispheres used some conflicting strategies. With practice on the pseudoword task, an early asymmetry first reversed and later was augmented. And, Mason, Prat, and Just (2013) document dynamic adjustment and reconfiguration of hemispheric contributions to language comprehension after rTMS to Wernicke's area.

Attending to individual differences also remains crucial. Mason and Just (2007), for instance, underscore RH activation differences related to their reading span measure of working memory. Lower-span readers were more apt to engage the RH in processing lexical ambiguities, but higher-span readers were more likely to maintain both meanings. Prat and Just (2011) report that the neural networks of higher-span readers were more adaptable and remained better synchronized in the face of increasing task demands, and that frontal brain activity—interpreted as a sign of neural efficiency—was related to vocabulary knowledge.

Finally, "embodied" or "situated" perspectives on cognition offer a fresh lens with which to examine lexical-semantic processing in RHD, particularly with respect to the types of representations that incoming words may activate other than semantic fields or associations. Although these views have multiple variants, the basic idea is that cognition is critically determined by some degree of sensory/perceptual and motor/action processing or simulation of past experience[6] (for reviews, see Kiefer & Pulvermüller, 2012; Meteyard, Cuadrado, Bahrami, & Vigliocco, 2012; see also Chatterjee, 2010, for a nuanced perspective). Binder and Desai (2011) add that affective experience also permeates concept knowledge and semantic processing. While these reviews identify controversy over both the necessity and exact nature of influence of perceptual/motor/affective representations for comprehension, the Lincoln et al. (2008) study of priming for perceptual representations is a nice example of work motivated by this type of perspective.

Discourse Processing

RHD language disorders are particularly evident in the domain of pragmatics (for recent reviews and perspectives, see Blake, 2007, 2015; Johns, Tooley, & Traxler, 2008; Tompkins, Kleposnioutou, & Scott, 2012), which involves the context-appropriate social use of language. Much of the relevant research focuses on discourse processing as a manifestation of pragmatic functioning. A growing literature suggests that some adults with RHD may have impairments in building, extracting, or applying the mental structures that guide discourse processing. These problems seem especially marked when the communicative task requires adults with RHD to revise mental models in order to update or repair initial interpretations, or to construct a coherent model by linking multiple or disparate representations of text elements, internal knowledge, and external contexts.

One frequently investigated aspect of discourse and conversation in RHD is that of supplying sufficiently informative content. Sherratt and Bryan (2012) recently summarized the contradictory findings related to relevance, usage of elements of discourse grammar, clarity disruptions, productivity, and cohesion, with some work identifying deficits and other work finding none (see also Blake, 2015; Cummings, 2007). Discourse content may or may not be sparse and insufficient, excessive, tangential, related only in broad strokes, or replete with disruptions. There also is much variability by task (Dressler, Stark, Vassilakou et al., 2004; Sherratt & Bryan, 2012). Some discourse processing problems may be less apparent in more natural interactions (Rousseaux, Daveluy, & Kozlowski, 2010), though adults with RHD may use fewer conversational speech acts than healthy control subjects (i.e., question, assertions, requests, commands; Soroker, Kasher, Giora et al., 2005) or may continue talking even after their communication partner has moved to close the conversation (Kennedy, 2000).

Other potential difficulties in creating, manipulating, or using discourse structure include (1) conveying, and perhaps appreciating, central themes of single discourse units (Dressler et al., 2004; Hough, 1990; Sherratt & Bryan, 2012) or of several related ones (Lojek-Osiejuk, 1996); (2) organizing and ordering elements of discourse structure (Lojek-Osiejuk, 1996; Sherratt & Bryan, 2012), though perhaps only or especially with anterior lesions (Marini, 2012); and (3) drawing certain kinds of inferences (e.g., Beeman, 1993; Hamel & Joanette, 2007), though perhaps only in cognitively demanding processing conditions (e.g., Dresseler et al., 2004; Tompkins, Blake, Baumgaertner, & Jayaram, 2004), including situations with insufficient contextual support (e.g., Blake, 2009a, 2009b).

While limited by its sample of four participants, Dressler et al.'s (2004) comprehensive analysis of multiple tasks, based on a theoretical model of text-pragmatic deficits, suggests that discourse impairments that do occur may be related to (1) difficulty with figure-ground distinctions (e.g., foregrounding relevant, central or essential information; assuming an appropriate perspective); (2) reduction in pragmatic inferences; and (3) a tendency toward description and self-evaluative comment rather than integrated discourse. The authors also relate these difficulties to level of processing demands. In their comprehensive, small sample study of men with RHD, Sherratt and Bryan (2012) note similar problems with choosing what is relevant to convey and marking it to reflect priority and given/new status.

A final area of potential difficulty with manipulating or using discourse structure is assimilating elements into a conceptual whole (e.g., Blake & Lesniewicz, 2005; Brownell, Carroll, Rehak, & Wingfield, 1992; Myers & Brookshire, 1995; Wapner, Hamby, & Gardner, 1981). The extent and nature of this problem, often described as a difficulty with integrating various sources of information in discourse processing, has been examined more fully in investigations of specific types of discourse units or processing operations. This literature describes potential impairments of the following.

(a) *Relating mental representations of stimuli and their associated contexts to determine or convey nonliteral intended meanings.* Problems of this sort have been reported on various metalinguistic tasks involving nonliteral forms and intents, such as selecting punchlines for jokes (Brownell, Michel, Powelson, & Gardner, 1983); recognizing conversational irony and its implications (Cutica, Bucciarelli, & Bara, 2006; Kaplan, Brownell, Jacobs, & Gardner, 1990); choosing connotative meanings of words (Schmitzer, Strauss, & DeMarco, 1997); interpreting idioms (Myers & Linebaugh, 1981; Papagno, Curti, Rizzo, Crippa, & Colombo, 2006); associating metaphors to sentence or picture representations (Rinaldi, Marangolo, & Baldassarri, 2004); and linking indirect speech acts to a broader context (Cutica et al., 2006; Stemmer, Giroux, & Joanette, 1994; Weylman, Brownell, Roman, & Gardner, 1989). However, similar difficulties can occur with nonliteral material, as when adults with RHD are asked explicitly to relate direct speech acts to a communicative context (Cutica et al., 2006). In addition, RHD does not seem to affect the activation or representation of nonliteral intended meanings (Stemmer, Giroux, & Joanette, 1994; Tompkins, 1990, 1991a; Tompkins, Boada, & McGarry, 1992; Tompkins et al., 2004) or their canonical structures (Bihrle, Brownell, & Powelson, 1986; Rehak, Kaplan, & Gardner, 1992), and adults with RHD can represent relevant elements of the (verbal) stimulus contexts in nonliteral processing tasks (Brownell, Pincus, Blum, Rehak, & Winner, 1997; Myers & Brookshire, 1994, 1996; Stemmer et al., 1994). Thus, the problem primarily seems to be one of the effortful synthesis of knowledge representations, including, perhaps, selecting from competing possibilities that are activated by the ambiguity inherent in many aspects of language (Tompkins et al., 2000, 2001; 2004).

(b) *Reconciling multiple, seemingly incongruent inferences to arrive at a full understanding of a discourse unit.* Adults with RHD have particular difficulty in contexts that support or induce conflicting interpretations (e.g., Brownell, Potter, Bihrle, & Gardner, 1986; Frederiksen & Stemmer, 1993; see also Tompkins, 2008), including those that violate canonical expectations (e.g., Rehak et al., 1992; Stemmer et al., 1994). Together with other work (e.g., Blake & Lesniewicz, 2005; Lehman-Blake & Tompkins, 2001; Myers & Brookshire, 1994) this observation suggests that inference generation *per se* is not a primary interpretive roadblock for adults with RHD. Again, the problem seems to be one of effortful integration, as would be needed to revise or repair interpretations based on ostensibly competing inferences (e.g., Blake & Lesniewicz, 2005; Stemmer & Joanette, 1998; Tompkins & Lehman, 1998; Tompkins et al., 2004).

(c) *Reasoning from a theory of mind.* RHD may affect the ability to understand the ways in which knowledge, beliefs, and motivations guide one's own behavior and that of others (e.g., Griffin, Friedman, Ween, Winner, Happé, & Brownell, 2006; Leigh, Oishi, Hsu et al., 2013; Winner, Brownell, Happé, Blum, & Pincus, 1998). Adults with RHD are less likely, for example, to use knowledge about communication partners' shared familiarity with a third party to determine how formally to address that person (Brownell et al., 1997); to provide explanatory remarks that mitigate the imposition of indirect requests (Brownell & Stringfellow, 1999); or to appreciate the implications of and motivations for conversational tangents and redundancies (Rehak et al., 1992). Again, these difficulties cannot be attributed to a failure to understand or represent individual elements of the scenarios in question (Brownell et al., 1997; Rehak et al., 1992; Winner et al., 1998). Tompkins, Scharp, Fassbinder, Meigh, and Armstrong (2008), after deconfounding stimulus materials often used to assess theory of mind, suggest that these difficulties may reflect, at least in part, problems with complex inferencing rather than inferences about mental states *per se*. Weed, McGregor, Nielsen, Roepstorff, and Frith (2010) also report that adults with RHD impute mental states to interacting shapes, but often underattribute relative to healthy control subjects.

We now turn to accounts of these discourse/pragmatic impairments. Many findings like those above are difficult to interpret, due to confounds introduced by the typically explicit, metalinguistic assessment tasks. However, such results seem to implicate primarily a set of attention-demanding, effortful integrative and organizational mental operations that are involved in discourse processing. As noted earlier, deficits of discourse representation and integration are not absolute. Adults with RHD perceive and represent many elements of both given and inferred information. They use explicit connectors to integrate components of a text (Brownell et al., 1992) and do well when interpretation is straightforward, as is the case for consistent passages (Brownell, Potter, Bihrle, & Gardner, 1986; Lehman-Blake & Tompkins, 2001; Tompkins, Bloise, Timko, & Baumgaertner, 1994) and canonical forms (Brownell & Stringfellow, 1999; Hough, 1990; Rehak et al., 1992; Stemmer et al., 1994). They can make lower-order theory of mind inferences (Siegal, Carrington, & Radel, 1996; Winner et al., 1998) and empathy judgments (Rehak et al., 1992) and determine appropriate personal reference from status information (Brownell et al., 1997). They profit from contexts that bias intended interpretations (e.g., Tompkins, 1990, 1991a, 1991b), making even optional inferences such as predictions when context is sufficiently constraining (Blake, 2009a, 2009b; Lehman-Blake & Tompkins, 2001).

These kinds of findings are consistent with other evidence that nonlanguage variables related to cognitive effort and/or task processing demands contribute importantly to observed performances of adults with RHD (for further discussion, see Tompkins et al., 2012). Because the expression of deficits in each of these domains seems to be moderated by processing abilities and demands as described above (see also Cherney, Drimmer, & Halper, 1997; Coslett, Bowers, & Heilman, 1987; Monetta & Joanette, 2003; Myers & Brookshire, 1994, 1996; Tompkins et al., 1994), general factors related to processing capacity and processing load need to be considered in any full account of RHD impairments and skills. Investigators of normal function also have attributed elevated RH activation to attentional demands, such as those associated with relative novelty (Martin, 1999), increased syntactic complexity (Just, Carpenter, Keller, Eddy, & Thulborn, 1996; Keller, Carpenter, & Just, 2001), lower reading skill (Prat, Mason, & Just, 2011), or greater processing difficulty (Guzzetti & Daini, 2014).

A lexical-level deficit in coarse semantic coding has been suggested to account for some problems in discourse comprehension (e.g., Beeman, 1993, 1998; Jung-Beeman, 2005). The only direct test of that premise indeed reports that the degree of impaired processing of particularly distant features of words[7] predicts narrative comprehension (Tompkins, Scharp, Meigh, & Fassbinder, 2008). The effects of treatment designed to facilitate coarse coding generalize to narrative comprehension, as well (Blake et al., 2015; Tompkins, Scharp, Meigh, Blake, & Wambaugh, 2012).

Other theoretical accounts of RHD discourse processing deficits center on concepts like effortful inference and integration,[8] social cognition, and/or suppression of contextually inappropriate alternatives. The accounts overlap in specifying, to some extent, the nature of RHD difficulties in constructing coherent, integrated mental structures to enable discourse production and comprehension. For example, Brownell and Martino (1998) refer to problems with "self-directed inference" (p. 325). This concept refers to comprehenders' efforts to discover and elaborate an interpretive framework when overlearned interpretive routines are inadequate and a text provides insufficient guidance as to how its elements fit together. Reasoning from a theory of mind also has gained popularity as an explanatory construct, per above (see also Brownell & Martino, 1998; Sabbagh, 1999; Weed et al., 2010), as has social cognition more generally. For instance, Sherratt and Bryan (2012) relate discourse production difficulties to an impaired appreciation of the listener's needs. To sharpen their early "cognitive resources" account of processing difficulties, Tompkins and colleagues (2000, 2001, 2004) appeal to suppression, a general psycholinguistic mechanism that is central to building an integrated discourse representation (Gernsbacher, 1990), and that requires attention to function effectively (Tompkins, Lehman-Blake, Baumgaertner, & Fassbinder, 2002). Their work shows that suppression function, or the ability to dampen mental activations that are contextually incompatible, predicts some aspects of narrative comprehension performance by adults with RHD. Beyond the lexical-level deficits reviewed previously, some adults with RHD have difficulty suppressing contextually inappropriate meanings of ambiguous inferences (Tompkins et al., 2001, 2004) or information from a prior narrative time frame that is normally suppressed in ongoing comprehension (Scharp & Tompkins, 2013). The suppression deficit hypothesis accommodates a variety of existing data, and intersects in interesting ways with the other accounts of RHD discourse processing deficits (Tompkins et al., 2000; Tompkins & Lehman, 1998). Suppression deficits also could contribute to a difficulty with constructing and integrating new conceptual models, a unifying explanation proposed by Stemmer and Joanette (1998) and more recently invoked by Marini, Carlomagno, Caltagirone, and Nocentini (2005).

Brownell's group (Brownell & Martino, 1998; Brownell et al., 1997) contends that difficulties in creating or using coherent discourse representations are insufficient to explain discourse processing in RHD. An additional essential ingredient, they suggest, is that adults with RHD experience a kind of social disconnection or diminished interest in people. As partial evidence of this affective dimension to the RHD communicative profile, Brownell and colleagues note that RHD adults infrequently invoke internal attributions for a character's actions, though they can integrate textual information and stored knowledge to generate plausible external attributions (Brownell, Blum, & Winner, 1994). This kind of evidence might be at least partly subsumable under the suppression or cognitive resources accounts. If, for example, external attributions are in some way more straightforward, more automatically accessible, or more strongly activated than internal attributions, particularly in a metalinguistic task, a dearth of the latter might be related to a difficulty inhibiting the former. However, other potentially relevant observations are not easily linked to suppression or cognitive resources. For instance, Brownell and colleagues' ascription also may be consistent with reports that adults with RHD may use fewer common social conventions (e.g., "How are you?") in conversation (Sidtis, Canterucci, & Katsnelson, 2009).

Potential explanatory constructs derive from a growing cognitive neuroscience literature, as well. Some of this work attributes to the RH some specialized computations or unique modes of operation that, when disrupted, might produce the kinds of discourse processing problems assumed to be typical of adults with RHD. These mechanisms, often characterized in opposition with presumed LH mechanisms, revolve around concepts like coarse (versus fine) semantic activation (e.g., Beeman, 1998), selection, and integration (Jung-Beeman, 2005); more (vs. less) veridical representation and maintenance of discourse information in long-term memory (Long, Johns, & Jonathan, 2012); or contextually integrative (vs. predictive) processing (Federmeier, 2007). A number of investigators conclude that the right and left hemispheres rely on different kinds of constraints to achieve meaning integration (e.g., Federmeier, 2007; Federmeier & Kutas, 1999; Titone, 1998). Some current views, however, suggest that both hemispheres use similar constraints but in differently graded manners or spanning different scopes. For example, Wlotko and Federmeier (2013) update Federmeier's (2007) influential LH prediction/RH integration proposal, reporting similar N400 patterns for highly expected and extremely unpredictable stimulus items in both hemispheres, but with the LH sensitive to a fuller range of predictability.

Linked to the notion of predictability, Giora (1997) argues that the processing of linguistic expressions differs depending on their salience—a concept very much related to novelty—which is a composite of frequency, familiarity, conventionality, and enhancement by prior context. She further proposes that the RH may be particularly suited to process or derive nonsalient, novel interpretations (Giora, 2007; see also Bohrn, Altmann, & Jacobs, 2012; Rapp, Mutschler, & Erb, 2012; Schmidt, DeBuse, & Seger, 2007, but not Mashal & Faust, 2008) rather than figurativity *per se*.

Thus far, evidence of RH contribution to language processing frequently seems to be related to more cognitively demanding or more complex semantic or conceptual selection and integration (e.g., Vigneau et al., 2011; Xu, Kemeny, Park, Frattali, & Braun, 2005), as when generating novel interpretations of language (Cardillo, Watson, Schmidt, Kranjec, & Chatterjee, 2012; Coulson & van Petten, 2007; Diaz, Barrett, & Hogstrom, 2011; Ferstl, Neumann, Bogler, & von Cramon, 2008; Giora, 2007; Schmidt et al., 2007) or maintaining, integrating, and updating mental models of what is happening in a narrative (Whitney, Huber, Klann et al., 2009; Yarkoni, Speer, & Zacks, 2008). This effortful selection, which can be aligned with the concept of "unification" (Nieuwland, 2012) of context and world knowledge, further characterizes RH involvement in processing counterfactual statements (Nieuwland, 2012), in dealing with information that is incongruent with context-pragmatic constraints (Jiang et al., 2013), and in generating discourse coherence (Mason & Just, 2007). Other work implicates the flexibility afforded by RH contributions to language processing, as when assimilating contextually unexpected or unusual information (Coulson & Williams, 2005; Federmeier, 2007; Meyer & Federmeier, 2007, 2008), retaining alternative meanings (Kacinik & Chiarello, 2007), or reevaluating plans (Shears, Hawkins, Varner, et al., 2008).

The "dynamic spillover" hypothesis (Prat et al., 2011) addresses flexibility more broadly. Prat and colleagues propose that RH regions—mostly homologous with the LH language network—are dynamically recruited, as needed for more difficult processing operations and/or to enable language comprehension for lower-skilled readers or for those with less cognitive resource capacity (see also Guzzetti & Daini, 2014). Although considerable work remains to specify the conditions under which this recruitment occurs (e.g., see Tremblay, Monetta, & Joanette, 2009), this explanatory construct could accommodate much of the existing literature. Also importantly, this approach again underscores the necessity of accounting for individual differences in building and testing models and hypotheses about RH contributions to language functioning, and about language disorders caused by RHD.

Various RH regions also have been implicated in the bilateral brain processing of theory of mind and social attribution (e.g., Ferstl et al., 2008; Mason & Just, 2009). These regions contribute to independent, spatiotemporally linked systems for face processing, mental state inferencing, and self-reflection or cognitive simulation (Wolf, Dziobek, & Heekeren, 2010).

More detailed hypotheses also can be drawn from a rapidly expanding functional neuroimaging literature that is identifying interconnected networks that support language processing, ascertaining how they work together, and discovering how they adapt in changing circumstances. For instance, the concept of dual-processing streams —that is, ventral "what" and dorsal "where" pathways that connect posterior and anterior brain regions—has recently been extended from vision to auditory language processing (e.g., Hickok, 2009), semantic memory (Binder & Desai, 2011), and lexical representation (Gow, 2012). The bilateral contributions of these streams to the integration of multiple sensory, perceptual, and cognitive processes, including those involved in language, provide seeds for hypothesizing about RHD lesion sites that may impair particular language processes, components, or systems. As another example, growing evidence from the field of connectomics (e.g., Duffau, 2013) can profitably inform lesion-function hypotheses.

Simulation, as noted previously, is a major component of perspectives that emphasize the role of sensory, motor, and affective experience in semantic representation and language processing (e.g., Binder & Desai, 2011; Kiefer & Pulvermüller, 2012; Meteyard et al., 2012). Bilateral brain networks subserve these representations (e.g., Binder & Desai, 2011), and as illustrated in Lincoln et al. (2008), hypotheses derived from these perspectives have the potential to add significantly to the explanatory landscape on the nature of RHD language disorders.

It would be surprising if any single explanatory concept could account for RHD discourse deficits, and combined attributions have appeared in the literature (see, e.g., Brownell & Marino, 1998; Champagne-Lavau, & Joanette, 2009; Myers, 1999; Tompkins & Lehman, 1998; Tompkins et al., 2002). Two long-range challenges are to sort out how potential explanatory constructs interact with one another to produce the picture(s) of strength, weakness, and performance variation that typify the RHD population, and to construct an integrated framework that captures the range of phenomena that support social communication. To approach these goals will require a great deal of work to develop existing accounts so that specific, *a priori* predictions can be derived and tested. These efforts, in turn, will benefit from more research that examines component processes and their interactions as set out in relevant models, including those of social communication (e.g., Lagarde, 2013; Liu, Chua, & Stahl, 2010; Pezzulo, Donnarumma, & Dindo, 2013; Swaab, Galinsky, Medvec, & Diermeier, 2012), discourse processing (e.g., Barbey, Colom, & Grafman, 2014; Dressler et al., 2004; Mar, 2004), and other aspects of pragmatic functioning (e.g., Bergen & Grodner, 2012; Prinz, 2013; Regel, Coulson, & Gunter, 2010; Stemmer, 1999a). Also, it will be important to continue to track multiple sources of performance variability. Such pursuits will help determine the extent to which nonlanguage cognitive functions (e.g., individual differences in attentional or working memory processes) are responsible for observed impairments, and the ways in which such functions intersect with hemispheric contributions to generate normal and disordered language performances. Furthermore, online investigations are needed, with systematic manipulation of stimulus features and demands, to evaluate RHD adults' real-time representation and use of crucial elements of internal knowledge and external context.

Correspondence in Literatures on Normal and Disordered Right Hemisphere Language Function

This volume contains many examples of the ways in which different sources of data on language and the brain inform one another and contribute to clinical decisions. Evidence of impaired and preserved performance in neurological language disorders supports inferences about the nature of intact language representation and processing systems; evidence and perspectives on normal language are used to predict and explain language difficulties that result from brain damage; and theories of both deficient and normal function have implications for assessment and treatment.

For RH language processes and disorders, efforts to hypothesize and evaluate mutual constraints, and to apply the results in rehabilitation, have barely begun. RHD language capacities and deficits have been a focus of systematic study for only about 30 years, and while studies of normal RH language function have exploded over the past 15–20 years, few labs are studying RHD language disorders, making for slow progress. In addition, investigations of normal and disordered RH language functioning have not often evaluated the same phenomena and mental computations, so generalizations between the two literatures usually are not directly tested.

Theory-driven research in RHD language is not only crucial for understanding the nature of RHD language deficits, but also helps identify dissociations that can fuel hypotheses about how the intact RH contributes to language. While there are few explicit and testable theories of the cognitive and linguistic underpinnings of social communication, RHD language research has increasingly consulted available models to guide the investigation of some of the cognitive and communicative processes of interest. Examples are found in work on inferencing (Dipper, Bryan, & Tyson, 1997; Lehman-Blake & Tompkins, 2001), indirect requests (Brownell & Stringfellow, 1999), and interpretation of jokes (Brownell et al., 1983) and metaphors (Lundgren, Brownell, Cayer-Meade, Milione, & Kearns, 2011), and as well as in other aspects of discourse processing (Dressler et al., 2004; Lojek-Osiejuk, 1996; Tompkins et al., 2000, Tompkins, Fassbinder et al., 2008), pragmatic functioning (Brownell et al., 1997; Kennedy, 2000; Soroker et al., 2005), and social attribution (Brownell & Martino, 1998). Such models can help unify the accumulating observations, circumscribe and operationalize key phenomena to investigate, and identify central premises to test.

Beyond the need to use theoretical models at all lies the question of what kinds of models ultimately will best inform our efforts. RHD language disorders presumably reside at a complex intersection of multiple linguistic, affective, and cognitive operations, levels, and domains that enable the social interactive use of language. Efforts to investigate RHD language disorders systematically have been hampered by a dearth of theoretical frameworks that address the range of, and interactions among, potentially relevant computations, dimensions, and systems. Ongoing research has led to useful hypotheses about the nature of RHD language disorders, but these proposals are largely unconnected to broader theoretical perspective(s). Thus, an integrated conceptual framework is needed to provide a structure for understanding the interactions among processing components and levels, and for clarifying the relationships among seemingly diverse results and hypotheses. Building such a model is a long-range enterprise, but some outlines have emerged to move us along this path. For example, Stemmer and Joanette (1998) describe the utility of a multilayer model of discourse that incorporates conceptual, propositional, and linguistic levels of representation and processing (Frederiksen, Bracewell, Breuleux, & Renaud, 1990), and which Dressler et al. (2004) profitably used to guide their investigation.[9] Stemmer (1999b) also advocates situating research on RHD communicative exchange within a broad framework that addresses the way in which any action is shaped by the synergistic interplay between the characteristics of an individual and his or her environment.

Another thorny source of difficulty for linking the RHD and intact RH language literatures, though neither new nor specific to RH research, relates to the unknown nature of the inferential bridge between normal and disordered hemisphere function. As noted earlier, many who generalize between these literatures assume, and sometimes propose explicitly, that performance after RHD reflects a diminution or loss of RH contributions to the processes in question, and a consequent overreliance on LH modes or operations (Beeman, 1993, 1998; Burgess & Simpson, 1988; Chiarello, 1998; Molloy, Brownell, & Gardner, 1990). This assumption is rather tenuous, for several reasons.

First, the interconnectedness of the cerebral hemispheres, whether only one or both are functioning normally, creates a major question mark in mapping results between damaged and normal brains. The two intact hemispheres interact in ways that are not predictable from the processing of either one alone (e.g., Banich & Nicholas, 1998; Rutherford & Lutz, 2004). Also, while newer technologies are allowing investigators to begin to address this question (e.g., Doron, Basset, & Gazzaniga, 2012), it is still unclear how the hemispheres coordinate, cooperate, facilitate, and/or inhibit one another when one is damaged, as Tucker (1981) noted long ago. For example, if a brain lesion releases some RH process from inhibition, the output of that process may be exaggerated rather than diminished.

Another complication for the direct mapping assumption is that performance after brain damage reflects dynamics other than those owing to the directly disrupted neural tissue. These include electrical and chemical changes in regions remote from the structural lesion (e.g., Andrews, 1991; Prabhakaran et al., 2007; Witte & Stoll, 1997), recruitment of undamaged portions of the damaged hemisphere (e.g., Turkeltaub et al., 2011), and intentional and incidental compensations that the language user develops as she or he tries to navigate the world with an altered system. These dynamics likely change over time as well, further obscuring the picture to be obtained from adults with RHD.

Finally, this uncertain state of affairs is evident in data that do not align easily with predictions that assume a direct mapping between normal and disordered performance. As described earlier, in people with intact brains, activation of the subordinate meanings of lexical ambiguities is rapidly suppressed by the LH, and may be maintained by the RH for a longer period of time (Burgess & Simpson, 1988). As a result, many investigators (e.g., Beeman, 1993, 1998; Burgess & Lund, 1998; Chiarello, 1988, 1998; Molloy et al., 1990) suggest that adults with RHD should not be able to activate and/or maintain alternative interpretations over prolonged periods. This kind of reasoning does not accord with evidence from RHD adults summarized above, demonstrating preserved activation and representation of nonliteral meanings (Rehak et al., 1992; Stemmer et al., 1994; see also Tompkins & Lehman, 1998) and sustained interference from activated alternative inferences (Tompkins et al., 2001, 2004). Even a more direct generalization, to lexical-level processing by adults with RHD, does not accord with data that documents priming of the metaphoric interpretations of lexical ambiguities at a point when the intact LH should have been able to inhibit them (Tompkins, 1990). This rather inexact correspondence of RHD and normal RH literatures has received little attention (though see also Griffin et al., 2006), and a better fit may remain elusive until more progress is made in understanding the nature of interactions between intact and damaged hemispheres, as well as physiological and psychological mechanisms of brain damage and recovery.

Functional neuroimaging studies of people with intact brains present some similar challenges for inferring the links between normal and disordered function. For instance, Griffin et al. (2006)

noted that damage to areas associated with theory of mind in the normal imaging literature may not impair theory of mind. In addition, normal variability is insufficiently addressed in neuroimaging studies of language, though it can be vast (Crozier et al., 1999). This variation, along with infrequent attention to individual attributes that may modulate hemispheric contributions to language functioning, renders even more problematic the process of generalizing between "normal" and "disordered" literatures. In sum, until there is a better understanding of the nature of the problem in mapping between intact and damaged brain systems, it will not be particularly surprising when predictions from one of these sources of RH language data are not borne out in the other.

A subsidiary issue involves the validity of generalizing between younger and older brains. The research on RH language processing in intact brains almost exclusively investigates the former, but RHD studies overwhelmingly evaluate the latter. This, along with evidence of aging-related differences in RH engagement in language (e.g., Guzzetti & Daini, 2014; Stites, Federmeier, & Stine-Morrow, 2013), dictates caution in applying to one population the theories, methods, or evidence that were developed with the other.

Considerations for Clinical Management of RHD Language Disorders

Clinical practice in RHD language disorders is primarily symptom driven and atheoretical. Furthermore, common clinical practice often is empirically tenuous or may even run counter to existing findings. For instance, if an adult with RHD has difficulty suppressing information that is irrelevant to a current context, the widespread practice of asking that client to generate multiple meanings of words or phrases may well be counterproductive. A theoretically oriented approach to clinical management offers the opportunity to identify and capitalize on processes that may underlie various communicative strengths and weaknesses, potentially enhancing generalization of treatment gains to a range of skills and contexts that rely on those processes. Thus, well-substantiated hypotheses about facilitators of and barriers to communication become a key ingredient in assessment and treatment planning. To illustrate, we consider several clinical implications from the evidence and hypotheses described above.

Of immediate clinical relevance, the manipulation of task processing demands can induce substantial performance variations in adults with RHD, particularly in relation to each individual's attentional or working memory capacity. Thus, regardless of whether facilitation or compensation is the primary treatment goal, a variety of processing factors potentially can be modified to make things more or less difficult for any given patient (see Tompkins, 1995, for suggestions). More generally, research that clarifies the extent to which language performance after RHD reflects attentional, working memory, or other nonlanguage cognitive impairments, rather than language deficits *per se*, will have direct implications for the assumptions underlying the development of treatment approaches.

As another illustration, we (Blake et al., 2015; Tompkins, Blake, Scharp, Meigh, & Wambaugh, 2013; Tompkins, Blake, Wambaugh, & Meigh, 2011; Tompkins, Scharp et al., 2012) have developed a novel, theoretically and empirically based treatment for language comprehension deficits after RHD. Contextual Constraint Treatment is designed to facilitate coarse coding or suppression processes by using biasing contexts to prestimulate the intended features or interpretations of words. The treatment is highly novel in being implicit rather than explicit, and in targeting partially domain-general processes that have been postulated and/or demonstrated to underlie a wide range of language comprehension abilities (e.g., Beeman, 1998; Tompkins et al., 2000). Most importantly, the treatment yields generalization well beyond trained and untrained items, to narrative comprehension, to suppression of contextually inappropriate meanings of ambiguous inferences, and to measures of patient- or surrogate-reported social communicative function.

Despite the potential clinical utility of a theory of deficient (or preserved) language perfor-mance, theory is far from sufficient as a basis for treatment planning. Even for an exquisitely defined deficit, no theory can prescribe what should happen in treatment, in either general or specific terms (Caramazza, 1989; Hillis, 1994). A theory of a deficit provides only a pointer to potential assessment or remediation goals and strategies. It is also unknown whether theory-driven treatment results in better outcomes than time-tested atheoretical approaches (Hillis, 1998). Fur-thermore, deficit-oriented therapy can run the risk of missing the bigger picture, which largely equates the therapeutic benefit for any particular client with its effects on consequences that go beyond the "impairment" itself (see, e.g., Frattali, 1998). These include the client's ability to perform specific daily life activities and to handle potential psychological, social, economic, and environmental repercussions of the condition under treatment.

For adults with RHD language disorders, a multifaceted and long-range program of research will be required to establish what kinds of treatments work best (see discussion in Tompkins et al., 1998). Research that investigates a full range of outcomes of RHD language disorders, and that ascertains the nature of interactions among these different outcomes, will be central to understand-ing how we might achieve meaningful treatment results. Unfortunately, nearly no work of this sort exists. Rigorous treatment studies also are desperately needed. Beyond incorporating design param-eters that maximize internal validity (Kearns, 1992), such investigations should use an assortment of measures at a variety of levels of outcome, evaluate evidence of maintenance and generalization to meaningful tasks and contexts, and include social validation or other consumer satisfaction assessments for patients and family members (see Tompkins et al., 1998). Treatment studies also are needed to investigate the value of targeting variables that mediate, moderate, or modify the relation-ships among deficits and higher-level outcomes, in addition to or rather than targeting the deficits themselves. More generally, intervention planning for anyone with a neurologically based language disorder ultimately will benefit from efforts to understand the "how" of treatment, with reference to the variety of cognitive, neurophysiological, and psychosocial processes that produce a favorable climate for adaptive learning and generalization after brain damage (see, e.g., Berthier, Pulvermüller, Dávila, Casares, & Gutiérrez, 2011; Danzl, Etter, Andreatta, & Kitzman, 2012; Godwin & Kreutzer, 2013; Jones & Jefferson, 2011; Lo, 2014; Overman & Carmichael, 2013; Whyte, 2009).

Acknowledgment

This work was supported in part by grants DC01820 and DC010182 from the National Institute on Deafness and Other Communication Disorders.

Notes

1 These results of course reflect the nature of the test, which, as Côté et al. noted, omits or underemphasizes several potentially important aspects of RHD language processing. The test's explicit, metalinguistic assess-ment format also must be considered.

2 These results again may reflect the metalinguistic semantic sorting task, but evidence from less cognitively demanding tasks, considered below, also suggests some RHD effect on processing alternate aspects of meaning.

3 Klepousniotou and Baum (2005a) suggest that their single word priming results are not entirely consistent with the suppression deficit hypothesis. By definition, however, suppression operates in context.

4 This result also could reflect a suppression deficit if adults with RHD were sensitive to perceptual infor-mation but deficient at selecting what best fit the pictorial context.

5 This result comes from an effortful semantic retrieval task—deciding whether word pairs that describe object features (e.g., *desert, humps*) combine to retrieve an object—and is likely to differ for different processes.

6 Being built around individual experience, these perspectives also capture the importance of inter-individual differences in language representation and processing.

7 However, these results may reflect instead some difficulty in using perceptual representations (see prior section on Lexical-Semantic Processing).

8 Recall that Jung-Beeman (2005) revised the coarse semantic coding model to include semantic integration and selection.

9 See Joanette and Goulet (1994) for some of the model's limitations.

References

Anaki, D., Faust, M., & Kravetz, S. (1998). Cerebral hemisphere asymmetries in processing lexical metaphors. *Neuropsychologia, 36*, 691–700.

Andrews, R.J. (1991). Transhemispheric diaschisis: A review and comment. *Stroke, 22*, 943–949.

Assaf, M., Jagannathan, K., Calhoun, V., Kraut, M., Hart Jr, J., & Pearlson, G. (2009). Temporal sequence of hemispheric network activation during semantic processing: A functional network connectivity analysis. *Brain and Cognition, 70*, 238–246.

Banich, M.T., & Nicholas, C.D. (1998). Integration of processing between the hemispheres in word recognition. In M. Beeman & C. Chiarello (Eds.), *Right hemisphere language comprehension: Perspectives from cognitive neuroscience.* Mahwah, NJ: Lawrence Erlbaum.

Barbey, A.K., Colom, R., & Grafman, J. (2014). Neural mechanisms of discourse comprehension: A human lesion study. *Brain, 137*(1), 277–287.

Baum, S.R., & Pell, M.D. (1999). The neural bases of prosody: Insights from lesion studies and neuroimaging. *Aphasiology, 13*, 581–608.

Baynes, K., & Eliassen, J.C. (1998). The visual lexicon: Its access and organization in commissurotomy patients. In M. Beeman & C. Chiarello (Eds.), *Right hemisphere language comprehension: Perspectives from cognitive neuroscience.* Mahwah, NJ: Lawrence Erlbaum.

Beeman, M. (1993). Semantic processing in the right hemisphere may contribute to drawing inferences from discourse. *Brain and Language, 44*, 80–120.

Beeman, M. (1998). Coarse semantic coding and discourse comprehension. In M. Beeman & C. Chiarello (Eds.), *Right-hemisphere language comprehension: Perspectives from cognitive neuroscience.* Mahwah, NJ: Lawrence Erlbaum.

Beeman, M., & Chiarello, C. (Eds.). (1998). *Right-hemisphere language comprehension: Perspectives from cognitive neuroscience.* Mahwah, NJ: Lawrence Erlbaum.

Benton, E., & Bryan, K. (1996). Right cerebral hemisphere damage: Incidence of language problems. *International Journal of Rehabilitation Research, 19*(1), 47–54.

Bergen, L., & Grodner, D.J. (2012). Speaker knowledge influences the comprehension of pragmatic inferences. *Journal of Experimental Psychology: Learning, Memory, and Cognition, 38*(5), 1450.

Berthier, M.L., Pulvermüller, F., Dávila, G., Casares, N.G., & Gutiérrez, A. (2011). Drug therapy of post-stroke aphasia: A review of current evidence. *Neuropsychology Review, 21*(3), 302–317.

Bihrle, A.M., Brownell, H.H., & Powelson, J.A. (1986). Comprehension of humorous and nonhumorous materials by left and right brain-damaged patients. *Brain and Cognition, 5*, 399–411.

Binder, J.R., & Desai, R.H. (2011). The neurobiology of semantic memory. *Trends in Cognitive Sciences, 15*(11), 527–536.

Blake, M.L. (2007). Perspectives on treatment for communication deficits associated with right hemisphere brain damage. *American Journal of Speech-Language Pathology, 16*, 331–342.

Blake, M.L. (2009a). Inferencing processes after right hemisphere brain damage: Maintenance of inferences. *Journal of Speech, Language and Hearing Research, 52*, 359–372.

Blake, M.L. (2009b). Inferencing processes after right hemisphere brain damage: Effects of contextual bias. *Journal of Speech, Language and Hearing Research, 52*, 373–384.

Blake, M.L. (2015). Cognitive-communication deficits associated with right hemisphere brain damage. In M.L. Kimbarow (Ed.), *Cognitive communication disorders* (2nd ed.). San Diego: Plural Publishing.

Blake, M.L., Duffy, J.R., Myers, P.S., & Tompkins, C.A. (2002). Prevalence and patterns of right hemisphere cognitive/communicative deficits: Retrospective data from an inpatient rehabilitation unit. *Aphasiology, 16*, 537–548.

Blake, M.L., & Lesniewicz, K. (2005). Contextual bias and predictive inferencing in adults with and without right hemisphere brain damage. *Aphasiology, 19*, 423–434.

Blake, M.L., Tompkins, C.A., Scharp, V.L., Meigh, K.M., & Wambaugh, J.L. (2015). Contextual Constraint Treatment for coarse coding deficit in adults with right hemisphere brain damage: Generalization to narrative discourse comprehension. *Neuropsychological Rehabilitation, 25*(1), 15–52.

Blonder, L.X., Burns, A.F., Bowers, D., Moore, R.W., & Heilman, K. M. (1993). Right hemisphere facial expressivity during natural conversation. *Brain and Cognition, 21*, 44–56.

Bohrn, I.C., Altmann, U., & Jacobs, A.M. (2012). Looking at the brains behind figurative language: A quantitative meta-analysis of neuroimaging studies on metaphor, idiom, and irony processing. *Neuropsychologia, 50*(11), 2669–2683.

Borod, J.C., Andelman, R., Olber, L.K., Tweedy, J.R., & Welkowitz, J. (1992). Right hemisphere specialization for the identification of emotional words and sentences: Evidence from stroke patients. *Neuropsychologia, 30*, 827–844.

Bouaffre, S., & Faita-Ainseba, F. (2007). Hemispheric differences in the time-course of semantic priming processes: Evidence from event-related potentials (ERPs). *Brain and Cognition, 63*(2), 123–135.

Brownell, H.H., Blum, A., & Winner, E. (1994). Attributional bias in RHD patients with impaired discourse comprehension. *Brain and Language, 43*, 121–147.

Brownell, H.H., Carroll, J.J., Rehak, A., & Wingfield, A. (1992). The use of pronoun anaphora and speaker mood in the interpretation of conversational utterances by right hemisphere brain-damaged patients. *Brain and Language, 43*, 121–147.

Brownell, H.H., & Martino, G. (1998). Deficits in inference and social cognition: The effects of right hemisphere brain damage on discourse. In M. Beeman & C. Chiarello (Eds.), *Right hemisphere language comprehension: Perspectives from cognitive neuroscience*. Mahwah, NJ: Lawrence Erlbaum.

Brownell, H.H., Michel, D., Powelson, J., & Gardner, H. (1983). Surprise but not coherence: Sensitivity to verbal humor in right-hemisphere patients. *Brain and Language, 18*, 20–27.

Brownell, H.H., Pincus, D., Blum, A., Rehak, A., & Winner, E. (1997). The effects of right-hemisphere brain damage on patients' use of terms of personal reference. *Brain and Language, 57*, 60–79.

Brownell, H.H., Potter, H.H., Bihrle, A.M., & Gardner, H. (1986). Inference deficits in right brain-damaged patients. *Brain and Language, 27*, 310–321.

Brownell, H.H., Potter, H.H., Michelow, D., & Gardner, H. (1984). Sensitivity to lexical denotation and connotation in brain-damaged patients: A double dissociation. *Brain and Language, 22*, 253–265.

Brownell, H.H., Simpson, T.L., Bihrle, A.M., Potter, H.H., & Gardner, H. (1990). Appreciation of metaphoric alternative word meanings by left and right brain damaged patients. *Neuropsychologia, 28*, 375–383.

Brownell, H. H., & Stringfellow, A. (1999). Making requests: Illustrations of how right-hemisphere brain damage can affect discourse production. *Brain and Language, 68*, 442–465.

Burgess, C., & Lund. K. (1998). Modeling cerebral asymmetries in high-dimensional space. In M. Beeman & C. Chiarello (Eds.), *Right hemisphere language comprehension: Perspectives from cognitive neuroscience*. Mahwah, NJ: Lawrence Erlbaum.

Burgess, C., & Simpson, G. (1988). Cerebral hemispheric mechanisms in the retrieval of ambiguous word meanings. *Brain and Language, 33*, 86–103.

Caramazza, A. (1989). Cognitive neuropsychology and rehabilitation: An unfulfilled promise? In X. Seron & G. DeLoche (Eds.), *Cognitive approaches to rehabilitation*. Hillsdale, NJ: Lawrence Erlbaum.

Cardillo, E.R., Watson, C.E., Schmidt, G.L., Kranjec, A., & Chatterjee, A. (2012). From novel to familiar: Tuning the brain for metaphors. *NeuroImage, 59*(4), 3212–3221.

Champagne-Lavau, M., & Joanette, Y. (2009). Pragmatics, theory of mind and executive functions after a right-hemisphere lesion: Different patterns of deficits. *Journal of Neurolinguistics, 22*(5), 413–426.

Chatterjee, A. (2010). Disembodying cognition. *Language and Cognition, 2*, 79–116.

Cherney, L., Drimmer, D., & Halper, A. (1997). Informational content and unilateral neglect: A longitudinal investigation of five subjects with right hemisphere damage. *Aphasiology, 11*, 351–364.

Chiarello, C. (1988). Semantic priming in the intact brain: Separate roles for the right and left hemispheres? In C. Chiarello (Ed.), *Right hemisphere contributions to lexical semantics*. New York: Springer Verlag.

Chiarello, C. (1998). On codes of meaning and the meaning of codes: Semantic access and retrieval within and between hemispheres. In M. Beeman & C. Chiarello (Eds.), *Right hemisphere language comprehension: Perspectives from cognitive neuroscience*. Mahwah, NJ: Lawrence Erlbaum.

Chiarello, C., & Church, K.L. (1986). Lexical judgments after right or left-hemisphere injury. *Neuropsychologia, 24*, 623–630.

Chiarello, C., Kacinik, N., Shears, C., Arambel, S., Halderman, L., & Robinson, C. (2006). Exploring cerebral asymmetries for the verb generation task. *Neuropsychology, 20*, 88–104.

Chieffi, S., Carlomagno, S., Silveri, M.C., & Gainotti, G. (1989). The influence of semantic and perceptual factors on lexical comprehension in aphasic and right brain-damaged patients. *Cortex, 25*, 591–598.

Coney, J. (2002). The effect of associative strength on priming in the cerebral hemispheres. *Brain and Cognition, 50*(2), 234–241.

Coslett, H.B., Bowers, D., & Heilman, K.M. (1987). Reduction in cerebral activation after right hemisphere stroke. *Neurology, 37*, 957–962.

Côté, H., Payer, M., Giroux, F., & Joanette, Y. (2007). Towards a description of clinical communication impairment profiles following right-hemisphere damage. *Aphasiology, 21*, 739–749.

Coulson, S., & Van Petten, C. (2007). A special role for the right hemisphere in metaphor comprehension? ERP evidence from hemifield presentation. *Brain Research, 1146*, 128–145.

Coulson, S., & Williams, R.F. (2005). Hemispheric asymmetries and joke comprehension. *Neuropsychologia, 43*, 128–141.

Coulson, S., & Wu, Y.C. (2005). Right hemisphere activation of joke-related information: An event-related brain potential study. *Journal of Cognitive Neuroscience, 17*, 494–506.

Crozier, S., Sirigu, A., Lehericy, S., van de Moortele, P., Pillon, B., Grafman, J., Agid, Y., Dubois, B., & LeBihan, D. (1999). Distinct prefrontal activations in processing sequence at the sentence and script level: An fMRI study. *Neuropsychologia, 37*, 1469–1476.

Cummings, L. (2007). Pragmatics and adult language disorders: Past achievements and future directions. *Seminars in Speech and Language, 28*(2), 96–110.

Cutica, I., Bucciarelli, M., & Bara, B.G. (2006). Neuropragmatics: Extralinguistic pragmatic ability is better preserved in left-hemisphere-damaged patients than in right-hemisphere-damaged patients. *Brain and Language, 98*, 12–25.

Danzl, M.M., Etter, N.M., Andreatta, R.D., & Kitzman, P.H. (2012). Facilitating neurorehabilitation through principles of engagement. *Journal of Allied Health, 41*, 35–41.

de Lima Müller, J., & de Salles, J.F. (2013). Studies on semantic priming effects in right hemisphere stroke. *Dementia and Neuropsychologia, 7*, 155–163.

Diaz, M.T., Barrett, K.T., & Hogstrom, L.J. (2011). The influence of sentence novelty and figurativeness on brain activity. *Neuropsychologia, 49*, 320–330.

Dipper, L.T., Bryan, K.L., & Tyson, J. (1997). Bridging inference and relevance theory: An account of right hemisphere inference. *Clinical Linguistics and Phonetics, 11*, 213–228.

Donnelly, K.M., Allendorfer, J.B., & Szaflarski, J.P. (2011). Right hemispheric participation in semantic decision improves performance. *Brain Research, 1419*, 105–116.

Doron, K.W., Bassett, D.S., & Gazzaniga, M.S. (2012). Dynamic network structure of interhemispheric coordination. *Proceedings of the National Academy of Sciences, 109*(46), 18661–18668.

Dressler, W.U., Stark, H.K., Vassilakou, M., Rauchensteiner, D., Tosic, J., Weitzenauer, S.M., . . . & Brunner, G. (2004). Textpragmatic impairments of figure-ground distinction in right-brain damaged stroke patients compared with aphasics and healthy controls. *Journal of Pragmatics, 36*(2), 207–235.

Duffau, H. (2013). The huge plastic potential of adult brain and the role of connectomics: New insights provided by serial mappings in glioma surgery. *Cortex*. doi: http://dx.doi.org/10.1016/j.cortex.2013.08.005

Duffy, J.R., & Myers, P.S. (1991). Group comparisons across neurologic communication disorders: Some methodological issues. *Clinical Aphasiology, 19*, 1–14.

Evans, K.M., & Federmeier, K.D. (2009). Left and right memory revisited: Electrophysiological investigations of hemispheric asymmetries at retrieval. *Neuropsychologia, 47*, 303–313.

Fassbinder, W., and Tompkins, C. A. (2001). Slowed lexical activation in right hemisphere brain damage? *Aphasiology, 15*, 1079–1090.

Federmeier, K.D. (2007). Thinking ahead: The role and roots of prediction in language comprehension. *Psychophysiology, 44*(4), 491–505.

Federmeier, K.D., & Kutas, M. (1999). Right words and left words: Electrophysiological evidence for hemispheric differences in meaning processing. *Cognitive Brain Research, 8*, 373–392.

Ferré, P., Fonseca, R.P., Ska, B., & Joanette, Y. (2012). Communicative clusters after a right-hemisphere stroke: Are there universal clinical profiles? *Folia Phoniatrica et Logopaedica, 64*(4), 199–207.

Ferstl, E.C., Neumann, J., Bogler, C., & Von Cramon, D.Y. (2008). The extended language network: A meta-analysis of neuroimaging studies on text comprehension. *Human Brain Mapping, 29*(5), 581–593.

Forgács, B., Bohrn, I., Baudewig, J., Hofmann, M.J., Pléh, C., & Jacobs, A.M. (2012). Neural correlates of combinatorial semantic processing of literal and figurative noun noun compound words. *NeuroImage, 63*(3), 1432–1442.

Frattali, C. (1998). *Measuring outcomes in speech-language pathology.* New York: Thieme.

Frederiksen, C.H., Bracewell, R.J., Breuleux, A., & Renaud, A. (1990). The cognitive representation and processing of discourse: Function and dysfunction. In Y. Joanette & H. H. Brownell (Eds.), *Discourse ability and brain damage: Theoretical and empirical perspectives.* New York: Springer Verlag.

Frederiksen, C.H., & Stemmer, B. (1993). Conceptual processing of discourse by a right hemisphere brain damaged patient. In H.H. Brownell & Y. Joanette (Eds.), *Narrative discourse in neurologically impaired and normal aging adults.* San Diego, CA: Singular Publishing Group.

Frishkoff, G.A. (2007). Hemispheric differences in strong versus weak semantic priming: Evidence from event-related brain potentials. *Brain and Language, 100*, 23–43.

Gagnon, J., Goulet, P., & Joanette, Y. (1989). Activation automatique et contrôlée du savoir lexico-sémantique chez les cérébrolésés droits. *Langages, 96*, 95–111.

Gainotti, G., Caltagirone, C., Miceli, G., & Masullo, C. (1983). Selective impairment of semantic-lexical discrimination in right-brain-damaged patients. In E. Perecman (Ed.), *Cognitive processing in the right hemisphere.* New York: Academic Press.

Gernsbacher, M.A. (1990). *Language comprehension as structure building.* Hillsdale, NJ: Lawrence Erlbaum.

Giora, R. (1997). Understanding figurative and literal language: The graded salience hypothesis. *Cognitive Linguistics, 8,* 183–206.

Giora, R. (2007). Is metaphor special? *Brain and Language, 100,* 111–114.

Godwin, E.E., & Kreutzer, J.S. (2013). Embracing a new path to emotional recovery: Adopting resilience theory in post-TBI psychotherapy. *Brain Injury, 27*(6), 637–639.

Gouldthorp, B., & Coney, J. (2011). Integration and coarse coding: right hemisphere processing of message-level contextual information. *Laterality, 16,* 1–23.

Goulet, P., Joanette, Y., Sabourin, L., & Giroux, F. (1997). Word fluency after a right-hemisphere lesion. *Neuropsychologia, 35,* 1565–1570.

Gow, D.W. (2012). The cortical organization of lexical knowledge: A dual lexicon model of spoken language processing. *Brain and Language, 121,* 273–288.

Grindrod, C.M., & Baum, S.R. (2003). Sensitivity to local sentence context information in lexical ambiguity resolution: Evidence from left-and right-hemisphere-damaged individuals. *Brain and Language, 85*(3), 503–523.

Grindrod, C.M., & Baum, S.R. (2005). Hemispheric contributions to lexical ambiguity resolution in a discourse context: Evidence from individuals with unilateral left and right hemisphere lesions. *Brain and Cognition, 57*(1), 70–83.

Griffin, R., Friedman, O., Ween, J., Winner, E., Happé, F., & Brownell, H. (2006). Theory of mind and the right cerebral hemisphere: Refining the scope of impairment. *Laterality: Asymmetries of Body, Brain and Cognition, 11,* 195–225.

Guzzetti, S., & Daini, R. (2014). Inter-hemispheric recruitment as a function of task complexity, age and cognitive reserve. *Aging, Neuropsychology, and Cognition,* 1–24. doi: 10.1080/13825585.2013.874522

Hagoort, P., Brown, C.M., & Swaab, T.Y. (1996). Lexical-semantic event-related potential effects in patients with left hemisphere lesions and aphasia, and patients with right hemisphere lesions without aphasia. *Brain, 119,* 627–649.

Hamel, C., & Joanette, Y. (2007). Logical and pragmatic inferencing abilities after left-and right-hemisphere lesions. *Brain and Language, 103*(1), 43–44.

Harpaz, Y., Lavidor, M., & Goldstein, A. (2013). Right semantic modulation of early MEG components during ambiguity resolution. *NeuroImage, 82*(15), 107–114.

Harpaz, Y., Levkovitz, Y., & Lavidor, M. (2009). Lexical ambiguity resolution in Wernicke's area and its right homologue. *Cortex, 45,* 1097–1103.

Heilman, K.H. (2009). Right hemispheric neurobehavioral syndromes. In J. Stein, R.L. Harvey, R.F. Macko, C.J. Winstein, & R.D. Zorowitz (Eds.), *Stroke recovery and rehabilitation* (pp. 201–212). New York: Demos Medical.

Henik, A., Dronkers, N.F., Knight, R.T., & Osimani, A. (1993). Differential effects of semantic and identity priming in patients with left and right hemisphere lesions. *Journal of Cognitive Neuroscience, 5,* 45–55.

Hickok, G. (2009). The functional neuroanatomy of language. *Physics of Life Reviews, 6*(3), 121–143.

Hillis, A.E. (1994). Contributions from cognitive analyses. In R. Chapey (Ed.), *Language intervention strategies in adult aphasia* (3rd ed.). Baltimore: Williams & Wilkins.

Hillis, A.E. (1998). Treatment of naming disorders: New issues regarding old therapies. *Journal of the International Neuropsychological Society, 4,* 648–660.

Hough, M.S. (1990). Narrative comprehension in adults with right and left hemisphere brain-damage: Theme organization. *Brain and Language, 38,* 253–277.

Howes, D., & Boller, F. (1975). Evidence for focal impairment from lesions of the right hemisphere. *Brain, 98,* 317–332.

Ingalhalikar, M., Smith, A., Parker, D., Satterthwaite, T.D., Elliott, M.A., Ruparel, K., . . ., Verma, R. (2014). Sex differences in the structural connectome of the human brain. *Proceedings of National Academy of Sciences USA, 111,* 823–828.

Jiang, X., Li, Y., & Zhou, X. (2013). Even a rich man can afford that expensive house: ERP responses to construction-based pragmatic constraints during sentence comprehension. *Neuropsychologia, 51,* 1857–1866.

Joanette, Y., & Ansaldo, A.I. (1999). Clinical note: Acquired pragmatic impairments and aphasia. *Brain and Language, 68,* 529–534.

Joanette, Y., & Goulet, P. (1989). Hémisphère droit et langage: Au-delà d'une certaine compétence lexico-sémantique. *Langages, 96,* 83–94.

Joanette, Y., & Goulet, P. (1994). Right hemisphere and verbal communication: Conceptual, methodological, and clinical issues. *Clinical Aphasiology, 22*, 1–24.

Johns, C. L., Tooley, K. M., & Traxler, M. J. (2008). Discourse impairments following right hemisphere brain damage: A critical review. *Language and Linguistics Compass, 2*(6), 1038–1062.

Jones, T. A., & Jefferson, S. C. (2011). Reflections of experience-expectant development in repair of the adult damaged brain. *Developmental Psychobiology, 53*(5), 466–475.

Jung-Beeman, M. (2005). Bilateral brain processes for comprehending natural language. *Trends in Cognitive Sciences, 9*, 512–518.

Just, M. A., Carpenter, P. A., Keller, T. A., Eddy, W. F., & Thulborn, K. E. (1996). Brain activation modulated by sentence comprehension. *Science, 274*, 114–116.

Kacinik, A. N., & Chiarello, C. (2007). Understanding metaphors: Is the right hemisphere uniquely involved? *Brain and Language, 100*, 188–207.

Kandhadai, P., & Federmeier, K. D. (2008). Summing it up: Semantic activation processes in the two hemispheres as revealed by event-related potentials. *Brain Research, 1233*, 146–159.

Kaplan, J. A., Brownell, H. H., Jacobs, J. R., & Gardner, H. (1990). The effects of right hemisphere damage on the pragmatic interpretation of conversational remarks. *Brain and Language, 38*, 315–333.

Kapur, N. (1996). Paradoxical functional facilitation in brain-behaviour research. *Brain, 119*, 1775–1790.

Kasher, A., Batori, G., Soroker, N., Graves, D., & Zaidel, E. (1999). Effects of right and left-hemisphere damage on understanding conversational implicatures. *Brain and Language, 68*, 566–590.

Kearns, K. P. (1992). Methodological issues in aphasia treatment research: A single-subject perspective. In J. A. Cooper (Ed.), *Aphasia treatment: Vol. 2. Current approaches and research opportunities.* Bethesda, MD: National Institutes of Health.

Kennedy, M. R. T. (2000). Topic scenes in conversations with adults with right-hemisphere brain damage. *American Journal of Speech-Language Pathology, 9*, 72–86.

Keller, T. A., Carpenter, P., & Just, M. A. (2001). The neural bases of sentence comprehension: An fMRI examination of syntactic and lexical processing. *Cerebral Cortex, 11*, 223–237.

Kiefer, M., & Pulvermüller, F. (2012). Conceptual representations in mind and brain: Theoretical developments, current evidence and future directions. *Cortex, 48*(7), 805–825.

Klepousniotou, E., & Baum, S. R. (2005a). Unilateral brain damage effects on processing homonymous and polysemous words. *Brain and Language, 93*(3), 308–326.

Klepousniotou, E., & Baum, S. R. (2005b). Processing homonymy and polysemy: Effects of sentential context and time-course following unilateral brain damage. *Brain and Language, 95*(3), 365–382.

Koivisto, M., & Laine, M. (2000). Hemispheric asymmetries in activation and integration of categorical information. *Laterality, 5*, 1–21.

Lagarde, J. (2013). Challenges for the understanding of the dynamics of social coordination. *Frontiers in Neurorobotics, 7*, 1–9.

Lehman-Blake, M. T., & Tompkins, C. A. (2001). Predictive inferencing in adults with right hemisphere brain damage. *Journal of Speech, Language, and Hearing Research, 44*, 639–654.

Lesser, R. (1974). Verbal comprehension in aphasia: An English version of three Italian tests. *Cortex, 10*, 247–263.

Lincoln, A. E., Long, D. L., Swick, D., Larsen, J., & Baynes, K. (2008). Hemispheric asymmetries in the perceptual representations of words. *Brain Research, 1188*, 112–121.

Liu, L. A., Chua, C. H., & Stahl, G. K. (2010). Quality of communication experience: Definition, measurement, and implications for intercultural negotiations. *Journal of Applied Psychology, 95*(3), 469.

Lo, E. H. (2014). 2013 Thomas Willis award lecture: Causation and collaboration for stroke research. *Stroke, 45*(1), 305–308.

Lojek-Osiejuk, E. (1996). Knowledge of scripts reflected in discourse of aphasics and right-brain-damaged patients. *Brain and Language, 29*, 68–80.

Long, D. L., Johns, C. L., & Jonathan, E. (2012). Hemispheric differences in the organization of memory for text ideas. *Brain and Language, 123*, 145–153.

Lovseth, K., & Atchley, R. A. (2010). Examining lateralized semantic access using pictures. *Brain and Cognition, 72*(2), 202–209.

Lundgren, K., Brownell, H. H., Cayer-Meade, C, Milione, J., & Kearns, K. P. (2011). Treating metaphor interpretation deficits subsequent to right hemisphere brain damage: Preliminary results. *Aphasiology, 25*, 456–474.

Mar, R. A. (2004). The neuropsychology of narrative: Story comprehension, story production and their interrelation. *Neuropsychologia, 42*(10), 1414–1434.

Marini, A. (2012). Characteristics of narrative discourse processing after damage to the right hemisphere. *Seminars in Speech and Language, 33*, 68–78.

Marini, A., Carlomagno, S., Caltagirone, C., & Nocentini, U. (2005). The role played by the right hemisphere in the organization of complex textual structures. *Brain and Language, 93*, 46–54.

Mashal, N., & Faust, M. (2008). Right hemisphere sensitivity to novel metaphoric relations: Application of the signal detection theory. *Brain and Language, 104*(2), 103–112.

Mason, R.A., & Just, M.A. (2007). Lexical ambiguity in sentence comprehension. *Brain Research, 1146*, 115–127.

Mason, R.A., & Just, M.A. (2009). The role of the theory-of-mind cortical network in the comprehension of narratives. *Language and Linguistics Compass, 3*(1), 157–174.

Mason, R.A., Prat, C.S., & Just, M.A. (2013). Neurocognitive brain response to transient impairment of Wernicke's area. *Cerebral Cortex.* doi: 10.1093/cercor/bhs423

Martin, A. (1999). Automatic activation of the medial temporal lobe during encoding: Lateralized influences of meaning and novelty. *Hippocampus, 9*, 62–70.

Meteyard, L., Cuadrado, S.R., Bahrami, B., & Vigliocco, G. (2012). Coming of age: A review of embodiment and the neuroscience of semantics. *Cortex, 48*(7), 788–804.

Meyer, A.M., & Federmeier, K.D. (2007). The effects of context, meaning frequency, and associative strength on semantic selection: Distinct contributions from each cerebral hemisphere. *Brain Research, 1183*, 91–108.

Meyer, A.M., & Federmeier, K.D. (2008). The divided visual world paradigm: Eye tracking reveals hemispheric asymmetries in lexical ambiguity resolution. *Brain Research, 1222*, 166–183.

Molloy, R., Brownell, H.H., & Gardner, H. (1990). Discourse comprehension by right-hemisphere stroke patients: Deficits of prediction and revision. In Y. Joanette & H.H. Brownell (Eds.), *Discourse ability and brain damage.* New York: Springer Verlag.

Monetta, L., & Joanette, Y. (2003). The specificity of the contribution of the right hemisphere to verbal communication: The cognitive resources hypothesis. *Journal of Speech-Language Pathology, 11*, 203–211.

Myers, P.S. (1999). *Right hemisphere damage: Disorders of communication and cognition.* San Diego, CA: Singular Publishing Group.

Myers, P.S., & Brookshire, R.H. (1994). The effects of visual and inferential complexity on the picture descriptions of non-brain-damaged and right-hemisphere-damaged adults. *Clinical Aphasiology, 22*, 25–34.

Myers, P.S., & Brookshire, R.H. (1995). Effects of noun type on naming performance of right-hemisphere-damaged and non-brain-damaged adults. *Clinical Aphasiology, 23*, 195–206.

Myers, P.S., & Brookshire, R.H. (1996). Effect of visual and inferential variables on scene descriptions by right-hemisphere-damaged and non-brain-damaged adults. *Journal of Speech and Hearing Research, 39*, 870–880.

Myers, P.S., & Linebaugh, C.W. (1981). Comprehension of idiomatic expressions by right-hemisphere-damaged adults. In R.H. Brookshire (Ed.), *Clinical aphasiology: Vol. 11.* Minneapolis, MN: BRK.

Nakagawa, A. (1991). Role of anterior and posterior attention networks in hemispheric asymmetries during lexical decisions. *Journal of Cognitive Neuroscience, 3*, 313–321.

Nieuwland, M.S. (2012). Establishing propositional truth-value in counterfactual and real-world contexts during sentence comprehension: Differential sensitivity of the left and right inferior frontal gyri. *NeuroImage, 59*(4), 3433–3440.

Overman, J.J., & Carmichael, S.T. (2013). Plasticity in the injured brain more than molecules matter. *The Neuroscientist.* doi: 10.1177/1073858413491146

Papagno, C., Curti, R., Rizzo, S., Crippa, F., & Colombo, M.R. (2006). Is the right hemisphere involved in idiom comprehension? A neuropsychological study. *Neuropsychology, 20*, 598–606.

Peretz, Y., & Lavidor, M. (2013). Enhancing lexical ambiguity resolution by brain polarization of the right posterior superior temporal sulcus. *Cortex, 49*(4), 1056–1062.

Pezzulo, G., Donnarumma, F., & Dindo, H. (2013). Human sensorimotor communication: A theory of signaling in online social interactions. *PloS ONE, 8*(11), e79876.

Prabhakaran, V., Raman, S.P., Grunwald, M.R., Mahadevia, A., Hussain, N., Lu, H., . . . Hillis, A.E. (2007). Neural substrates of word generation during stroke recovery: The influence of cortical hypoperfusion. *Behavioural Neurology, 18*(1), 45–52.

Prat, C.S., & Just, M.A. (2011). Exploring the neural dynamics underpinning individual differences in sentence comprehension. *Cerebral Cortex, 21*(8), 1747–1760.

Prat, C.S., Mason, R.A., & Just, M.A. (2011). Individual differences in the neural basis of causal inferencing. *Brain and Language, 116*, 1–13.

Prinz, W. (2013) Action representation: Crosstalk between semantics and pragmatics. *Neuropsychologia.* doi: http://dx.doi.org/10.1016/j.neuropsychologia.2013.08.015

Rapp, A.M., Mutschler, D.E., & Erb, M. (2012). Where in the brain is nonliteral language? A coordinate-based meta-analysis of functional magnetic resonance imaging studies. *NeuroImage, 63*, 600–610.

Regel, S., Coulson, S., & Gunter, T.C. (2010). The communicative style of a speaker can affect language comprehension? ERP evidence from the comprehension of irony. *Brain Research, 1311*, 121–135.

Rehak, A., Kaplan, J.A., & Gardner, H. (1992). Sensitivity to conversational deviance in right-hemisphere-damaged patients. *Brain and Language, 42,* 203–217.

Rehak, A., Kaplan, J. A., Weylman, S.T., Kelly, B., Brownell, H.H., & Gardner, H. (1992). Story processing in right-hemisphere brain-damaged patients. *Brain and Language, 42,* 320–336.

Rinaldi, M.C., Marangolo, P., & Baldassarri, F. (2004). Metaphor comprehension in right brain-damaged patients with visuo-verbal and verbal material: A dissociation (re)considered. *Cortex, 40*(3), 479–490.

Ross, E.D., & Monnot, M. (2011). Affective prosody: What do comprehension errors tell us about hemispheric lateralization of emotions, sex and aging effects, and the role of cognitive appraisal. *Neuropsychologia, 49*(5), 866–877.

Rousseaux, M., Daveluy, W., & Kozlowski, O. (2010). Communication in conversation in stroke patients. *Journal of Neurology, 257,* 1099–1107.

Rutherford, B.J., & Lutz, K.T. (2004). Conflicting strategies and hemispheric suppression in a lexical decision task. *Brain and Cognition, 55*(2), 387–391.

Sabbagh, M.A. (1999). Communicative intentions and language: Evidence from right-hemisphere damage and autism. *Brain and Language, 70,* 29–69.

Sass, K., Krach, S., Sachs, O., & Kircher, T. (2009). Lion–tiger–stripes: Neural correlates of indirect semantic priming across processing modalities. *NeuroImage, 45*(1), 224–236.

Scharp, V.L., & Tompkins, C.A. (2013). Suppression and narrative time shifts in adults with right-hemisphere brain damage. *American Journal of Speech-Language Pathology, 22,* S256–S267.

Schmidt, G.L., Cardillo, E.R., Kranjec, A., Lehet, M., Widick, P., & Chatterjee, A. (2012). Not all analogies are created equal: Associative and categorical analogy processing following brain damage. *Neuropsychologia, 50*(7), 1372–1379.

Schmidt, G.L., DeBuse, C.J., & Seger, C.A. (2007). Right hemisphere metaphor processing? Characterizing the lateralization of semantic processes. *Brain and Language, 100,* 127–141.

Schmitzer, A.B., Strauss, M., & DeMarco, S. (1997). Contextual influences on comprehension of multiple-meaning words by right hemisphere brain-damaged and non-brain-damaged adults. *Aphasiology, 11,* 447–460.

Shapleske, J., Rossell, S.L., Woodruff, P., & David, A. (1999). The planum temporale: A systematic, quantitative review of its structural, functional, and clinical significance. *Brain Research Reviews, 29,* 26–49.

Shears, C., Hawkins, A., Varner, A., Lewis, L., Heatley, J., & Twachtmann, L. (2008). Knowledge-based inferences across the hemispheres: Domain makes a difference. *Neuropsychologia, 46*(10), 2563–2568.

Sherratt, S., & Bryan, K. (2012). Discourse production after right brain damage: Gaining a comprehensive picture using a multi-level processing model. *Journal of Neurolinguistics, 25*(4), 213–239.

Sidtis, D., Canterucci, G., & Katsnelson, D. (2009). Effects of neurological damage on production of formulaic language. *Clinical Linguistics and Phonetics, 23,* 270–284.

Siegal, M., Carrington, J., & Radel, M. (1996). Theory of mind and pragmatic understanding following right hemisphere damage. *Brain and Language, 53,* 40–50.

Soroker, N., Kasher, A., Giora, R., Batori, G., Corn, C., Gil, M., & Zaidel, E. (2005). Processing of basic speech acts following localized brain damage: a new light on the neuroanatomy of language. *Brain and Cognition, 57*(2), 214–217.

Stemmer, B. (Ed.). (1999a). Pragmatics: Theoretical and clinical issues. [Special Issue]. *Brain and Language, 68*(3).

Stemmer, B. (1999b). Discourse studies in neurologically impaired populations: A quest for action. *Brain and Language, 68,* 402–418.

Stemmer, B., Giroux, F., & Joanette, Y. (1994). Production and evaluation of requests by right-hemisphere brain-damaged individuals. *Brain and Language, 47,* 1–31.

Stemmer, B., & Joanette, Y. (1998). The interpretation of narrative discourse of brain-damaged individuals within the framework of a multilevel discourse model. In M. Beeman & C. Chiarello (Eds.), *Right hemisphere language comprehension: Perspectives from cognitive neuroscience.* Mahwah, NJ: Lawrence Erlbaum.

Stites, M.C., Federmeier, K.D., & Stine-Morrow, E.A.L. (2013). Cross-age comparisons reveal multiple strategies for lexical ambiguity resolution during natural reading. *Journal of Experimental Psychology: Learning, Memory, and Cognition, 39,* 1823–1841.

Swaab, R.I., Galinsky, A.D., Medvec, V., & Diermeier, D.A. (2012). The communication orientation model explaining the diverse effects of sight, sound, and synchronicity on negotiation and group decision-making outcomes. *Personality and Social Psychology Review, 16,* 25–53.

Titone, D. (1998). Hemispheric differences in context sensitivity during lexical ambiguity resolution. *Brain and Language, 65,* 361–394.

Tompkins, C.A. (1990). Knowledge and strategies for processing lexical metaphor after right or left hemisphere brain damage. *Journal of Speech and Hearing Research, 33,* 307–316.

Tompkins, C.A. (1991a). Automatic and effortful processing of emotional intonation after right or left hemisphere brain damage. *Journal of Speech and Hearing Research, 34,* 820–830.

Tompkins, C.A. (1995). *Right hemisphere communication disorders: Theory and management.* San Diego, CA: Singular Publishing Group.

Tompkins, C.A. (2012). Rehabilitation for cognitive-communication disorders in right hemisphere brain damage. *Archives of Physical Medicine and Rehabilitation, 93,* S61–S69.

Tompkins, C.A., & Baumgaertner, A. (1998). Clinical value of online measures for adults with right hemisphere brain damage. *American Journal of Speech-Language Pathology, 7,* 68–74.

Tompkins, C.A., Baumgaertner, A., Lehman, M.T., & Fassbinder, W. (2000). Mechanisms of discourse comprehension impairment after right hemisphere brain damage: Suppression in lexical ambiguity resolution. *Journal of Speech, Language, and Hearing Research, 43,* 62–78.

Tompkins, C.A., Blake, M.T., Scharp, V.L., Meigh, K.M., & Wambaugh, J.L. (2013). Implicit treatment of underlying comprehension processes improves narrative comprehension in right hemisphere brain damage. In Clinical Aphasiology Conference: Clinical Aphasiology Conference (2013): 43rd. Tucson, AZ, May 28 through June 2.

Tompkins, C.A., Blake, M.T., Wambaugh, J.L., & Meigh, K.M. (2011). A novel, implicit treatment for language comprehension processes in right hemisphere brain damage: Phase I data. *Aphasiology, 25*(6–7), 789–799.

Tompkins, C.A., Bloise, C.G.R., Timko, M.L., & Baumgaertner, A. (1994). Working memory and inference revision in brain-damaged and normally aging adults. *Journal of Speech and Hearing Research, 37,* 896–912.

Tompkins, C.A., Boada, R., & McGarry, K. (1992). The access and processing of familiar idioms by brain damaged and normally aging adults. *Journal of Speech and Hearing Research, 35,* 626–637.

Tompkins, C.A., Fassbinder, W., Blake, M.L., Baumgaertner, A., & Jayaram, N. (2004). Inference generation during text comprehension by adults with right hemisphere brain damage: Activation failure vs. multiple activation? *Journal of Speech, Language, and Hearing Research, 47,* 1380–1395.

Tompkins, C.A., Fassbinder, W., Scharp, V.L., & Meigh, K. M. (2008). Activation and maintenance of peripheral semantic features of unambiguous words after right hemisphere brain damage in adults. *Aphasiology, 22,* 119–138.

Tompkins, C.A., Klepousniotou, E., & Gibbs Scott, A. (2012). Nature and assessment of right hemisphere disorders. In I. Papathanasiou, P. Coppens, & C. Potagas (Eds.), *Aphasia and related neurogenic communication disorders* (pp. 297–343). Sudbury, MA: Jones & Bartlett.

Tompkins, C.A., & Lehman, M.T. (1998). Interpreting intended meanings after right hemisphere brain damage: An analysis of evidence, potential accounts, and clinical implications. *Topics in Stroke Rehabilitation, 5,* 29–47.

Tompkins, C.A., Lehman, M.T., Wyatt, A., & Schulz, R. (1998). Functional outcome assessment of adults with right hemisphere brain damage. *Seminars in Speech and Language, 19,* 303–321.

Tompkins, C.A., Lehman-Blake, M.T., Baumgaertner, A., & Fassbinder, W. (2001). Mechanisms of discourse comprehension impairment after right hemisphere brain damage: Suppression in inferential ambiguity resolution. *Journal of Speech, Language, and Hearing Research, 44*(2), 400–415.

Tompkins, C.A., Lehman-Blake, M., Baumgaertner, A., & Fassbinder, W. (2002). Characterizing comprehension difficulties after right brain damage: Attentional demands of suppression function. *Aphasiology, 16,* 559–572.

Tompkins, C.A., Scharp, V.L., Meigh, K.M., Blake, M.L., & Wambaugh, J.L. (2012). Generalization of a novel, implicit treatment for coarse coding deficit in right hemisphere brain damage: A single subject experiment. *Aphasiology, 26*(5), 689–708.

Tompkins, C.A., Scharp, V.L., Meigh, K.M., & Fassbinder, W. (2008). Coarse coding and discourse comprehension in adults with right hemisphere brain damage. *Aphasiology, 22,* 204–223.

Tremblay, T., Monetta, L., & Joanette, Y. (2009). Complexity and hemispheric abilities: Evidence for a differential impact on semantics and phonology. *Brain and Language, 108,* 67–72.

Tucker, D.M. (1981). Lateral brain function, emotion, and conceptualization. *Psychological Bulletin, 89,* 19–46.

Turkeltaub, P.E., Messing, S., Norise, C., & Hamilton, R.H. (2011). Are networks for residual language function and recovery consistent across aphasic patients? *Neurology, 76,* 1726–1734.

Vigneau, M., Beaucousin, V., Hervé, P.Y., Jobard, G., Petit, L., Crivello, F., . . . & Tzourio-Mazoyer, N. (2011). What is right-hemisphere contribution to phonological, lexico-semantic, and sentence processing? Insights from a meta-analysis. *NeuroImage, 54*(1), 577–593.

Wapner, W., Hamby, S., & Gardner, H. (1981). The role of the right hemisphere in the apprehension of complex linguistic materials. *Brain and Language, 14,* 15–32.

Weed, E., McGregor, W., Nielsen, J.F., Roepstorff, A., & Frith, U. (2010). Theory of Mind in adults with right hemisphere damage: What's the story? *Brain and Language, 113*(2), 65–72.

Weltman, K., & Lavidor, M. (2013). Modulating lexical and semantic processing by transcranial direct current stimulation. *Experimental Brain Research, 226*, 121–135.

Weylman, S., Brownell, H.H., Roman, M., & Gardner, H. (1989). Appreciation of indirect requests by left- and right-brain-damaged patients: The effects of verbal context and conventionality of wording. *Brain and Language, 36*, 580–591.

Whitney, C., Huber, W., Klann, J., Weis, S., Krach, S., & Kircher, T. (2009). Neural correlates of narrative shifts during auditory story comprehension. *NeuroImage, 47*(1), 360–366.

Whyte, J. (2009). Directions in brain injury research: From concept to clinical implementation. *Neuropsychological Rehabilitation, 19*(6), 807–823.

Winner, E., Brownell, H., Happe, F., Blum, A., & Pincus, D. (1998). Distinguishing lies from jokes: Theory of mind deficits and discourse interpretation in right hemisphere brain-damaged patients. *Brain and Language, 62*, 89–106.

Witte, O.W., & Stoll, G. (1997). Delayed and remote effects of focal cortical infarctions: Secondary damage and reactive plasticity. *Advances in Neurology, 73*, 207–227.

Wlotko, E.W., & Federmeier, K.D. (2013). Two sides of meaning: The scalp-recorded N400 reflects distinct contributions from the cerebral hemispheres. *Frontiers in Psychology, 4*, 1–15.

Wolf, I., Dziobek, I., & Heekeren, H.R. (2010). Neural correlates of social cognition in naturalistic settings: A model-free analysis approach. *NeuroImage, 49*, 894–904.

Xu, J., Kemeny, S., Park, G., Frattali, C., & Braun, A. (2005). Language in context: Emergent features of word, sentence, and narrative comprehension. *NeuroImage, 25*, 1002–1015.

Yang, Y., Tompkins, C.A., Meigh, K.M., & Prat, C.S. (submitted). Voxel-based lesion symptom mapping of coarse coding and suppression deficits in right-hemisphere-damaged patients. *American Journal of Speech-Language Pathology.*

Yarkoni, T., Speer, N.K., & Zacks, J.M. (2008). Neural substrates of narrative comprehension and memory. *NeuroImage, 41*(4), 1408–1425.

Zaidel, E. (1998). Language in the right hemisphere following callosal disconnection. In B. Stemmer & H.A. Whitaker (Eds.), *Handbook of neurolinguistics.* San Diego, CA: Academic Press.

25

PROSODY AND THE APROSODIAS

Donna C. Tippett and Elliott Ross

Introduction

"You sound so happy!"
"I could hear it in his voice."
"What did she mean by that?"
"Don't use that tone with me."

Ordinary comments such as these reveal the profound understanding that human communication is more than semantics and syntax. Pitch, loudness, stress on syllables and words, and rate of speech, collectively known as prosody, infuse meaning into spoken messages and convey emotional information. It is not only what one says, but how one says it that matters. In fact, if the affective-prosodic message is not consistent with the language content, listeners will believe the affective intention (Ackerman, 1983; Bowers, Coslett, Bauer, Speedie, & Heilman, 1987; Mehrabian, 2007). The ability to recognize affective intention is vital for accurate perception of a communication partner's emotional state and generation of an appropriate response to this circumstance. Misinterpretation of affective intention can limit interpersonal relationships and result in social isolation (Blonder, Pettigrew, & Kryscio, 2012). In this chapter, the taxonomy and neurology of prosody, the aprosodic syndromes and their assessment, treatment, and functional implications will be discussed.

Although no longer tenable, language has been viewed traditionally as a dominant and lateralized function of the left cerebral hemisphere (Benson, 1979; Ross, 2010). This concept evolved from the study of aphasia and its associated lesions in the late 19th century by Dax (1936), Broca (1861; 1865), Wernicke (1874; 1881), and Lichtheim (1885). Their seminal publications led to many insights about the neural organization of language functions and that in strongly right-handed individuals damage to the left hemisphere was present in patients who had language impairments. These early observations established that language functions depend on specific regions of the left cerebral hemisphere and provided the groundwork for Geschwind's (1965) aphasia classification system.

A special role for the right hemisphere and the importance of the emotional aspects of communication, however, were recognized by Hughlings Jackson (1878–1915), who reported that even patients with severe aphasias were still able to communicate emotional information via vocalizations and gestural behaviors. Subsequently, an early study of functional imaging of the brain revealed bilateral, fairly homologous, activation of both cerebral hemispheres during speech production (Larson, Skinhøj, & Lassen, 1978), a finding that was robustly supported by subsequent functional imaging research (e.g., Mitchell & Ross, 2008; Ross & Monnot, 2008; Sidtis, 2007; Van Lancker Sidtis, 2006). The contemporary view is that language is a distributed process that actively engages both hemispheres. The definition of language is expanded accordingly to extend beyond its basic verbal-linguistic elements (i.e., vocabulary, lexicon, grammar) to encompass paralinguistic components (Ross, 2010). The prosodic elements of language are imposed on the propositional components to convey meaning, crucial for human interactions (Carton, Kessler, & Pape, 1999; Weintraub & Mesulam, 1983; Wymer, Lindman, & Booksh, 2002). In fact, the index cases that led to the initiation of research into the right hemisphere's role in language and communication beginning in the 1970s (Bowers, Bauer, & Heilman, 1993; Blonder, Bowers, & Heilman, 1991; Heilman, Scholes, & Watson, 1975; Ross, 1981; Ross & Mesulam, 1979; Tucker, Watson, & Heilman, 1977) all presented clinically because of psychosocial dissonance (Heilman, 2002; Ross, 1982).

Types of Prosody

Prosody is defined as the rhythm of language (Monrad-Krohn, 1947) and includes loudness, pitch, stress, juncture, and duration (Tompkins, 1995). Speakers vary these prosodic elements to convey linguistic and affective information to listeners to facilitate their communicative intent. *Linguistic* or *intrinsic prosody* differentiates declarative, interrogative, imperative, and exclamatory sentences and disambiguates words and phrases (Monrad-Krohn, 1947; Wong, 2002). A rise in pitch at the end of a sentence indicates a question, whereas a steady pitch indicates a statement or command (Ultan, 1978). Lexical or phonemic stress differentiates word meaning (Cruttenden, 1997), such as "**con**tent" (i.e., subject matter) versus "con**tent**" (i.e., satisfied) or "**rec**ord" as a noun versus "re**cord**" as a verb. Contrastive stress, or word emphasis (Cruttenden, 1997), clarifies meaning, such as the difference between "**I** walked your dog" (I, not others, walked your dog) versus "I walked **your** dog" (I walked your dog, not other dogs). In addition, word emphasis and pausing can make confusing syntax clear, for example, "The boy . . . and the **girl** carrying the books . . . walked to school" (only the girl is carrying the books) versus "The boy and the girl carrying the **books** . . . walked to school" (both are carrying the books). *Intellectual prosody* (Monrad-Krohn, 1947) conveys attitudinal information, such distinguishing sincerity ("This **is** delicious" spoken with emphasis on "is") versus sarcasm ("This is **delicious**" spoken with emphasis on "delicious" and rising terminal intonation). *Emotional prosody* (Monrad-Krohn, 1947) reveals the sentiment of the speaker, such as happiness, sadness, anger, or fear. Sadness can be conveyed in a quiet voice with a falling pitch contour; anger can be conveyed in a loud, harsh voice and fast rate of speech. *Affective* or *extrinsic prosody* refers to both attitudinal and emotional prosody (Ross, 2000). Other types of prosody include *inarticulate prosody* (e.g., sighing, grunting), *dialectal* or *regional prosody*, and *idiosyncratic prosody*, which is unique to an individual speaker (Monrad-Krohn, 1963; Ross, 2010).

Aprosodia

Aprosodia refers to deficits in language and communication produced by focal brain lesions that impair the production, comprehension, and/or repetition of affective prosody (Ross, 1981). An individual with "sensory" aprosodia may be able to understand the overt, propositional content of a message conveyed by words and syntax, but is unable to recognize the emotional subtext (Bowers, Coslett, Bauer, Speedie, & Heilman, 1987; Heilman, Scholes, & Watson, 1975; Ross, 1981; Weintraub, Mesulam, & Kramer, 1981). An individual with "motor" aprosodia may have a flat, monotone pattern of speech that does not convey emotional connotation, but is still able to comprehend the affective aspects of communication (Ross & Mesulam, 1979). This is distinct from prosodic production impairments due to dysarthria, such as the disordered prosody in ataxic and hypokinetic dysarthria (Duffy, 2005). Cognitive/language deficits, such as diminished processing and attention, and anosognosia, may compromise performance on tests of prosody and exacerbate emotional communication deficits, but are also distinct from aprosodia.

Ross (1981) proposed specific aprosodia syndromes, analogous to classic aphasia syndromes. The functional-anatomic organization of prosody in the right hemisphere appears to mirror that of propositional language in the left hemisphere. For example, loss of the ability to produce or repeat affective prosody with preserved comprehension is associated with lesions in right frontal operculum or homologue of Broca's area (Ross & Monnot, 2008). Loss of ability to comprehend affective prosody is associated with lesions in right temporal operculum or homologue of Wernicke's area (Ross & Monnot, 2008). These functional-anatomic relationships are valid only for acute brain injury immediately post onset, as recovery of function occurs with neural reorganization (Ross, 2010; Ross & Monnot, 2008).

Evidence regarding the functional-anatomic relationships of the aprosodic syndromes is mixed, with some studies providing support for this paradigm (e.g., Denes, Caldognetto, Semenza, Vagges, & Zettin, 1984; Gorelick & Ross, 1987; Ross & Monnot, 2008) and others raising reservations about these syndromes (e.g., Cancelliere & Kertesz, 1990; Wertz, Henschel, Auther, Ashford, & Kirshner, 1998). It is thought that this discrepancy is due to when and how individuals are examined post stroke (Ross, 2010; Ross & Monnot, 2008; Ross, Thompson, & Yenkosky, 1997). The aprosodic syndromes, similar to aphasic syndromes, show the best functional-anatomic relationships if studied within the first 4–6 weeks post stroke before recovery and long-term neural reorganization occurs.

In addition to stroke, other etiologies associated with aprosodic deficits include traumatic brain injury (Rosenbek, Rodriguez, Hieber, Leon, Crucian, Ketterson, Ciampitti, Singletary, Heilman, & Gonzalez Rothi, 2006), Alzheimer's disease (Testa, Beatty, Gleason, Orbelo, & Ross, 2001), autism spectrum disorders (Wymer, Lindman, & Booksh, 2002), fetal and early life exposure to alcohol (Monnot, Nixon, Lovallo, & Ross, 2001), schizophrenia (Mitchell & Crow, 2005; Ross, Orbelo, Cartwright, Hansel, Burgard, Testa, & Buck 2001) and posttraumatic stress disorder (Freeman, Hart, Kimbrell, & Ross, 2009).

Neurology of Prosody

The neurology of prosody comprehension and production is complex, and the type of prosody must be considered. Right hemisphere specialization for perception and production of emotions is a long-standing concept (Blonder, Bowers, & Heilman, 1991; Borod, 2000). The predominant role of the right hemisphere in processing *emotional prosody* is supported by a substantial and varied literature, including studies recording event-related brain potentials (Pihan, Altenmüller, Hertrich, & Ackermann, 2000); fMRI studies showing right hemisphere activation in association with prosody judgments (Beaucousin, Lacheret, Turbelin, Morel, Mazoyer, & Tzourio-Mazoyer, 2007; Buchanan, Lutz, Mirzazade, Specht, Shah, Zilles, & Jäncke, 2000); dichotic listening paradigms showing a left ear advantage for prosody (Grimshaw, Kwasny, Covell, & Johnson, 2003; Ley & Bryden, 1982), and lesion studies of judging emotional meaning from prosody (Adolphs, 2002; Blonder et al., 1991; Cancelliere, & Kertesz, 1990; Heilman, Scholes, & Watson, 1975; Pell, 2006; Ross & Monnot, 2008; Ross, Thompson, & Yenkosky, 1997). Dara, Bang, Gottesman, and Hillis (2014) found that impairment in comprehension of emotional prosody is a more sensitive indicator of acute right hemisphere dysfunction than unilateral spatial neglect. The authors recommended that acute stroke assessment include bedside assessment of affective-prosodic comprehension to detect right hemisphere dysfunction readily, and thus direct medical interventions to salvage right cortical function. Specific cerebral lesion sites have been associated with prosodic deficits. For example, affective prosody comprehension has been found to be associated with lesions involving the right temporal operculum and thalamus (Gorelick & Ross, 1987; Ross, 1981; Ross & Monnot, 2008; Wolf & Ross, 1987). Impairment of affective prosody production is associated with lesions involving the right frontal operculum and anterior insula (Gorelick & Ross, 1987; Ross, 1981; Ross & Mesulam, 1979; Ross & Monnot, 2008), and injury to the frontal operculum is associated with deficits in affective prosodic repetition (Ross & Monnot, 2008).

In addition to these observations regarding right hemisphere dominance for affective prosody, there are reports showing that left-brain hemisphere damage can disrupt modulation of affective prosody (Adolphs, Damasio, & Tranel, 2002; Cancelliere & Kertesz, 1990; Geigenberger & Ziegler, 2001; Ross, 2000; Ross, Thompson, & Yenosky, 1997). Disruption of affective prosody following left brain damage may be the result of loss of callosal integration of the dominant language functions represented in both the left and right hemispheres (Ross & Monnot, 2008; Ross, Thompson, & Yenkosky, 1997), whereas impairment following right brain damage is attributed to loss of affective-communicative representations (Blonder et al., 1991; Bowers et al., 1993). Furthermore, deficits in affective prosody production and comprehension can occur due to damage to the right basal ganglia and thalamus (Breitenstein, Daum, & Ackermann, 1998; Cancelliere & Kertesz, 1990; Cohen, Riccio, & Flannery, 1994; Gorelick & Ross, 1987; Karow & Connors, 2003; Ross, 1981; Ross, Harney, de Lacoste-Utamsing, & Purdy, 1981;Van Lancker Sidtis, Pachana, Cummings, & Sidtis, 2006;Wolfe & Ross, 1987). More recently, an "affective empathy network" has been proposed based on performance on affective empathy tasks, including comprehension of affective prosody, in individuals with acute right hemisphere stroke. This network includes the anterior insula and temporal pole, specifically the pole of the superior temporal gyrus (Leigh, Oishi, Hsu, Lindquist, Gottesman, Jarso, Crainiceanu, Mori, & Hillis, 2013). Leigh et al. (2013) found that those with impaired performance on an affective empathy task also had impaired recognition of affective prosody; impairment in the latter was not judged to be causative of impairment in the former as the affective empathy task did not require listening to tone of voice. Instead, the authors concluded that areas of the brain necessary for affective empathy may also be necessary for comprehension of affective prosody.

Hypotheses regarding hemispheric lateralization of emotions include the right hemisphere hypothesis, the valence hypothesis, and the emotion-type hypothesis. The right hemisphere hypothesis traditionally ascribes a greater role in emotion processing, regardless of valence, to the right hemisphere (Blonder et al., 1991; Borod, 2000). The valence hypothesis invokes involvement of both cerebral hemispheres in emotion processing, albeit differently. According to the valence-specific laterality concept, the left hemisphere is specialized for positive or pleasant emotions, whereas the right hemisphere is specialized for negative or unpleasant emotions (Heller, 1990; Silberman & Weingartner, 1986;Tucker & Williamson, 1984).The emotion-type hypothesis posits that the right hemisphere processes primary emotions (e.g., anger, disgust, fear, sadness, happiness), whereas the left hemisphere processes social types of emotions (e.g., envy, jealousy, admiration) (Ross, Homan, & Buck, 1994). Patterns of performance on tasks of comprehension and production of affective prosody by individuals with left and right brain damage appear to support the right hemisphere hypothesis (Ross & Monnot, 2008; Ross, Thompson, & Yenkosky, 1997). In left brain damaged individuals, if the verbal-articulatory demands are incrementally reduced, their performance on tests of affective prosody dramatically improve; in contrast, reducing verbal-articulatory demands in right-brain damaged patients does not improve their performance when using the Aprosodia Battery (see below). In addition, when the types of comprehension errors were studied in older versus younger normal subjects using the Aprosodia Battery (Ross & Monnot, 2011), older subjects showed increased error rates on comprehension of happy, sad, and angry prosody (primary emotions) but not pleasant-surprise or disinterest prosody (social emotions), lending support to the emotion-type hypothesis (Ross & Monnot, 2011). This finding is consistent with the classic right hemisphere aging effects on cognitive performance (Botwink, 1977; Hochnadel & Kaplan, 1984).

Similar to affective prosody, *linguistic prosody* appears to be modulated by both the left and right hemispheres (e.g., Balan & Gandour, 1999; Baum, Pell, Leonard, & Gordon, 1997; Gandour & Baum, 2001; Heilman, Bowers, Speedie, & Coslett, 1984; Schirmer, Alter, Kotz, & Friederici, 2001; Walker, Joseph, & Goodman, 2009; Walker, Pelletier, & Reif, 2004). There are hemispheric differences, however, with left hemisphere damage causing particular difficulty modulating temporal parameters and inconsistent difficulty modulating frequency-related parameters (Shah, Baum, & Dwivedi, 2006; Wong, 2002). Theoretical explanations for hemispheric specialization include the "task-dependent" or "functional" theory and the "cue-dependent" or "acoustic" theory. According to the task-dependent theory, more linguistic-type cues lateralize to the left hemisphere, and more affective-emotional–type cues lateralize to the right hemisphere (Van Lancker, 1980). Lateralization of prosody based on acoustic signal is proposed in the cue-dependent theory. If the cue is signaled by temporal features, then it lateralizes to the left hemisphere. If the cue is signaled by spectral features, then it lateralizes to the right hemisphere (Robin, Tranel, & Damasio, 1990; Van Lancker & Sidtis, 1992).

The neurology of *emphatic* or *contrastive stress* has been investigated to a lesser degree. Findings are not conclusive regarding whether perception and production of prosodic stress is lateralized in the brain (Baum 1998; Behrens, 1988; Bradvik, Dravins, Holtás, Rosên, Ryding, & Ingvar, 1991; Ouellett & Baum, 1994; Pell, 1998; 1999a; 1999b; Weintraub et al., 1981). However, a recent investigation of the neuroacoustic basis of prosodic stress in individuals with left and right brain damage robustly supports the task-dependent rather than the cue-dependent theory of lateralization (Ross, Shayya, & Rousseau, 2013).

Assessment of Prosody

Published measures for assessment of prosody include the Battery of Emotional Expression and Compression (Cancelliere & Kertesz, 1990), the Aprosodia Battery (Ross et al., 1997), and the Florida Affect Battery (Bowers, Bauer, & Heilman, 1999). Each of these measures has been used in prosody research, but could be employed for clinical purposes.

The Battery of Emotional Expression and Comprehension (Cancelliere & Kertesz, 1990) assesses the ability to express emotion via prosody and recognize the emotional valence of prosody, situations, and facial expressions. The Battery of Emotional Expression and Comprehension consists of five subtests: Elicitation of Emotional Prosody, Repetition of Emotional Prosody, Identification of Emotional Prosody, Identification of Emotional Situations, and Identification of Emotional Faces. Cancelliere and Kertesz (1990) administered this test to individuals with right hemisphere stroke and to control subjects to investigate the relationship between the intrahemispheric location of lesions and disturbances of emotional expression and comprehension. The basal ganglia lesions emerged most frequently in aprosodia syndromes, followed by anterior temporal lobe and insula lesions. However, their subjects were studied many months post stroke, and do not necessarily reflect acute localizations because of recovery and long-term neural reorganization (Ross & Monnot, 2008; Ross, 2010).

The Aprosodia Battery (Ross et al., 1997) assesses comprehension and production (spontaneous and repetition) of affective prosody and quantifies results to distinguish patterns of deficits associated with right versus left cerebral damage. Verbal-articulatory demands are reduced incrementally on the comprehension and repetition tasks. Patients select labeled drawings of faces, expressing different emotions, to match stimuli presented at the word, monosyllable, and asyllabic levels. Stimuli include sentences in which the emotion is conveyed by a sentence ("I am going to the other movies"), repeated monosyllables ("ba ba ba ba ba ba"), and an asyllabic articulation ("aaaaaahhhh"). Individuals are also asked to discriminate acoustically degraded paired stimuli to assess if they convey the same or a different emotion. For affective repetition, individuals are asked to mimic the previously described stimuli, and a sample of spontaneous speech is obtained when they discuss an emotional experience. Their performance is recorded and analyzed acoustically for their ability to vary intonation, which in English (a nontonal language) appears to be the most salient acoustic feature underlying affective prosody (Ross, Edmondson, Seibert, & Homan, 1988; Ross & Monnot, 2008; Ross, Thompson, & Yenkosky, 1997). The Aprosodia Battery has been used to study several different clinical populations with robust results, including patients with fetal and early life exposure to alcohol (Monnot et al., 2001; Monnot, Nixon, Lovallo, & Ross, 2002), Alzheimer's disease (Testa et al., 2001), leukoaraiosis (Ross, Hansel, Orbelo, & Monnot, 2005), multiple sclerosis (Beatty, Orbelo, Sococco, & Ross, 2003), posttraumatic stress disorder (Freeman et al., 2009), and schizophrenia (Ross et al., 2001). The Aprosodia Battery also has been administered to healthy adults to investigate maturational-aging effects (Orbelo, Grim, Talbott, & Ross, 2005; Ross & Monnot, 2008).

The Florida Affect Battery (Bowers et al., 1999) assesses the ability to identify spoken prosody as well as facial expression of emotional affects. This test was designed as a research tool for investigating disturbances in the perception and understanding of nonverbal communicative signals of emotion that can occur as part of neurologic or psychiatric disorders. The stimuli used in constructing the facial affect tasks include four different women, each displaying one of five different emotions. There are five subtests: Facial Identity Discrimination, Facial Affect Discrimination, Facial Affect Naming, Facial Affect Selection, and Facial Affect Matching. The prosody tasks are designed to complement the facial perception tasks. The first three prosodic subtests consist of a set of semantically neutral simple sentences spoken in various nonemotional or emotional tones of voice. The fourth prosody subtest involves affectively intoned sentences whose semantic content conflicts with or complements the prosodic message. Normative and psychometric properties are described (Bowers et al., 1999). The test has been administered to individuals with left and right hemisphere stroke (Blonder et al., 1991; Bowers, Blonder, Slomine, & Heilman, 1996) and temporal lobe epilepsy (Bowers et al., 1999).

Treatment of Aprosodia

In contrast to the number of studies investigating the neurology of prosody, relatively little attention has been directed to studies examining treatment options. Two current approaches to the treatment of aprosodia are imitative treatment and cognitive-linguistic treatment (Jones, Plowman-Prine, Rosenbek, Shrivastay, & Wu, 2009; Leon, Rosenbek, Crucian, Hieber, Holiway, Rodriguez, Ketterson, Ciampitti, Freshwater, Heilman, & Gonzalez Rothi, 2005; Rosenbek, Crucian, Leon, Hieber, Rodriguez, Holiway, Ketterson, Ciampitti, Heilman, & Gonzalez Rothi, 2004; Rosenbek et al., 2006). In imitative treatment, a clinician models the desired emotional utterance. The utterance is then produced in unison by the clinician and the patient. Subsequently, the patient produces targeted utterances after a delay, and eventually after imaging a situation appropriate to the emotional prosody of the utterance. The underlying rationale for this treatment is that aprosodia results from a disruption of motor planning, resulting in flattened intonation contours (Baum & Pell, 1999; van der Merwe, 1997).

In cognitive-linguistic treatment, the patient is given written descriptions of the characteristics of various tones of voice to express a variety of emotions. The patient matches cards listing different emotions to these descriptions of voice. The patient is eventually asked to produce a particular tone of voice. This therapy is based on the hypothesis that aprosodia results from a disruption of the nonverbal affect lexicon; that is, how an angry voice or sad voice sounds (Blonder et al., 1991; Bowers et al., 1993).

A phase I investigation showed a positive response to both the imitative and cognitive-linguistic approaches to treating aprosodia (Rosenbek et al., 2004). A follow-up study of three individuals with motor aprosodia post right hemisphere stroke also demonstrated that both therapies were active (Leon et al., 2005). Russell, Laures-Gore, and Patel (2010) reported both acoustic and perceptual changes in an individual with receptive and expressive aprosodia after bilateral strokes after imitative therapy.

Use of visual feedback, such as that provided by a computerized pitch feedback program, may be another treatment avenue. In a single-subject case report, an individual with aprosodia following traumatic brain injury demonstrated gain in affective prosody after treatment with a computerized pitch feedback program (Stringer, 1996). Incorporation of motor learning enhancement techniques may be used in combination with imitative and cognitive-linguistic therapy (Leon & Rodriguez, 2008), capitalizing on the theory that aprosodia is due to a motor planning deficit. Further study is needed to investigate whether the motor learning principles of "knowledge of results" (feedback about whether a response is correct or incorrect) and "knowledge of performance" (feedback about why a response is correct or incorrect) (Proctor & Dutta, 1995) can enhance aprosodia treatment.

Functional Implications of Aprosodia

Interpretation of a person's affective state guides the course of communication interaction and has implications for successful social interactions. Interpretation and use of prosodic elements are crucial for communicative interactions and for the well-being of speakers and communication partners (Carton et al.,1999; Heilman, 2002; Mitchell & Crow, 2005; Ross, 1997; Trauner, Ballantyne, Friedland, & Chase, 1996; Voeller, 1995; Weintraub & Mesulam, 1983; Wymer et al., 2002). Recognition of prosody is one means to judge emotional tenor, and thus evoke an appropriately empathetic response. Failure to recognize the emotional state of another can result in failed interpersonal interactions. In a study of 12 individuals with right hemisphere stroke, ability to decode the meaning of facial expression and prosody were associated with decreased marital satisfaction (Blonder et al., 2012). Profound social dysfunction of an individual with behavioral variant frontotemporal dementia was judged to be due in part to her difficulty in processing emotional facial and prosodic cues during human communication (Dara, Kirsch-Darrow, Ochfield, Slenz, Agranovich, Vasconcellos-Faria, Ross, Hillis, & Kortte, 2013).

Conclusion

Ability to understand and express emotion via prosody is as integral to communication as the comprehension of complex syntax and a varied lexicon. Impaired ability to express and understand emotions is debilitating to those with aprosodia, compromising integration into home, work, and community life. The implications of aprosodia also affect family members and friends, as the individual with aprosodia may be seen as being unable to empathize—that is, understand and share in the feelings of others. The results of a recent study from our Stroke Prevention and Recovery Center (SPARC) revealed that 50% of spouses or adult children of right hemisphere stroke survivors reported the stroke survivor's difficulty understanding the feelings of other people (loss of emotional empathy) to be among most important residual symptoms following stroke (Hillis & Tippett, 2014). These important functional implications point to an obvious need for treatment studies to investigate therapy options. Novel therapies to improve affective perspective-taking in general and prosody specifically, such as transcranial magnetic stimulation or transcranial direct current stimulation, and effective patient and family education programs, are fertile ground for research (Hillis, 2014). Our expanding understanding of the etiologies and cognitive processes underlying prosody is essential to the development of evidence-based practice to treat aprosodia.

References

Ackerman, B.P. (1983). Form and function in children's understanding of ironic utterances. *Journal of Experimental Child Psychology, 35*, 487–508. doi:10.1023/A:1005120109296

Adolphs, R. (2002). Neural systems for recognizing emotion. *Current Opinion in Neurobiology, 12*, 169–177. doi:10.1016/S0959-4388(02)00301-X

Adolphs, R., Damasio, H., & Tranel, D. (2002). Neural systems for recognition of emotional prosody: A 3-D lesion study. *Emotion, 2*, 23–51. doi:10.1037/1528-3542.2.1.23

Balan, A., & Gandour, J. (1999). Effect of sentence length on the production of linguistic stress by left- and right-hemisphere-damaged patients. *Brain and Language, 67*, 73–94. doi:10.1006/brln.1998.2035

Baum, S.R. (1998). The role of fundamental frequency and duration in the perception of linguistic stress by individuals with brain damage. *Journal of Speech, Language, and Hearing Research, 41*, 31–40. doi:10.1044/jslhr.4101.31

Baum, S.R., & Pell, M.D. (1999). The neural bases of prosody: Insights from lesion studies and neuroimaging. *Aphasiology, 13*, 581–608. doi:10.1080/026870399401957

Baum, S.R., Pell, M.D., Leonard, C.L., & Gordon, J.K. (1997). The ability of right- and left- hemisphere-damaged individuals to produce and interpret prosodic cues marking phrasal boundaries. *Language and Speech, 40*, 313–330.

Beaucousin, V., Lacheret, A., Turbelin, M. R., Morel, M., Mazoyer, B., & Tzourio-Mazoyer, N. (2007). fMRI study of emotional speech comprehension. *Cerebral Cortex, 17*, 339–352. doi:10.1093/cercor/bhj151

Beatty, W.W., Orbelo, D.M., Sococco, K.H., & Ross, E.D. (2003). Comprehension of affective prosody in multiple sclerosis. *Multiple Sclerosis, 9*, 148–153. doi:10.1191/1352458503ms897oa

Behrens, S.J. (1988). The role of the right hemisphere in linguistic stress. *Brain and Language, 33*, 104–127.

Benson, D.F. (1979). *Aphasia, alexia, and agraphia.* New York: Churchill Livingstone.

Blonder, L.X., Bowers, D., & Heilman, K.M. (1991). The role of the right hemisphere in emotional communication. *Brain, 114*, 1115–1127. doi:10.1093/brain/114.3.1115

Blonder, L.X., Pettigrew, L.C., & Kryscio, R.J. (2012). Emotion recognition and martial satisfaction in stroke. *Journal of Clinical and Experimental Neuropsychology, 34*, 634–642. doi:10.1080/13803395.2012.667069

Borod, J.C. (2000). *The neurophysiology of emotion.* New York: Oxford University Press.

Botwink, J. (1977). Intellectual abilities. In J.E. Birren & K.W. Schaie (Eds.), *Handbook of the psychology of aging.* New York: Van Nostrand Reinhold.

Bowers, D., Bauer, R.M., & Heilman, K.M. (1993). The non-verbal affect lexicon: Theoretical perspectives from neurological studies of affect perception. *Neuropsychology, 7*, 433–444. doi:10.1037/0894-4105.7.4.433

Bowers, D., Blonder, L.X., & Heilman, K.M. (1999). *The Florida Affect Battery.* Gainesville: University of Florida Brain Institute. Available at: http://neurology.ufl.edu/files/2011/12/Florida-Affect-Battery-Manual.pdf.

Bowers, D., Blonder, L.X., Slomine, B., & Heilman, K.M. (1996). *Nonverbal emotional signals: Patterns of impairment following hemispheric lesions using the Florida Affect Battery.* San Francisco: American Academy of Neurology.

Bowers, D., Coslett, H.B., Bauer, R.M., Speedie, L.J., & Heilman, K.M. (1987). Comprehension of emotional prosody following unilateral hemispheric lesions: Processing defect versus distraction defect. *Neuropsychologia, 25*, 317–328. doi:10.1016/0028-3932(87)90021-2

Bradvik, B., Dravins, C., Holtás, S., Rosên, I., Ryding, E., & Ingvar, D.H. (1991). Disturbances of speech prosody following right brain infarcts. *Acta Neurologica Scandinavica, 8*, 114–126. doi:10.1111/j.1600-0404.1991.tb04919.x

Breitenstein, C., Daum, I., & Ackermann, H. (1998). Emotional processing following cortical and subcortical brain damage: Contribution of the fronto-striatal circuitry. *Behavioral Neurology, 11*, 29–42. doi:10.1155/1998/579029

Broca, P. (1861). Perte de la parole: ramollissement chronique et destruction partielle du lobe anterieur gauche du cerveau. *Bulletins de la Société d'anthropologie, 2*, 235–238.

Broca, P. (1865). Sur le siège de la faculté du langage articulé. *Bulletins de la Société d'anthropologie, 6*, 337–393.

Buchanan, T.W., Lutz, K., Mirzazade, S., Specht, K., Shah, N.J., Zilles, K., & Jäncke, L. (2000). Recognition of emotional prosody and verbal components of spoken language: an fMRI study. *Cognitive Brain Research, 9*, 227–238. doi:10.1016/S0926-6410(99)00060-9

Cancelliere, A.E.B., & Kertesz, A. (1990). Lesion localization in acquired deficits of emotional expression and comprehension. *Brain and Cognition, 13*, 133–147. doi:10.1016/0278-2626(90)90046-Q

Carton, J.S., Kessler, E.A., & Pape, C.L. (1999). Nonverbal decoding skills and relationship well-being in adults. *Journal of Nonverbal Behavior, 23*, 91–100. doi:10.1023/A:1021339410262

Cohen, M.J., Riccio, C.A., & Flannery, A.M. (1994). Expressive aprosodia following stroke to the right basal ganglia: A case report. *Neuropsychology, 8*, 242–245. doi:10.1037/0894-4105.8.2.242

Cruttenden, A. (1997). *Intonation*. Cambridge: Cambridge University Press.

Dara, C., Bang, J., Gottesman, R.F., & Hillis, A.E. (2014). Right hemisphere dysfunction is better predicted by emotional prosody impairments as compared to neglect. *Journal of Neurology and Translational Neuroscience, 2*, 1037.

Dara, C., Kirsch-Darrow, L., Ochfield, E., Slenz, J., Agranovich, A., Vasconcellos-Faria, A., Ross, E., Hillis, A.E., & Kortte, K.B. (2013). Impaired emotion processing from vocal and facial cues in frontotemporal dementia compared to right hemisphere stroke. *Neurocase: The Neural Basis of Cognition, 19*, 521–529. doi:10.1080/13554794.2012.701641

Dax, M. (1936). Lésions de la moitié gauche de l'encéphale coincedent avec l'oublie des signes de la pensée. Montpelier. *Gazette Hebdomadaire de Medecine et de Chirurgie, 17*, 259–260.

Denes, G., Caldognetto, E.M., Semenza, C., Vagges, K., & Zettin, M. (1984). Discrimination and identification of emotions in human voice by brain-damaged subjects. *Acta Neurologia Scandinavia, 69*, 154–162. doi:10.1111/j.1600–0404.1984.tb07794.x

Duffy, J.R. (2005). *Motor speech disorders: Substrates, differential diagnosis, and management*. St. Louis, MO: Mosby.

Freeman, T.W., Hart, J., Kimbrell, T., & Ross, E.D. (2009). Comprehension of affective prosody in veterans with chronic posttraumatic stress disorder. *Journal of Neuropsychiatry and Clinical Neuroscience, 21*, 52–58. doi:10.1176/appi.neuropsych.21.1.52

Gandour, J., & Baum, S.R. (2001). Production of stress retraction by left- and right-hemisphere-damaged patients. *Brain and Language, 79*, 482–494. doi:10.1006/brln.2001.2562

Geigenberger, A., & Ziegler, W. (2001). Receptive prosodic processing in aphasia. *Aphasiology, 15*, 1169–1188. doi:10.1080/02687040143000555

Geschwind, N. (1965). Disconnexion syndromes in animals and man. *Brain, 88*, 237–294, 585–644. doi:10.1093/brain/88.2.237

Gorelick, P.B., & Ross, E.D. (1987). The aprosodias: Further functional-anatomical evidence for the organization of affective language in the right hemisphere. *Journal of Neurology, Neurosurgery, and Psychiatry, 50*, 553–560. doi:10.1136/jnnp.50.5.553

Grimshaw, G.M., Kwasny, K.M., Covell, E., & Johnson, R.A. (2003). The dynamic nature of language lateralization: Effects of lexical and prosodic factors. *Neuropsychologia, 41*, 1008–1019. doi:10.1016/S0028-3932(02)00315-9

Heilman, K.M. (2002). *Matter of mind: A neurologist's view of brain-behavior relationships*. New York: Oxford University Press, pp. 53–63.

Heilman, K.M., Bowers, D., Speedie, L., & Coslett, H.B. (1984). Comprehension of affective and nonaffective prosody. *Neurology, 34*, 917–921.

Heilman, K.M., Scholes, R., & Watson, R.T. (1975). Auditory affective agnosia: Disturbed comprehension of affective speech. *Journal of Neurology, Neurosurgery, and Psychiatry, 38*, 69–72. doi:10.1136/jnnp.38.1.69

Heller, W. (1990). The neuropsychology of emotion: Developmental patterns and implication for psychopathology. In N. Stein, B.L. Leventhal, & T. Trabasso (Eds.), *Psychological and biological approaches to emotion* (pp. 167–211). Hillsdale, NJ: Lawrence Erlbaum.

Hillis, A.E. (2014). Inability to empathize: Brain lesions that disrupt sharing and understanding another's emotions. *Brain, 137*, 981–997. doi:10.1093/brain/awt317

Hillis, A.E., & Tippett, D.C. (2014). Stroke recovery: Surprising influences and residual consequences. *Advances in Medicine*. doi.org/10.1155/2014/378263

Hochnadel, G., & Kaplan, E. (1984). Neuropsychology of normal aging. In M.L. Albert (Ed.), *Clinical neurology of aging* (pp. 231–244). New York: Oxford University Press.

Jackson, J.H. (1874/1915). On the nature of duality of the brain. *Brain, 38*, 96–103. (Original work published 1874). doi:10.1093/brain/ 38.1–2.96

Jones, H.N., Plowman-Prine, E.K., Rosenbek, J.C., Shrivastay, R., & Wu, S.S. (2009). Fundamental frequency and intensity mean and variability before and after two behavioral treatments for aprosodia. *Journal of Medical Speech-Language Pathology, 17*, 45–52.

Karow, C.M., & Connors, E.C. (2003). Affective communication in normal and brain-damaged adults: An overview. *Seminars in Speech and Language, 24*, 69–91. doi:10.1055/s-2003–38900

Larsen, B., Skinhøj, E., & Lassen, N.A. (1978). Variations in regional cortical blood flow in the right and left hemispheres during automatic speech. *Brain, 101*, 193–209. doi:10.1093/brain/101.2.193

Leigh, R., Oishi, K., Hsu, J., Lindquist, M., Gottesman, R.F., Jarso, S., Crainiceanu, C., Mori, S., & Hillis, A.E. (2013). Acute lesions that impair affective empathy. *Brain, 136*, 2539–2549. doi:10.1093/brain/awt177

Leon, S.A., & Rodriguez, A.D. (2008). Aprosodia and its treatments. Perspectives on *Neurophysiology and Neurogenic Speech and Language Disorders, 18*, 66–72. doi:10.1044/nnsld18.2.66

Leon, S.A., Rosenbek, J.C., Crucian, G.P., Hieber, B., Holiway, B., Rodriguez, A.D., Ketterson, T.U., Ciampitti, M.Z., Freshwater, S., Heilman, K.M., & Gonzalez Rothi, L.J. (2005). Active treatments for aprosodia secondary to right hemisphere stroke. *Journal of Rehabilitation Research and Development, 42*, 93–101.

Ley, R.G., & Bryden, M.P. (1982). A dissociation of right and left hemisphere effects for recognizing emotional tone and verbal content. *Brain and Cognition, 1*, 3–9. doi:10.1016/0278–2626(82)90002–1

Lichtheim, L. (1885). On aphasia. *Brain, 7*, 433–484.

Mehrabian, A. (2007). *Nonverbal communication*. Edison, NJ: Transaction Publishers.

Mitchell, R.L., & Crow, T.J. (2005). Right hemisphere language functions and schizophrenia: The forgotten hemisphere? *Brain, 128*, 963–978.

Mitchell, R.L.C., & Ross, E.D. (2008). fMRI evidence for the effect of verbal complexity on lateralization of the neural response associated with decoding prosodic emotion. *Neuropsychologia, 46*, 2880–2887. doi:10.1016/j.neuropsychologia.2008.05.024

Monnot, M., Lovallo, W., Nixon, S., & Ross, E.D. (2002). Neurological basis of deficits in affective prosody: Comprehension among alcoholics and fetal alcohol exposed adults. *Journal of Neuropsychiatry and Clinical Neuroscience, 14*, 321–328.

Monnot, M., Nixon, S., Lovallo, W., & Ross, E. (2001). Altered emotional perception in alcoholics: Deficits in affective prosody comprehension. *Alcoholism: Clinical and Experimental Research, 25*, 362–369. doi:10.1111/j.1530–0277.2001.tb02222.x

Monrad-Krohn, G. (1947). The prosodic quality of speech and its disorders. *Acta Psychologia Scandinavia, 22*, 225–265.

Monrad-Krohn, G.H. (1963). The third element of speech: Prosody and its disorders. In I. Halpern (Ed.), *Problems in dynamic neurology* (pp. 101–118). Jerusalem: Hebrew University Press.

Orbelo, D.M., Grim, M.A., Talbott, R.E., & Ross, E.D. (2005). Impaired comprehension of affective prosody in elderly subjects is not explained by age-related hearing or age-related cognitive decline. *Journal of Geriatric Neurology and Psychiatry, 18*, 25–32. doi:10.1177/0891988704272214

Ouellette, G.P., & Baum, S.R. (1994). Acoustic analysis of prosodic cues in left- and right-hemisphere-damaged patients. *Aphasiology, 8*, 257–283.

Pell, M.D. (1998). Recognition of prosody following unilateral brain lesion: Influence of functional and structural attributes of prosodic contours. *Neuropsychologia, 36*, 701–715.

Pell, M.D. (1999a). Fundamental frequency encoding of linguistic and emotional prosody by right-hemisphere damaged speakers. *Brain and Language, 69*, 161–192. doi:10.1006/brln.1999.2065

Pell, M.D. (1999b). The temporal organization of affective and non-affective speech in patients with right-hemisphere infarcts. *Cortex, 35*, 435–477. doi:10.1016/S0010-9452(08)70813-X

Pell, M.D. (2006). Cerebral mechanisms for understanding emotional prosody in speech. *Brain and Language, 96*, 221–234. doi:10.1016/j.bandl.2005.04.007

Pihan, H., Altenmüller, E., Hertrich, I., & Ackermann, H. (2000). Cortical activation patterns of affective speech processing depend on concurrent demands on the subvocal rehearsal system. A DC-potential study. *Brain, 123*, 2338–2349. doi:10.1093/brain/123.11.2338

Proctor, R.W., & Dutta, A. (1995). *Skill acquisition and human performance*. Thousand Oaks, CA: Sage Publications.

Robin, D.A., Tranel, D., & Damasio, H. (1990). Auditory perception of temporal and spectral events in patients with focal left and right cerebral lesions. *Brain and Language, 39*, 539–555.

Rosenbek, J.C., Crucian, G.P., Leon, S.A., Hieber, B., Rodriguez, A.D., Holiway, B., Ketterson, T.U., Ciampitti, M., Heilman, K.M., & Gonzalez Rothi, L.J. (2004). Novel treatments for expressive aprosodia: A phase I investigation of cognitive-linguistic and imitative interventions. *Journal of International Neuropsychological Society, 10*, 786–793. doi:10.1017/S135561770410502X

Rosenbek, J.C., Rodriguez, A.D., Hieber, B., Leon, S.A., Crucian, G.P., Ketterson, T.U., Ciampitti, M., Singletary, F., Heilman, K. M., & Gonzalez Rothi, L.J. (2006). Effects of two treatments for aprosodia secondary to acquired brain injury. *Journal of Rehabilitation Research and Development, 43*, 379–390. doi:10.1682/JRRD.2005.01.0029

Ross, E.D. (1981). The aprosodias: Functional-anatomic organization of the affective components of language in the right hemisphere. *Archives of Neurology, 38*, 561–569. doi:10.1001/archneur.1981.00510090055006

Ross, E.D. (1982). The divided self: Contrary to conventional wisdom, not all language is commanded by the brain's left side. *The Sciences, 22*, 8–12.

Ross, E.D. (1997). Right hemisphere syndromes and the neurology of emotions. In S.C. Schacter & O. Devinsky (Eds.), *Behavioral neurology and the legacy of Norman Geschwind* (pp. 183–184). Philadelphia: Lippincott-Raven.

Ross, E.D. (2000). Affective prosody and the aprosodias. In M.M. Mesulam (Ed.), *Principles of behavioral and cognitive neurology* (pp. 316–331). New York: Oxford University Press.

Ross, E.D. (2010). Cerebral localization of functions and the neurology of language: Fact versus fiction or is it something else? *Neuroscientist, 16*, 222–243. doi:10.1177/1073858409349899

Ross, E.D., Edmondson, J.A., Seibert, G.B., & Homan, R.W. (1988). Acoustical analysis of affective prosody during right-sided Wada test: A within subjects verification of the right hemisphere's role in language. *Brain and Language, 33*, 128–145.

Ross, E.D., Hansel, S.L., Orbelo, D.M., & Monnot, M. (2005). Relationship of leukoaraiosis to cognitive decline and cognitive aging. *Cognitive and Behavioral Neurology, 18*, 89–97.

Ross, E.D., Harney, J.H., de Lacoste-Utamsing, C., & Purdy, P.D. (1981). How the brain integrates affective and propositional language into a unified behavioral function: Hypothesis based on clinicoanatomic evidence. *Archives of Neurology, 38*, 745–748. doi:10.1001/archneur.1981.00510120045005

Ross, E.D., Homan, R.W., & Buck, R. (1994). Differential hemispheric lateralization of primary and social emotions. *Neuropsychiatry, Neuropsychology, and Behavioral Neurology, 7*, 1–9.

Ross, E.D., & Mesulam, M.-M. (1979). Dominant language functions of the right hemisphere? Prosody and emotional gesturing. *Archives of Neurology, 36*, 144–148. doi:10.1001/archneur.1979.00500390062006

Ross, E.D., & Monnot, M. (2008). Neurology of affective prosody and its functional-anatomic organization in right hemisphere. *Brain and Language, 104*, 51–74. doi:10.1016/j.bandl.2007.04.007

Ross, E.D., & Monnot, M. (2011). Affective prosody: What do comprehension errors tell us about hemispheric lateralization of emotions, sex, and aging effects, and the role of cognitive appraisal. *Neuropsychologia, 49*, 866–877. doi:10.1016/j.neuropsychologia.2010.12.024

Ross, E.D., Orbelo, D.M., Cartwright, J., Hansel, S., Burgard, M., Testa, J.A., & Buck, R. (2001). Affective-prosodic deficits in schizophrenia: Profiles of patients with brain damage and comparison with relation to schizophrenic symptoms. *Journal of Neurology, Neurosurgery and Psychiatry, 70*, 597–604. doi:10.1136/jnnp.70.5.597

Ross, E.D., Shayya, L., & Rousseau, J.F. (2013). Prosodic stress: Acoustic, aphasic, aprosodic and neuroanatomic interactions. *Journal of Neurolinguistics, 26*, 526–551. doi:10.1016/j.jneuroling.2013.02.003

Ross, E.D., Thompson, R.D., & Yenkosky, J.P. (1997). Lateralization of affective prosody in brain and the callosal integration of hemispheric language functions. *Brain and Language, 56*, 27–54. doi:10.1006/brln.1997.1731

Russell, S., Laures-Gore, J., & Patel, R. (2010). Treating expressive aprosodia: A case study. *Journal of Medical Speech-Language Pathology, 18*, 115–119.

Schirmer, A., Alter, K., Kotz, S.A., & Frederici, A.D. (2001). Lateralization of prosody during language production: A lesion study. *Brain and Language, 76*, 1–17. doi:10.1006/brln.2000.2381

Shah, A.P., Baum, S.R., & Dwivedi, V.D. (2006). Neural substrates of linguistic prosody: Evidence from syntactic disambiguation in the productions of brain-damaged patients. *Brain and Language, 96*, 78–89. doi:10.1016/j.bandl.2005.04.005

Sidtis, J.J. (2007). Some problems for representations of brain organization based on activation in functional imaging. *Brain and Language, 102*, 130–140. doi:10.1016/j.bandl.2006.07.003

Silberman, E.K., & Weingartner, H. (1986). Hemispheric lateralization of function related to emotion. *Brain and Cognition, 5*, 322–353. doi:10.1016/0278-2626(86)90035-7

Stringer, A.Y. (1996). Treatment of motor aprosodia with pitch biofeedback and expression modeling. *Brain Injury, 10*, 583–590. doi:10.1080/026990596124151

Testa, J.A., Beatty, W.W., Gleason, A.C., Orbelo, D.M., & Ross, E.D. (2001). Impaired affective prosody in Alzheimer disease: Relationship to aphasic deficits and emotional behaviors. *Neurology, 57*, 1474–1481. doi:10.1212/WNL.57.8.1474

Tompkins, C.A. (1995). *Right hemisphere communication disorders: Theory and management*. San Diego: Singular Publishing.

Trauner, D.A., Ballantyne, A., Friedland, S., & Chase, C. (1996). Disorders of affective and linguistic prosody in children after early unilateral brain damage. *Annals of Neurology, 39*, 361–367. doi:10.1002/ana.410390313

Tucker, D.M., Watson, R.T., & Heilman, K.M. (1977). Discrimination and evocation of affectively intoned speech in patients with right parietal disease. *Neurology, 27*, 947–950.

Tucker, D.M., & Williamson, P.A. (1984). Asymmetric neural control systems in human self-regulation. *Psychological Review, 91*, 185–215. doi:10.1037/0033-295X.91.2.185

Ultan, R. (1978). Some general characteristics of interrogative systems. In C.A. Ferguson, E.A. Moravcsik, & J.P. Greenberg (Eds.), *Universals of human language, vol. 4*. Palo Alto: Stanford University Press.

van der Merwe, A. (1997). A theoretical framework for the characterization of pathologic speech sensorimotor control. In M.R. McNeil (Ed.), *Clinical management of sensorimotor speech disorders* (pp. 1–25). New York: Thieme.

Van Lancker, D. (1980). Cerebral lateralization of pitch cues in the linguistic signal. *International Journal of Human Communication, 13*, 201–277. doi:10.1080/08351818009370498

Van Lancker, D., & Sidtis, J.J. (1992). The identification of affective prosody stimuli by left- and right-hemisphere-damaged subjects: All errors are not created equal. *Journal of Speech and Hearing Research, 35*, 963–970.

Van Lancker Sidtis, D. (2006). Does functional neuroimaging solve the questions of neurolinguistics? *Brain and Language, 98*, 276–290. doi:10.1016/j.bandl.2006.05.006

Van Lancker Sidtis, D., Pachana, N., Cummings, J.L., & Sidtis, J.J. (2006). Dysprosodic speech following basal ganglia insult: Toward a conceptual framework for the study of the cerebral representation of prosody. *Brain and Language, 97*, 135–153. doi:10.1016/j.bandl.2005.09.001

Voeller, K.K. (1995). Clinical neurologic aspects of the right-hemisphere deficit syndrome. *Journal of Child Neurology, 10*, S16–S22.

Walker, J.P., Joseph, L., & Goodman, J. (2009). The production of linguistic prosody in subjects with aphasia. *Clinical Linguistics and Phonetics, 23*, 529–549. doi:10.1080/02699200902946944

Walker, J.P., Pelletier, R., & Reif, L. (2004). The production of linguistic prosodic structures in subjects with right hemisphere damage. *Clinical Linguistics and Phonetics, 18*, 85–106.

Weintraub, S., & Mesulam, M.-M. (1983). Developmental learning disabilities of the right hemisphere: Emotional, interpersonal, and cognitive components. *Archives of Neurology, 40*, 463–468. doi:10.1001/archneur.1983.04210070003003

Weintraub, S., Mesulam, M.-M., & Kramer, L. (1981). Disturbances in prosody: A right-hemisphere contribution to language. *Archives of Neurology, 38*, 742–744. doi:10.1001/archneur.1981.00510120042004

Wernicke, C. (1874). *Der aphasische sSymptomenkomplex*. Breslau (Poland): Cohen and Weigert.

Wernicke, C. (1881). *Lehrbuch der gehirnkrankheiten*. Berlin: Theodor Fisher.

Wertz, R.T., Henschel, C.R., Auther, L.L., Ashford, J.R., & Kirshner, H.S. (1998). Affective prosodic disturbances subsequent to right hemisphere stroke: A clinical application. *Journal of Neurolinguistics, 11*, 89–102.

Wolf, G.I., & Ross, E.D., (1987). Sensory aprosodia with left hemiparesis from subcortical infarction. Right analogue of sensory-type aphasia with right hemiparesis? *Archives of Neurology, 44*, 661–671. doi:10.1001/archneur.1987.00520180082024

Wong, P.C.M. (2002). Hemispheric specialization of linguistic pitch patterns. *Brain Research Bulletin, 59*, 83–95. doi:10.1016/S0361–9230(02)00860–2

Wymer, J.H., Lindman, L.S., & Booksh, R.L. (2002). A neuropsychological perspective of aprosody: Feature, function, assessment, and treatment. *Applied Neuropsychology, 9*, 37–47.

INDEX